# Color Atlas of Equine Pathology

# Color Atlas of Equine Pathology

Claus D. Buergelt and
Fabio Del Piero

WILEY Blackwell

*Editorial offices:* 2121 State Avenue, Ames, Iowa 50014-8300, USA
The Atrium, Southern Gate, Chichester, West Sussex, PO19 8SQ, UK
9600 Garsington Road, Oxford, OX4 2DQ, UK

For details of our global editorial offices, for customer services and for information about how to apply for permission to reuse the copyright material in this book please see our website at www.wiley.com/wiley-blackwell.



*Library of congress cataloging-in-publication data*
Color atlas of equine pathology / Claus D. Buergelt and Fabio Del Piero.
p. ; cm.
Includes bibliographical references and index.
ISBN 978-0-470-96284-8 (hbk. : alk. paper) – ISBN 978-1-118-52089-5 – ISBN 978-1-118-52095-6 – ISBN 978-1-118-52098-7 – ISBN 978-1-118-69510-4
I. Buergelt, Claus D. II. Del Piero, Fabio.
[DNLM: 1. Horse Diseases–pathology–Atlases. 2. Autopsy–veterinary–Atlases. SF 951]
SF951
636.1'089892–dc23

2013007456

A catalogue record for this book is available from the British Library.

Wiley also publishes its books in a variety of electronic formats. Some content that appears in print may not be available in electronic books.

Cover design by Nicole Teut

Set in Sabon 10.5/13 pt by Toppan Best-set Premedia Limited

1 2014

# Contents

# Contributors

Julia A. Conway, DVM, DACVP
Clinical Assistant Professor
Department of Infectious Diseases and Pathology
University of Florida
Gainesville, FL 32611-0880

Julie B. Engiles, VMD, DACVP
Assistant Professor of Pathology
School of Veterinary Medicine
University of Pennsylvania
Kennett Square, PA 19348

Pamela Eve Ginn, DVM, DACVP
Associate Dean
Office of Students & Instructions
College of Veterinary Medicine
University of Florida
Gainesville, FL 32611-0125

Ingeborg Maria Langohr, DVM, PhD, DACVP
Associate Professor
Department of Pathobiological Sciences
College of Veterinary Medicine
Louisiana State University
Baton Rouge, LA 70803

Donald J. Meuten, DVM, PhD, DACVP
Professor Department of Population, Health and Pathobiology
College of Veterinary Medicine
North Carolina State University
Raleigh, NC 27606

# Preface

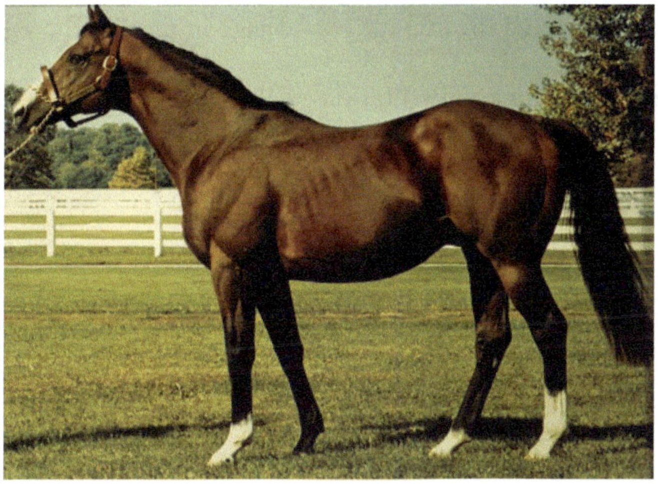

Native Dancer, 1950–1967, most celebrated and successful Thoroughbred racehorse and stallion.

The atlas is intended as a reference for readers interested in the pathology of equine diseases. It features macroscopic digital images of equine diseases supplemented by microscopic transparencies and a text highlighting the main aspects of equine diseases and disorders. The atlas is structured according to different body systems and emphasizes pathologic aspects of diseases in the neonate, juvenile, and adult horse. While attempting to incorporate as many diseases for which information and illustrations were available, the editors are aware that some may have been omitted by chance. Not all images are of best quality as these are from historic entities for which better examples were not available. For very unique equine diseases, contributions from colleagues in the field were solicited. We gratefully acknowledge their willingness to share their material and knowledge.

As editors professionally engaged in a high number of equine necropsies and tissue biopsies, we acquired a substantial knowledge base and collected a plethora of pathologic illustrations during our careers. We would like to convey this richness of professional experience to the readership. We are thankful for having enjoyed the opportunity to first share the equine pathology with veterinary students, trainees in veterinary pathology, and clinicians at our institutions. With this volume, we strive to make our material and expertise available to a wider veterinary and equine community, especially general practitioners, farm managers, and veterinary pathologists. Although we attempted to keep most illustrations at the macroscopic pathologic level, we saw the need for microscopic, immunohistochemistry, and graphic support in disease entities where gross changes are usually absent or overlap and when morphologic aspects for differential diagnoses had to be clarified. We selected chapter contributors as experts in the field where we felt incomplete in our image collection and knowledge base. We also solicited individual transparencies from individual sources and made every effort to obtain their permission as copyright owners. We are aware that some diseases are incompletely covered and that we did not expand the geographic scope of our work beyond North America. We refer to other resources describing global equine diseases in more details. Resources to complement disease aspects in the atlas are available on the website as Dr. John M. King's Necropsy Show and Tell, Cornell University or Noah's Arkive, University of Georgia.

Finally we are grateful to our equine patients for providing us a large range of disease examples and the stimulus to engage in putting the atlas together.

Claus D. Buergelt, Gainesville, Florida
Fabio Del Piero, Baton Rouge, Louisiana

# Acknowledgments

The core collection presented in this atlas is derived from the files of our institutions: Louisiana State University, the University of Florida, and the University of Pennsylvania. We thank our educational institutions for providing the cases.

Many people from other institutions around the world have generously contributed to the contents of the atlas. Our thanks and appreciation go to their support starting foremost with those who contributed chapters to the atlas: Julia Conway, Pamela Ginn, Julie Engiles, Ingeborg Langohr, and Donald Meuten.

In addition, with utmost appreciation and gratitude, we acknowledge Ted Clark (Canada), Perry Habecker (USA), John M. King (USA), and John Roberts (USA) for their enthusiasm for this work and for providing images from their files.

From the following individual educational institutions and practices we received contributions.

United States: R. Alleman, N. Allison, T.A. Banner, A. Boone, M. Calderwood Mays, W. Carlton, J. Cooley, S. Diab, M. Drost, J. Edwards, P. Hambleton, J. Harvey, T. Haskett, A. Hattel, P. Isenbarg, J. Kennedy-Peters, M. Law, D. Meuten, S.A. Montgomery, J. Neel, L. Perryman, S. Petersen-Jones, M. Pozor, D. Richardson, L. Roth-Johnson, M. Sebastian, F. Shahriar, R. Smedley, P. Stromberg, F. Uzal, B. Valentine, B. Williams, N. Williams.

Brazil: D. Driemeier and R. Fighera.

Canada: S. Ashburner and R. Foster.

Italy: C. Cantile and R. Rossi.

United Kingdom: D.T. Blunden and E. Milne.

Switzerland: F. Ehrensperger.

M. Kiupel, Diagnostic Center for Population and Animal Health, Michigan State University, performed and provided the immunostaining of mesothelioma and hepatoblastoma cases.

The editors of the *Journal of the American Veterinary Association*, Cambridge University Press, and Elsevier gave us permission to use several illustrations. The Animal Technology Institute Taiwan granted permission to reprint images originally published in an *Atlas of Alimentary Tract Pathology*, by C.D. Buergelt, R.M. Chu, and R.C.T. Lee.

We thank Ingeborg Langohr, Michigan State University, for reviewing the manuscript and for ideas and suggestions for improvement; J. Abbot for improving images; Nancy Buergelt for encouragement, patience, computer help, and sharing interest in the project; and Susan Engelken and Erica Judisch at Wiley Blackwell for their advice, support, and patience in helping make this atlas possible.

C.D.B.
F.D.P.

# 1 The Equine Necropsy



*Color Atlas of Equine Pathology*, First Edition. Claus D. Buergelt and Fabio Del Piero.

# I. General considerations

A necropsy can be defined as the orderly, systematic dissection of a cadaver. It should have as its objective to determine the cause of death or nature of a disease process. A necropsy always should be thorough and complete to obtain the best possible answer to the cause of disease or death. A partial necropsy yields only partial answers. Gross examination alone frequently provides an incomplete diagnosis. Additional microscopic, toxicologic, parasitologic, bacteriologic, virology, or molecular biologic assays are ancillary tests to obtain the most accurate final diagnosis. There are many methods to perform a complete necropsy. Regardless of the choice, to generate the most accurate outcome, the approach should always be the same so that no organs or tissues are overlooked.

Equine necropsies can be divided into three types: the disease-oriented necropsy, the insurance necropsy, and the medicolegal necropsy, each of them requiring a modified approach. The events of a necropsy should be documented by records of the physical findings and by photography, radiographs, collected specimens, and laboratory findings. Protective attire and the right set of instruments are important prerequisites for the adequate performance of a necropsy, so is the optimal environment under field conditions. The necropsy should be conducted within a reasonable time frame after death to avoid tissue decomposition. If euthanasia is performed, the animal should be bled out before the postmortem examination is begun to avoid spilling of blood into organs to be examined.

At the end of the necropsy, all observations should be written down or recorded. All findings should be documented objectively because the signed necropsy record becomes a legal document. The results of all ancillary tests including histopathology should be accompanied by a narrative and interpretation of the findings.

The necropsy procedure described in this chapter is taught at the University of Florida. Other methods are described elsewhere.

# II. Techniques

### *1. Positioning, examining, and opening of the carcass*

After the body weight is determined or estimated, the animal is positioned in left lateral recumbency. For identification purposes, a whole-body photograph is taken. If there is a tattoo or brand, these are recorded. The external examination involves all body orifices, mucous membranes including the lining, ocular sclera, the hooves, ears, eyes, and the condition of the hair coat. Valuable information concerning disease of internal organs can be obtained by observing color changes of visible mucous membranes. The gross examination should also include the nutritional status of the animal.

A ventral midline incision extending from the pelvis to the head facilitates the subsequent skinning of the carcass and reflection of the right front leg and hind leg. In the male horse the prepuce is reflected and testes removed from the scrotal sac. This is followed by opening of the abdominal cavity by incision through the abdominal wall.

## 2. *Evisceration of the abdominal, pelvic, and thoracic organs*

The abdominal viscera, in particular the intestinal tract, are checked for expected anatomic position. The amount and character of the peritoneal fluid (100–200 mL normal, clear, and straw colored) is assessed. After examination of the cranial mesenteric root, the entire gastrointestinal tract is removed to inspect and remove the remaining organs from the abdominal cavity. Individual organs are assessed for color, consistency, symmetry, and, where appropriate, aspect of the cut surface. Individual organs can be weighed and measured under certain circumstances.

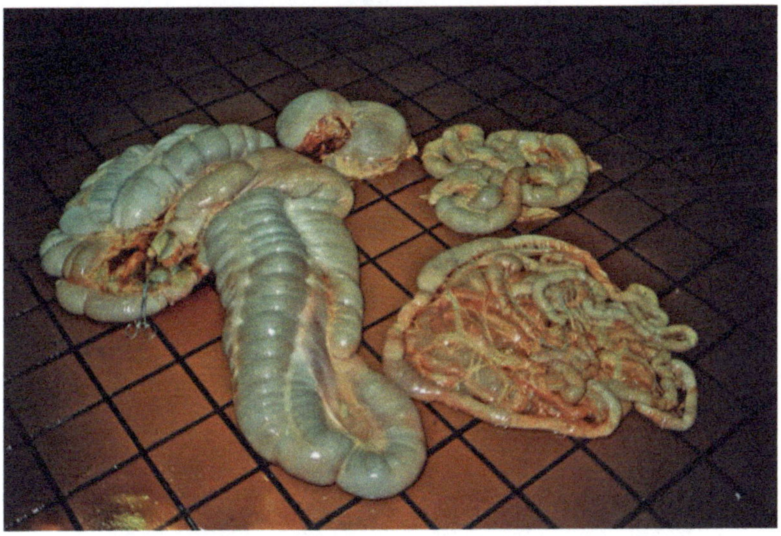

**Figure 1.1.** Horse. Gastrointestinal Tract. The length of the gastrointestinal tract requires separation into four segments: stomach, small intestinal loops, large colon, cecum, and transverse small colon. (Reprinted with permission from *Equine Medicine and Surgery*, Colahan et al., Figure 3-55, Page 122, Copyright Elsevier, 1999.)

The bones of the pelvic cavity are cut with a handsaw for removal of the organs of the pelvic cavity including the urinary bladder, rectum, and genital tract.

The right rib cage is removed from the chest using strong rib cutters. The entire pluck is removed en bloc, starting with loosening of the tongue from the oral cavity. The tongue is left attached to the esophagus, which is cut at the diaphragmatic hiatus and removed from the opened thorax together with trachea, lungs, and the heart. Trachea, lungs, and heart are separately examined.

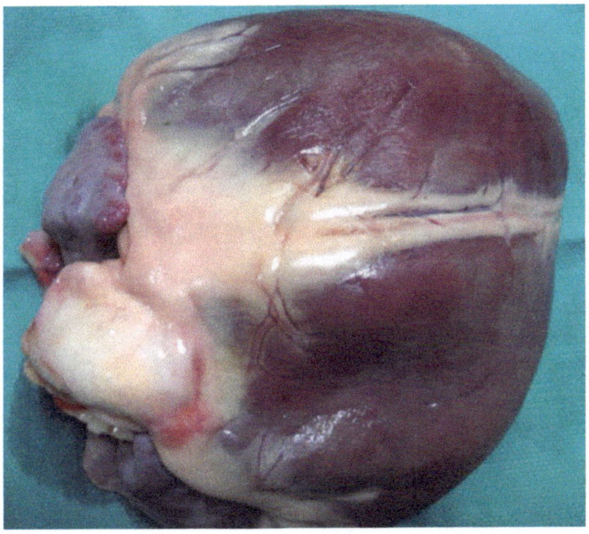

**Figure 1.2.** Horse. Normal Heart. There are several methods of orderly dissection of the heart. Care should be taken not to mutilate major anatomic structures and pathologic alterations of the heart. The left and right heart sides should be identified before the atria and ventricles are opened. The pointed apex is entirely formed by the left ventricle.

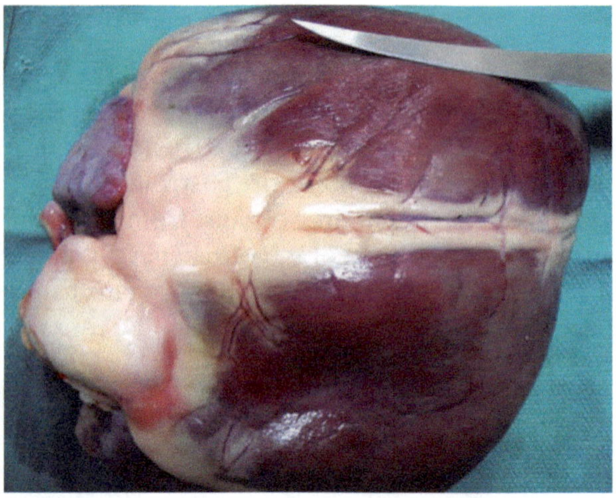

**Figure 1.3.** Horse. Opening of the Left Heart. The left ventricle is opened longitudinally by placing the cutting knife at the free lateral side. The cut is directed toward the left atrium, the tip of the instrument passing underneath the mitral valve leaflet toward the aortic ostium.

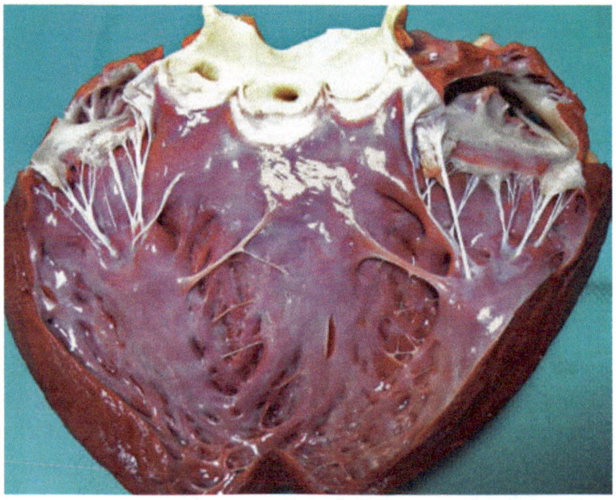

**Figure 1.4.** Horse. Opening of the Left Heart. The mitral valve leaflet is cut and the ascending aorta is opened. Rinsing with water facilitates the assessment of various internal structures of the left heart. The entire heart is weighed and measurements of valvular circumferences and ventricular and atrial muscular thickness can be taken.

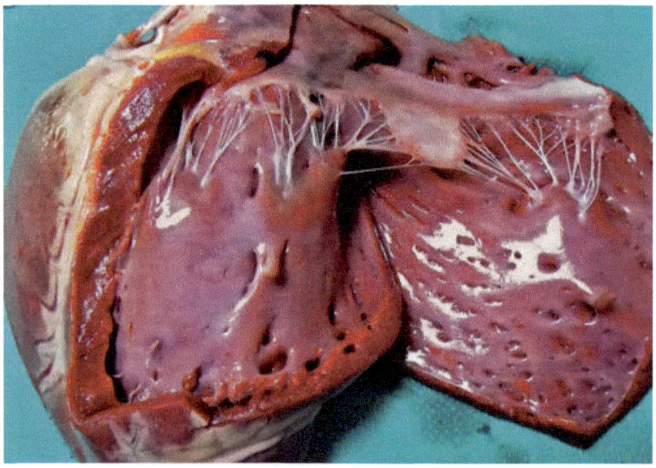

**Figure 1.5.** Horse. Opening of the Right Heart. An incision is made by knife following the ventricular septum. The instrument is turned along the ventricular septum into the right atrium. Inspection of the internal structures is similar to the procedure listed for the left heart.

*a. Cranial mesenteric artery*

After dissection of the perivascular tissue, the vascular branch is opened with scissors. The mesenteric arterial root lumen is checked for patency and smoothness of its intima to rule out the presence of *Strongylus vulgaris* larvae.

## 3. *Removal of the brain and spinal cord*

Before removing the head, cerebrospinal fluid can be collected by syringe from the atlanto-occiptal cistern for analysis to aid in the diagnosis of central nervous system disease. Decapitation is performed at the level of the atlanto-occipital joint. The guttural pouches near the occipital condyles are inspected. The cranial cervical ganglion is located next to the carotid artery in the dorsocaudal aspect of the medial compartment of the guttural pouches and can be felt as a bulge in the fold of tissue at that site.

The severed head is placed tightly into a vice or on a solid surface against a rigid object such as a wall or raised table corner.

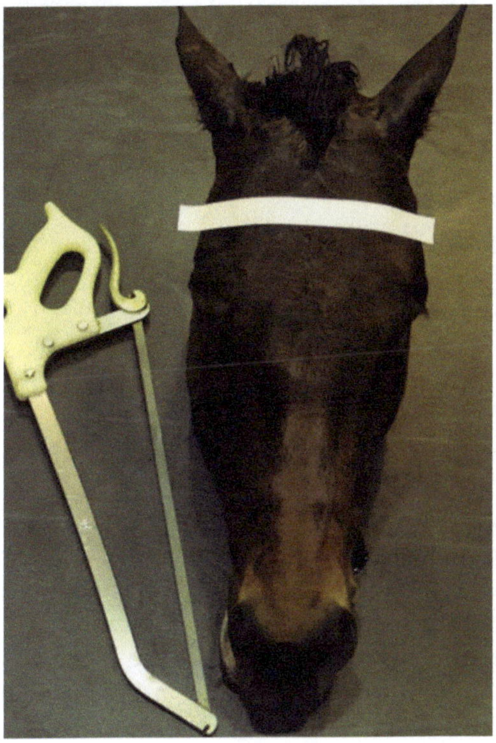

**Figure 1.6.** Horse. Head. For a field necropsy, a simple method to access the brain is to perform a transverse craniotomy via handsaw through the middle of the head caudal to the last visible molar tooth toward the palatine bone and oral cavity, thus splitting the head into rostral and caudal parts.

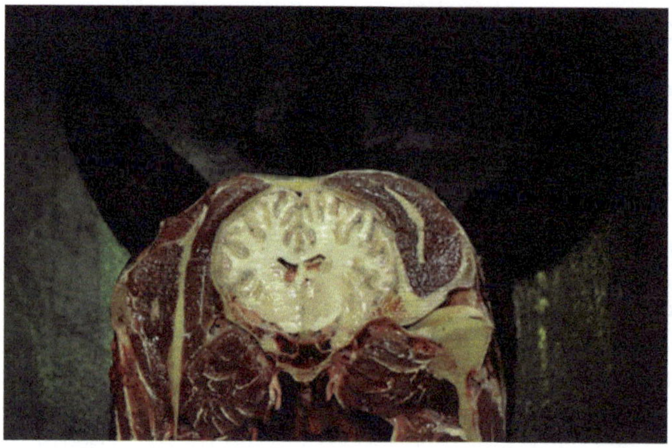

**Figure 1.7.** Horse. With the cranium open, both rostral and caudal portions of the brain can be removed with a gentle push. This technique is easier to perform if the mandible is removed at the temporomandibular joints and across the pterygomandibular folds to reduce the bulkiness of the equine head.

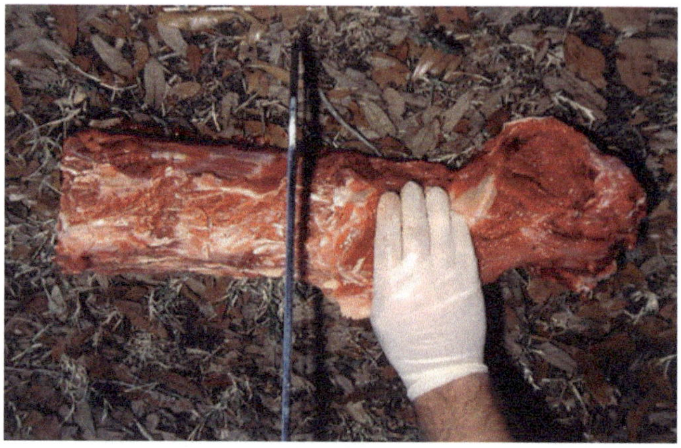

**Figure 1.8.** Horse. Spinal Cord. Removal. Field Technique. (Reprinted from Equine Medicine and Surgery, Colahan et al., Figure 3-65, page 127, Copyright Elsevier, 1999.)

For the removal of the spinal cord, institutional facilities use an electric band saw. The spinal cord can also be safely harvested with a handsaw under field conditions. After fleshing, it is preferred to divide the vertebral column into three to four major segments (cervical, two thoracic, lumbar). Depending on the suspected location of the pathologic process, one or all of these segments are cut transversely through the arches and bodies of adjacent vertebrae, leaving the intervertebral articulations intact.

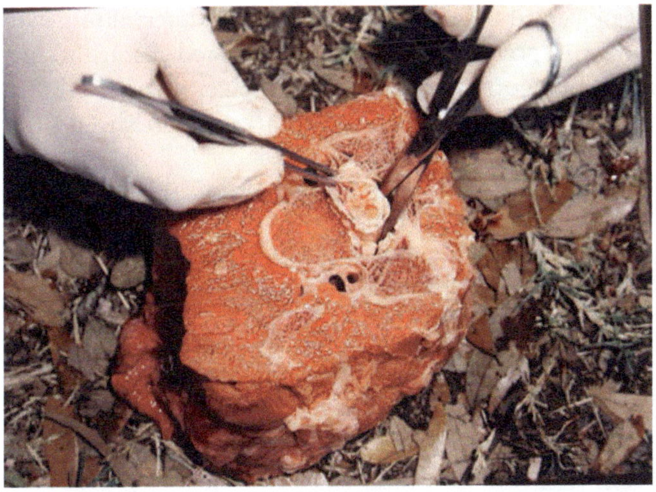

**Figure 1.9.** Horse. Spinal Cord. The vertebral canal is exposed and the spinal cord segment is removed with scissors. This can be repeated on as many vertebrae as necessary.

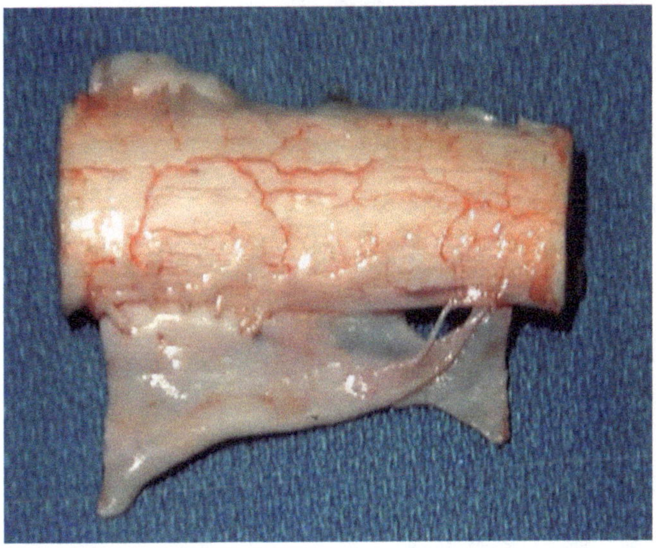

**Figure 1.10.** Horse. Spinal Cord. Normal. This piece measures the length of one vertebra and has the dura mater removed for better fixation.

### *4. Examination of the locomotor system*

As part of a routine necropsy, one should open a regular set of joints. This examination should be extended when clinical history identifies their involvement in lameness. Similarly, muscles and tendons are examined when indicated. Knowledge of joint anatomy facilitates a direct, safe approach to any joint. The skin over the selected joint should be removed to guarantee better visibility and sterility should there be the need to collect joint fluid for culture. Under normal condition, a slight amount of viscous straw-colored fluid oozes from an opened joint. A healthy articular cartilage has a moist, smooth, light bluish-white surface. The synovial fossae vary in size depending on joint location and age of the animal. In cases of laminitis, the hooves are separated proximal to the coronary band and the pedal bone can be exposed by splitting the hooves into halves with a handsaw or electric bandsaw.

### *5. Examination of the placental membranes and the fetus*

Placentation in the mare is classified at the gross level as diffuse. The placenta is composed of chorioallantois, allantoamnion, and the umbilical cord. The examination of placental membranes is critical in determining events that led to abortion, stillbirth, premature birth, or prolonged gestation. Ideally, intact, noncontaminated, and completely preserved placental membranes are needed for meaningful diagnostic analysis. The total placenta should be weighed.

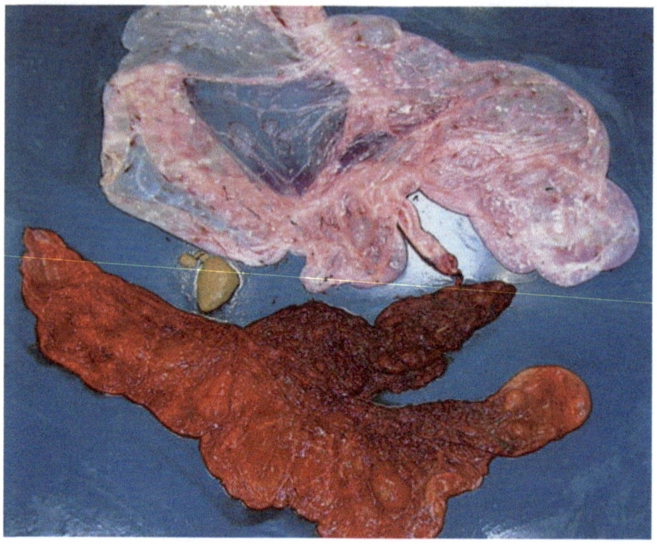

**Figure 1.11.** Horse. Placental Membranes. Both membranes are spread out; the chorionallantois as an "F" and the amnion as a flat membrane to which a small portion of umbilicus is attached. The visible chorionic surface on the bottom is velvety and reddened because it is rich in vasculature. The amnion on the top is normally thin and translucent and contains coiled muscular arteries. A yellow hippomane (allantoic calculus) is present between the placental membranes. Hippomanes contain lipids, cellular debris of desquamated fetal membranes, and mineral deposits. Their function is unclear.

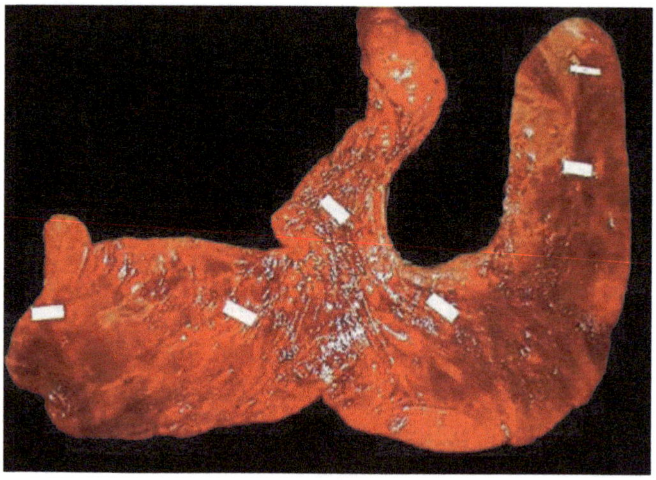

**Figure 1.12.** Horse. Placental Membranes. Several sites of tissue collection for histologic evaluation should be chosen from both placental membranes. (Courtesy Dr. J. Roberts, National Zoo, Washington DC.) (See also Chapter 12, "Diseases of the Reproductive Tract.")

The umbilicus severed from its attachment contains the urachus, two arteries, and, depending on the segment, covered by amnion or allantois, one or two veins, respectively. The length of the umbilicus should be measured. The umbilicus normally contains several twistings that should not be confused with pathologic twists.

The fetus should be weighed, its gender determined, and a crown-rump length established. A complete necropsy should be performed regardless of gestational age and tissue freshness. Autolysis rapidly occurs in kidneys and liver; lung and heart tissues stay relatively viable for some time.

## III. Tissue collection

Depending on how much the complete necropsy reveals at the gross level, ancillary tests are required to determine the cause of death or nature of disease. These tests include histopathology, virology, bacteriology, toxicology, parasitology, serology, molecular biology, or postmortem radiology. Each test requires special handling of the selected specimen. Regarding histopathology, the collection of tissue should take into account sample size, fixation type, fixation time, and volume of fixative. There should be 10 times as much fixative as tissue volume.

## IV. Recording of findings of routine cases

All observations should be recorded or written down at the end of the necropsy and ideally before the carcass and its remaining organs are disposed of. Gross abnormalities should be recorded in an objective and descriptive manner to allow the reader a mental image of what the prosector saw. The necropsy report should incorporate weights and measurements of organs as well as shape, color, texture, and aspect of the cut surface. The diagnoses should be listed in order of importance. At the end of the report, a comment should interpret the cause of death or nature of disease and explain possible inconsistencies between clinical history and pathologic findings. It should incorporate and interpret the results of all ancillary tests performed. Incidental findings, background pathology, or postmortem changes should be listed as such.

### Equine necropsy – Fact sheet

#### Definition

Orderly dissection of a cadaver

#### Types

- Disease oriented
- Insurance
- Medicolegal

#### Objective

Performance of a complete necropsy to obtain a complete answer for the cause of death or nature of disease.

### Equine necropsy – Fact sheet continued

**Special techniques for**

- Brain and spinal cord
- Heart
- Placental membranes

**Tissue collection**

- Histopathology
- Ancillary tests

**Recording**

Dated and signed necropsy report

## Selected reference

King R, Dodd N. 2009. *The Necropsy Book*. 5th ed. Guernee, IL: Charles Louis Davis DVM Foundation.

# 2 Diseases of Foals and Juveniles



*Color Atlas of Equine Pathology*, First Edition. Claus D. Buergelt and Fabio Del Piero.

In this text, a foal is defined as up to 4 weeks of age from the time of birth. Juveniles are defined as age 1 month to 12 months.

## I. Foal Disorders and Diseases

### *1. Congenital abnormalities*

Congenital abnormalities affect many organ systems. Many are life threatening. Only the most important are presented in this chapter. Less common abnormalities are listed at the end of the chapter.

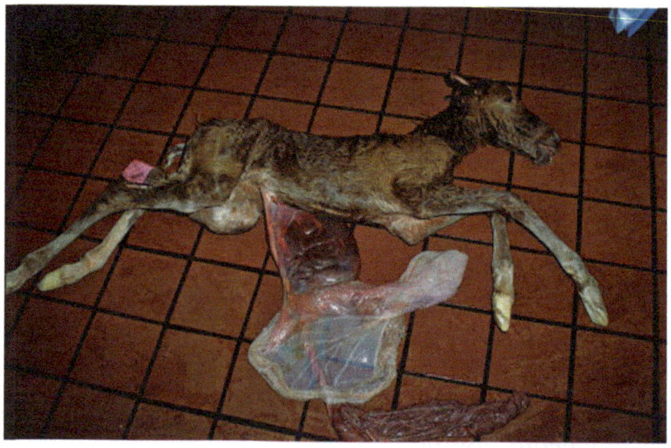

**Figure 2.1.** Neonatal Foal. Body. Umbilical Hernia. This abnormality displays an open abdomen and eviscerated abdominal organs along the ventral midline.

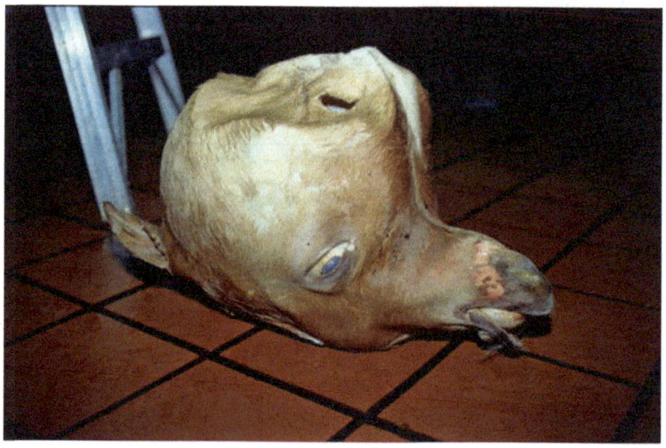

**Figure 2.2.** Neonatal Foal. Head. Hydrocephalus. The head is disfigured from protruding brain markedly filled with central nervous system (CNS) fluid.

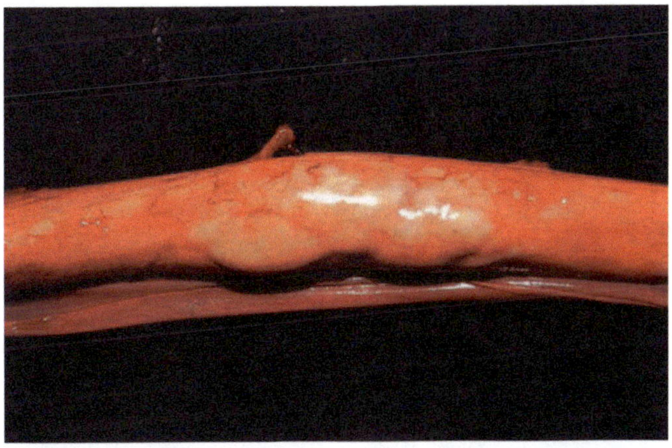

**Figure 2.3.** Foal. Spinal Cord. Hamartomatous Myelodysplasia. A spinal cord tissue protrusion at the laterodorsal aspect of L1 resulted in cord compression. (Courtesy Dr. J. Roberts, National Zoo, Washington DC.)

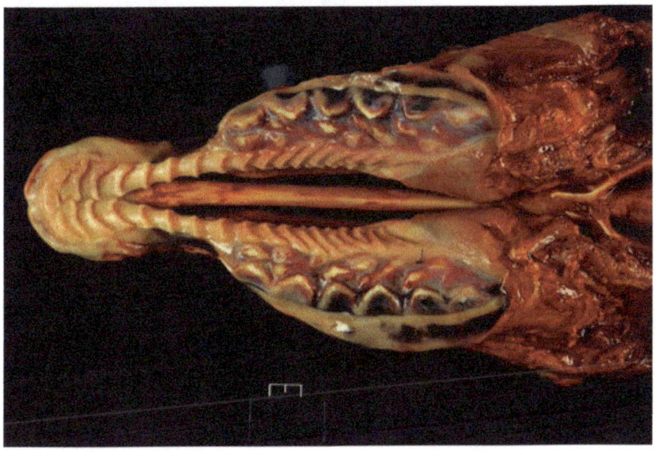

**Figure 2.4.** Foal. Mouth. Cleft Palate (Palatoschisis). Both the soft and hard palates are open and directly connected with the nasal cavity. The large size of the cleft leads to aspiration of ingesta and subsequent aspiration pneumonia.

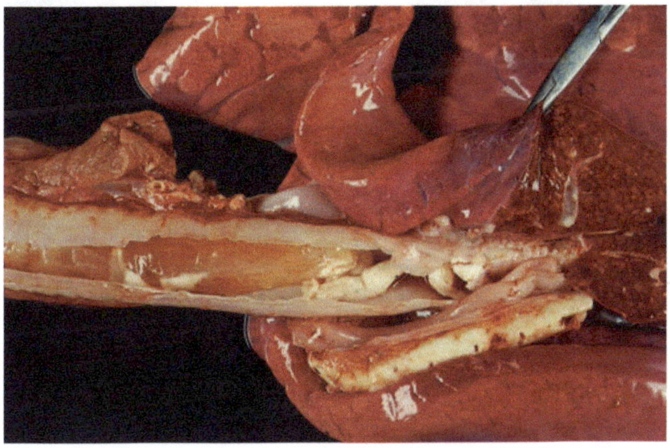

**Figure 2.5.** Foal. Trachea. Cleft Palate. Milk Aspiration. The distal trachea in this foal with cleft palate is filled with milk.

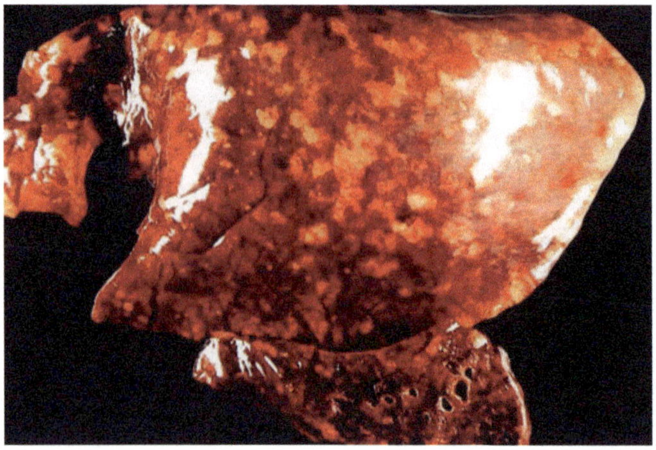

**Figure 2.6.** Foal. Lung. Aspiration Pneumonia. Secondary to cleft palate. The lungs are mottled, and major portions are consolidated.

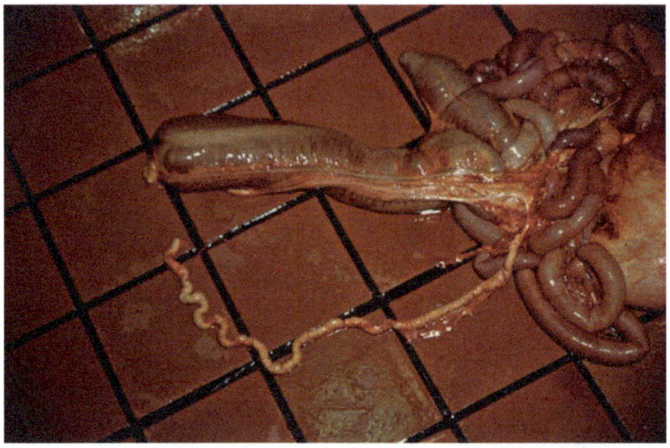

**Figure 2.7.** Foal. Large Intestine. Atresia Coli. The tubular misconnection of colonic segments resulted in a distal thin and empty colon with portions of the right and left ventral colons markedly distended with feces.

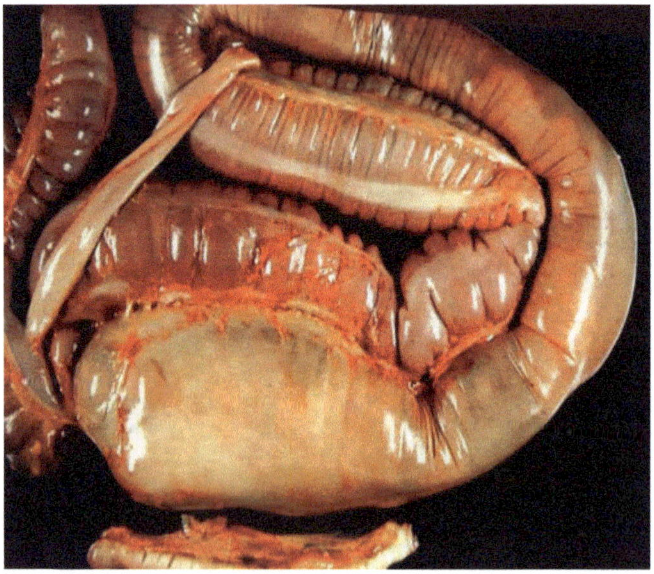

**Figure 2.8.** Foal. Large Intestine. Atresia Coli. Atresia occurred at the site of the transverse colon distending the entire large colon with feces. (Reprinted with permission from Animal Technology Institute Taiwan, Republic of China.)

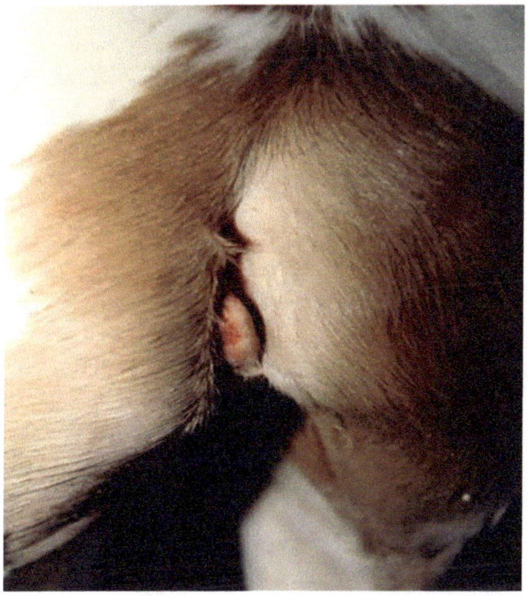

**Figure 2.9.** Foal. Rear. Atresia Ani. Absence of tail.

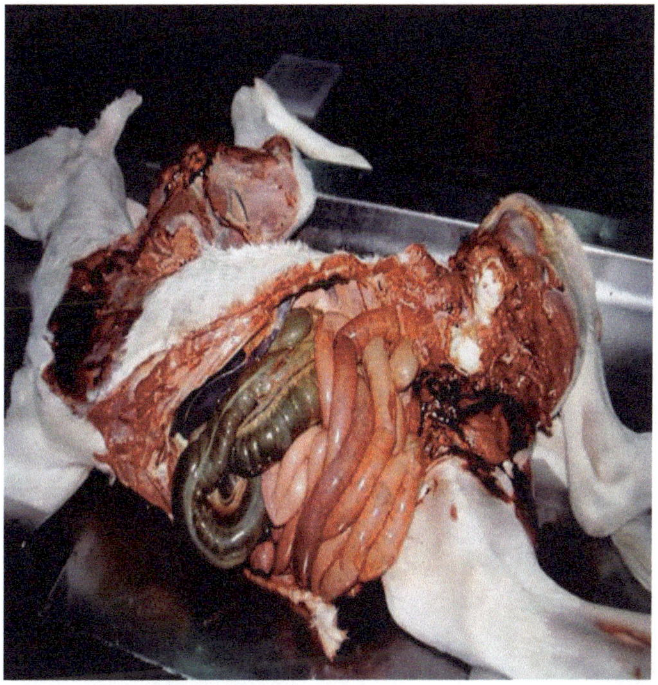

**Figure 2.10.** Overo Foal. Large Intestine. Intestinal Aganglionosis. The absence of myenteric ganglia in the terminal ileum, cecum, and entire colon in white foals born to overo spotted parents is known as lethal white syndrome. The large intestinal tract is impacted by green meconium.

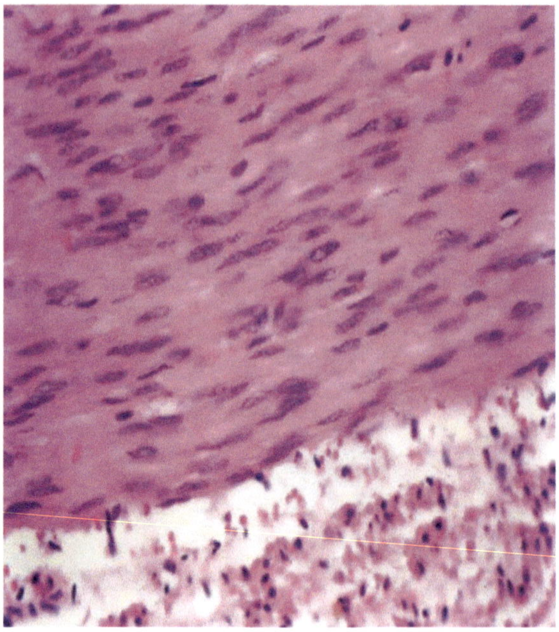

**Figure 2.11.** Overo Foal. Colon. Aganglionosis. Myenteric plexus ganglia are missing between the two layers of the tunica muscularis. (H&E)

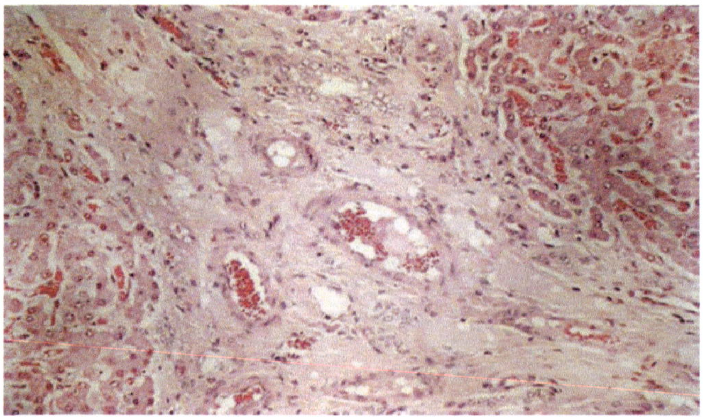

**Figure 2.12.** Foal. Liver. Portosystemic Shunt. Microscopic findings include fibrosis and duplication of arterioles in portal triads. (H&E)

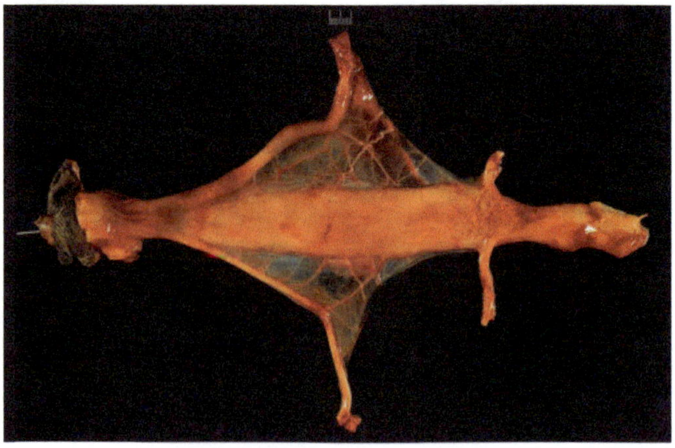

**Figure 2.13.** Foal. Urachus. Patent Urachus. Failure of the urachus to involute after birth leads to dribbling of urine. The condition is susceptible to infection and rupture leading to uroperitoneum.

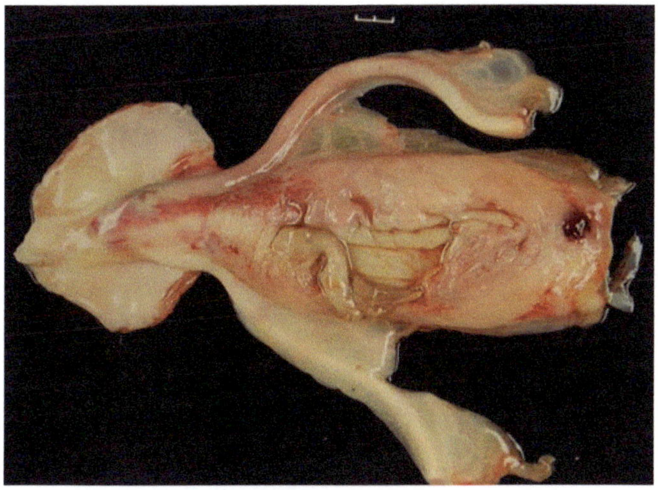

**Figure 2.14.** Foal. Urinary Bladder. Rupture. This condition occurs typically in newborn male foals. The site of rupture is the dorsal aspect of the urinary bladder. The condition has been postulated to result from weakness of the musculature at this site, which is particularly susceptible to trauma during birth. Uroperitoneum is the fatal outcome.

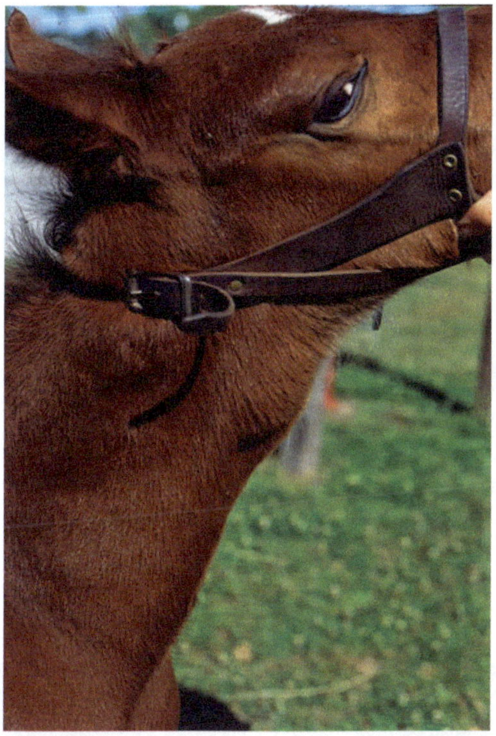

**Figure 2.15.** Foal. Thyroid Gland. Hyperplasia/Goiter. The round contour of an enlarged thyroid gland is visible protruding the skin of the lateral cranial neck. The condition has been reported to lead to mandibular prognathism, skeletal malformations (contraction of forelimbs), and dysmaturity in carpal and tarsal bone ossification and is known as thyroid hyperplasia-musculoskeletal deformity syndrome or hypothyroidism and dysmaturity syndrome. It may be diet related in a mare deficient in iodine or due to toxic plants like locoweed (*Astragalus mollissimus*) or fescue.

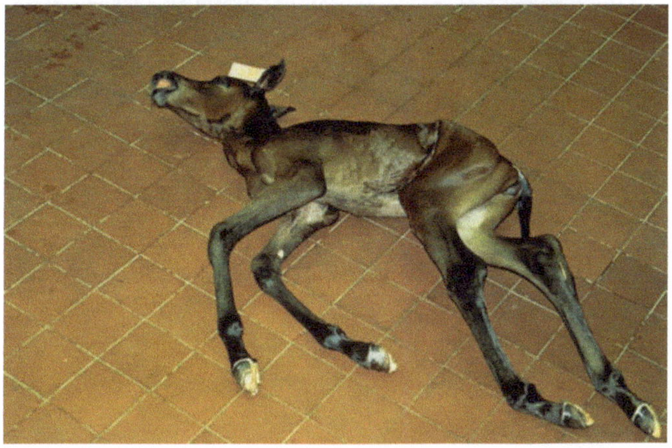

**Figure 2.16.** Foal. Skeletal System. Thyroid Hyperplasia and Skeletal Deformities. There is evidence of deformities of the limbs. Nasal bones and the spine may also be involved.

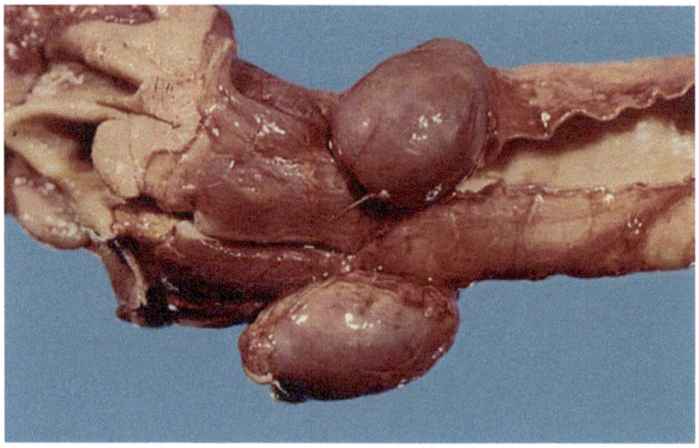

**Figure 2.17.** Foal. Thyroid Glands. Hyperplasia. Both thyroid glands are bilaterally and symmetrically enlarged. This condition can be seen in iodine deficiency.

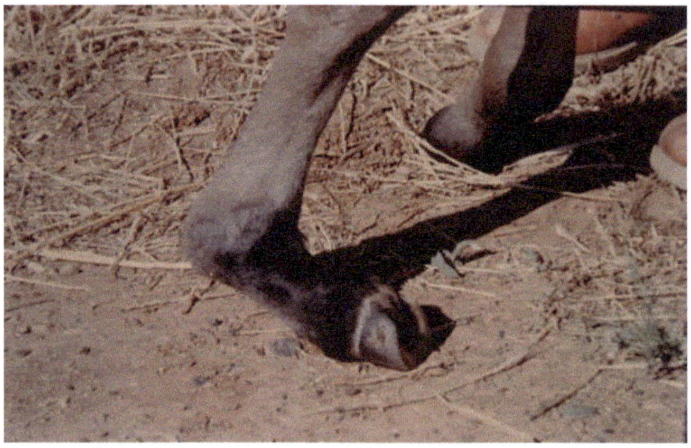

**Figure 2.18.** Foal. Fore Leg. Distal Limb. Joint and Tendon Laxity. The distal limb is deviated and held in palmar flexion position (angular deformity). There are two forms of deformity: deep flexor contracture and superficial flexor contracture. The congenital tendon contractures usually are the result of uterine malpositioning. They can also be acquired, such as from trauma.

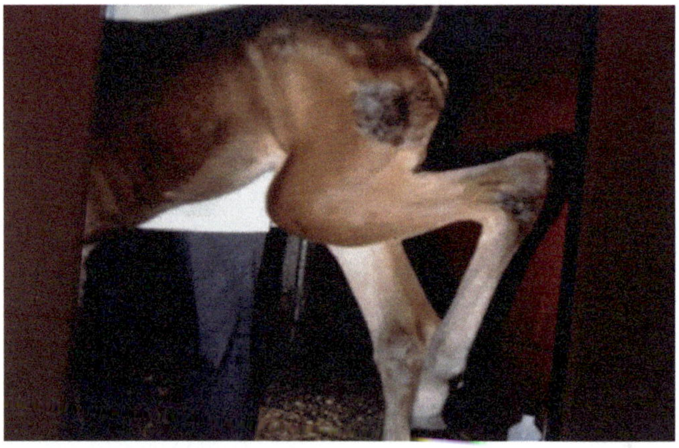

**Figure 2.19.** Foal. Luxation Patella. The foal exhibits a spastic leg.

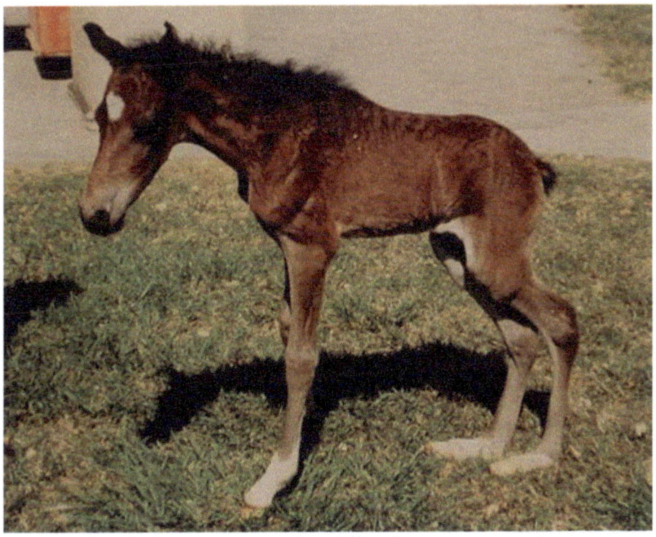

**Figure 2.20.** Foal. Extremities. Segmental Hypoplasia of Distal Phalanx and Angular Limb Deformity of Hind Legs. Fetlocks are involved. The front limbs are overextended.

## 2. Acquired diseases

*a. Neonatal isoerythrolysis*

Mares sensitized to fetal incompatible alloantigens develop alloantibodies such as agglutinins and hemolysins in the serum and colostrum. When colostrum is ingested by suckling foals during the first 2 days postpartum, isoimmune hemolytic disease develops in the foal. It may occur in newborn mules as well. Characteristic gross findings are shown in the accompanying figures.

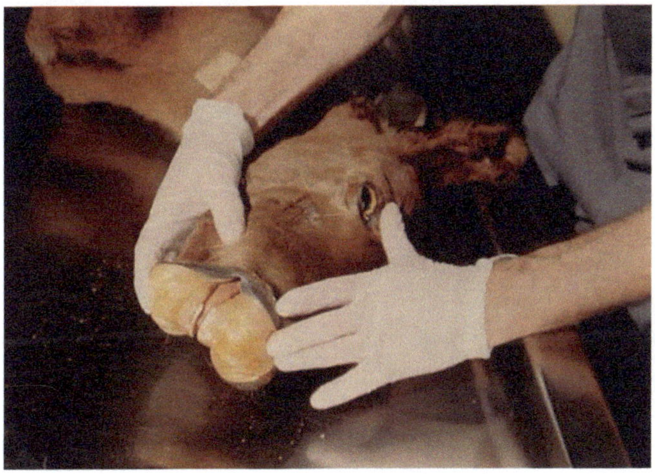

**Figure 2.21.** Foal. Oral Cavity. Mucous Membranes. Neonatal Isoerythrolysis. These are yellow from bilirubinemia secondary to hemolysis.

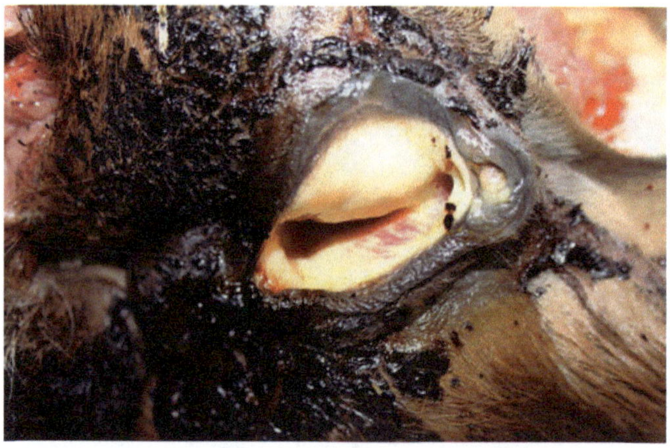

**Figure 2.22.** Foal. Vulva. Mucous Membranes. Neonatal Isoerythrolysis. These are yellow from bilirubinemia secondary to hemolysis.

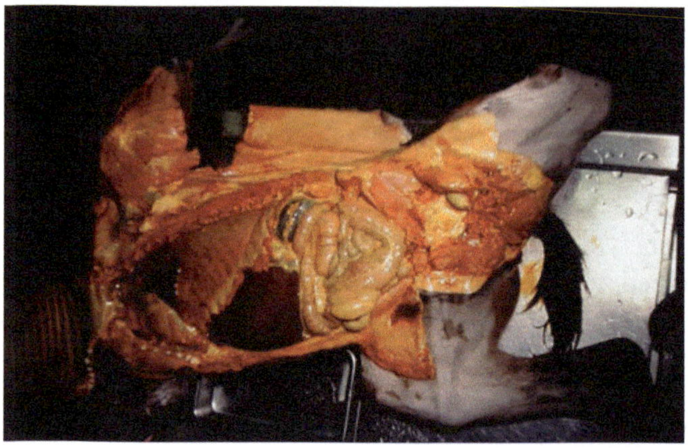

**Figure 2.23.** Foal. Body as Whole. Neonatal Isoerythrolysis. Icterus. Abdominal and subcutaneous fat are diffusely yellow, and the kidney is a deep blue color suggesting pigmentary nephrosis from hemolysis.

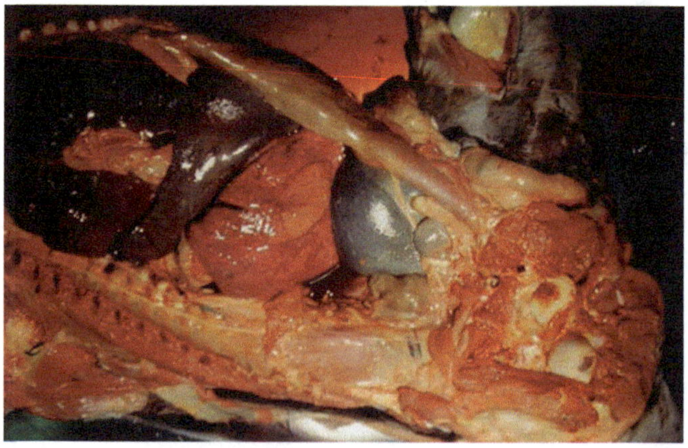

**Figure 2.24.** Foal. Abdominal Organs. Neonatal Isoerythrolysis. The spleen is enlarged, the urinary bladder is distended by burgundy-red urine suggesting hemoglobinuria, and the thoracic vertebrae and aorta are yellowish discolored.

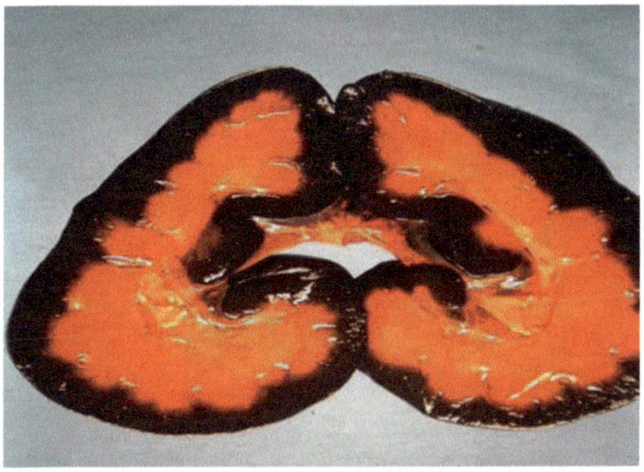

**Figure 2.25.** Foal. Kidney. Neonatal Isoerythrolysis. Pigmentary Nephrosis. The cortex is deep red from hemolysis and the medulla yellow from icterus.

*b. Actinobacillosis*

The multisystem disease caused by *Actinobacillus equuli* is also known as "navel ill," shigellosis, or sleepy foal syndrome. The bacterium is one of the causes of neonatal septicemia and usually enters through an open and inappropriately cared for umbilicus to typically shower the lung, kidneys, and multiple joints. Failure of passive transfer is an important predisposing factor.

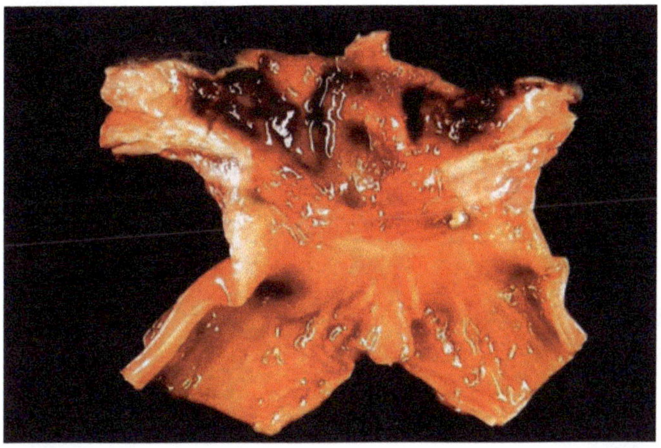

**Figure 2.26.** Foal. Umbilicus. Abscess. The wall of the opened umbilicus is covered by clotted blood admixed with fibrin and pus.

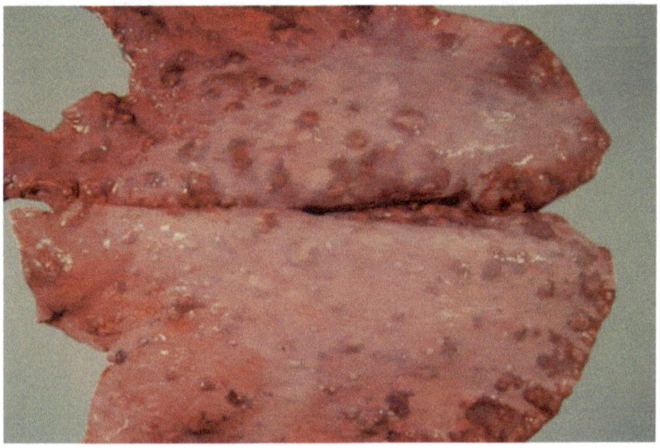

**Figure 2.27.** Foal. Lung. Multifocal Suppurative Pneumonia. *Actinobacillus equuli* bacterial emboli caused these multiple brownish abscesses via capillary colonization.

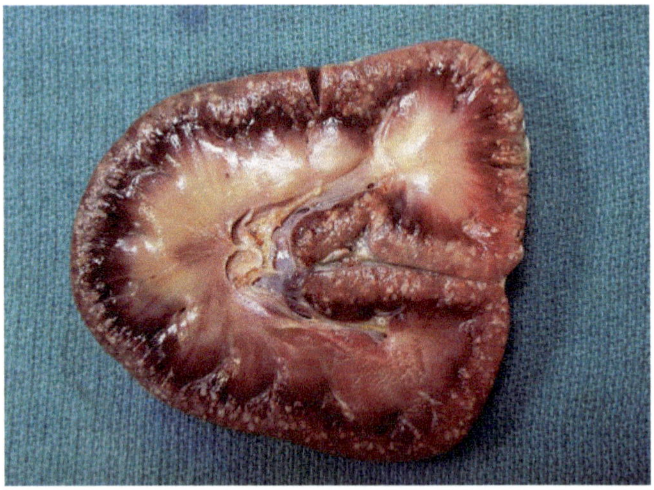

**Figure 2.28.** Foal. Kidney. Embolic Glomerulonephritis. Multiple microabscesses. *Actinobacillus equuli* showering into the capillary bed of glomeruli caused multifocal embolic glomerulonephritis. Differential bacterial etiologies include *Staphylococcus* sp., *E. coli, Streptococcus equi* subsp. *zooepidemicus*, or *Klebsiella pneumoniae.*

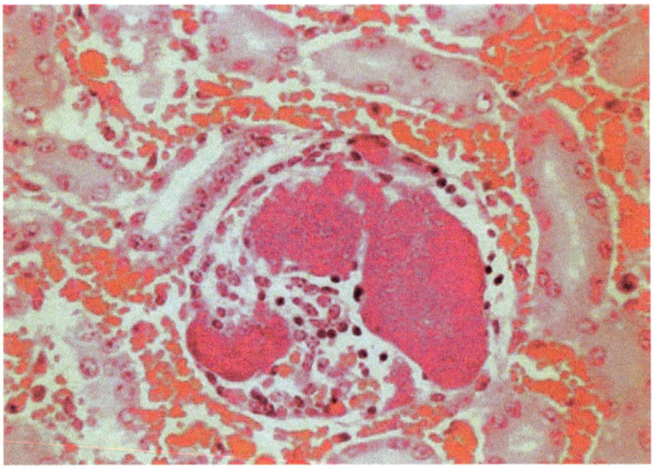

**Figure 2.29.** Foal. Kidney. Bacterial Emboli. Myriads of *A. equuli* bacteria are entrapped within glomerular capillaries. (H&E)

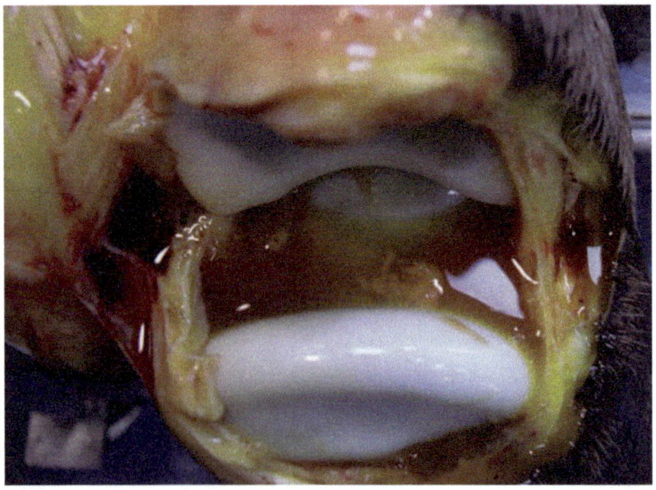

**Figure 2.30.** Foal. Hock Joint. Fibrinopurulent Synovitis. Although causing lameness, it may resolve if the foal survives because there is no damage to the articular cartilage.

### *c. Tyzzer's disease*

This liver disease of foals is caused by *Clostridium piliforme* with rodents and adult horses serving as the reservoir. The organism is obligatory intracellular and transmitted through the fecal-oral route from a contaminated environment.

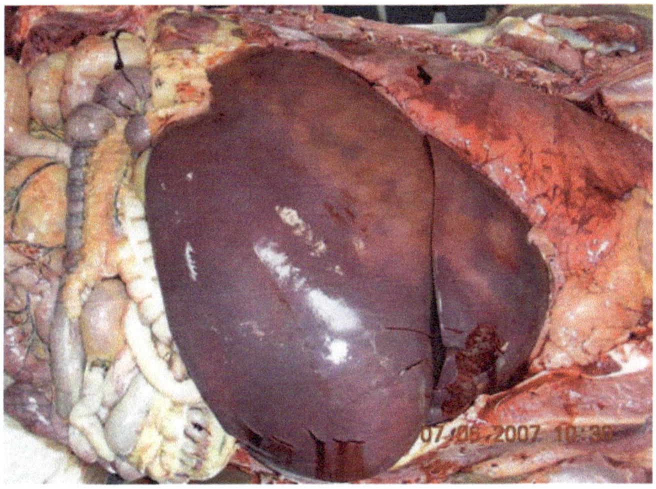

**Figure 2.31.** Foal. Liver. Tyzzer's Disease. Hepatic Necrosis. The liver is markedly enlarged.

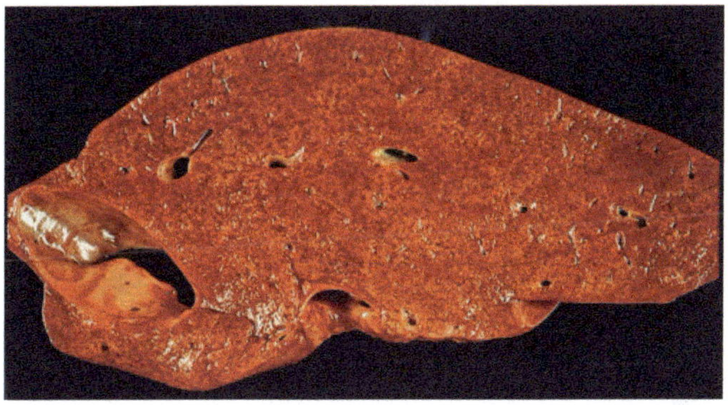

**Figure 2.32.** Foal. Liver. Tyzzer's Disease. On cross section, multiple small, white, and yellowish coalescing areas are present suggesting necrosis and inflammation.

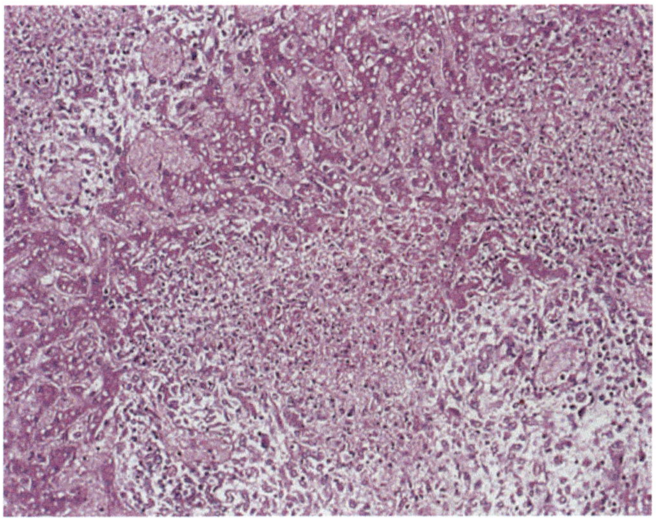

**Figure 2.33.** Foal. Liver. Tyzzer's Disease. Foci of coagulation necrosis are intermingled with mixed inflammatory cells. (H&E)

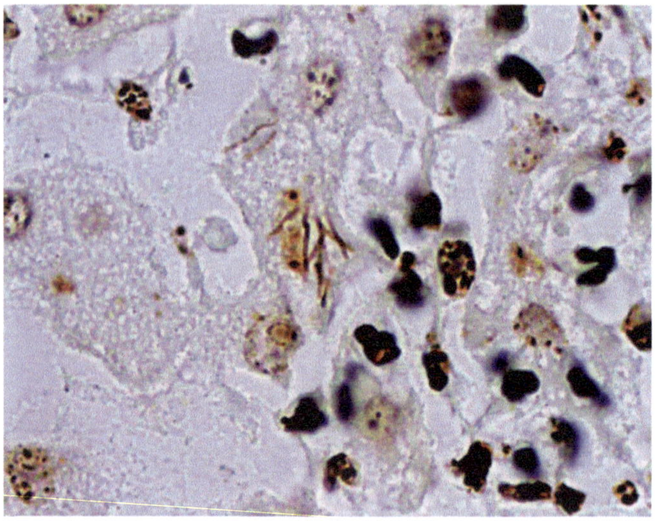

**Figure 2.34.** Foal. Liver. Tyzzer's Disease. A silver stain demonstrates filamentous brown bacilli within hepatocytes with an "Asian Letter" arrangement. (Warthy-Starry)

Other causes of bacterial hepatitis are *A. equuli, Rhodococcus equi*, and *S. equi* subsp. *zooepidemicus*.

### *d. Clostridial enteritis*

Foals with colic and bloody diarrhea may develop a necrotizing hemorrhagic enterocolitis caused by both pathogenic *Clostridium perfringens* and *Clostridium difficile*. Both produce enterotoxins responsible for the clinical and pathologic changes.

Five strains (types A–E) of *C. perfringens* are classified according to the enterotoxins produced by them. These are alpha, beta, epsilon, and/or iota enterotoxins. In foals, *C. perfringens* type C is generally associated with diarrhea. A commercial enzyme-linked immunosorbent assay (ELISA) is used to identify the enterotoxins in feces. It should be mentioned that *C. perfringens* type A can reside in the normal intestinal flora of horses.

As for *C. difficile*, an emerging enteric pathogen, toxins produced are toxin A, an enterotoxin, and toxin B, a cytotoxin. Most toxigenic strains producing disease secrete both toxins. The toxins are analyzed by fecal ELISA.

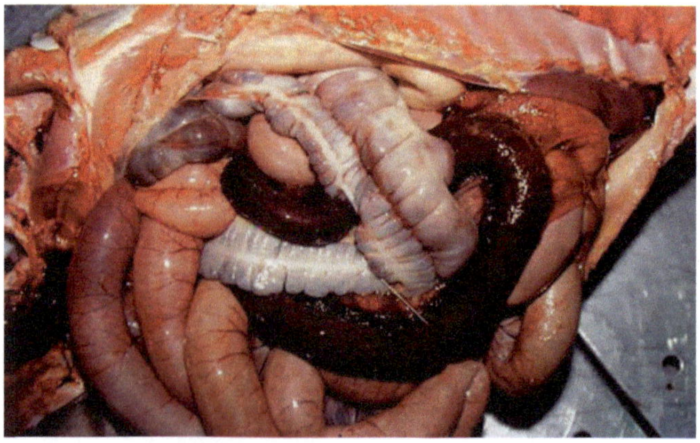

**Figure 2.35.** Foal. Abdominal Cavity. Clostridial Disease. Loops of the jejunum are markedly reddened. *C. perfringens* should be considered as cause. Small intestinal volvulus and *C. difficile* should be considered in the differential diagnosis.

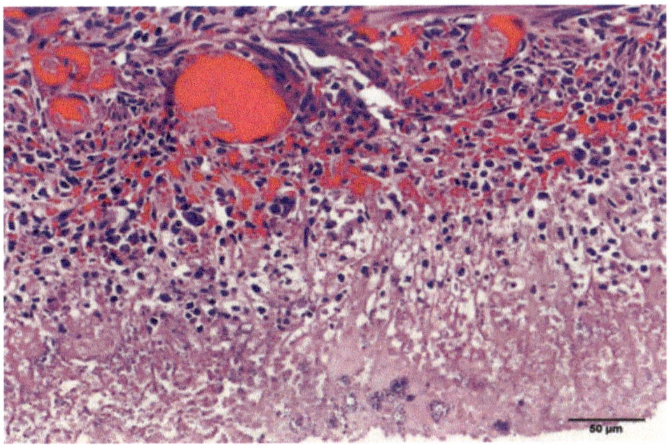


**Figure 2.36.** Foal. Small Intestine. Clostridial Disease. The superficial mucosa has undergone diffuse necrosis, whereas the adjacent lamina propria is hyperemic and contains fibrin thrombi in some blood vessels. (H&E).

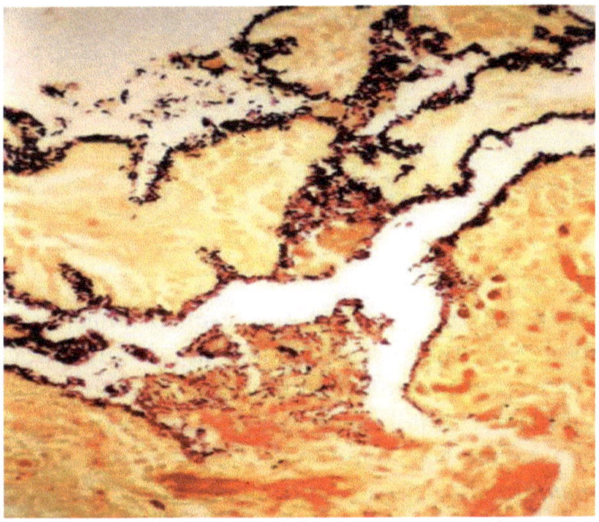

**Figure 2.37.** Foal. Small Intestine. Clostridial Disease. A gram stain will reveal gram-positive rods colonizing the necrotic mucosa as a dense monotonous layer. (Brown & Brenn).

Other enteric pathogens in foals include *Salmonella, Campylobacter* sp., *R. equi, E. coli, Streptococcus durans, Aeromonas hydrophila, Lawsonia intracellularis*, coronavirus, rotavirus, *Cryptosporidium parvum*, and *Strongyloides westeri.*

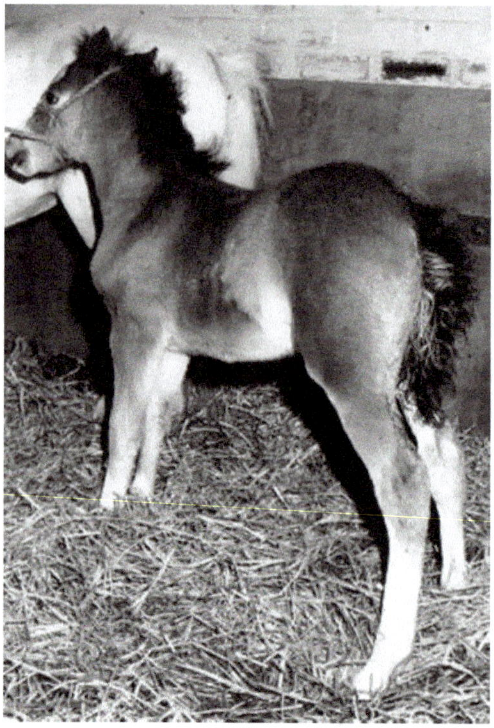

**Figure 2.38.** Foal. Pony Body. Rotavirus. Diarrhea is the main complaint clinically. The virus predisposes to bacterial enteric pathogens. The diagnosis of rotavirus diarrhea is made by ELISA or by transmission electron microscopic examination of negatively stained feces.

*e. Salmonellosis and foal sepsis*

Epizootic outbreaks of foal sepsis are the result of infection by a variety of bacteria and involve multiple organs and tissues. Many septicemias develop from infection by opportunistic bacilli taking advantage of immunocompromised foals or of foals with failure of passive transfer of colostral antibodies. Frequent bacteria isolated in septic foals are *A. equuli*, *S. equi* var. *zooepidemicus*, *K. pneumoniae*, *E. coli*, and *Salmonella*. The age of the foal is important as to the likelihood of which bacterium may be involved.

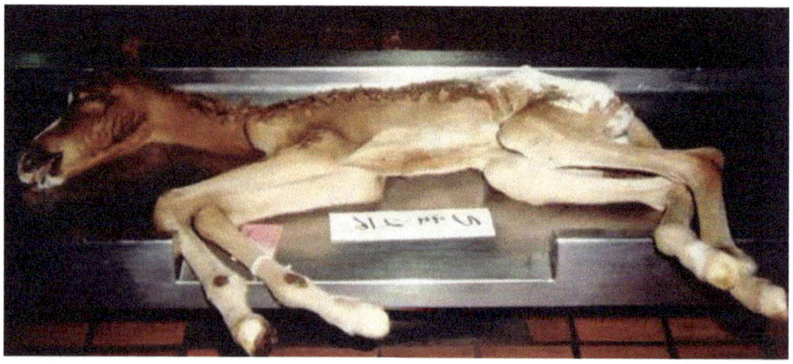

**Figure 2.39.** Foal. Whole Body. Sepsis. Stunted growth, emaciation, and especially dehydration can be external signs of foal sepsis.

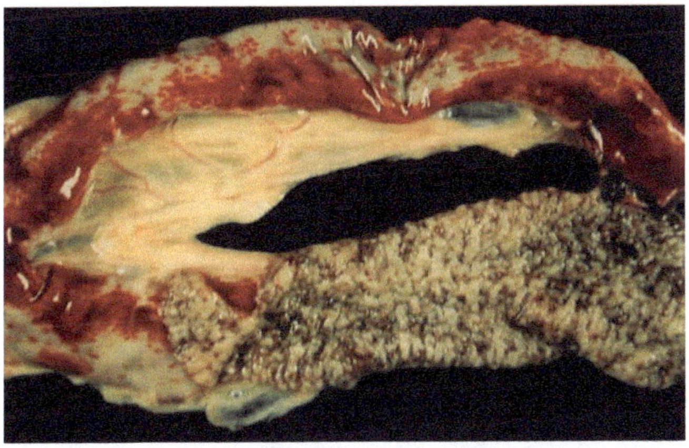

**Figure 2.40.** Foal. Small Intestine. Salmonella Enteritis. The opened mucosa exhibits fibrinonecrotic diffuse enteritis with ecchymotic hemorrhage on the serosal surface indicating septicemia. Septicemic salmonellosis can occur between 1 and 3 months of age.

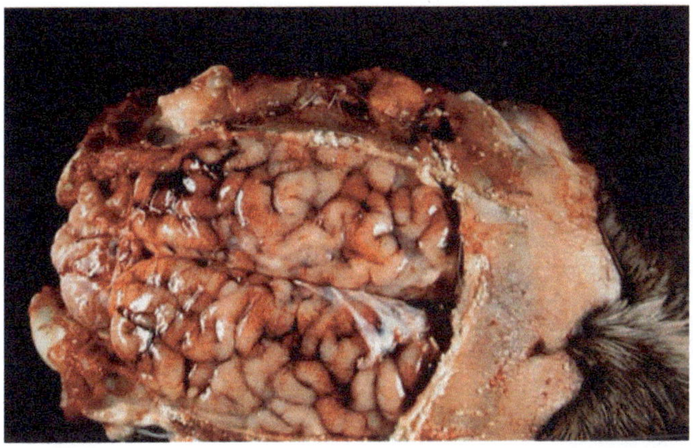

**Figure 2.41.** Foal. Meninges. Salmonella Septicemia. The meningeal surface exhibits ecchymotic hemorrhage and a faint cloudy exudate suggesting fibrinopurulent inflammation.

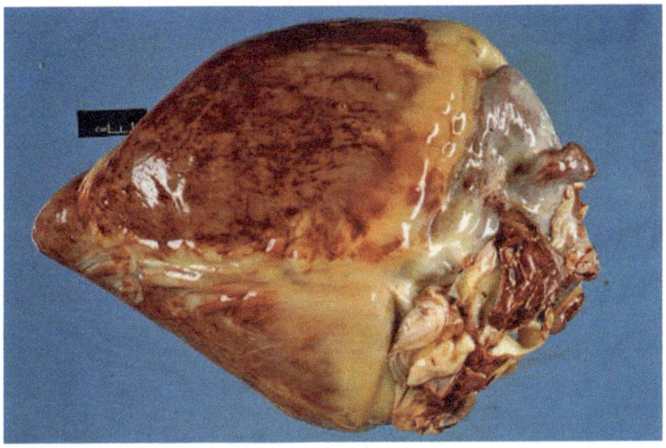

**Figure 2.42.** Foal. Heart. Salmonella Septicemia. The epicardium shows petechial and ecchymotic hemorrhage. Differential diagnosis: purpura hemorrhagica.

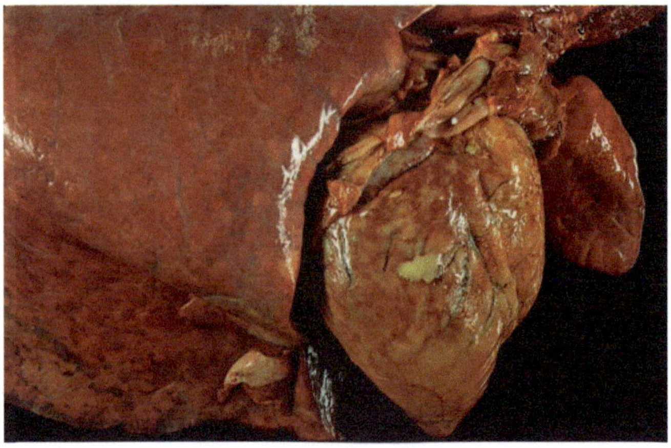

**Figure 2.43.** Foal. Heart and Lung. Salmonella Septicemia. The epicardium is covered by a fibrin clot. The lungs are wet from edema.

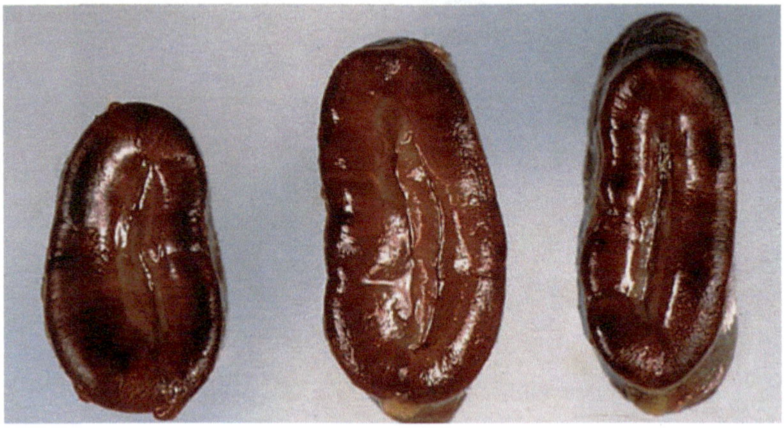

**Figure 2.44.** Foal. Adrenal Glands. Salmonella Septicemia. Typically, the cortex is hemorrhagic or ecchymotic. The condition is known as Waterhouse-Friderichsen syndrome in septic human infants.

## Foal septicemia – Fact sheet

**Definition:** Inflammatory response of various organs to embolic dissemination of bacteria from a primary source (nidus)

### Primary source

- Umbilicus
- Digestive
- Respiratory

### Organ systems involved in pathology

Frequent

- Lung
- Kidney
- Joints
- Lymphoid system

Less Frequent

- Central nervous system
- Liver

### Infectious agents isolated

Frequent

- *Actinobacillus equuli*
- *Coliforms*
- *Klebsiella pneumoniae*
- *Salmonella*
- *Streptococcus* sp.

## Foal septicemia – Fact sheet continued

### Infectious agents isolated

Less frequent

- *Listeria monocytogenes*
- *Candida albicans*
- *Aspergillus fumigatus*

### Risk factors

- **Poor umbilical hygiene**
- **Colostrum deprivation**
- **Nutritional imbalance**
- **Management practices**

*f. Toxic hepatopathy*

In the early 1980s, a paste probiotic product introduced to the market for stimulating appetite in neonatal foals was found to cause clinical signs of liver failure and subsequent death. Further investigations incriminated iron fumarate overload as responsible for the liver failure due to severe panhepatic necrosis.

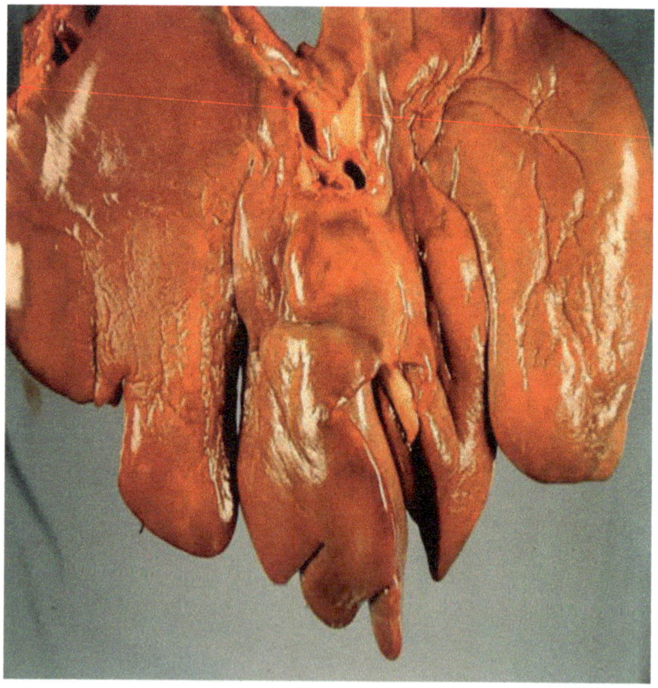

**Figure 2.45.** Foal. Liver. Degeneration and Necrosis. Iron Toxicosis. Discoloration and decrease in liver size. The liver surface appears flattened in the center of the lobes.

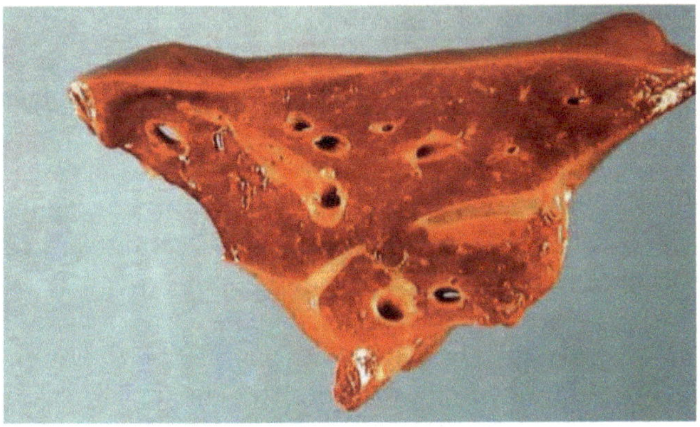

**Figure 2.46.** Foal. Liver. Degeneration and Necrosis. Iron Toxicosis. On cross section, the parenchyma appears reduced because the vascular and biliary structures are relatively prominent. Yellow discoloration is the result of icterus.

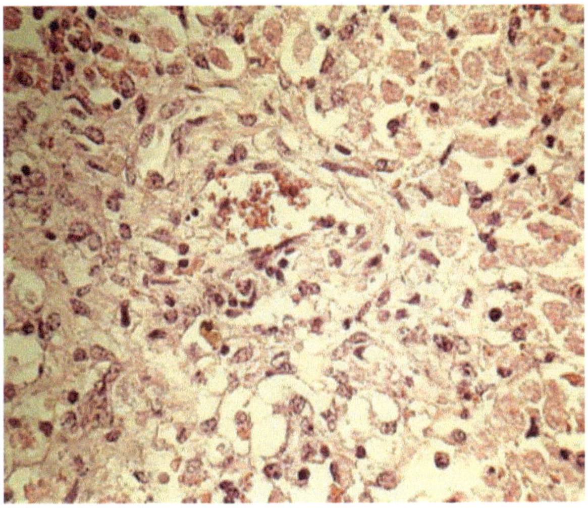

**Figure 2.47.** Foal. Liver. Hepatocellular Collapse. Iron Toxicosis. Hepatic cords are in disarray. Hepatocytes are vacuolated and disintegrated (necrosis). Sinusoids are dilated. (H&E)

Other acutely lethal toxins in foals to consider as differential diagnoses for sudden death are mycotoxins, organophosphates, ethionine, gentamicin, cantharidin, red maple leaf, and *Indigofera* plants.

*g. Immunodeficiency disease of Arabian foals*

Severe combined immunodeficiency disease (SCID) of Arabian Foals affects both the cellular and humoral immune systems of these animals at a young age. The disease is inherited by a non–sex-linked gene in an autosomal recessive mode. Of such affected animals 25% may be carriers of the defective mutated gene. The deficiency affects both T and B lymphocyte lineages blocking their development. Affected foals suffer from secondary adenoviral pneumonia, sometimes complicated by superimposed infection with *Pneumocystis jiroveci* (formerly *carinii)* or *Rhodococcus equi*. Affected animals have a largely reduced or even grossly inapparent thymus, small lymph nodes, and a small spleen indicating hypoplastic lymphoid tissue. The disease has been largely eliminated by genetic testing and selective breeding. Clinical and morphologic parameters for the diagnosis of SCID include hypogammaglobulinemia, lymphopenia of peripheral blood, and hypoplasia of lymphoid tissues, particular the thymus.

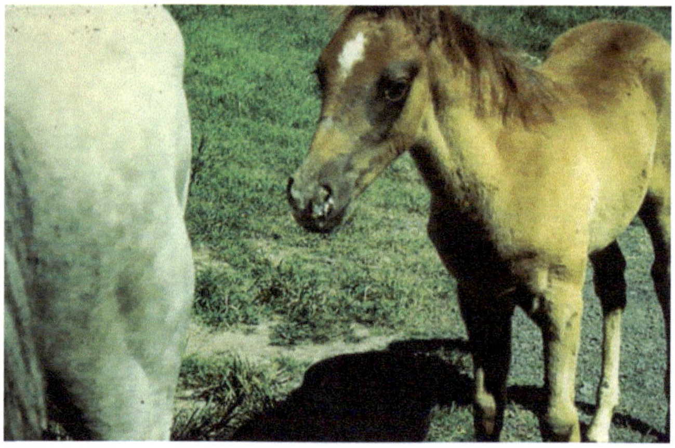

**Figure 2.48.** Arabian Foal. Head. SCID. Nasal and ocular discharges are indicators of a respiratory problem (pneumonia) in affected Arabian foals.

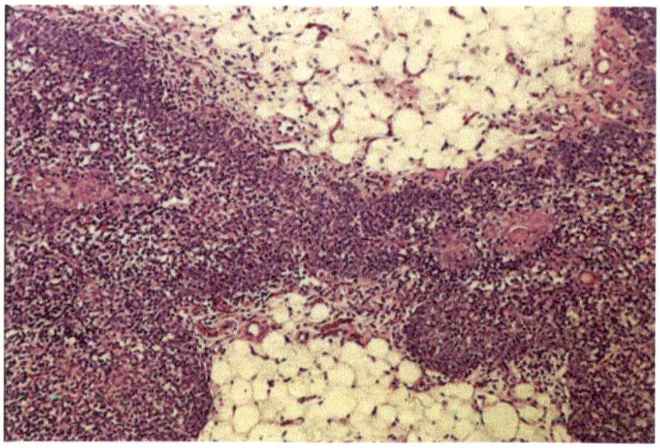

**Figure 2.49.** Arabian Foal. Thymus. SCID. Hypoplasia. The thymus will be difficult to find grossly. Microscopically, it is characterized by paucity of lymphocytes in cortex and medulla. (H&E). (Courtesy Dr. L. Perryman, Colorado State University.)

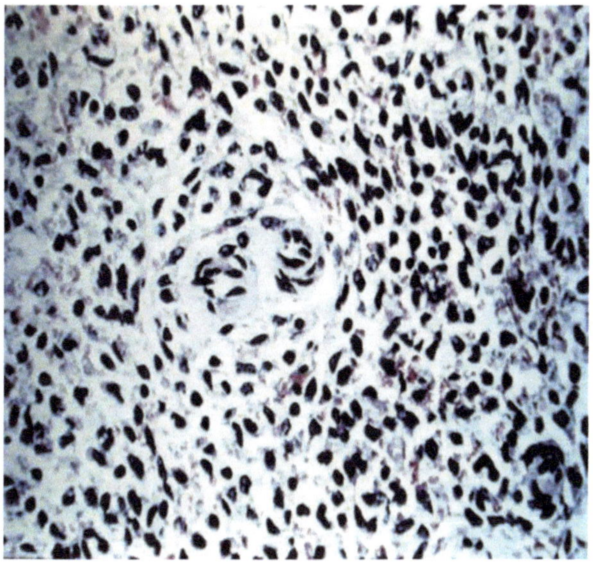

**Figure 2.50.** Arabian Foal. Spleen. SCID. Hypoplasia. The number of lymphocytes is reduced around the splenic arteriole because there is evidence of lack of connective tissue framework at the site of lymphoid follicles when compared to lymphoid atrophy of different etiology. (H&E)

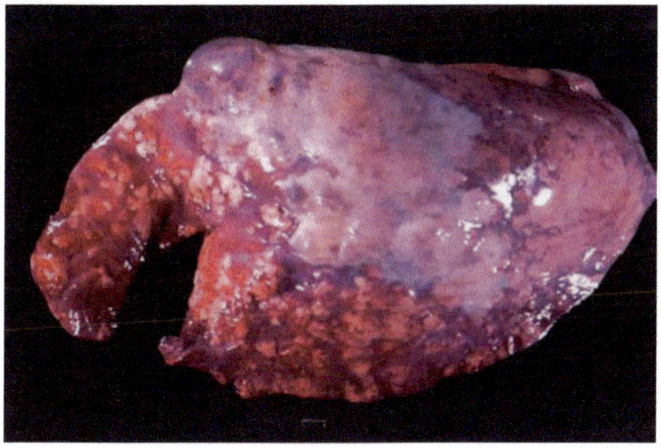

**Figure 2.51.** Arabian Foal. Lung. SCID. Adenovirus. Cranioventral Pneumonia. Plum-red discoloration of the cranioventral lung is suggestive of bronchointerstitial pneumonia by adenovirus infection.

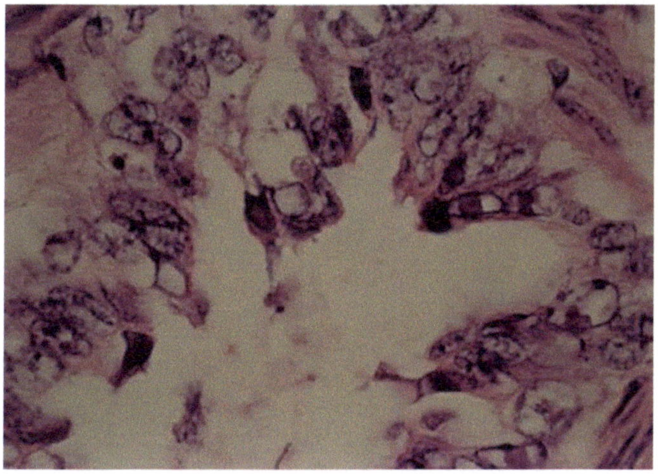

**Figure 2.52.** Arabian Foal. Lung. SCID. Bronchiolitis. Necrotizing bronchiolitis with intranuclear amphophilic viral inclusions. Intraluminal neutrophils can be observed. Adenoviral bronchiolitis is characterized by the presence of basophilic intranuclear viral inclusions in epithelial cells. (H&E)

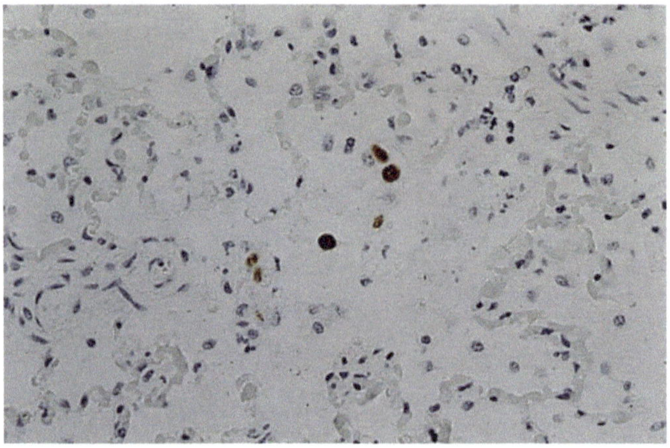

**Figure 2.53.** Arabian Foal. Lung. SCID. Adenovirus. Indirect immunohistochemistry demonstrates intranuclear adenovirus antigen within endothelial cells. (IHC)

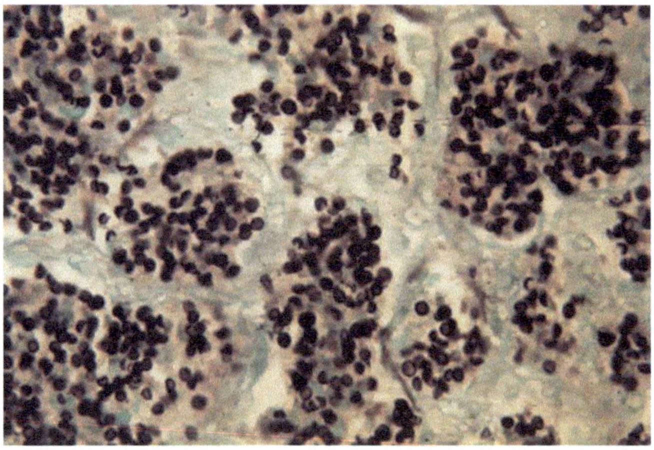

**Figure 2.54.** Arabian Foal. Lung. SCID. Pneumocystosis. *Pneumocystis jiroveci* is a frequent concomitant pathogen in SCID foals and can be detected by a special stain in alveoli markedly distended by highly proteinaceous fluid. (GMS). (Courtesy Dr. L. Perryman, Colorado State University.)

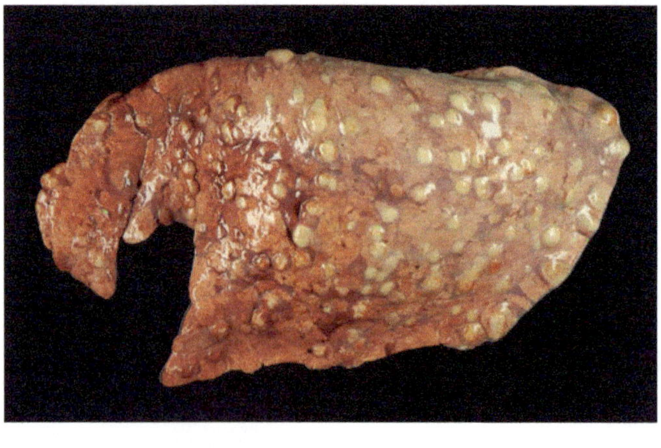

**Figure 2.55.** Arabian Foal. Lung. SCID. Multifocal Caseous and Pyogranulomatous Pneumonia. *P. jiroveci* was detected microscopically in addition to *R. equi*.

### Hemogram of SCID foal obtained on three different days

| | Day 1 | Day 2 | Day 3 | Normal |
|---|---|---|---|---|
| WBC | 4100 | 2728 | 3100 | 10,450 µL |
| Neutrophils | 3772 | 2728 | 3772 | 4600 µL |
| Lymphocytes | 0 | 31 | 176 | 5330 µL |
| Monocytes | 283 | 341 | 264 | 340 µL |
| Basophils | 41 | 0 | 44 | 0 µL |
| Eosinophils | 0 | 0 | 44 | 140 µL |

WBC = white blood cells.

*h. Patterns and comparison of foal lung diseases*

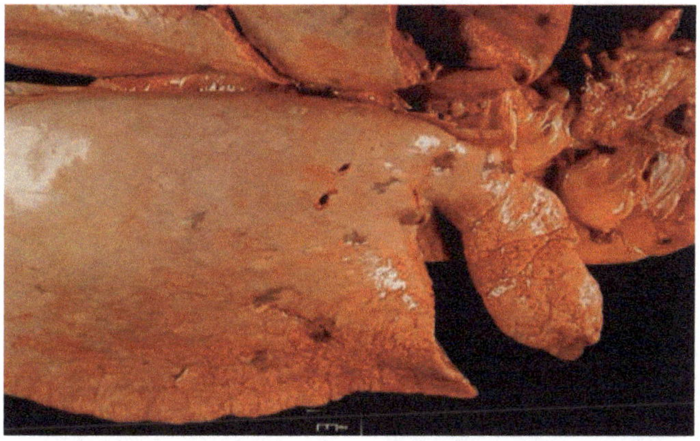

**Figure 2.56.** Foal. Lung. Normal.

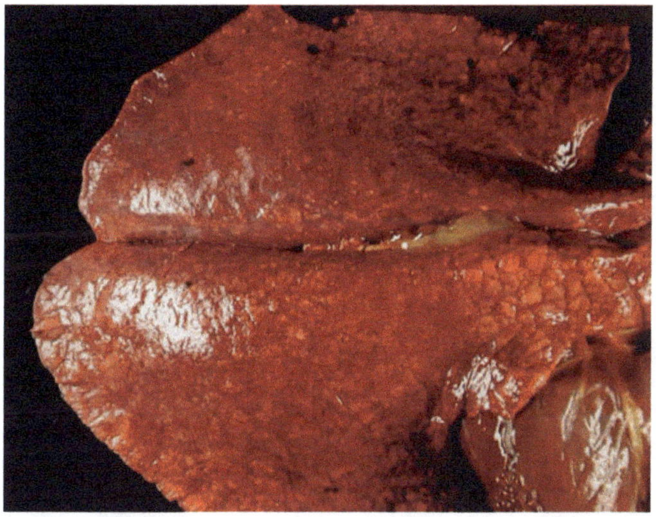

**Figure 2.57.** Foal. Lung. Diffuse Atelectasis. The lung shows a uniform collapsed profile and brown color due to underperfusion and nonaeration.

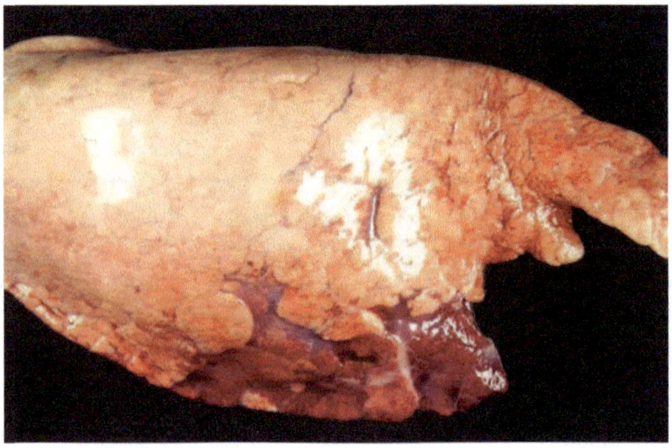

**Figure 2.58.** Foal. Lung. Cranioventral Necrosuppurative Bronchopneumonia. Consolidation of the cranial lung suggests aspiration or bacteria as causes.

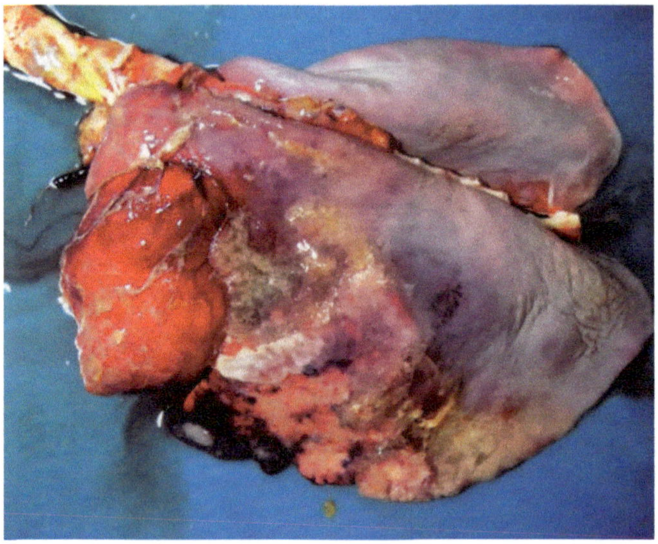

**Figure 2.59.** Foal. Lung. Locally Extensive Pneumonia. *S. equi* subsp. *zooepidemicus* was the cause.

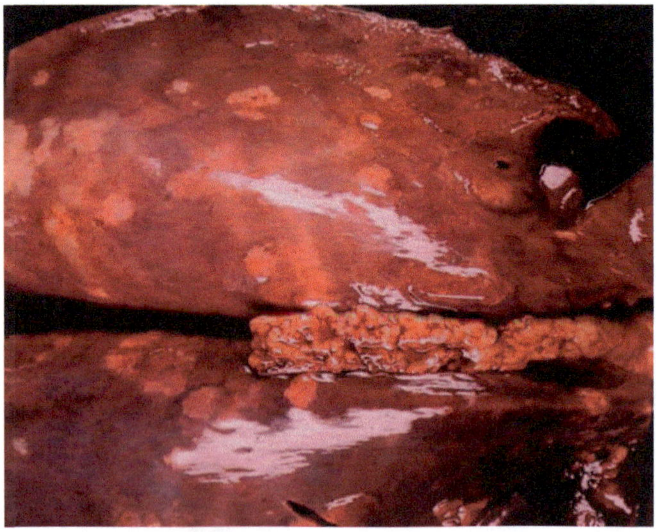

**Figure 2.60.** Foal. Lung. Abscesses. Hematogenous spread of bacteria such as *A. equuli* should be considered as the cause.

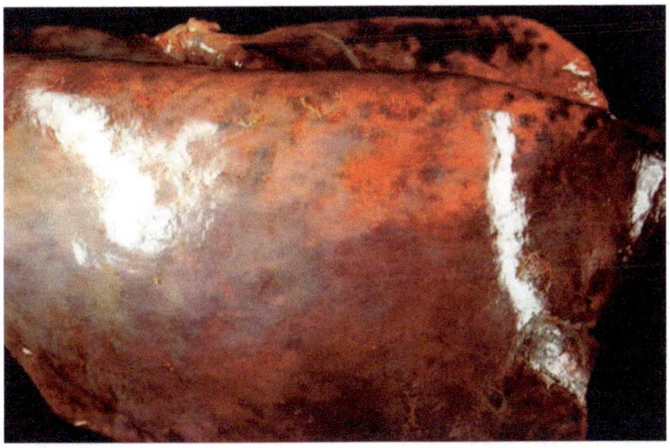

**Figure 2.61.** Foal. Lung. Interstitial Pneumonia. Diffuse consolidation is present in all lobes. Such a lung feels firm on touch. The disorder results from type 2 pneumocyte proliferation and is of viral, bacterial, and/or toxic etiology.

*i. Tumors*

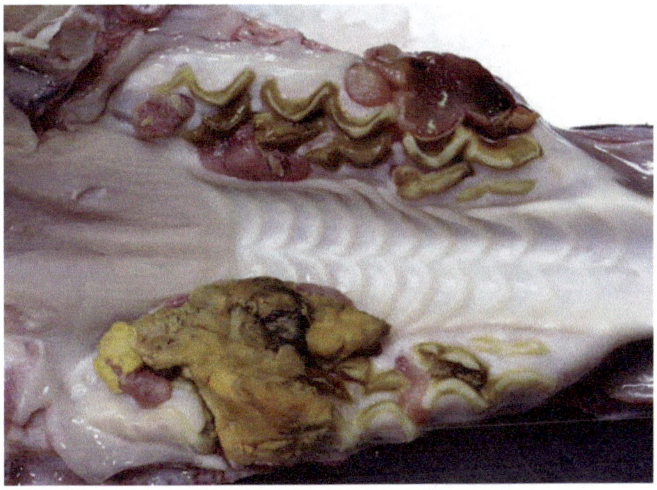

**Figure 2.62.** Foal. Gum. Oral Congenital Hemangiosarcoma. There are small irregular fleshy growths in the gum next to the molars of the maxilla.

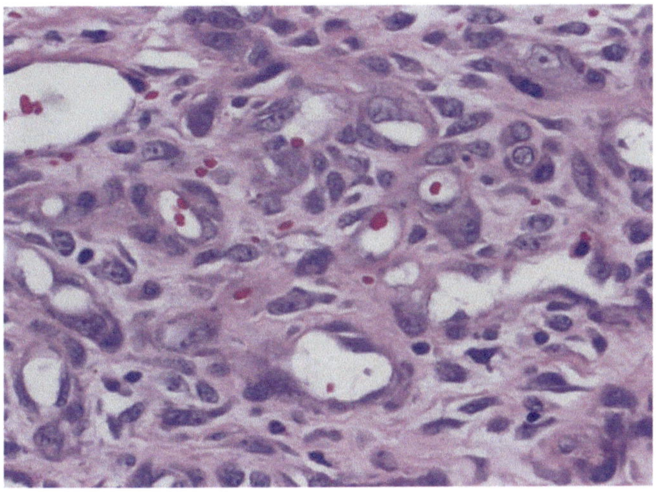

**Figure 2.63.** Foal. Gum. Oral Congenital Hemangiosarcoma. Microscopic features that qualify for the diagnosis of hemangiosarcoma are bundles of spindled cells and plump and irregular endothelial cells lining small channels partially filled with red blood cells. (H&E)

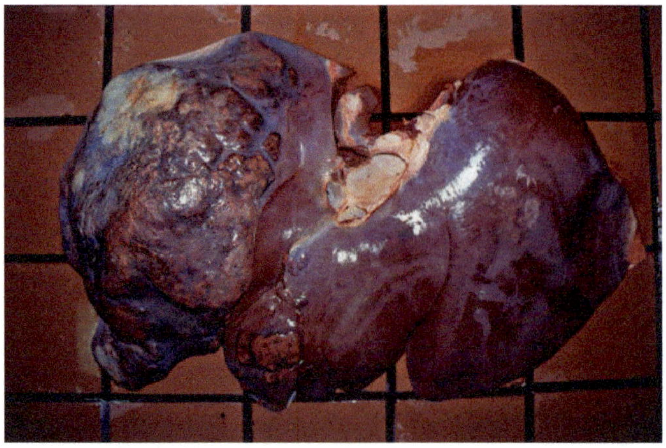

**Figure 2.64.** Foal. Liver. Hepatoblastoma. Multifocal, semi-firm brown/tan raised nodular growths extend throughout the liver lobes replacing the hepatic parenchyma.

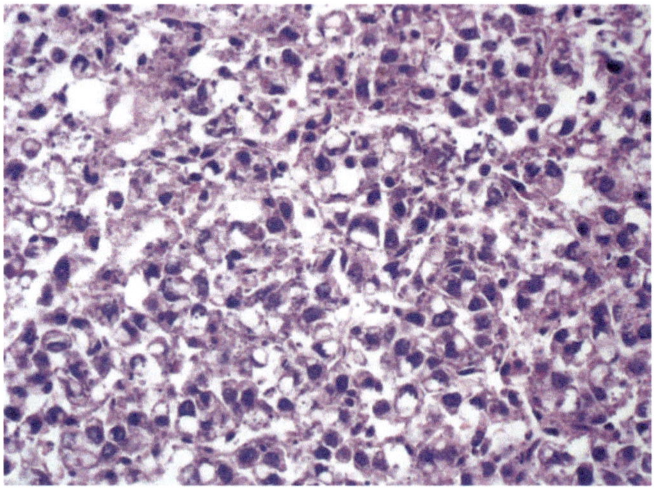

**Figure 2.65.** Foal. Liver. Hepatoblastoma. Microscopic features of the nodular tissue are packages of neoplastic round to polygonal hepatoid cells with no special histologic arrangement. Many of these cells have a vacuolar cytoplasm displacing the nuclei peripherally. Nuclei are round to ovoid to reniform with hyperchromatic chromatin. (H&E)

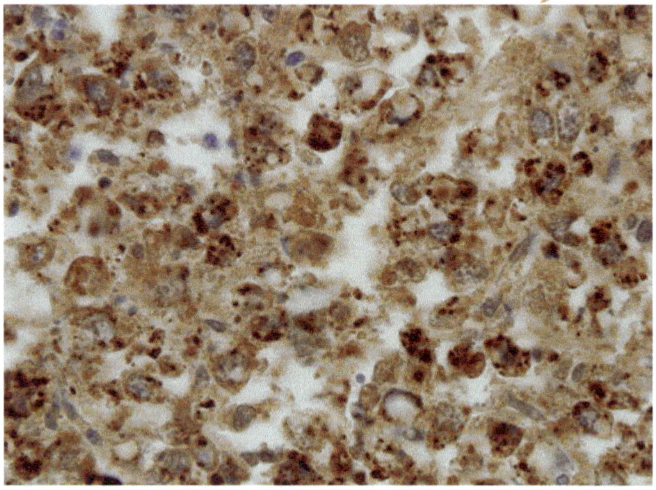

**Figure 2.66.** Foal. Liver. Foal. Hepatoblastoma. The neoplastic cells show strong labeling for hepatocyte paraffin 1. (IHC)

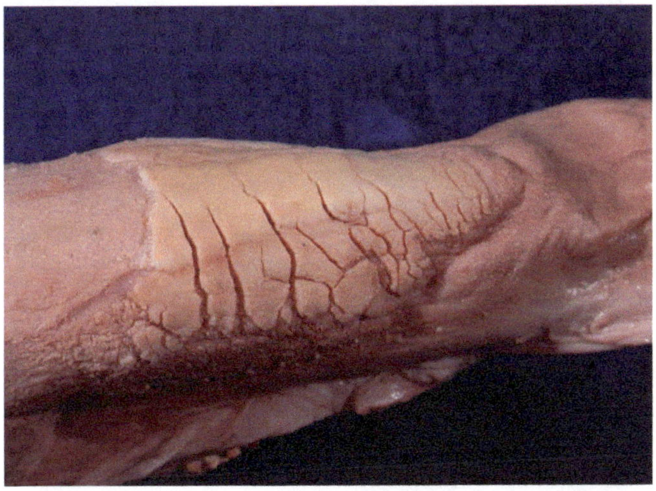

**Figure 2.67.** Foal. Tongue. Parakeratosis. Candidiasis (Thrush). The surface of the tongue is affected by severe parakeratosis. Infection by the yeast *Candida albicans* is the cause of this lesion in immunocompromised animals. Bacteria such as *S. equi* subsp. *zooepidemicus* are differential agents in nonimmunocompromised foals.

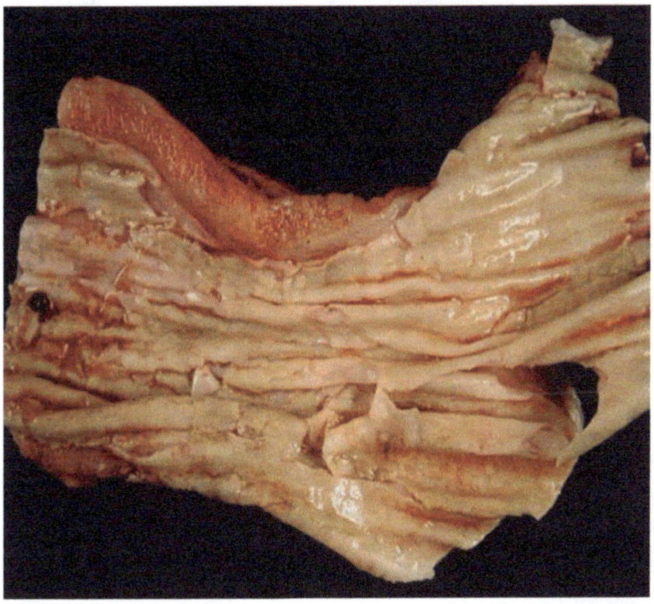

**Figure 2.68.** Foal. Esophagus. Parakeratosis. Candidiasis (Thrush). White plaques are suggestive of *C. albicans* infection.

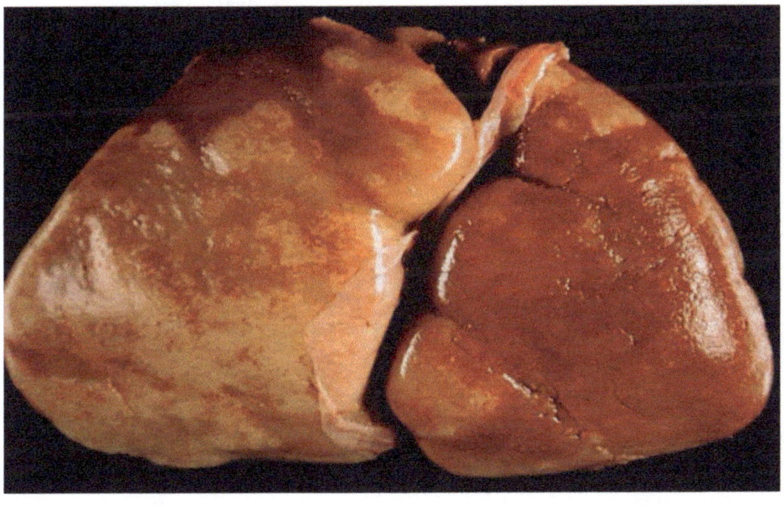

**Figure 2.69.** Foal. Kidney. Multifocal, Necrotizing Nephritis. Candidiasis. Areas of tan bulging tissue representing yeasts are spread within the kidneys.

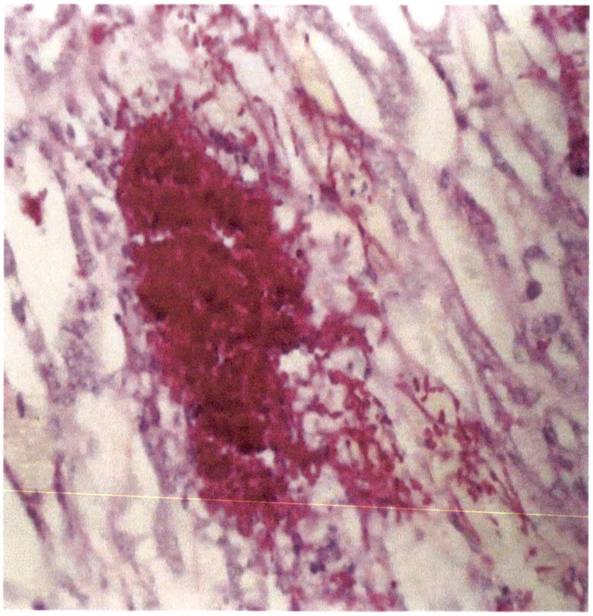

**Figure 2.70.** Foal. Kidney. Intralesional *Candida* sp. A cluster of yeasts positive for periodic acid-Schiff is located within tubules. (PAS)

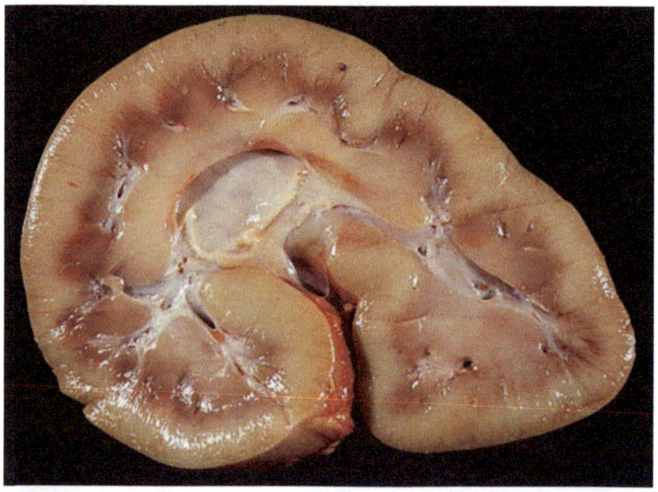

**Figure 2.71.** Foal. Kidney. Nephrosis. The pale kidney is moist and swollen. The animal was treated with aminoglycosides.

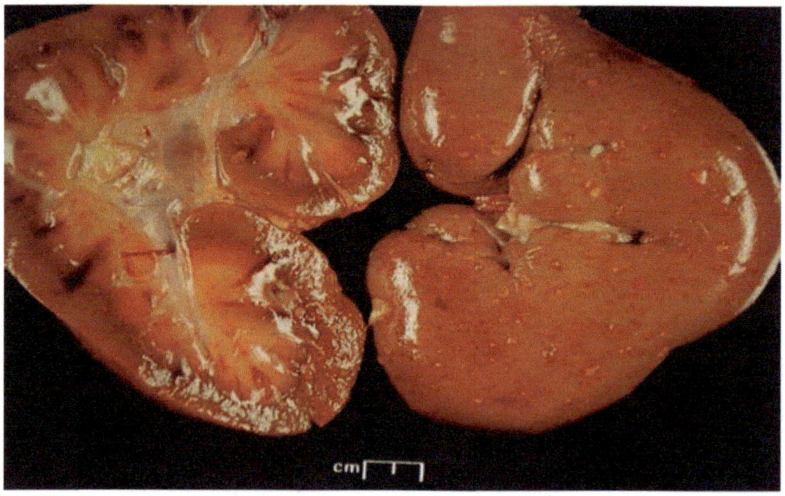


**Figure 2.72.** Foal. Kidney. Microabscesses. Hematogenously spread and bacterial in origin. *Streptococcus equi* subsp. *zooepidemicus* was isolated.

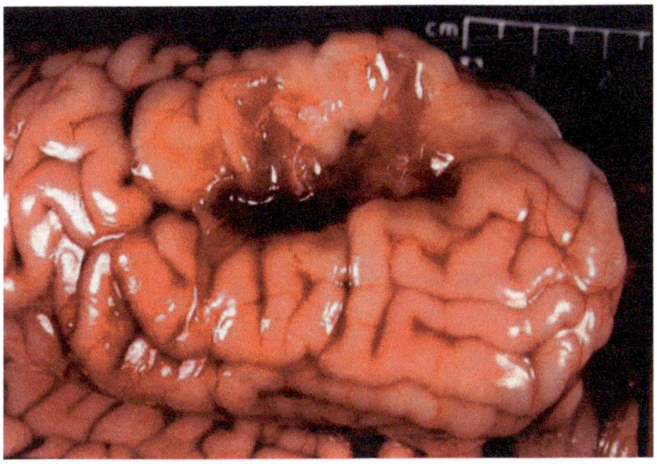


**Figure 2.73.** Foal. Brain. Focal Cerebral Encephalopathy. Area of malacia. Affected foals may become lethargic, dummies, or wanderers. Focal lesions may result from peripartum trauma or asphyxia-hypoxia during parturition.

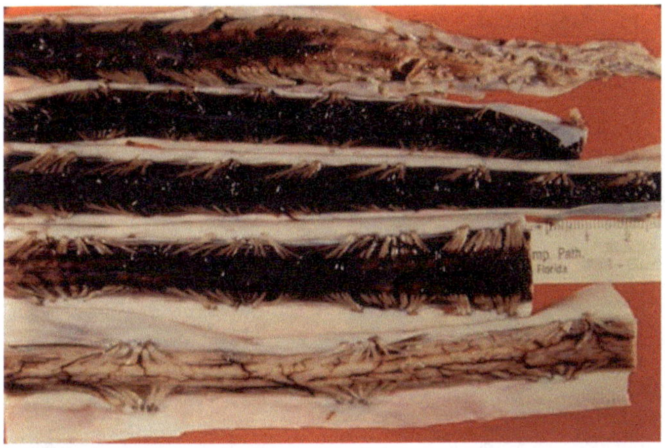

**Figure 2.74.** Foal. Spinal Cord. Hypoxic Ischemic Encephalopathy (Neonatal Maladjustment Syndome). Severe frank subdural and intramedullary spinal cord hemorrhage may result from dystocia or fetal stress during or after birth. The affected animals are incoordinated, unable to stand, unable to nurse, stuporous or hyperexcitable. Similar changes may be present in the brain.

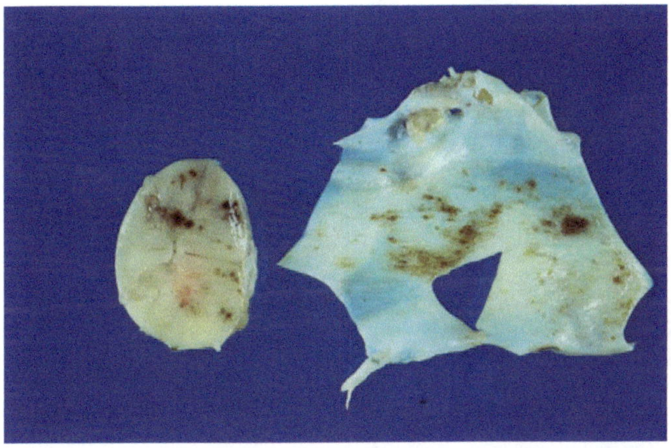

**Figure 2.75.** Foal. Brainstem and Dura. Multifocal Hemorrhage. Eastern Equine Encephalitis (EEE). Multiple petechiae and ecchymoses are the indirect result of EEE alphavirus infection.

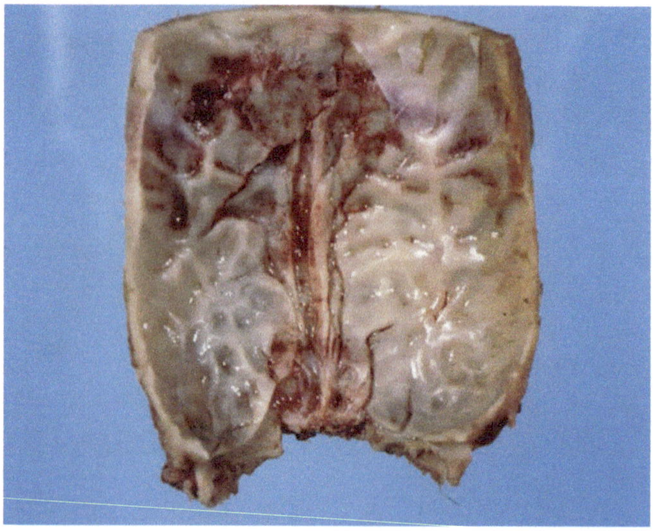

**Figure 2.76.** Foal. Skull. Fracture. Traumatic.

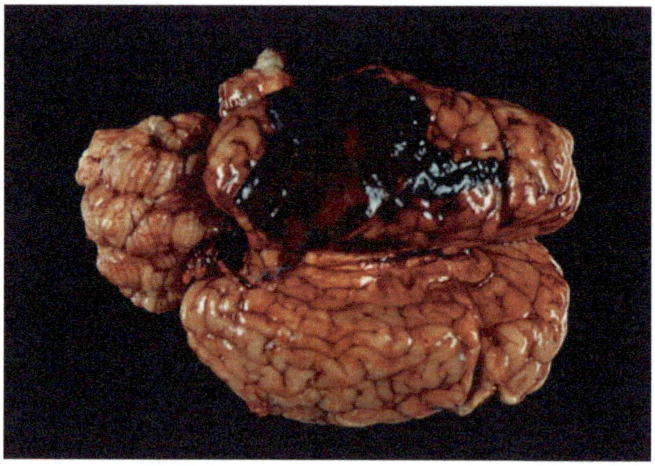

**Figure 2.77.** Foal. Brain. Hematoma. Traumatic.

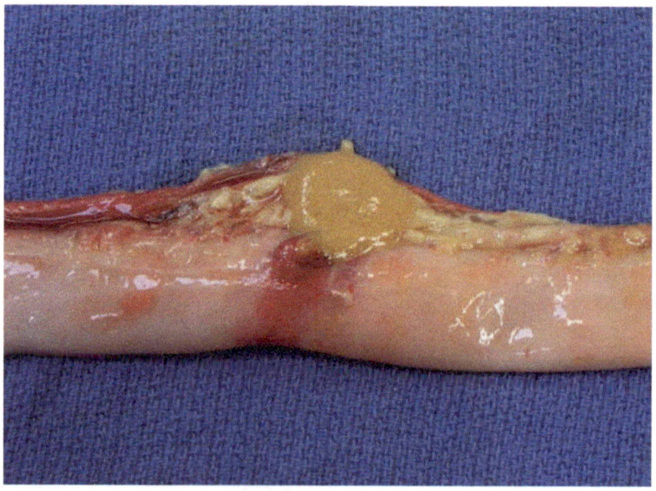

**Figure 2.78.** Foal. Intestine. Perforation. Focal necrosis due to thrombosis resulted in perforation and septic peritonitis.

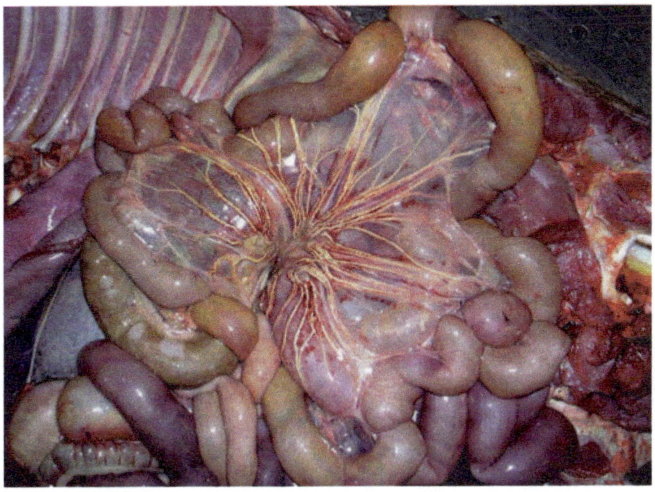

**Figure 2.79.** Foal. Mesentery. Postprandial lymphangiectasia.

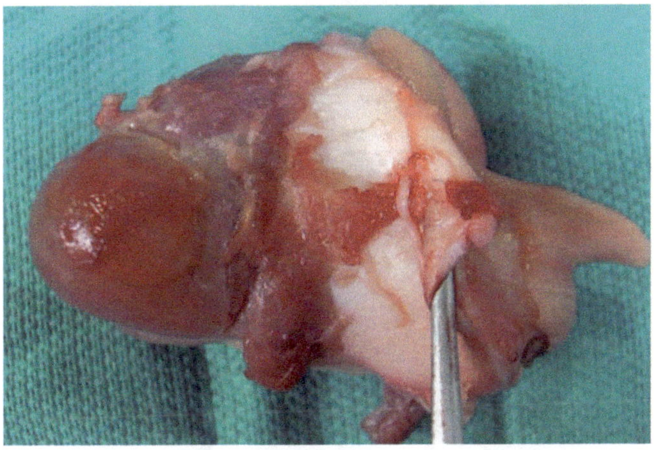

**Figure 2.80.** Foal. Larynx. Perilaryngeal Cyst deforming Larynx. (Courtesy Dr. P. Habecker, University of Pennsylvania.)

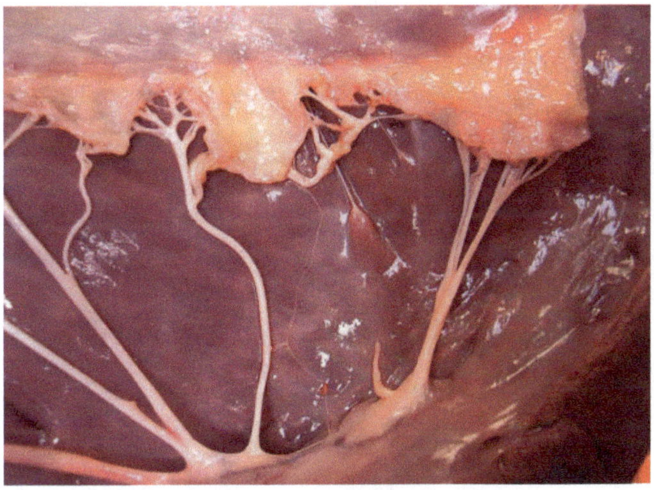

**Figure 2.81.** Foal. Heart. Mitral Valve. Ruptured Chorda Tendinea. The rupture had occurred at the papillary muscle insertion site. Pulmonary edema is a fatal complication.

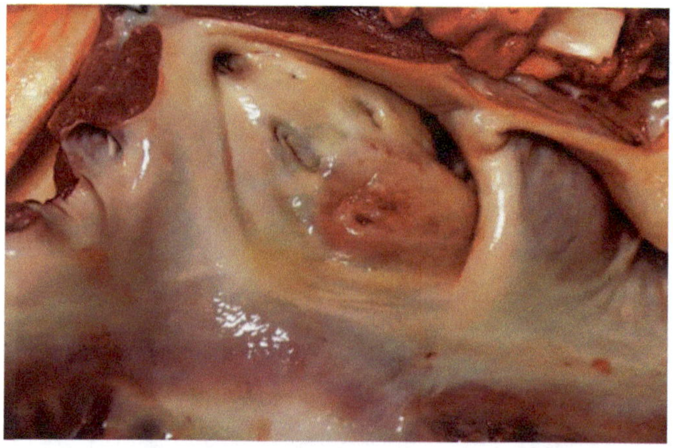

**Figure 2.82.** Foal. Heart. Atrial Septum. Valvula Foraminis Ovalis.

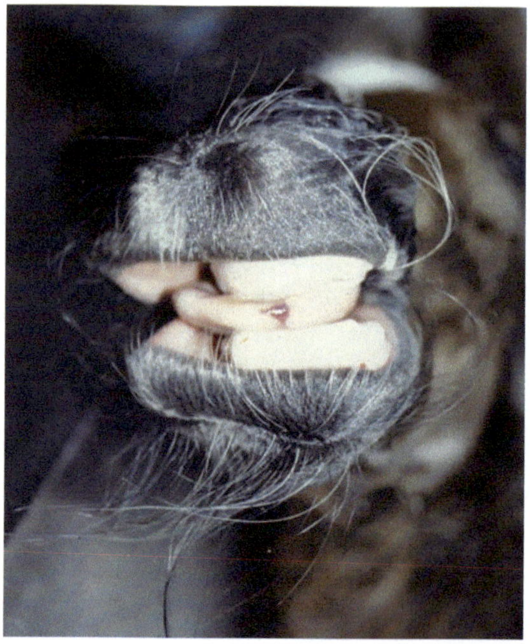

**Figure 2.83.** Foal. Neonate. Head. Vibrissae. Prolonged hair around lips indicates hypermaturity.

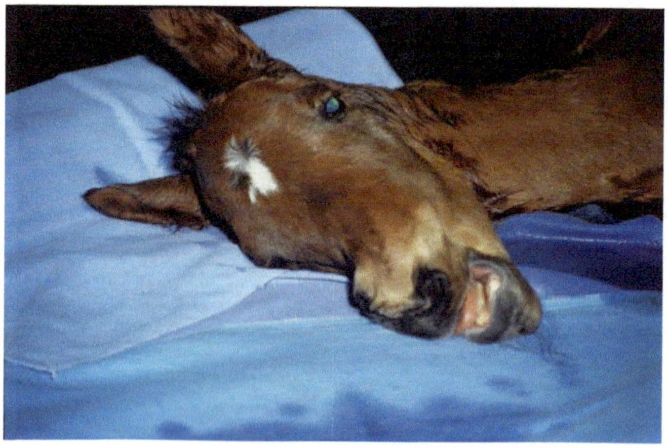

**Figure 2.84.** Foal. Neonate. Head. Nasal Deformity. Traumatic or body pregnancy.

## Congenital abnormalities of foals

### Central nervous system

- Hydrocephalus
- Cerebellar abiotrophy
- Optic nerve hypoplasia/aplasia

### Cardiovascular

- Ventricular septal defect (VSD)
- Truncus arteriosus
- Tetralogy of Fallot
- Patent ductus arteriosus (PDA)
- Persistent right aortic arch

### Respiratory

- Tracheal dysplasia
- Wry nose
- Diaphragmatic hernia

### Gastrointestinal

- Palotoschisis
- Megaesophagus
- Intestinal atresia
- Atresia ani
- Aganglionosis
- Meckel's diverticulum
- Mesodiverticular band

### Liver

- Portal shunts
- Hepatic fibrosis

### Urinary tract

- Horseshoe kidney
- Renal aplasia/hypoplasia
- Polycystic kidneys
- Persistent urachus

## Common congenital abnormalities – continued

**Reproductive tract**

- Turner syndrome
- Parovarian cysts
- Segmental aplasia of the uterus
- Umbilical hernia
- Cryptorchidism

**Skeleton**

- Atlanto-occipital malformation
- Lordosis, kyphosis, scoliosis
- Inferior brachygnathism

**Tendons**

- Contractions
- Angular deformities
- Arthrogryposis

**Skin**

- Congenital porphyria
- Hyperelastosis cutis
- Lavender foal syndrome
- Presumptive chronic progressive lymphedema in draft horses

**Hematopoietic**

- Immunodeficiency

**Eye**

- Microphthalmia
- Dermoids
- Iris hypoplasia

**Ear**

- Aplasia/hypoplasia of external ear

## II. Diseases of juveniles

This section addresses the diseases of those organ systems primarily involved in the age group of 1 to 12 months. Affected organ systems to be discussed include respiratory, digestive, and locomotor systems. Specific individual diseases presented are *R. equi* pneumonia and enteritis, juvenile interstitial pneumonia, gastroduodenal ulcer disease, bacterial hemorrhagic enteric diseases, and septic polyarthritis.

### 1. *Acquired diseases*

#### *a.* Rhodococcus equi

Typically, the infection by this bacterium is recognized in horses between 3 and 6 months of age, occasionally older. Organ systems involved in *R. equi* infection are respiratory or digestive. Rarely does the infection simultaneously involve both. The pulmonary variant is the more frequent one. Dissemination of *R. equi* to other organs such as liver, CNS, bones, placenta, or eyes can occur.

*R. equi* infection is endemic in stud farms where it causes significant morbidity. The bacillus is gram-positive and facultative intracellular. Regarding the respiratory disease, environmental soil-borne *R. equi* is inhaled and phagocytized by macrophages of the lung. Although the bacterium can be killed by neutrophils, *R. equi* multiplies and eventually destroys alveolar macrophages. Plasmids recovered from isolates are crucial for virulence. All strains of *R. equi* isolated from clinical cases have a large 80–90 kb plasmid and express virulence-associated protein A antigens. Control of infectivity is largely monitored by cell-mediated immunity.

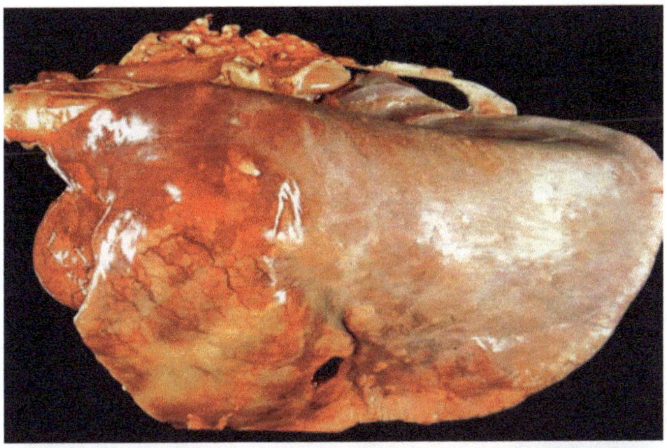

**Figure 2.85.** Juvenile. Lung. Chronic Cranioventral Caseous and Pyogranulomatous Bronchopneumonia. A large plum-colored area of consolidation is present in the cranial lung.

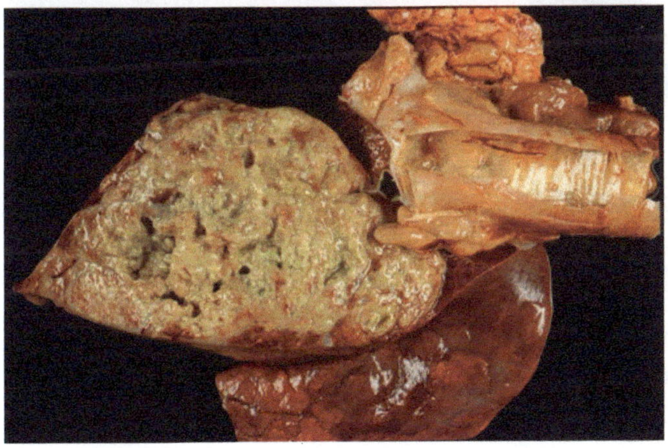

**Figure 2.86.** Juvenile. Lung. Pyogranulomatous Bronchopneumonia. The same area in cross section demonstrates caseous necrosis.

Figure 2.87. Juvenile. Lung. Pulmonary Abscesses and Interstitial Pneumonia. Multiple elevated nodules represent pulmonary abscesses. These may become confluent. The brown zones at the periphery of the nodules and in the dorsal diaphragmatic part represent interstitial pneumonia, which may become quite extensive in some cases and need to be differentiated from the primary form of juvenile interstitial pneumonia discussed in the next section. Above form of interstitial pneumonia is associated with the presence of *R. equi* bacilli.

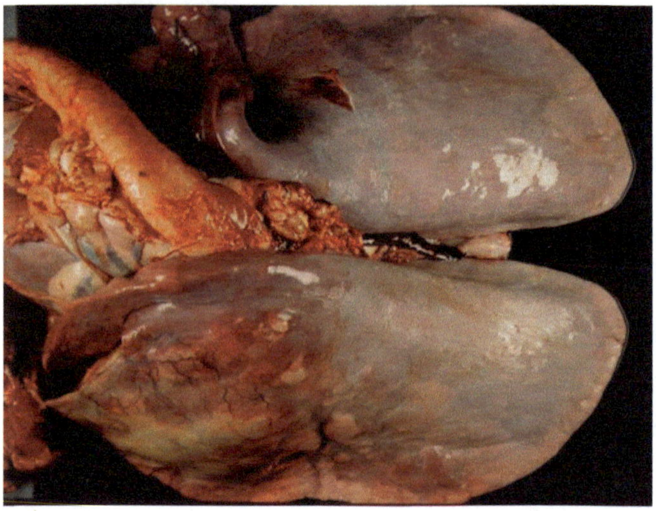

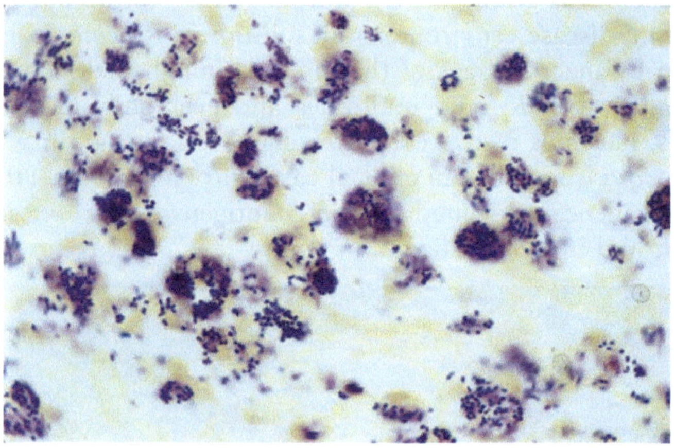

Figure 2.88. Juvenile. Lung. Abscess. A Gram stain reveals intralesional, positive intracellular (macrophages) bacilli compatible with *R. equi*. (Brown and Brenn)

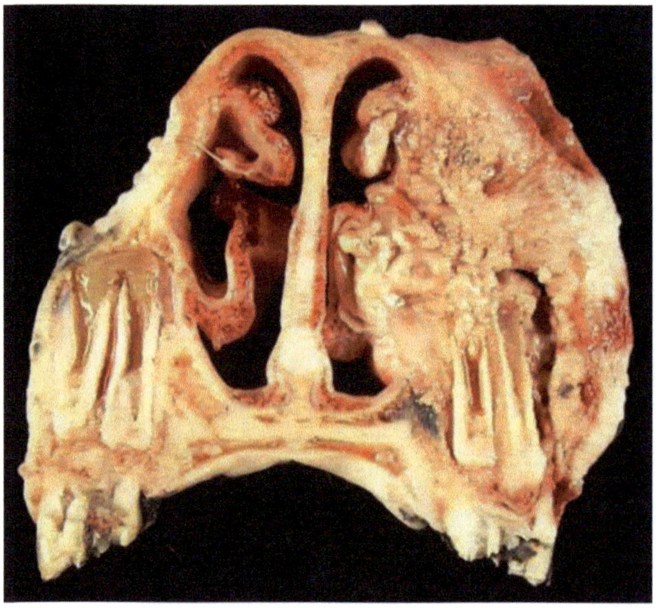

Figure 2.89. Juvenile. Maxilla. Pyogranulomatous Osteomyelitis. The maxillary bones and nasal turbinates are distorted by a dry granular exudate from which *R. equi* was isolated. Portal of entry was likely inhalation.

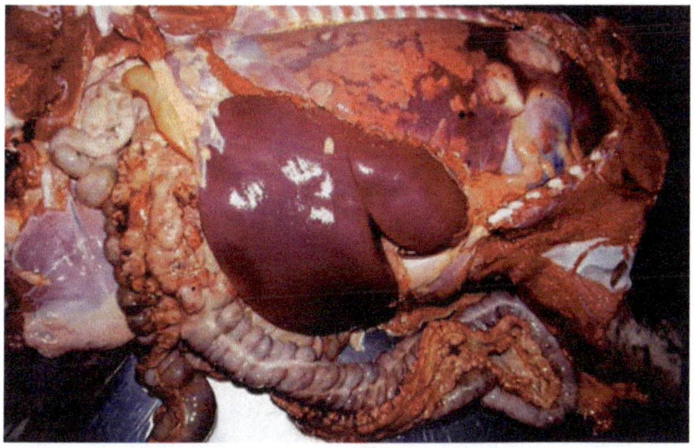

**Figure 2.90.** Juvenile. Intestine. *R. equi* Pyogranulomatous Lymphadenitis. Colonic lymph nodes are markedly enlarged representing the alimentary form of *R. equi* infection. A cranioventral pneumonia is also present.

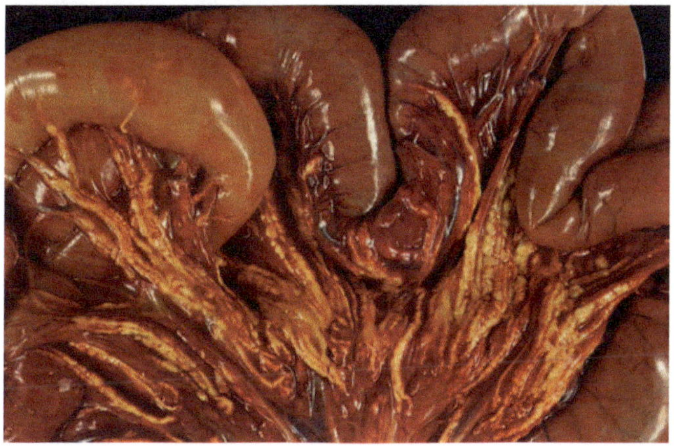

**Figure 2.91.** Juvenile. Mesenteric Lymphatics. *R. equi* Pyogranulomatous Lymphangitis. Mesenteric lymphatics are string-like thickened. Differential diagnosis: *Actinobacillus equuli* subsp. *hemolyticus* infection.

*b. Interstitial pneumonia*

Juvenile interstitial pneumonia can occur between 1 and 7 months of age. It is defined as type 2 pneumocyte hyperplastic reaction following damage to the alveolar-capillary unit of the lung. During the acute phase, alveolar walls denuded from type 1 pneumocytes become covered by hyaline membranes. Type 2 pneumocyte hyperplasia and interstitial thickening due to accumulation of lymphoid cells and fibrous tissue as well as various mononuclear inflammatory cells such as neutrophils, macrophages, and lymphocytes in the intra-alveolar lumen characterize the chronic phase. Chemical/toxic, allergic, or infectious factors are possible causes. Infectious etiologies are postulated to be equine herpesvirus-1 and -4, influenza virus, equine viral arteritis virus, *R. equi*, and *P. jiroveci*. However, the etiology of most cases of juvenile interstitial pneumonia remains undetermined.

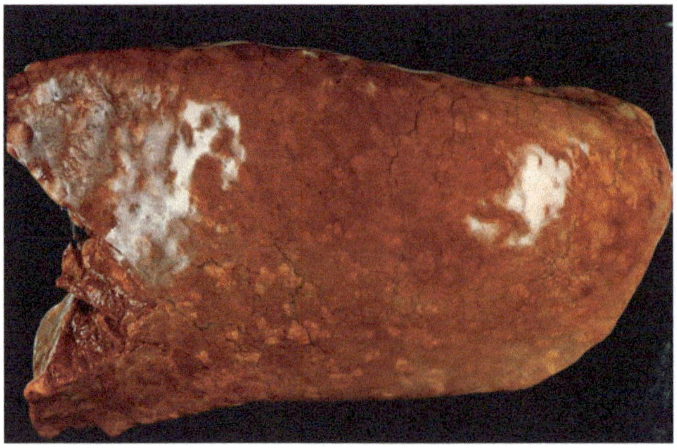

**Figure 2.92.** Juvenile. Lung. Interstitial Pneumonia. The entire lung is turgid, mottled brown, and firm. Yellow foci remain aerated.

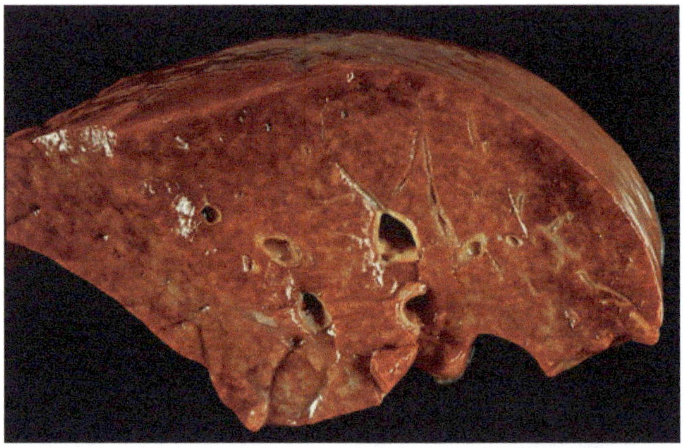

**Figure 2.93.** Juvenile. Lung. Interstitial Pneumonia. On cross section, the brown parenchyma is dry and bulges slightly. The yellow foci are aerated.

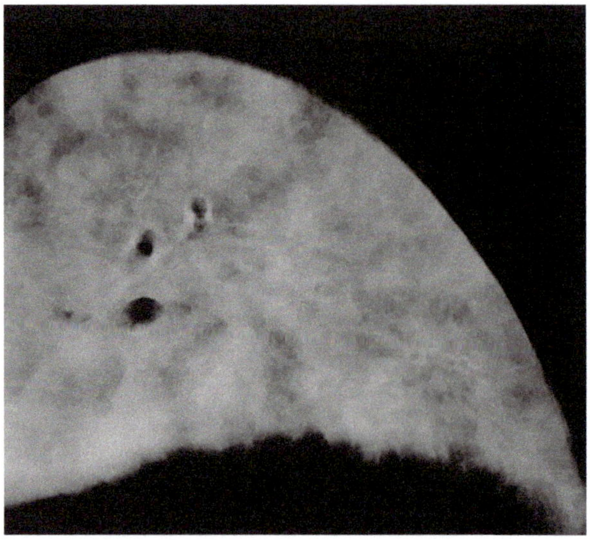

**Figure 2.94.** Juvenile. Lung. Interstitial Pneumonia. Radiographically, an alveolar-interstitial pattern of increased densities is appreciated.

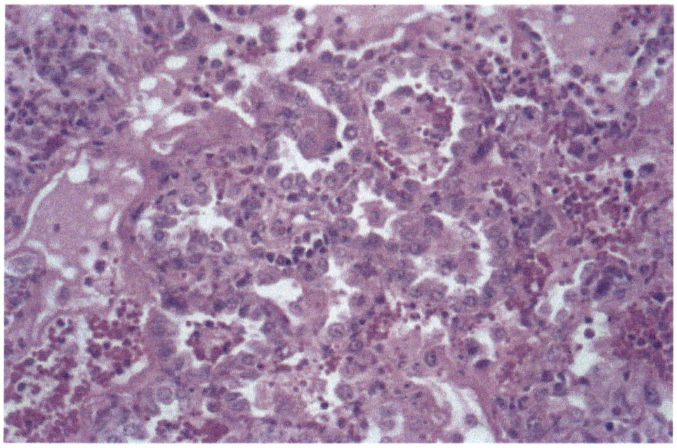

**Figure 2.95.** Juvenile. Lung. Chronic Interstitial Pneumonia. At the microscopic level, diffuse proliferation of type 2 pneumocytes has resulted in an adenomatoid pattern of alveolar thickening. (H&E)

The identification of herpesvirus intranuclear inclusions determined to represent equine herpesvirus-5 can be noticed in a small percentage of the cases in adult horse infection with multinodular pulmonary fibrosis. Evidence for this agent in the pathogenesis is presently missing in juvenile horses.

## Juvenile interstitial pneumonia – Fact sheet

**Definition:** Primary damage to alveolar-capillary unit

**Age of Affected Animals:** 1–7 months

### Etiology considerations

**Infectious Agents**

- Equine influenza virus
- Equine viral arteritis virus
- Equine herpesviruses
- *Rhodococcus equi*
- *Klebsiella pneumoniae*
- *Streptococcus* sp.
- *Pneumocystis jiroveci*

**Toxic/chemical causes**

- Crofton weed
- Perilla mint
- Paraquat
- Pyrrolizidine alkaloids
- Oxygen

## Juvenile interstitial pneumonia – Fact sheet continued

### Pathologic findings

**Gross**

- Diffuse consolidation of all lung lobes

**Microscopic**

- Alveolar necrosis
- Hyaline membrane formations in alveoli in acute phase
- Type 2 pneumocyte hyperplasia in chronic phase
- Neutrophils and monocytes in alveolar spaces

*c. Gastroduodenal ulcer disease*

The syndrome has almost exclusively been confined to sucklings and early weanlings. Gastroduodenal ulcer disease (GDUD) syndrome reached its peak in the mid-1980s, but it is still an occasional problem in intensive mare/foal operations. The most severe lesion in affected animals is in the anterior duodenum. The cause of GDUD in young horses remained largely unknown until experimental induction of the disorder incriminated excessive dosing with nonsteroidal anti-inflammatory drugs interfering with local gastric production of cytoprotective prostaglandin E. Rotavirus diarrhea has been discussed but has not been proven to be involved as a precipitating factor.

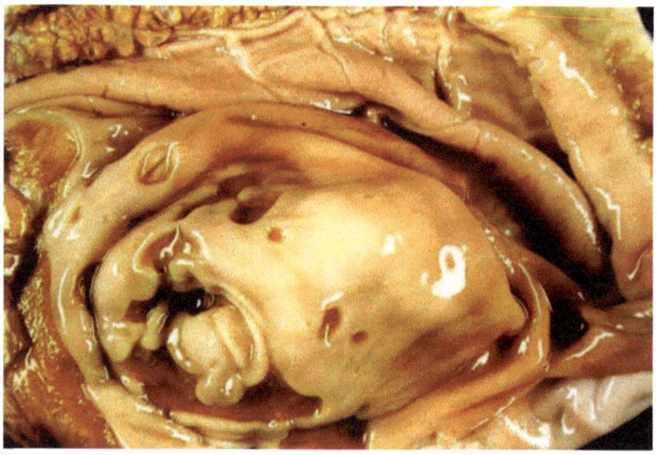

**Figure 2.96.** Juvenile. Glandular Stomach. Ulcers. Large deep but nonperforating ulcers are present in the glandular mucosa of the pyloric antrum.

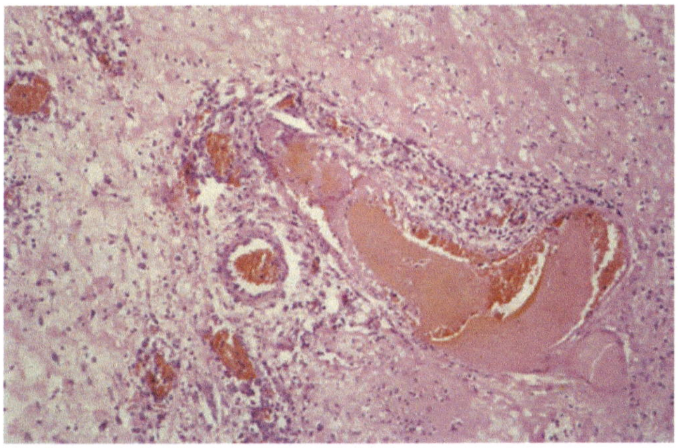

**Figure 2.97.** Juvenile. Glandular Stomach. Thrombotic Vein. A large submucosal vein is thrombosed with perivascular edema and red blood cell extravasation. It is responsible for the gastric ulcer in the overlying mucosa. (H&E)

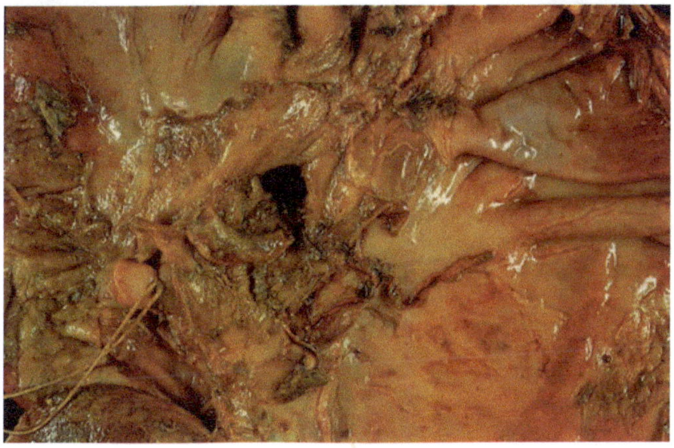

**Figure 2.98.** Juvenile. Glandular Stomach. Perforating Ulcer. A large solitary mucosal ulcer led to perforation.

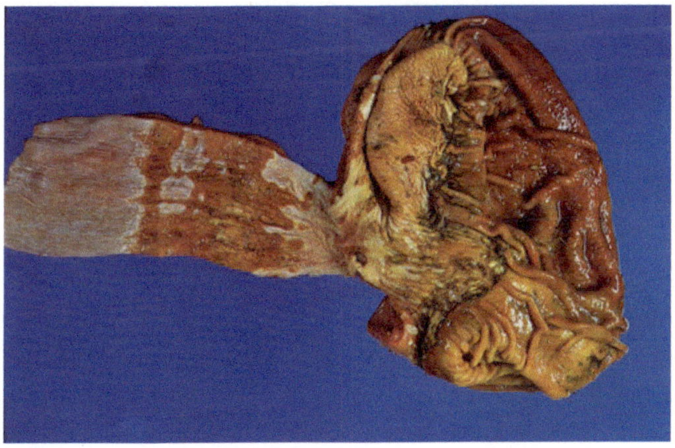

**Figure 2.99.** Juvenile. Esophagus and Nonglandular Stomach. Mucosal Erosions. The mucosa of the distal esophagus shows patchy areas of inflammation and erosions. Differential diagnosis: reflux esophagitis. Several erosions and shallow ulcers are present in the nonglandular stomach.

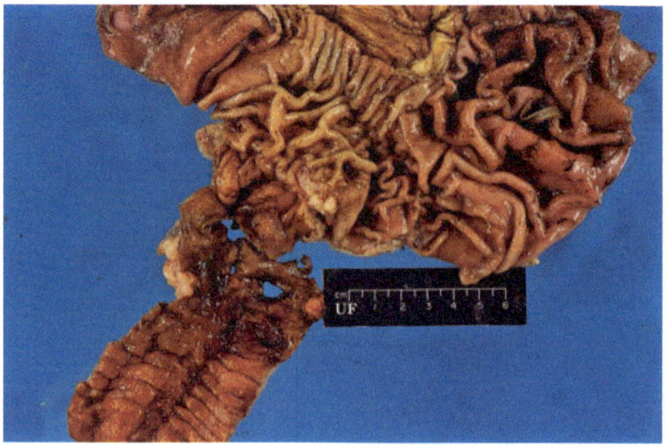


**Figure 2.100.** Juvenile. Duodenum. Perforating Ulcers. These are present close to the pylorus. Severe peritonitis is the outcome.

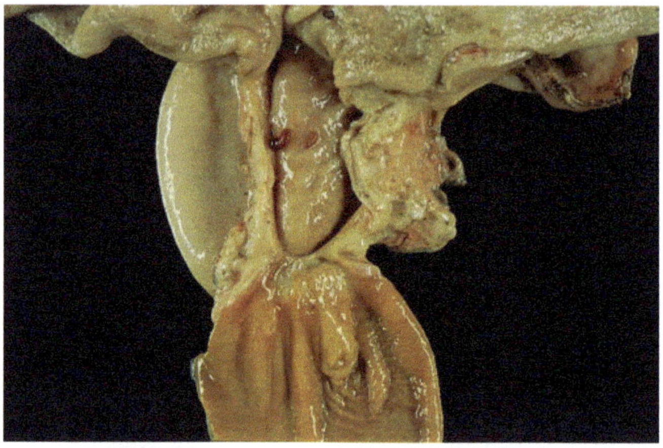

**Figure 2.101.** Juvenile. Duodenum. Stricture. The stricture is a complication from healing attempts of chronic duodenal ulceration. It may result in proximal duodenal obstruction, sometimes with ascending pancreatitis and severe cholangiohepatitis and prominent bile duct fibrosis, dilatation, and bile accumulation.

### *d. Enteric bleeding events*

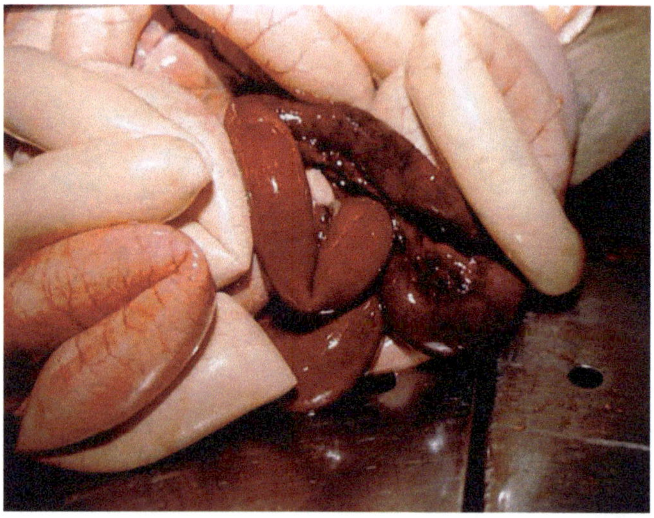

**Figure 2.102.** Juvenile. Small Intestine. Volvulus. Rotation of segments of small intestinal loops around the mesenteric axis resulted in severe venous compression, congestion, and extravasation of red blood cells.

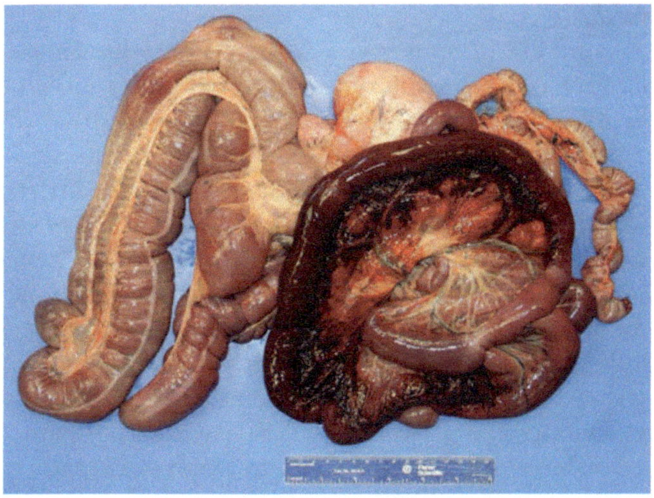

**Figure 2.103.** Juvenile. Small Intestine. Clostridial Disease. A segment of small intestinal loops is reddish and distended. *C. perfringens* type C was isolated. (Courtesy Dr. F. Shariar, Tustin, CA.)

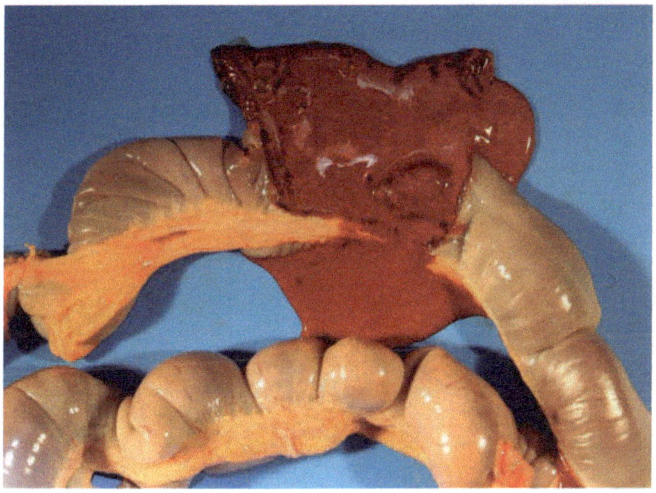

**Figure 2.104.** Juvenile. Large Intestine. Clostridial Disease. The reddening of the opened intestinal segment is the result of mucosal hemorrhage. Toxin A from *C. difficile* was identified in this case. (Courtesy Dr. S. Diab, San Bernadino, CA.)

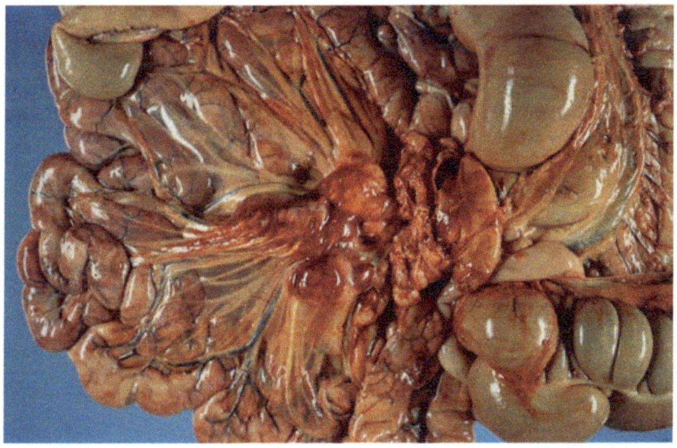

**Figure 2.105.** Juvenile. Small Intestine and Mesenteric Lymph Nodes. Pyogranulomatous Lymphadenitis. Acute Salmonellosis. The serosal surface of the small intestine is slightly reddened, whereas the mesenteric lymph nodes are markedly reddened suggesting drainage of extravasated red blood cells. *Salmonella* serotype B was isolated from the feces.

*e. Septic polyarthritis*

This disease is common in foals younger than 4 months. Single or multiple joints may be affected. The condition can have a devastating life-threatening outcome. It is likely multifactorial but mainly the result of disseminating gram-negative bacteria. Starting from poor umbilical hygienic management (less common these days) to failure of passive colostral transfer, poor nutritional and environmental management, and bacterial overgrowth in target organs such as the digestive tract and lung, bacteria will hematogenously reach synovial membranes, articular surfaces, physes, and bone marrow of mainly long bones to induce painful and treatment-resistant septic polyarthritis. The stifle joints appear most frequently involved, but any limb joint can be affected. Articular lesions can be classified by duration, nature of inflammatory exudate, and anatomic structure within the joint.

Systemically disseminating bacteria are gram-negative pathogens, in particular *E. coli*, *Proteus*, *Pseudomonas aeruginosa*, *Salmonella*, and *K. pneumoniae*, but also *Streptococcus* sp. and *Staphylococcus* sp. can be isolated on occasion.

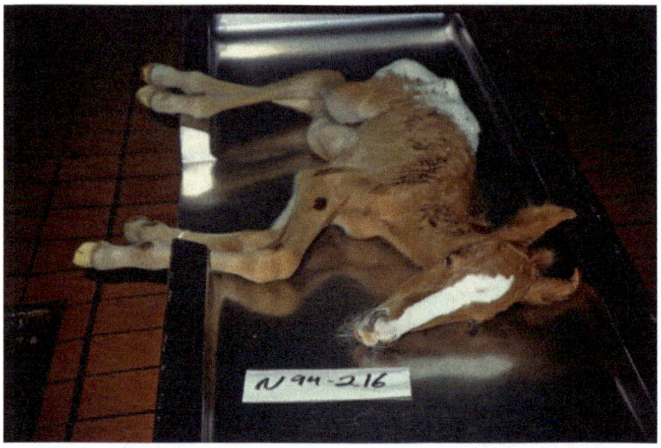

**Figure 2.106.** Foal. Body. Emaciation and Septic Polyarthritis. Osseous protuberances reflect a poor nutritional plane. Swollen joints of both front and hind legs are clinically associated with pain and lameness.

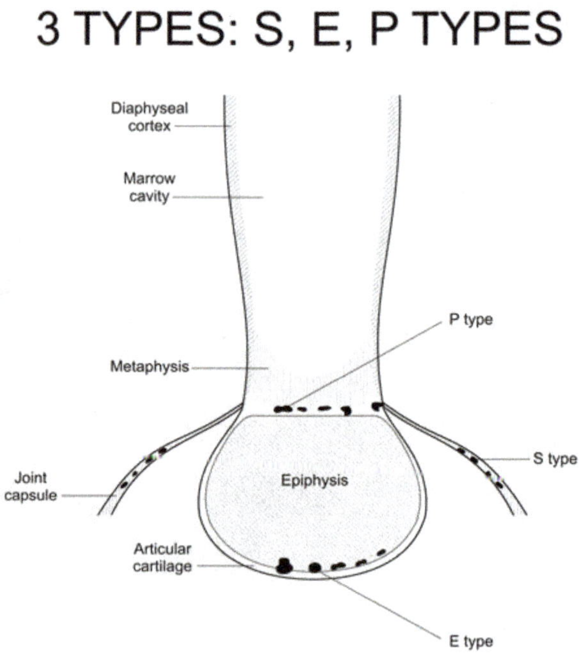


**Diagram.** Concept of Various Phases of Septic Joint Disease in Foals. (Modified according to Dr. E. Firth, College of Veterinary Medicine, Massey University, New Zealand.) In this concept joint diseases are classified according to anatomic location, duration, and severity. Accordingly, joint diseases are divided into three phases: S-phase affecting the synovial membranes only, being mainly acute and less severe, but causing lameness and swelling nonetheless; E-phase, describing the involvement of the epiphysis, and P-phase describing the involvement of the physis in inflammation. The latter is prognostically the most unfavorable as to outcome and the least treatable as to choice of medication. Recently, a fourth form has been added: T-form (Tarsal).

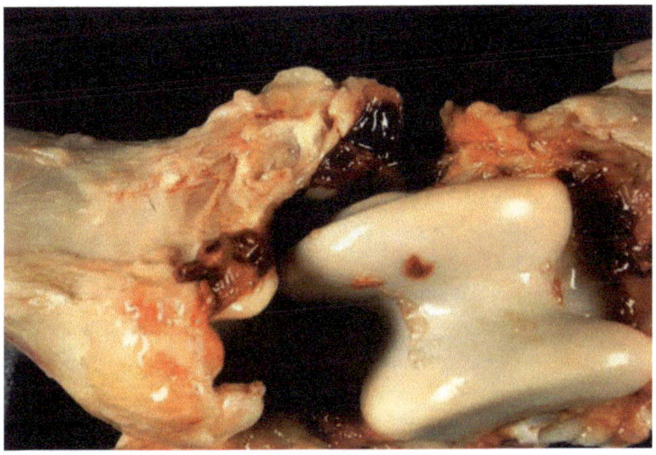

**Figure 2.107.** Juvenile. Hock Joint. S-Phase Arthritis. Synovial membranes are slightly thickened and reddened. Joint fluid escaped at the joint opening but was increased and straw colored. The articular surface remains smooth and glistening.

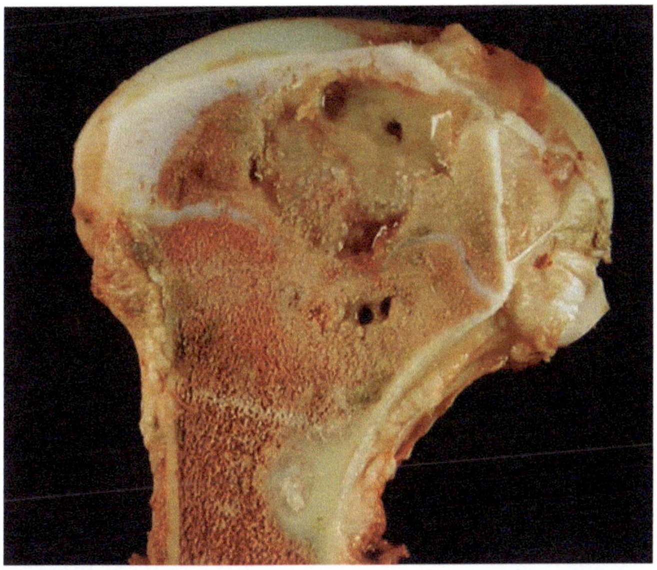

**Figure 2.108.** Juvenile. Midsagittal Section. Femur. E-Phase Arthritis. The entire epiphysis is eroded and has been replaced by yellow exudate. The inflammation extended toward the physis. Such involvement leads to collapse of the articular surface. *Salmonella* group B was isolated from the synovial fluid.

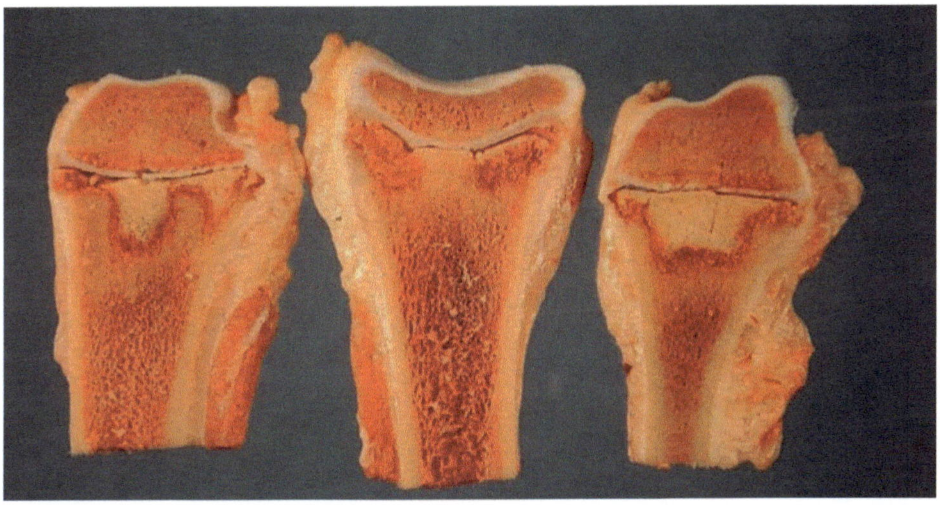

**Figure 2.109.** Juvenile. Midsagittal Sections. Distal Tibia, Distal Metatarsus, Distal Metacarpus. P-Phase. The physes of several bones have a yellow exudate sharply demarcated by a red ring suggesting sequestration. No growth was obtained from the synovial fluid.

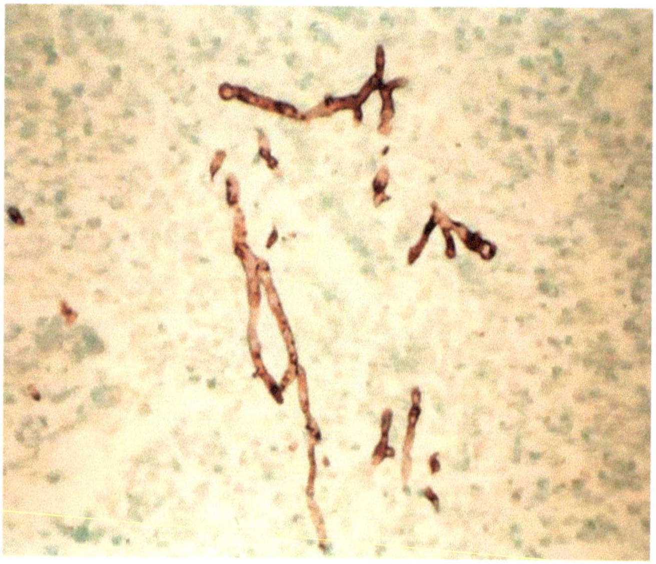

**Figure 2.110.** Juvenile. Long Bone. Physis. Arthritis. Histologically, a fungal stain identified the presence of intralesional hyphae of *Aspergillus* sp. (GMS)

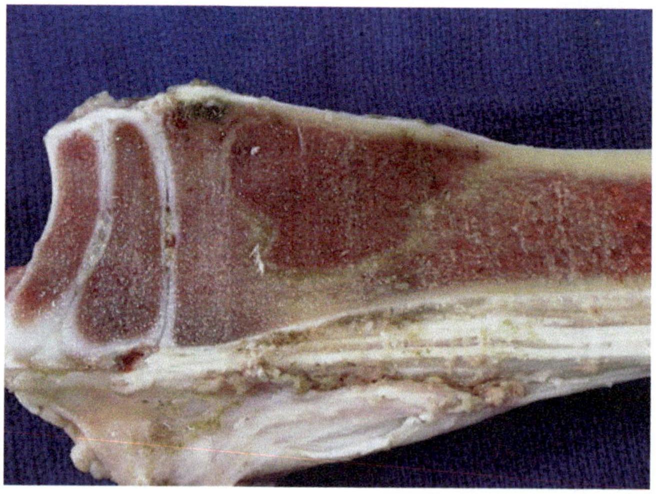

**Figure 2.111.** Juvenile. Midsagittal Section. Distal Tarsus. T-Phase Arthritis. Focal subphyseal necrosis and sequestrum.

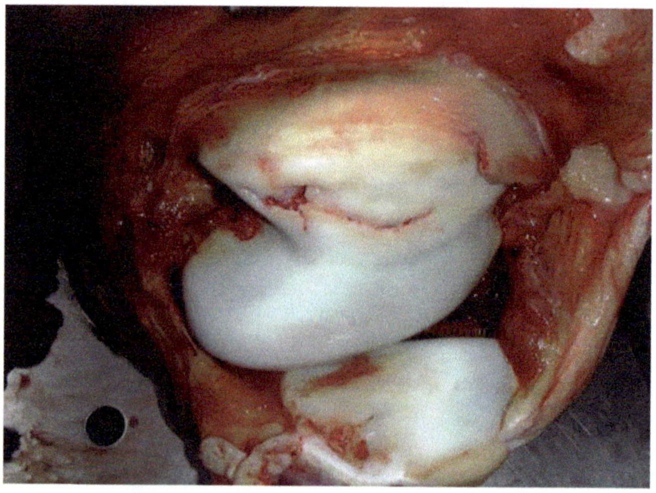

**Figure 2.112.** Juvenile. Stifle Joint. Osteochondrosis Dissecans (OCD). Erosion of the medial condyle and patella represents OCD of a juvenile Clydesdale.

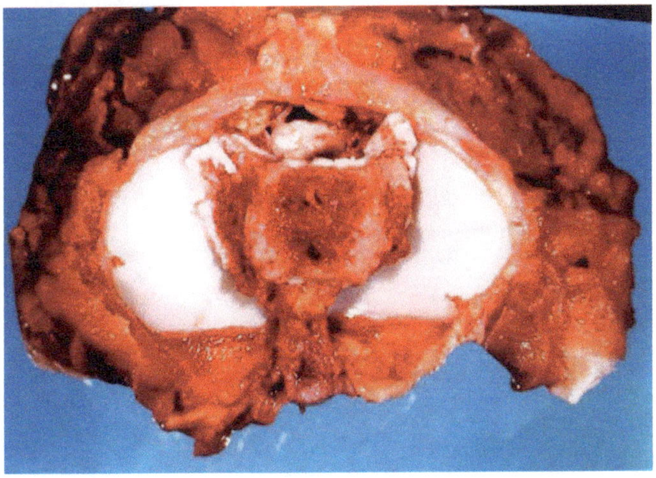

**Figure 2.113.** Juvenile. Dens. Atlanto-occipital Joint. Fracture. This traumatic event led to compression of the overriding spinal cord.

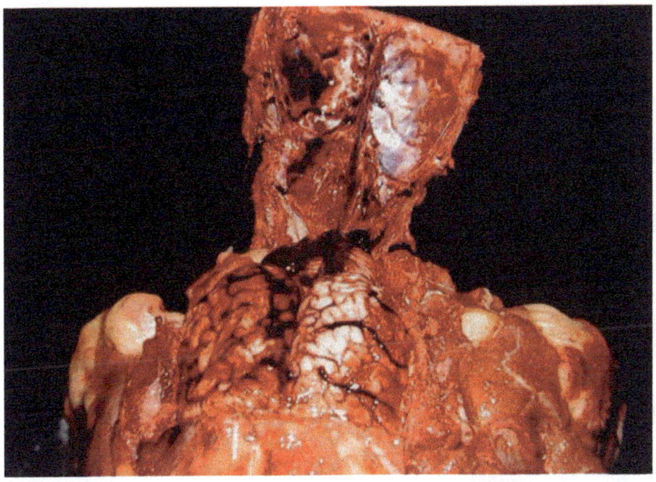

**Figure 2.114.** Juvenile. Skull. Fracture. This traumatic event resulted in diffuse meningeal hemorrhage.

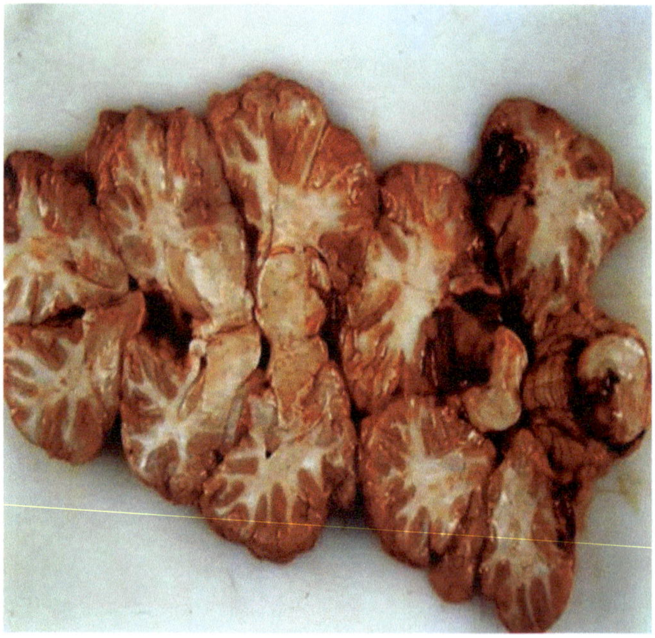

**Figure 2.115.** Juvenile. Brain. Hemorrhage. Multiple foci of parenchymal hemorrhage into the caudal brain were the result of intracarotid injections of a straining foal.

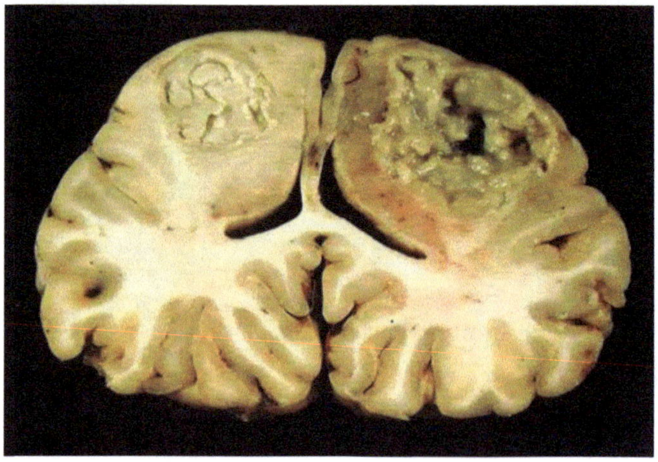

**Figure 2.116.** Juvenile. Brain. Cerebral Abscess. *Streptococcus equi* subsp. *equi* was isolated from a large abscess within the cerebral hemisphere.

## Selected references

Ainsworth DM, Weldon AD, Beck KA, Rowland PH. 1993. Recognition of *Pneumocystis carinii* in foals with respiratory distress. *Equine Vet J* 25(2):103–108.

Barr BS. 2003. Pneumonia in weanlings. *Vet Clin North Am Equine Pract* 19(1):35–49.

Dawson TR, Horohov DW, Meier WG, Muscatello G. 2010. Current understanding of the equine immune response to *Rhodococcus equi*. An immunological review of *R. equi* pneumonia. *Vet Immunol Immunopathol* 135(1–2):1–11.

Del Piero F, Wilkens PA, Lopez JW, et al. 1997. Equine viral arteritis in newborn foals: clinical, pathological, serological, microbiological and immunohistochemical observations. *Equine Vet J* 29(3):178–185.

Diab SS, Kinde H, Moore J, et al. 2012. Pathology of *Clostridium perfringens* type C enterotoxemia in horses. *Vet Pathol* 49(2):255–263.

Frederick J, Giguere S, Sanchez IC. 2009. Infectious agents detected in the feces of diarrheic foals: a retrospective study of 233 cases (2003–2008). *J Vet Intern Med* 23(6):1254–1260.

Genetzky RM, McNeel SV, Loparco FV. 1984. *Rhodococcus equi* pneumonia in foals. *Mod Vet Pract* 65(10):787–790.

Giguère S, Cohen ND, Chaffin MK, et al. 2011. Diagnosis, treatment, control and prevention of infection caused by *Rhodococcus equi* in foals. *J Vet Intern Med* 25(6):1209–1220.

Hollis AR, Wilkins PA, Palmer JE, Boston RC. 2008. Bacteremia in equine neonatal diarrhea: a retrospective study (1990–2007). *J Vet Intern Med* 22(5):1203–1209.

Johnson AL. 2010. Clinical commentary. Congenital malformations—uncommon but important causes of neurological signs in neonates. 2010. *Equine Vet Educ* 22(12):599–601.

Lakritz J, Wilson WD, Berry CR, Schrenzel MD, Carlson GP, Madigan JE. 1993. Bronchointerstitial pneumonia and respiratory distress in young horses: clinical, clinicopathologic, radiographic, and pathological findings in 23 cases (1984–1989). *J Vet Intern Med* 7(5):277–288.

Loehr CV, Polster U, Kuhnert P, Karger A, Rurangirwa FR, Teifke JP. 2012. Mesenteric lymphangitis and sepsis due to RTX toxin-producing *Actinobacillus* spp in 2 foals with hypothyroidism-dysmaturity syndrome. *Vet Pathol* 49(4):592–601.

McHuliffe SB, Slovis NM. 2008. *Color Atlas of Diseases and Disorders of the Foal*. Edinburgh, UK: Saunders Elsevier.

Meijer WG, Prescott JF. 2004. *Rhodococcus equi*. *Vet Res* 35(4):383–396.

Page P, Parker R, Harper C, Cuthrie A, Neser J. 2006. Clinical, clinicopathologic, postmortem examination findings and familial history of 3 Arabians with lavender foal syndrome. *J Vet Intern Med* 20(6):1491–1494.

Page AE, Slovis NM, Gebhart CJ, Wolfsdorf K, Mapes SM, Pusterla N. 2011. Serial use of serologic assays and fecal PCR assays to aid in identification of subclinical *Lawsonia intracellularis* infection for targeted treatment of thoroughbred foals and weanlings. *J Am Vet Med Assoc* 238(11):1482–1489.

Patterson-Kane JC, Carrick JB, Axon JE, Wilkie I, Begg AP. 2008. The pathology of bronchointerstitial pneumonia in young foals associated with the first outbreak of equine influenza in Australia. *Equine Vet J* 40(3):199–203.

Platt H. 1973. Septicemia in the foal. A review of 61 cases. *Br Vet J* 129(3):221–229.

Raisis AL, Hodgson JL, Hodgson DR. 1996. Equine neonatal septicemia: 24 cases. *Aust Vet J* 73(4):137–140.

Reilly JK, Palmer JE. 1994. Systemic candidiasis in four foals. *J Am Vet Med Assoc* 205(3):464–466.

Robinson JA, Allen GK, Green EM, Fales WH, Loch WE, Wilkerson CG. 1993. A prospective study of septicaemia in colostrum-deprived foals. *Equine Vet J* 25(93):214–219.

# 3 Diseases of the Nervous System and Peripheral Nerves

- I. Central nervous system
  1. Removal and examination of the brain and spinal cord
  2. Malformations
     a. Hydrocephalus
     b. Meningocele
  3. Degeneration
     a. Equine leukoencephalomalacia (ELEM)
     b. Nigropallidal encephalomalacia
     c. Cerebellar abiotrophy
     d. Grove poisoning
     e. Equine degenerative myelopathy (EDM)
     f. Lower motor neuron disease (EMND)
     g. Cervical stenotic compressive myelopathy
     h. Postanesthetic myelopathy
  4. Inflammation
     a. Viral
     b. Protozoal: Equine protozoal encephalomyelitis
     c. Bacterial
     d. Mycotic
     e. Parasitic
  5. Traumatic injuries
  6. Neoplastic
  7. Miscellaneous
     a. Choroid plexus cholesteatoma
     b. Epidural synovial cyst
- II. Peripheral nervous system
  1. Polyneuritis equi (polyradiculitis, cauda equina neuritis)
  2. Grass sickness
  3. Peripheral neuropathies

*Color Atlas of Equine Pathology*, First Edition. Claus D. Buergelt and Fabio Del Piero.

# I. Central nervous system

## 1. Removal and examination of the brain and the spinal cord

The goal for safe brain removal through an opened calvarium is to avoid mutilation via uncontrolled cuts. It is therefore recommended to observe standard techniques for calvarium removal. Several methods have been described to open the calvarium. The safe removal of the spinal cord is a challenging task but is manageable even under field condition. Guidelines are offered in Chapter 1, "The Equine Necropsy." Sections of both sciatic nerves should be added to the routine central nervous system (CNS) tissue collection at necropsy.

## 2. Malformations

### a. Hydrocephalus

Hydrocephalus is defined as excessive accumulation of cerebrospinal fluid (CSF) in ventricles resulting in compression atrophy of the neuropile. It is the consequence of obstruction to the path of CSF circulation. Hydrocephalus can be congenital or acquired.

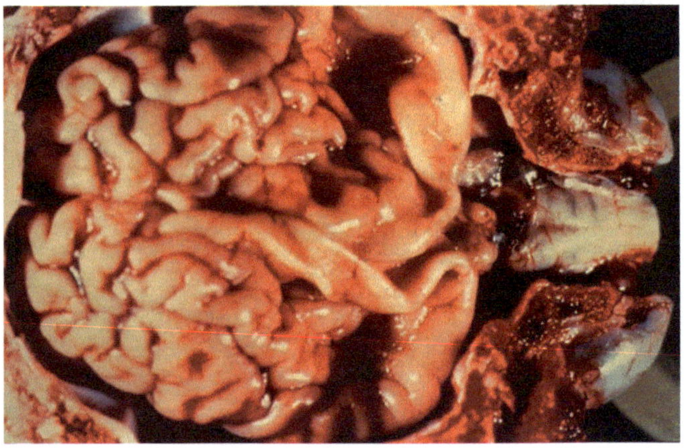

**Figure 3.1.** Horse. Brain. Hydrocephalus. The caudal cerebral hemispheres are collapsed. An abscess obstructed the lateral apertures of the fourth ventricle.

### b. Meningocele

This is a rare condition in the horse.

## 3. Degeneration

### a. Equine leukoencephalomalacia (ELEM)

Substantial random necrosis of the white matter substance is the result of the consumption of moldy corn contaminated by *Fusarium verticilloides* (formerly *F. moniliforme*). Hay may also be contaminated with *Fusarium*. The major toxin involved is fumonisin B1. The toxin inhibits the enzyme ceramide synthase and interferes with the synthesis of sphingolipids. Clinical signs include dysphagia, ataxia, and blindness.

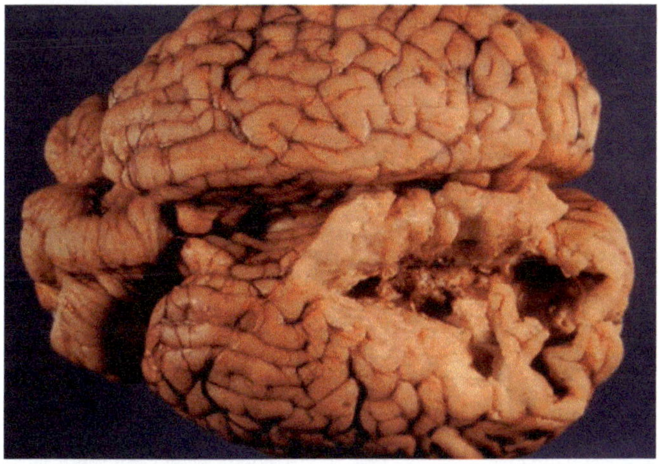

**Figure 3.2.** Horse. Brain. Leukoencephalomalacia. The frontal lobe unilaterally reveals massive malacia (cavitation).

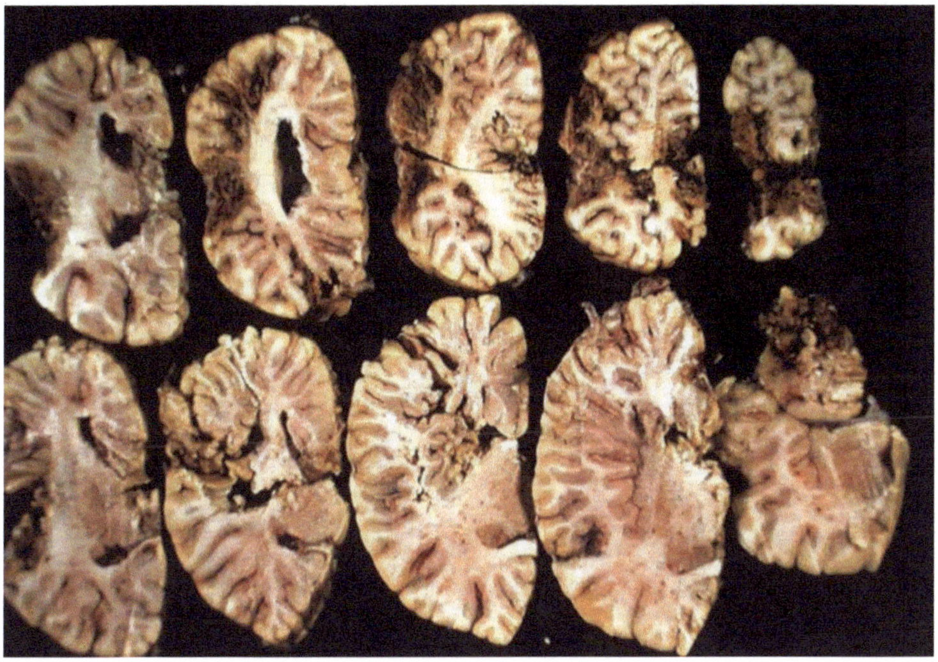

**Figure 3.3.** Horse. Brain. Leukoencephalomalacia. Coronal sections are characterized by cavitations in the white matter substance.

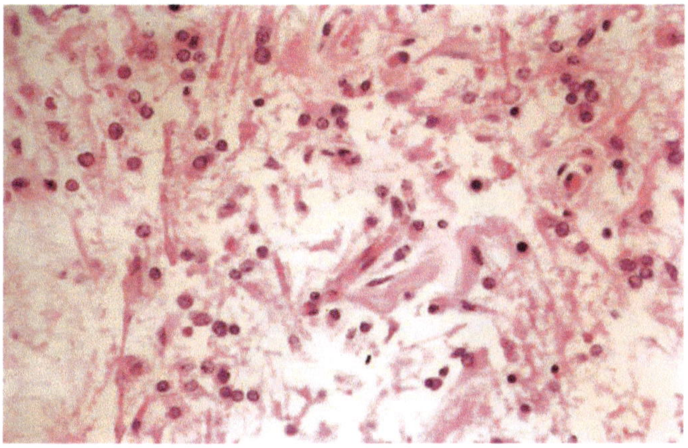

**Figure 3.4.** Horse. Brain. Leukoencephalomalacia. There is evidence of loss of neuropile with disarray of neurofilaments, gliosis, and some mononuclear cell inflammation, including foamy macrophages. (H&E)

*b. Nigropallidal encephalomalacia*

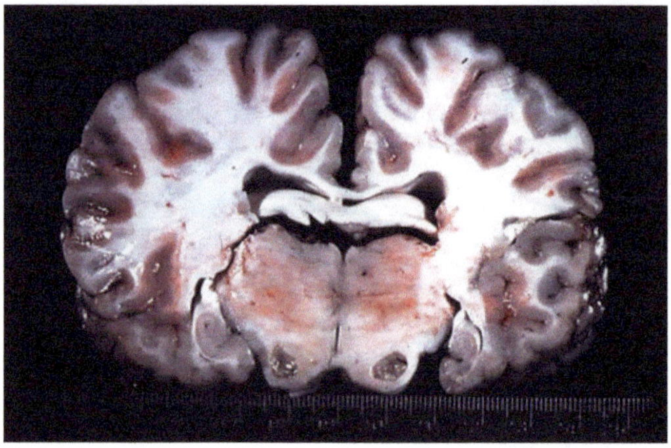

**Figure 3.5.** Horse. Brain. Nigropallidal Encephalomalacia. The consumption of yellow star thistle (*Centaurea solstitialis*) and Russian knapweed (*Centaurea* (*Reponticum*) *repens*) results in bilateral symmetric malacia and yellow-tan discoloration in the substantia nigra and anterior globus pallidus. The toxic compounds are lactones and pyrones, effective in 30–90 days of eating the plant on a daily basis. The toxins have a dopaminergic effect and damage cell membranes. (Courtesy Dr. J. King, Cornell University.)

*c. Cerebellar abiotrophy*

The condition is defined as loss of organization of certain tissue substance of the cerebellum during fetal life and up to 6 months of age leading to progressive symmetric atrophy and occurs primarily in Arabian horses. The disorder can also be seen in Oldenburg horses, Miniature horses, and ponies. The determination of the weight correlation between cerebrum and cerebellum (reduced weight) and microscopic confirmation of deranged orientation of Purkinje cells and loss of granular cells in the cerebellum establish the specific diagnosis.

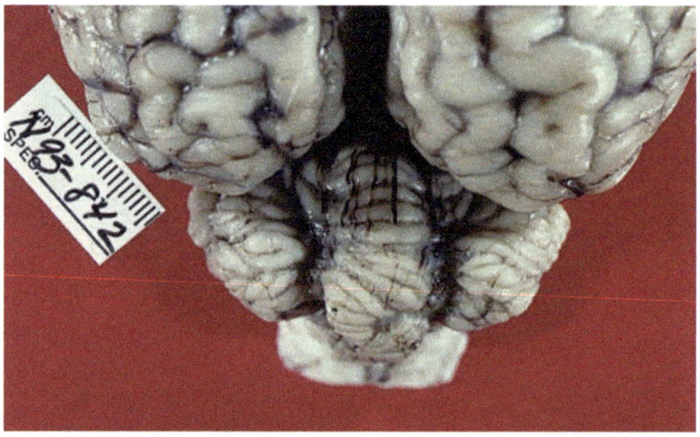

**Figure 3.6.** Horse. Cerebellum. Abiotrophy. Grossly, the reduction of the cerebellum may be subtle in some cases. The sulci between the vermis and the cerebellar hemispheres should not be present, and the cerebellum is reduced in weight when compared with the rest of the brain (less than 8% of the whole brain weight).

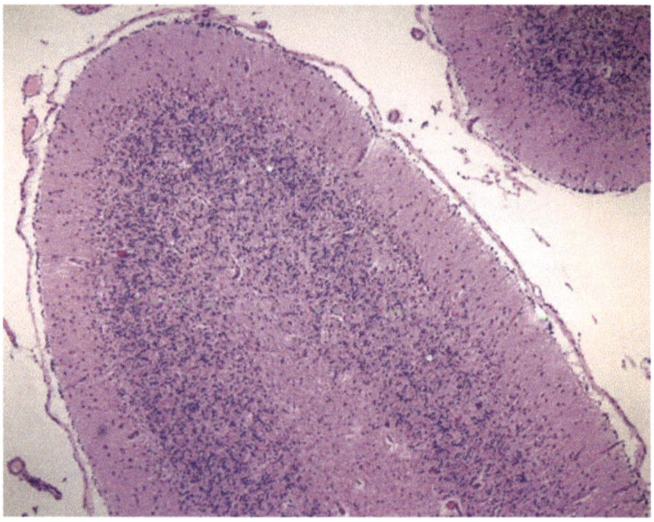

**Figure 3.7.** Horse. Cerebellum. Abiotrophy. The granular cell layer is hypocellular microscopically. (H&E)

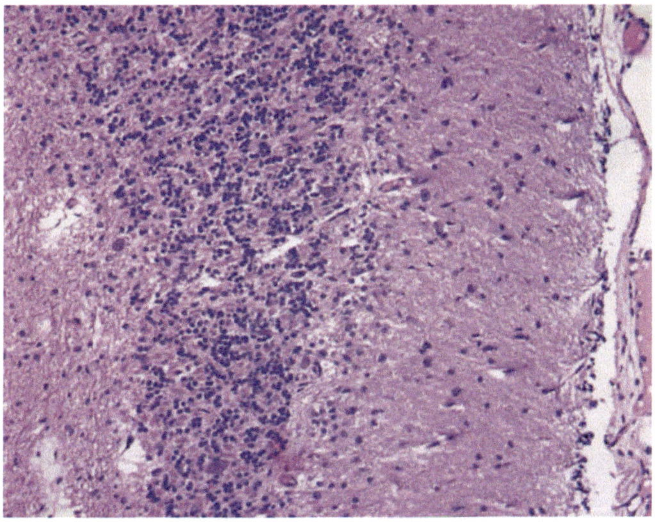

**Figure 3.8.** Horse. Cerebellum. Abiotrophy. On higher magnification, the Purkinje cells are decreased and poorly aligned next to the granular cell layer. (H&E)

*d. Grove poisoning*

The plant *Indigofera spicata* (creeping indigo) produces indospicine, a liver and nervous tissue toxin. A single peptide, it inhibits protein synthesis as an antagonist to the amino acid arginine. When consumed by horses, the toxin induces hepatic encephalopathy and recumbence due to CNS involvement.

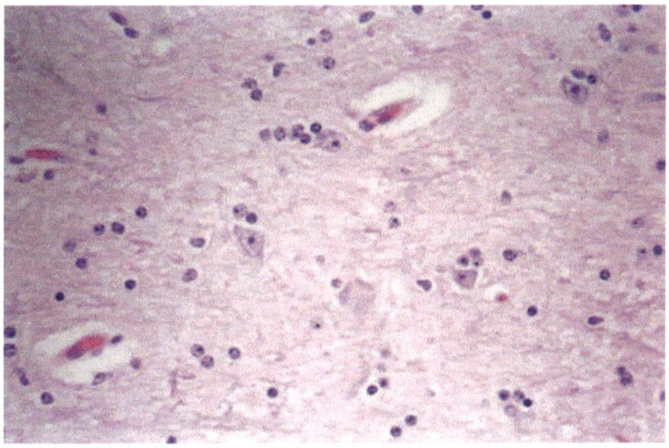

**Figure 3.9.** Horse. Brain. Grove Poisoning. There is microscopic evidence of gliosis and astrocytosis. (H&E)

*e. Equine degenerative myelopathy (EDM)*

Studies have implicated vitamin E deficiency and a possible breed and familial disposition (Morgan horse) to this disease. Copper imbalance has also been speculated to be involved in the pathogenesis. The disorder is associated with neuroaxonal dystrophy. The dystrophy is present in the cerebellum, brainstem, medulla oblongata, and spinal cord and is characterized by a histologic pattern of axonal loss and secondary demyelination.

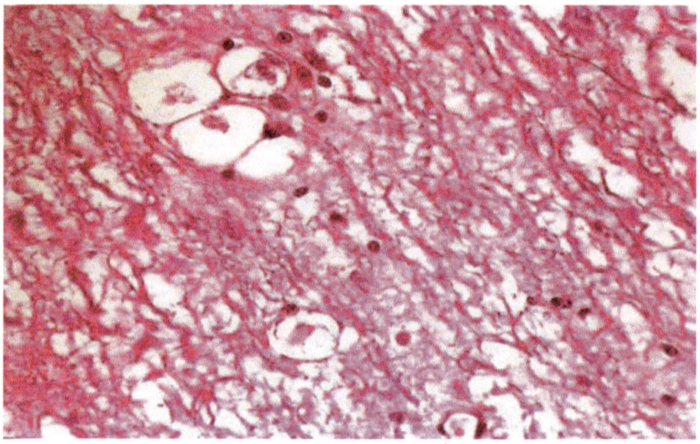

**Figure 3.10.** Horse. Spinal Cord. Equine Degenerative Myeloencephalopathy (EDM). Axonal spheroids and neuroaxonal dystrophy. (H&E)

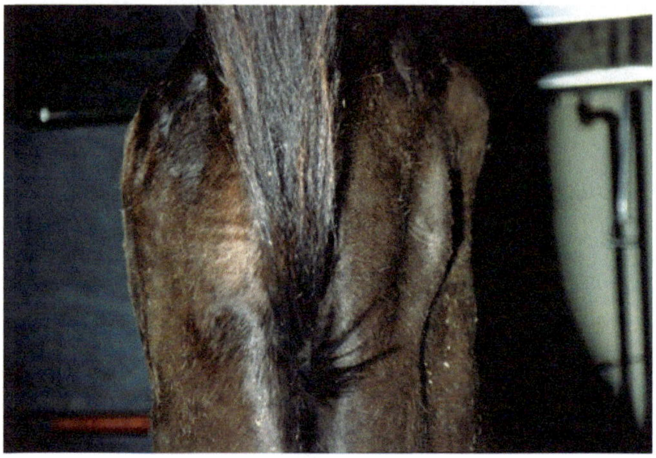

**Figure 3.11.** Horse. Hindquarter. Equine Degenerative Myeloencephalopathy (EDM). Atrophy of gluteal muscles, particularly evident on the right side.

*f. Lower motor neuron disease (EMND)*

This condition occurs sporadically in individual animals and rarely in outbreaks affecting the motor neurons located in the ventral horns of the spinal cord. Generalized weakness and coccygeal, triceps brachii, and femoral muscle neurogenic atrophy are clinical signs. The condition is responsive to treatment with vitamin E. An association with neurotoxins produced by blue-green algae or cyanobacteria has been hypothesized.

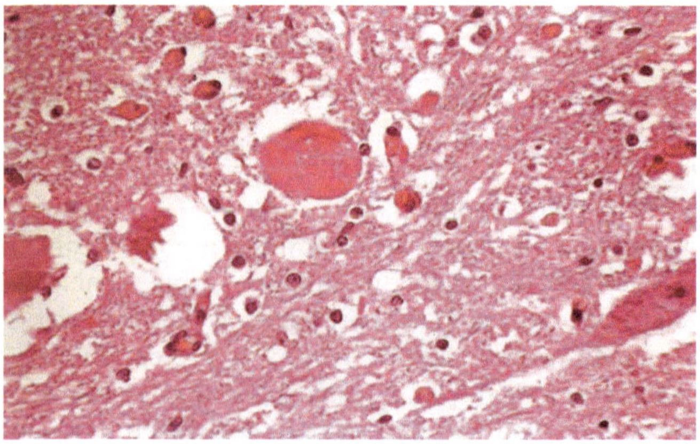

**Figure 3.12.** Horse. Spinal cord. Lower Motor Neuron Disease (EMND). There is neuronal chromatolysis. The neurons are swollen and have lost the nucleus. No inflammation is present. (H&E)

*g. Cervical stenotic compressive myelopathy*

Also known as "wobbler" syndrome, this is a disorder of young fast-growing thoroughbred and standardbred horses and is associated with the vertebrae of the cervical spinal cord. Compression of the cervical spinal cord from either narrowing of the epidural space or instability result in neuroaxonal degeneration (Wallerian degeneration) of ascending (above the lesion) and descending (below the lesion) nervous spinal tracts with clinical manifestations of lameness and ataxia. There are two forms: the static form affecting C5-C6 vertebrae and the dynamic stenotic form affecting C3-C4 vertebrae. Osteochondrosis of the articular facets is another differential cause as are healed fractures of vertebral facets. Thorough evaluation for vertebral dysplastic predisposing lesions necessitates disarticulation of affected vertebrae.

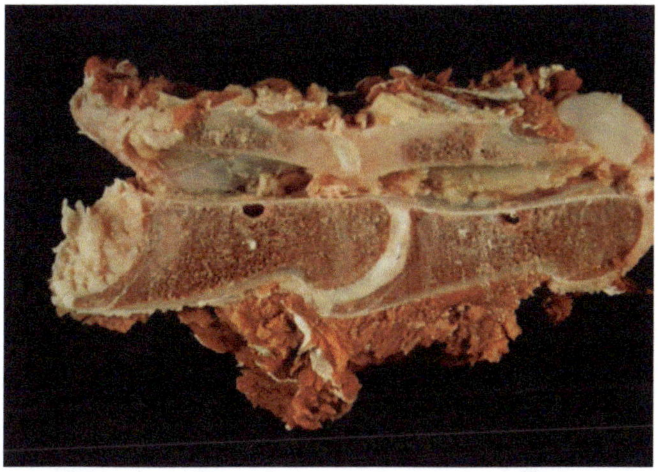

**Figure 3.13.** Horse. Cervical Vertebrae. Stenotic Myelopathy. There is evidence of severe stenosis of the spinal canal.

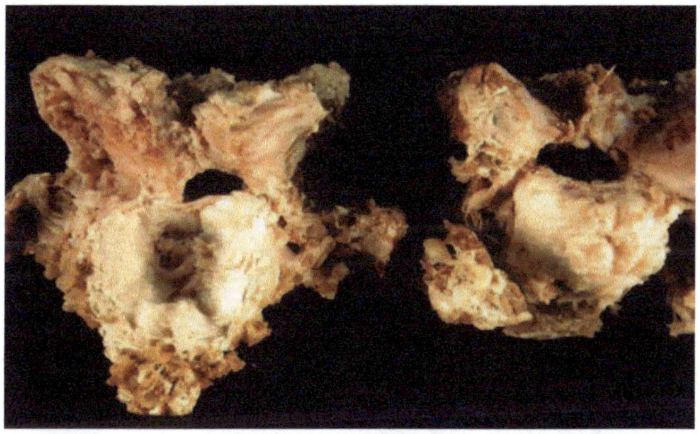

**Figure 3.14.** Horse. Cervical Vertebrae. Stenotic Myelopathy. Disarticulated vertebrae with focal narrowing of the spinal canal on left.

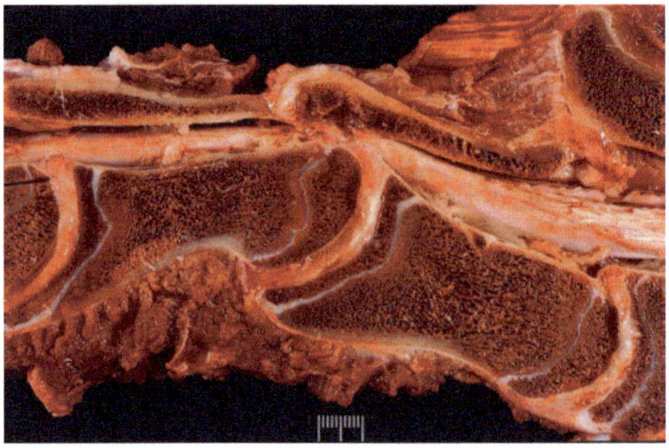

**Figure 3.15.** Horse. Cervical Vertebrae. Instability. Narrowing of the spinal canal results during flexion of the neck.

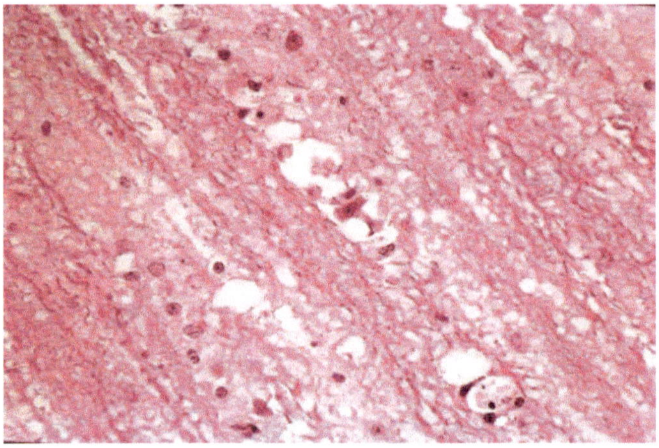

**Figure 3.16.** Horse. Spinal Cord ("Wobbler"). Neuroaxonal Degeneration (Wallerian Degeneration). There is microscopic evidence of axonal swelling, loss of myelin, and the presence of gitter cells. (H&E)

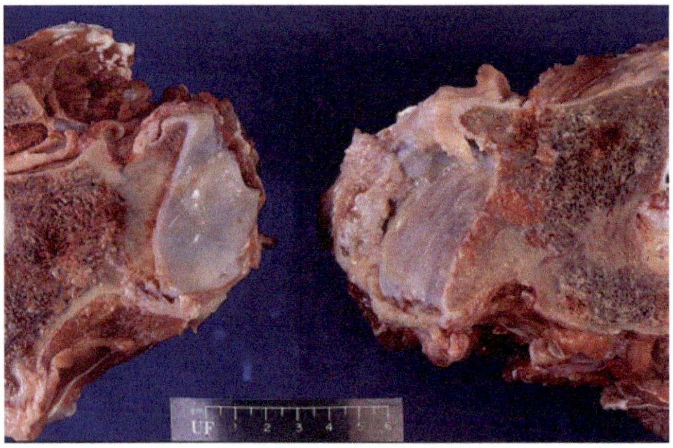


**Figure 3.17.** Horse. Articular Facets, Vertebrae. Osteochondrosis. There is evidence of crevices in the articular cartilage and asymmetry of articular facets.

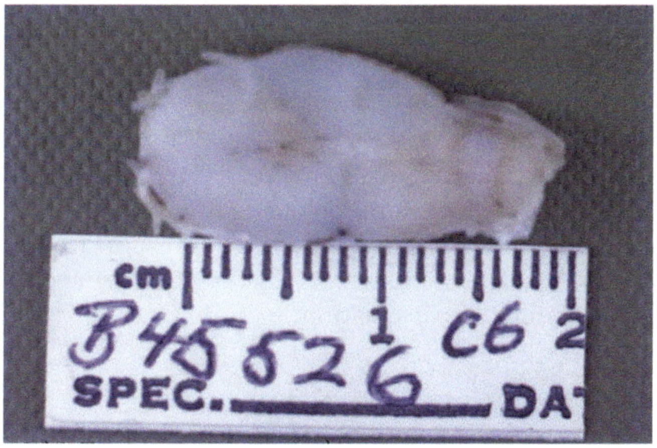


**Figure 3.18.** Horse. Spinal Cord. Cervical Myelopathy. The condition is characterized by asymmetric narrowing of the dorsolateral spinal canal resulting in unilateral compression atrophy of the spinal cord.

*h. Postanesthetic myelopathy*

In young heavy breed horses undergoing surgery in dorsal recumbency, hypotension induced by anesthesia (halothane) and increased pressure on the caudal vena cava by large abdominal, possibly impacted organs may lead to ischemic neuroaxonal degeneration and polycavitation of the spinal cord. Asymmetric or possibly symmetric lesions of malacia can be anywhere in the spinal cord.

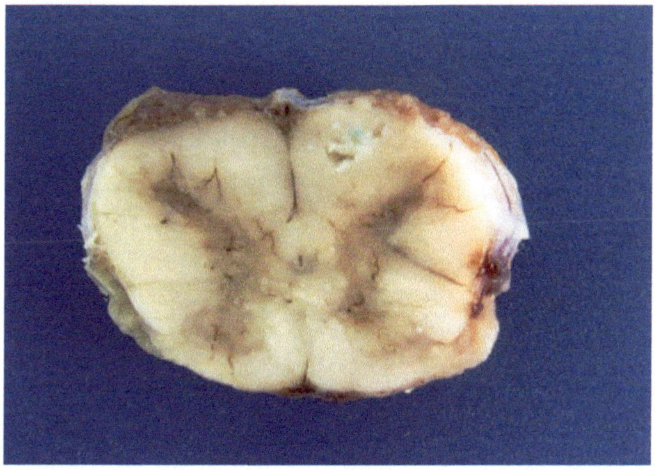

**Figure 3.19.** Horse. Spinal Cord. Hemorrhage, malacia, and cavitations are present on cut section affecting mainly the gray matter, but also white matter substance. Differential diagnosis: Fibrocartilagenous embolism from the nucleus pulposus to the vessels of the cervical intumescence of the spinal cord via ventral spinal artery. Seen in large equine breeds. (Courtesy Dr. A. Hattel, Pennsylvania State University.)

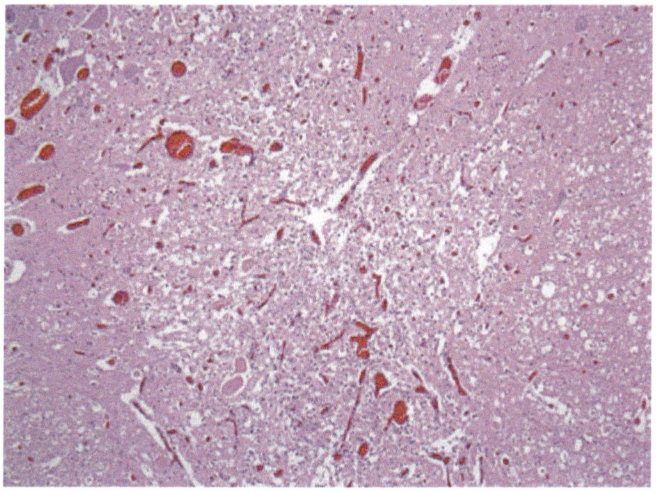

**Figure 3.20.** Horse. Spinal Cord. Microscopically myelomalacia is evident. (H&E) (Courtesy Dr. A. Hattel, Pennsylvania State University.)

## 4. *Inflammation*

### *a. Viral*

i. Rabies. A zoonotic disease affecting the CNS of many mammalian species is caused by a neurotropic RNA rhabdovirus. The clinical signs in affected horses are extremely variable. Both vicious and paralytic forms may occur. The virus reaches the CNS by retrograde axonal transport from bite wounds. Grossly, there may be a rare mild hemorrhage on the meningeal surface. The disease can be controlled by vaccination.

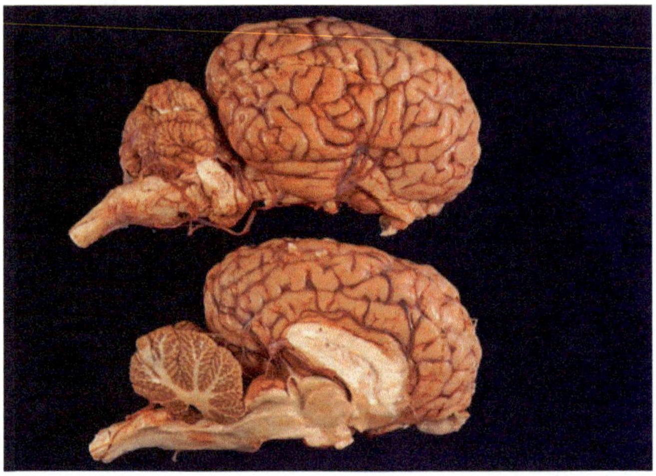

**Figure 3.21.** Horse. Brain. Rabies. Grossly, the appearance of the brain is usually unremarkable.

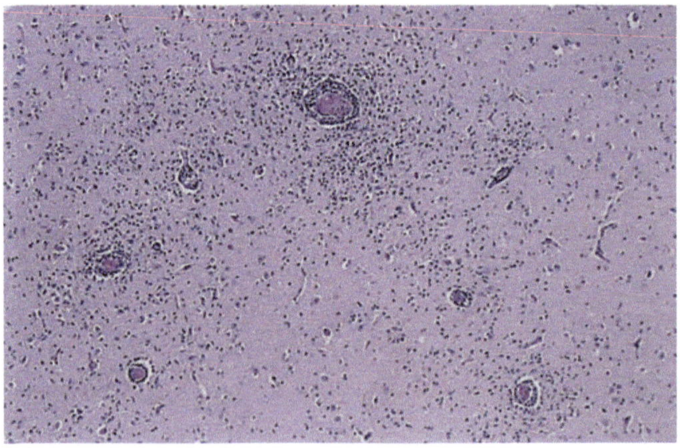

**Figure 3.22.** Horse. Brain. Rabies. The microscopic changes are perivascular lymphocytic polioencephalomyelitis indicative of viral etiology. (H&E)

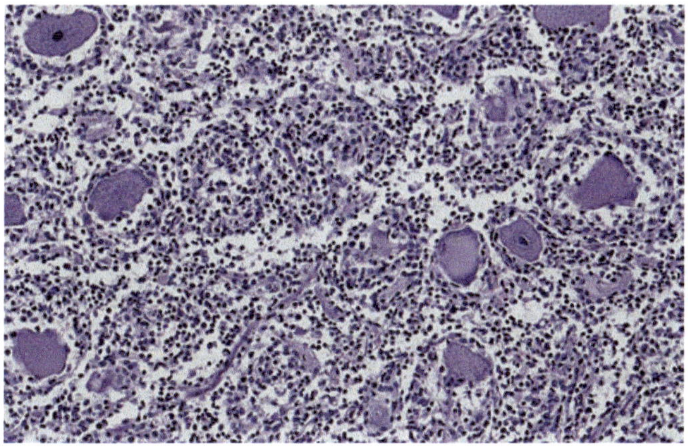

**Figure 3.23.** Horse. Brain. Rabies. There is lymphocytic trigeminal ganglionitis. (H&E) (Reprinted with permission from *Equine Infectious Diseases*, Selon-Long, Figure 19.11, Page 189, Copyright Elsevier, 2007.)

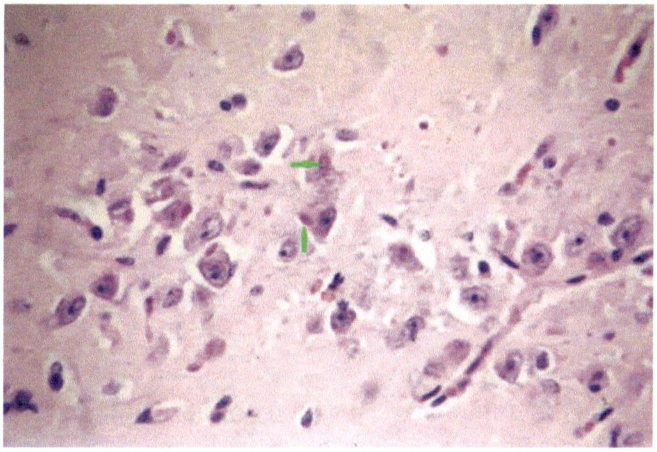

**Figure 3.24.** Horse. Brain. Rabies. The finding of magenta intracytoplasmic inclusion bodies, the so-called Negri bodies (arrows), is conclusive evidence for the diagnosis of rabies. (H&E)

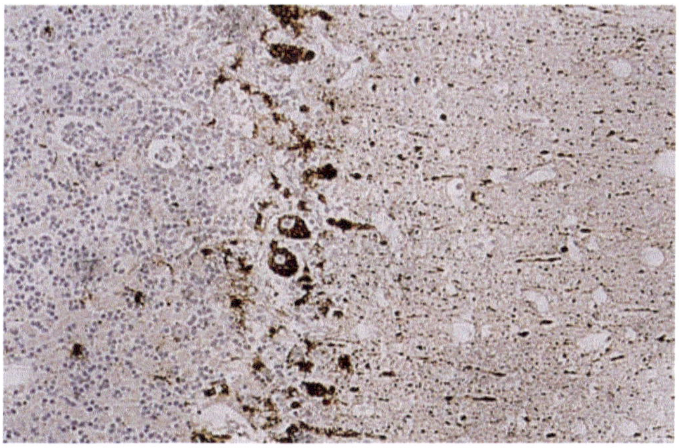

**Figure 3.25.** Horse. Cerebellum. Rabies. Viral antigen is demonstrated in the cytoplasm of Purkinje cells and cells of the granular cell layer by indirect immunohistochemistry. (IHC) (Reprinted with permission from *Equine Infectious Diseases*, Selon-Long, Figure 19.8, Page 188, Copyright Elsevier, 2007.)

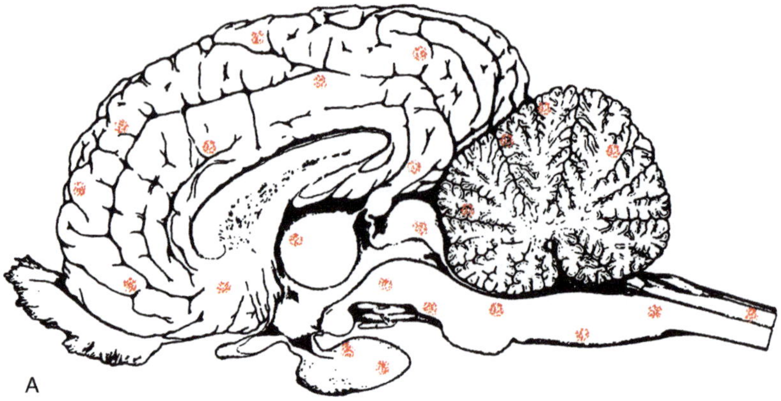

A

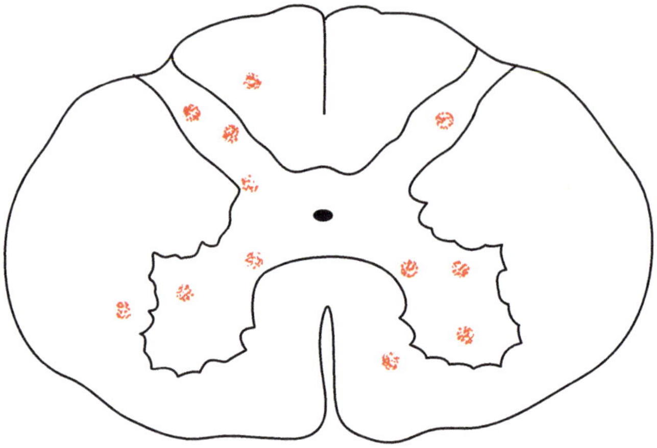

B

**Charts A and B.** Distribution of Rabies-Induced Encephalomyelitis in Equine Brain and Spinal Cord. (Courtesy Dr. Carlo Cantile, Pisa University.)

It has been suggested that cervical spinal cord and adjacent brainstem are optimal tissue regions for rabies testing in the horse.

ii. Equine alpha viral encephalomyelitis. Eastern equine encephalitis (EEE), Western equine encephalitis (WEE), and Venezuelan equine encephalitis (VEE) strains have been described for this family of Togaviridae, all arthropod-borne viruses. They primarily affect the gray matter substance of the brain and spinal cord inducing a polioencephalomyelitis. In the southeastern part of the United States, EEE is very prevalent. High fever is a hallmark clinical sign of EEE together with CNS disturbances such as depression and dementia. The virus initially spreads hematogenously to the bone marrow, lymph nodes, muscle and connective tissue, followed by a secondary cycle within the CNS. The virus has affinity to neurons, glial cells, cardiocytes, smooth muscle cells, and fibroblasts in the renal interstitium. The disease can be controlled by vaccination. Alphaviruses are a public health consideration in that they are transmitted to people via mosquitoes (e.g., *Culiseta* sp. and *Culex* sp.) and are listed as bioterror agents.

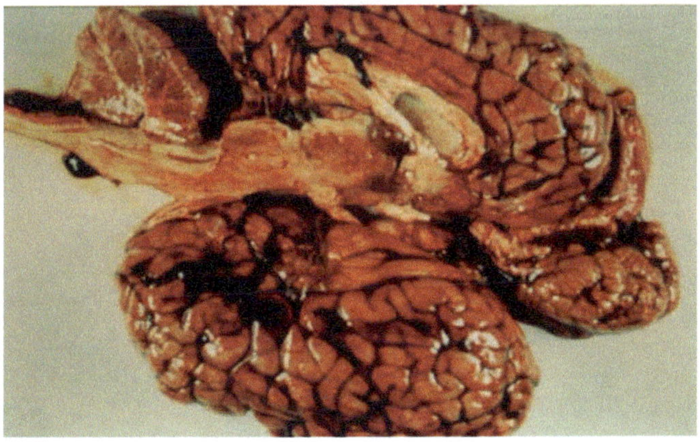

**Figure 3.26.** Horse. Brain. EEE. On rare occasions, cases of EEE exhibit diffuse hyperemia of the meningeal surface.

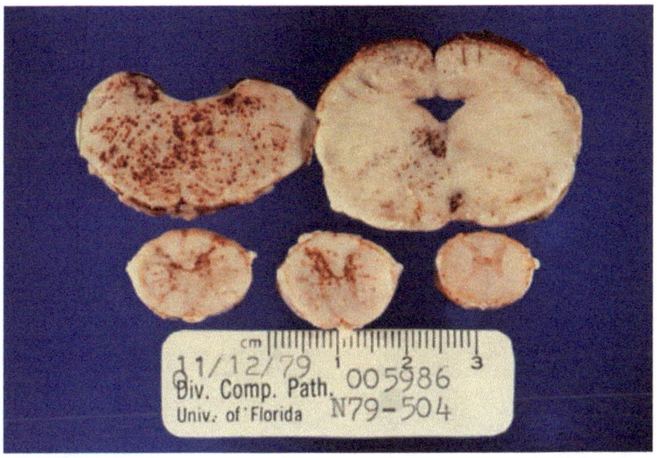


**Figure 3.27.** Horse. Brain. EEE. On cut section, the neuropile reveals petechiae and ecchymoses.

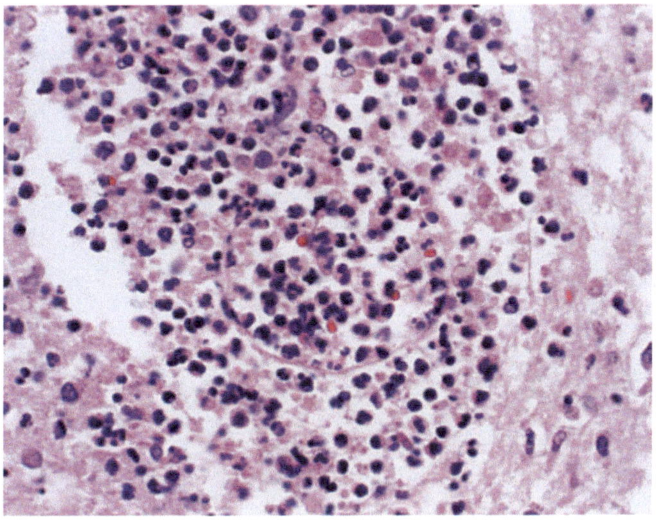

**Figure 3.28.** Horse. Brain. EEE. Histologically, depending on the strain and time course of the disease, a neutrophilic and/or lymphocytic meningoencephalitis can be expected. In this case, the neuropile is infiltrated by mainly neutrophils diapedesing from a vessel. (H&E)

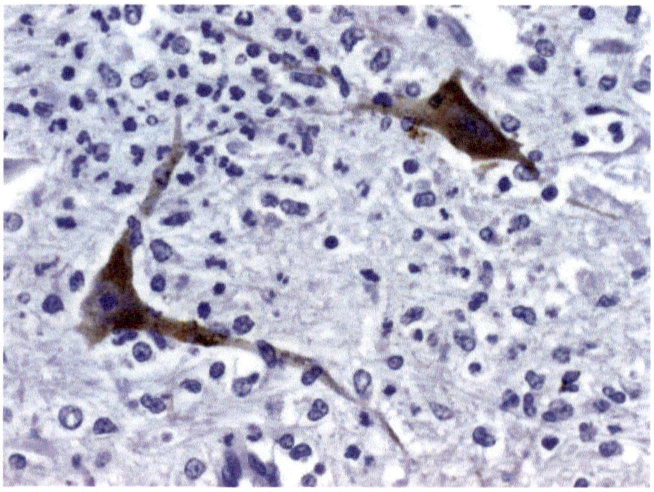

**Figure 3.29.** Horse. Brain. EEE. The distribution of viral antigen is demonstrated in the cytoplasm and axons of the neurons and dendrites by indirect immunohistochemistry. (IHC)

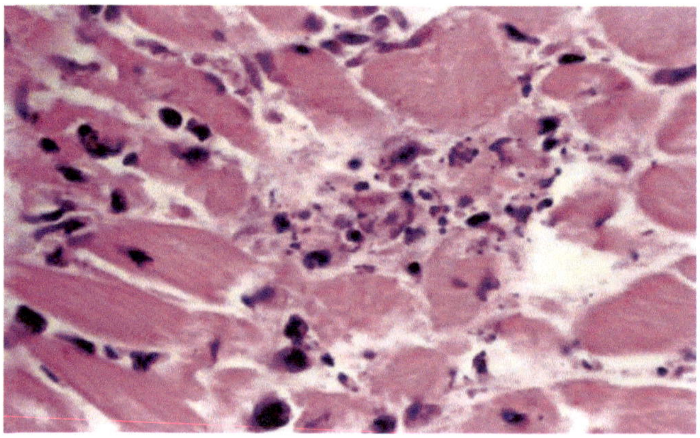

**Figure 3.30.** Horse. Heart. EEE. Another organ involved in EEE is the heart where multifocal necrotizing myocarditis develops. (H&E)

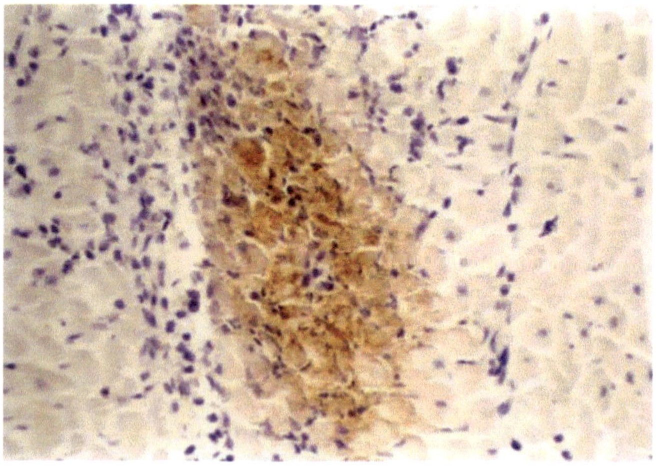

**Figure 3.31.** Horse. Heart. EEE is associated with a viral antigen as demonstrated within the cytoplasm of cardiocytes by indirect immunohistochemistry. (IHC)

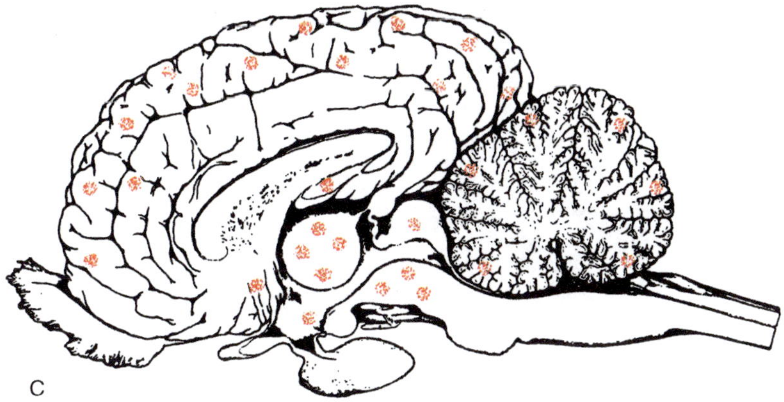

C

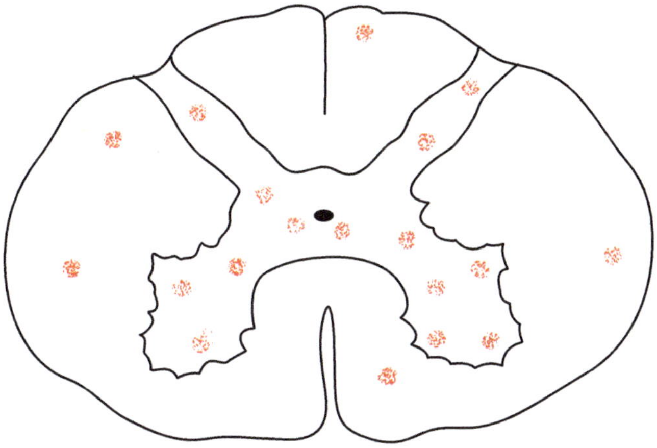

D

**Charts C and D.** Distribution of Equine Alpha Virus within the Brain and Spinal Cord. (Courtesy Dr. C. Cantile, Pisa University.)

iii. West Nile virus encephalomyelitis. West Nile virus (WNV) is a member of the genus *Flavivirus* originally isolated from the blood of a woman with fever in Uganda in 1937. The virus entered the North American continent in 1999 and progressively spread north and south. It reached South America (Argentina) in 2006. The virus is transmitted by many species of mosquitoes to susceptible mammals and birds. Mammals including the horse are considered dead-end hosts for this flavivirus. The virus causes rhombencephalitis and myelitis in the horse. Disease prevention in horses is achieved through vaccination.

WNV also infects humans and is therefore a zoonotic pathogen. Fewer than 1% of humans develop fatal menigoencephalitis.

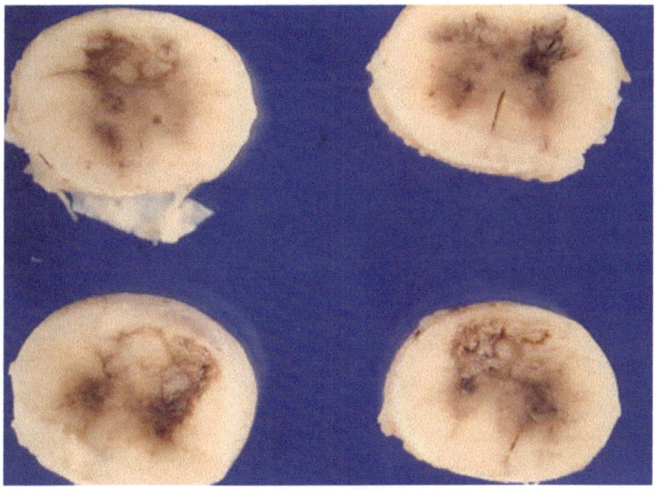

**Figure 3.32.** Horse. Spinal Cord. WNV. At times, hemorrhage can be observed in the gray matter of the rhombencephalon and brainstem and especially as segmentally confluent soft red foci within the spinal cord. Differential gross diagnoses: Equine protozoal myelitis (EPM); postanesthetic myelitis; fibrocartilaginous embolus.

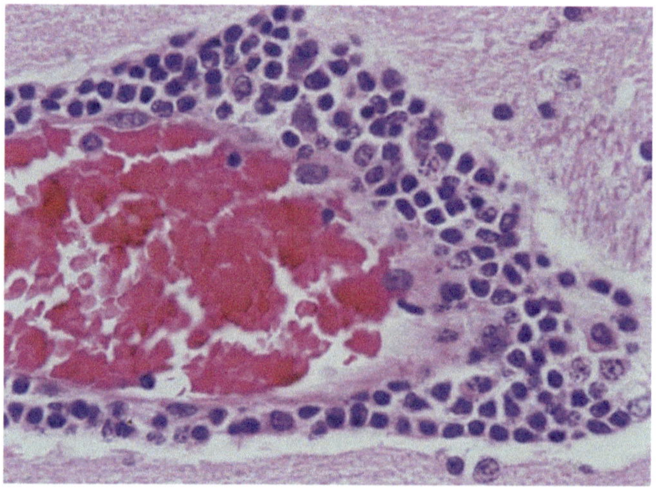

**Figure 3.33.** Horse. Spinal Cord. WNV. Histologic changes are compatible with a neurotropic viral etiology. The inflammatory response is mild to severe and mainly perivascular and lymphocytic with a few histiocytes. (H&E)

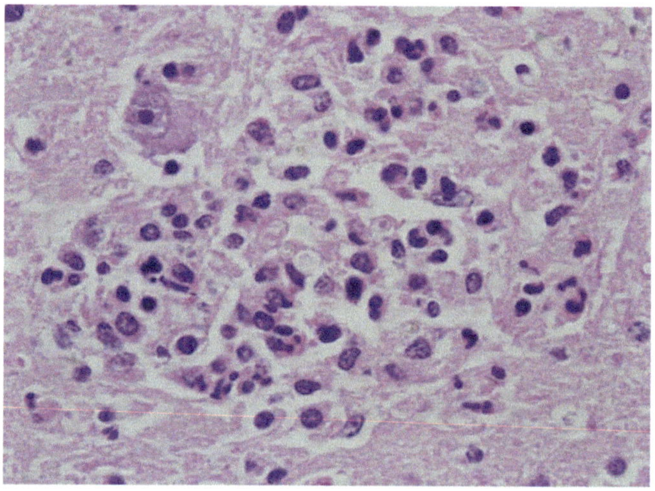

**Figure 3.34.** Horse. Spinal Cord. WNV. Glial nodules composed of activated glial cells and mixed inflammatory cells are supportive for the diagnosis of WNV infection. Glial nodules may also be present in some EEE cases. (H&E)

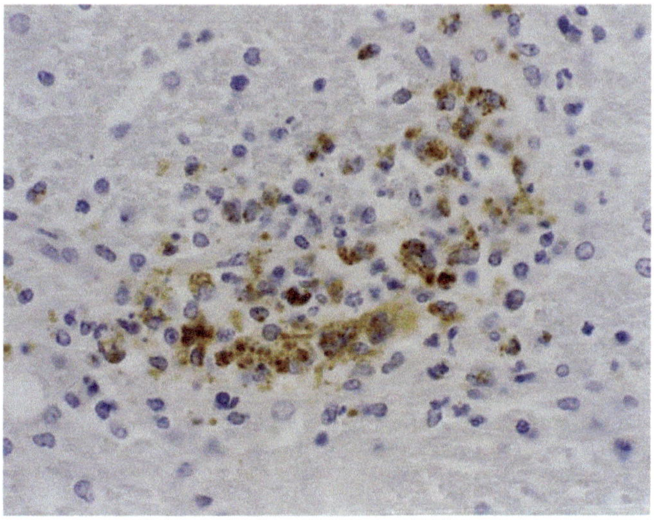

**Figure 3.35.** Horse. Spinal Cord. WNV. Glial Nodule. Detection of intracytoplasmic viral antigen. (IHC)

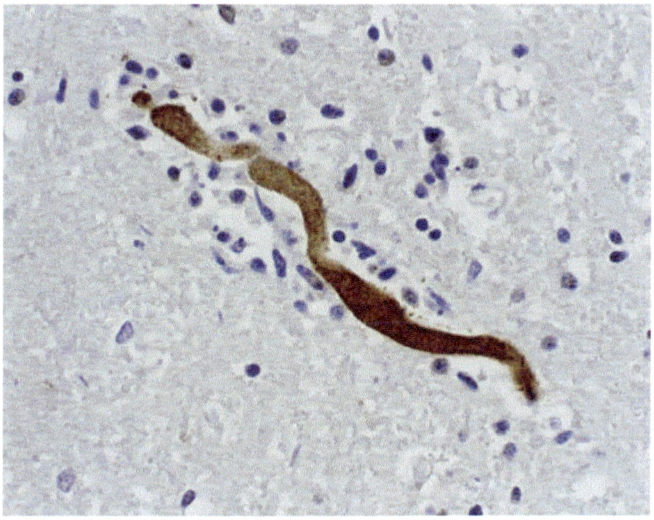

**Figure 3.36.** Horse. Spinal Cord. WNV. Flaviviral antigen within spinal cord fiber and with spheroids demonstrated by indirect immunohistochemistry. (IHC)

## West Nile virus encephalomyelitis – Fact sheet

### Definition

- Acute to subacute encephalomyelitis caused by a single-stranded RNA flavivirus

### Incidence

- Outbreaks in Africa, Europe, North America, and Latin America
- Distribution of disease depends on season and vector activity
- Potential reservoirs and hosts include mosquitoes and multiple avian species

### Gross findings

- Multifocal to confluent hemorrhages mainly through segments of the spinal cord
- Brainstem and rhombencephalon are affected by hemorrhage to a lesser degree

### Microscopic findings

- Mild to severe polioencephalomyelitis with perivascular small T lymphocytes, lesser perivascular macrophages, multifocal glial nodules, occasional neutrophils, and ring hemorrhage.

### Immunohistochemistry

- Scant viral antigen can be demonstrated within the cytoplasm of neurons, fibers and glial cells forming nodules.

### Differential diagnosis

- Equine protozoal myelitis (EPM)
- Rabies
- Borna disease
- Eastern equine encephalitis (and Western equine encephalitis and Venezuelan equine encephalitis)
- Equine herpesvirus (EHV)-1
- Equine infectious anemia (EIA)
- Halicephalobus gingivalis

### Public health concern

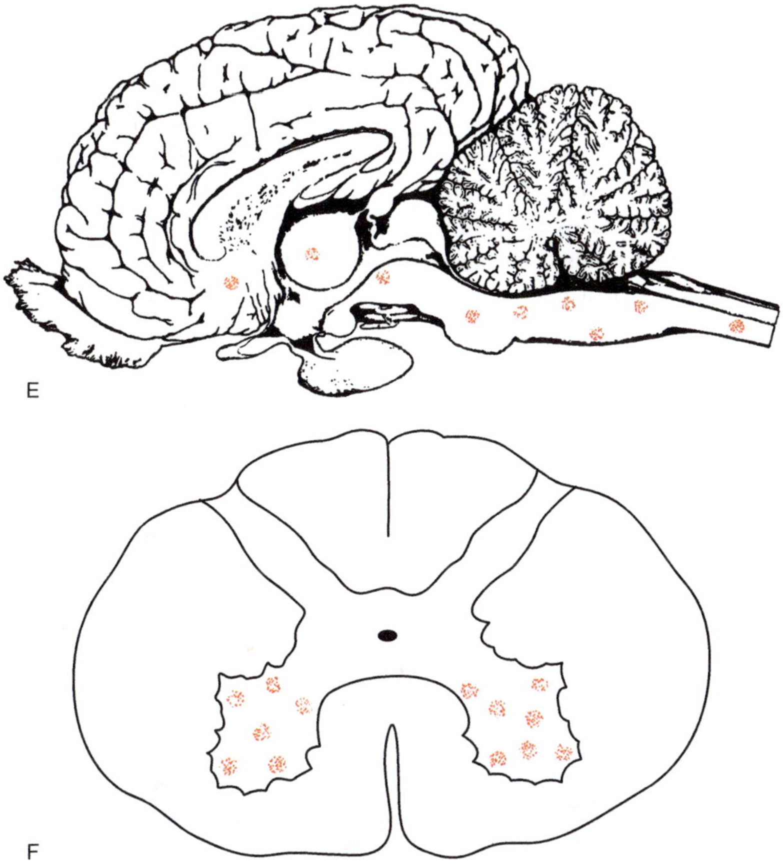


**Charts E and F.** Distribution of WNV lesions within Brain and Spinal Cord. (Courtesy of Dr. C. Cantile, Pisa University.)

iv. Equine herpesvirus encephalomyelitis. As a member of the *Alphaherpesvirinae* subfamily, the virus is highly contagious and potentially fatal when causing sporadic outbreaks of neurologic disease in horses. Horses can contract the herpesvirus from sneeze droplets of infected animals but also water, fences, and contaminated equipment. There is no threat to humans. Clinical signs reflect spinal cord involvement with paresis and ataxia. Recovery is possible. Mortality rates may range from 10% to 75%. Vaccination seems to be unprotective against the neurologic form of EHV-1.

As to the neuropathology of EHV-1, there may be gross evidence of linear perivascular hemorrhage to the spinal cord. Necrotizing vasculitis with thrombosis is a key histologic feature leading to malacia and hemorrhage in the gray matter substance. Viral inclusions should not be expected. This virus is not neurotropic like so many other herpesviruses. The virus replicates in endothelial cells, as well as in vascular myocytes and pericytes.

There seems to be a genetic difference of the herpesvirus that causes the CNS condition and the one that causes respiratory and reproductive disease.

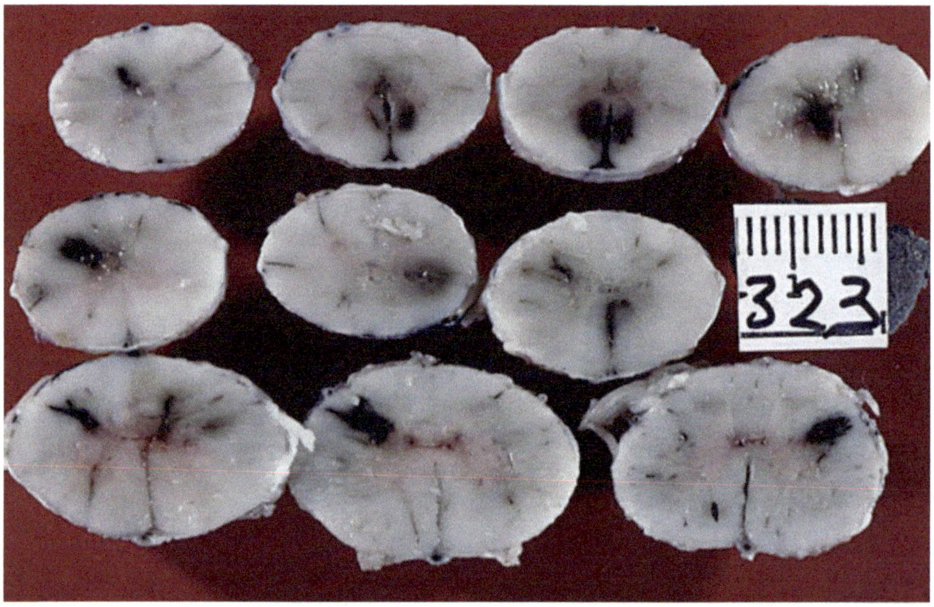


**Figure 3.37.** Horse. Spinal Cord. EHV-1. Several foci of perivascular radial hemorrhage are present in the ventral and lateral funiculi. Some of these are close to the ventral fissure. Differential diagnosis should include WNV and EPM.

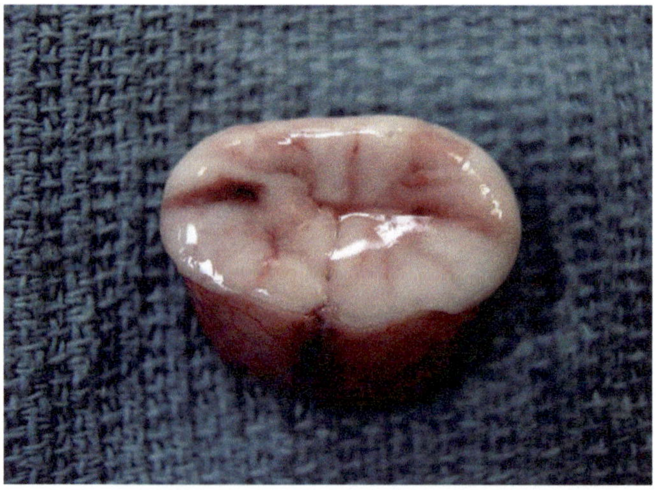

**Figure 3.38.** Horse. Spinal Cord. EHV-1. A focus of linear hemorrhage is present in the white matter substance.

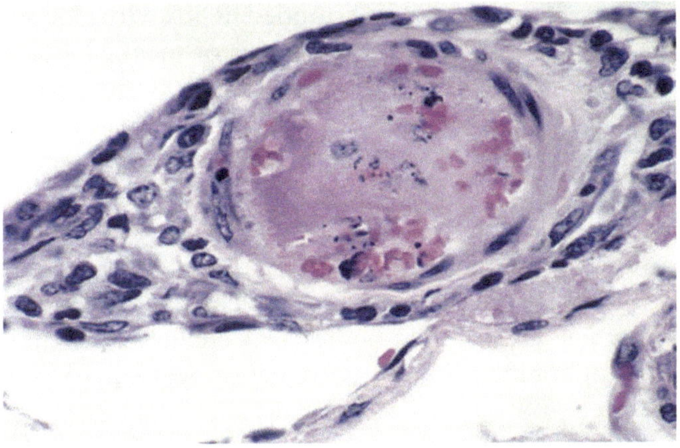

**Figure 3.39.** Horse. Spinal Cord. EHV-1. There is microscopic evidence of spinal cord vasculitis with thrombosis and lymphocytic cuffing. (H&E)

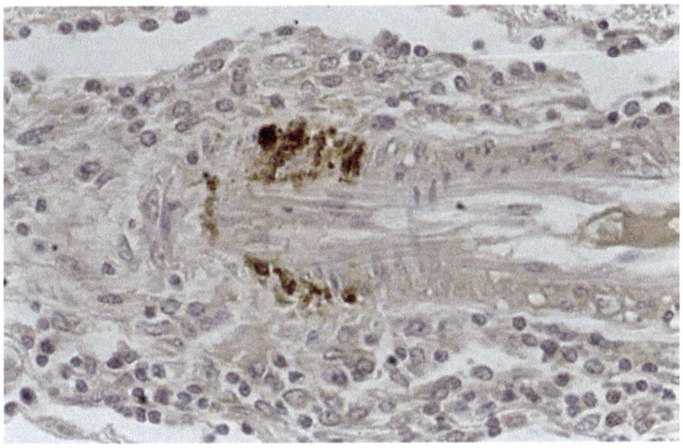

**Figure 3.40.** Horse. Spinal Cord. EHV-1. Viral antigen can be demonstrated by indirect immunohistochemistry in the nucleus and cytoplasm of endothelial cells, myocytes, and pericytes. (IHC)

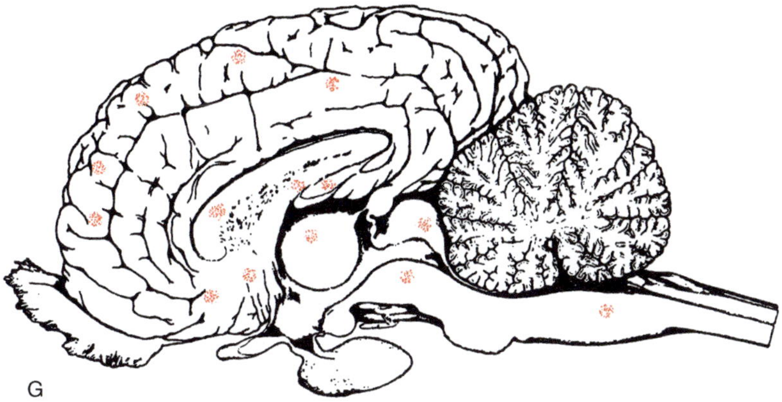

G

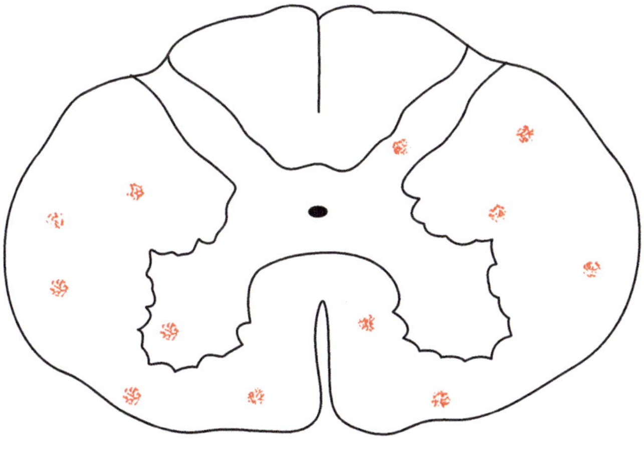

H

**Charts G and H.** Distribution of EHV-1 in Brain and Spinal Cord. (Courtesy Dr. C. Cantile, Pisa University.)

v. Equine Borna disease. This single-stranded RNA virus of undetermined classification is exotic to the United States. It is of focal geographic distribution in Western and Eastern Europe. Antibodies to the virus have been detected in human patients with mental illness in the United States. The virus is transmitted by ticks and infects sheep, cats, and rabbits. The European shrews are able to carry large amounts of the virus in numerous organs and cell types. Gross lesions may include meningeal petechiae. Microscopic features include perivascular, often prominent lymphocytic cuffing, neuronal necrosis, and sometimes glial nodules. Occasional intranuclear or intracytoplasmic inclusion bodies known as Joest-Degen bodies are conclusive for the diagnosis of Borna disease. Ganglionitis and optic nerve neuritis can also occur. Spinal cord involvement is rare.

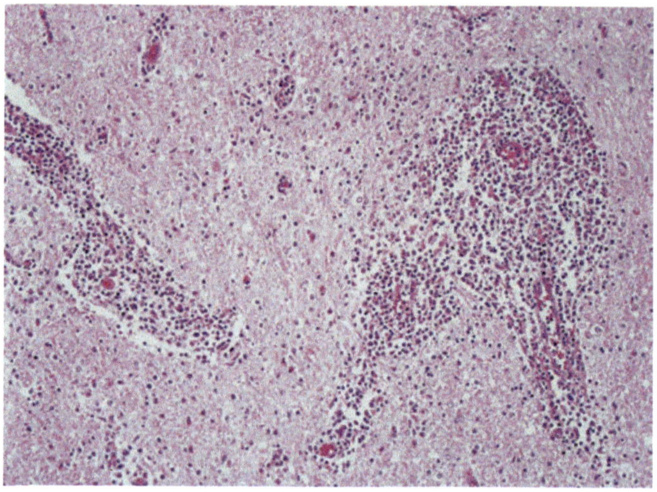

**Figure 3.41.** Horse. Brain. Borna Disease. There is microscopic evidence of disseminated nonsuppurative parenchymal polioencephalitis. The inflammation is characterized by large perivascular mononuclear cell cuffs containing mainly lymphocytes, but also plasma cells and macrophages with some cells expanding into the neuropil. In some cases, the cuffs are composed of dense aggregates of lymphoctes only. (H&E) (Courtesy Dr. F. Ehrensperger, University of Zurich.)

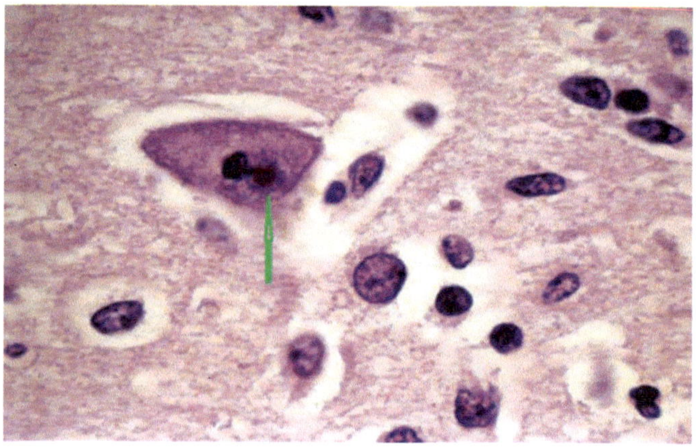

**Figure 3.42.** Horse. Brain. Borna Disease. Intracytoplasmic Joest-Degen inclusion in Borna disease (arrow). (H&E) (Courtesy Dr. F. Ehrensperger, University of Zurich.)

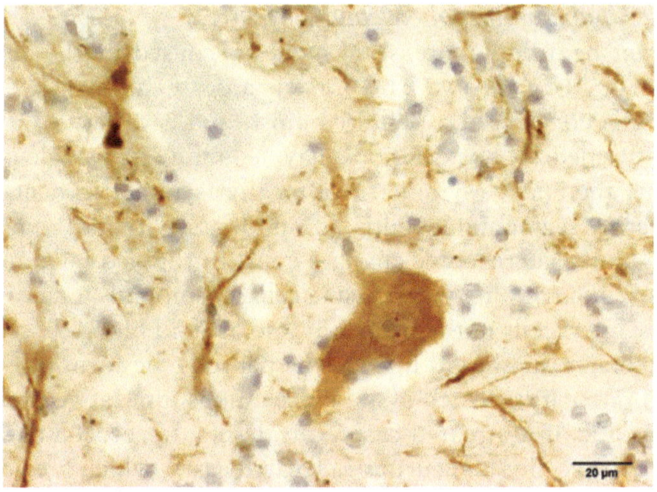


**Figure 3.43.** Horse. Brain. Borna Disease. Intracytoplasmic and intranuclear demonstration of Borna virus in neurons of the Ammon's horn by indirect immunohistochemistry. (IHC) (Courtesy Dr. F. Ehrensperger, University of Zurich.)

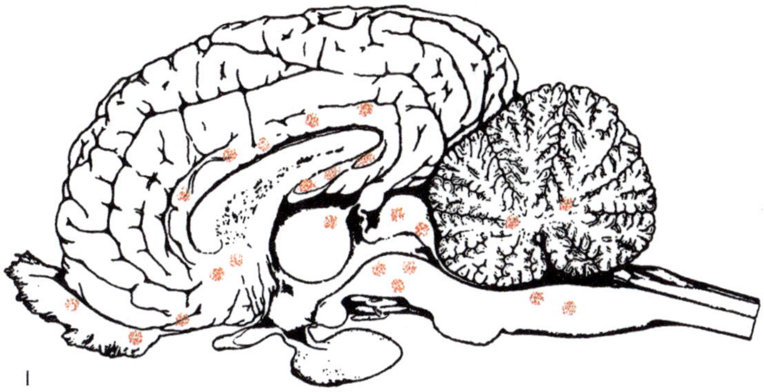

I

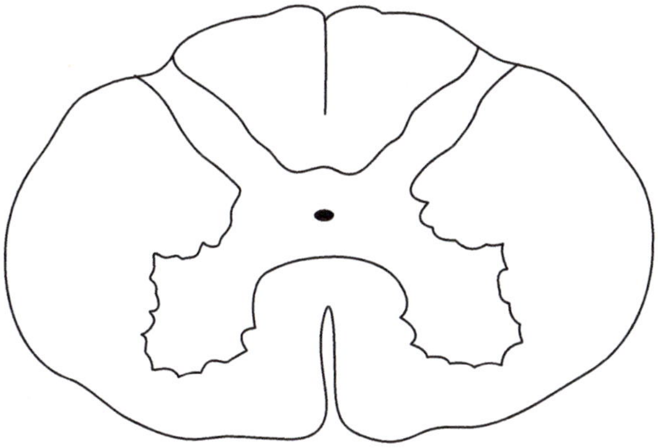

J

**Charts I and J.** Distribution of Borna Disease Virus in Brain and Spinal Cord. (Dr. C. Cantile, Pisa University.)

## vi. Equine infectious anemia

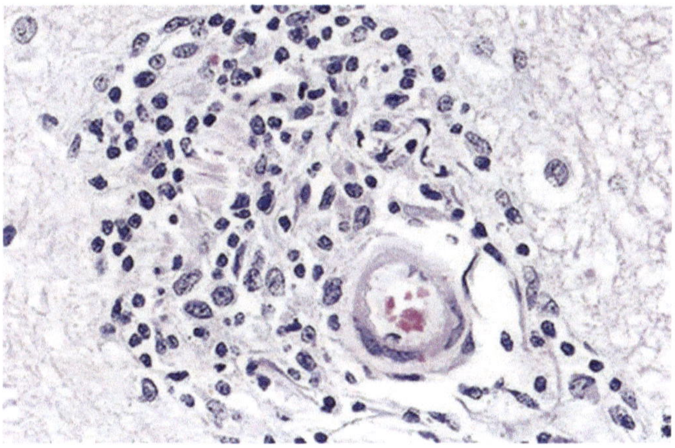

**Figure 3.44.** Horse. Brain. EIA. A lymphocytic infiltration can be present in the meninges and neuropile. The neurotropic strain of the equine infectious anemia virus can induce lymphocytic encephalitis, sometimes accompanied by giant cells. (H&E) (Courtesy Dr. B. Williams, Joint Pathology Center and former AFIP, Washington, DC.)

*b. Protozoal: Equine protozoal encephalomyelitis*

This important neurologic disease of horses is caused by the apicomplexan protozoa *Sarcocystis neurona*. The horse is a dead-end host for *S. neurona*. The opossum is considered a definitive host, and a variety of avian species serve as an intermediate host. Lesions may be limited to a single or few spinal cord segments and may be symmetric or focally asymmetric, hence the former descriptive term "segmental myelitis." Brain lesions are most common in the medulla and pons. Microscopic changes consist of mixed inflammatory infiltrates composed of lymphocytes, plasma cells, eosinophils, macrophages, and multinucleate giant cells in the neuropile and around blood vessels. Differential etiologic diagnosis should include the neurotropic form of equine infectious anemia retrovirus, which may induce a nonsuppurative granulomatous encephalomyelitis. In untreated cases, intralesional protozoa can be demonstrated in neurons or in the neuropile. Treated cases, which are very common these days, often do not contain protozoa, and the inflammation can be reduced to mild perivascular lymphocytic infiltration. In these cases the final diagnosis is obtained by ruling out the other infectious diseases of the equine CNS. Testing for EPM can be done on the CSF (e.g., by Western blot).

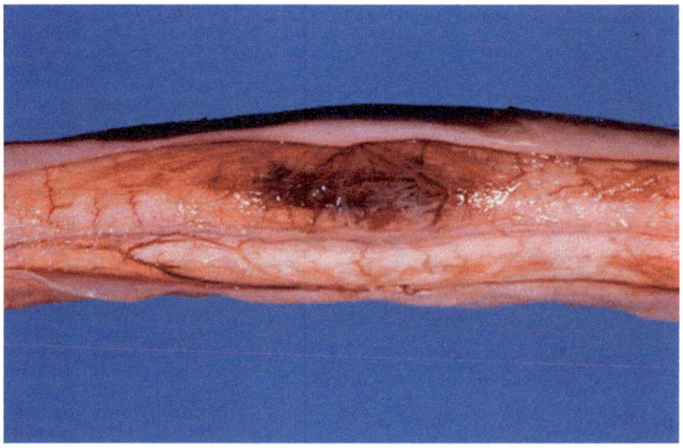

**Figure 3.45.** Horse. Spinal Cord. EPM. Segmental hemorrhage is present on the leptomeningeal surface of the spinal cord after removal of the dura mater.

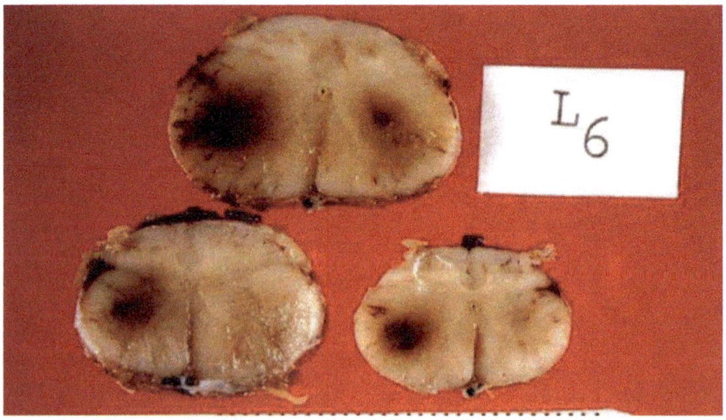


**Figure 3.46.** Horse. Spinal Cord. EPM. Coronal sections of the spinal cord show multiple foci of hemorrhage within the white matter.

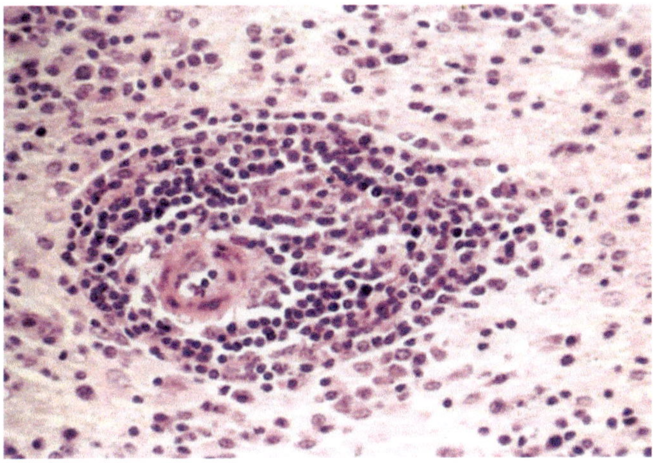

**Figure 3.47.** Horse. Spinal Cord. EPM. Marked inflammation composed of lymphocytes and histiocytes around blood vessels and within the neuropile. (H&E)

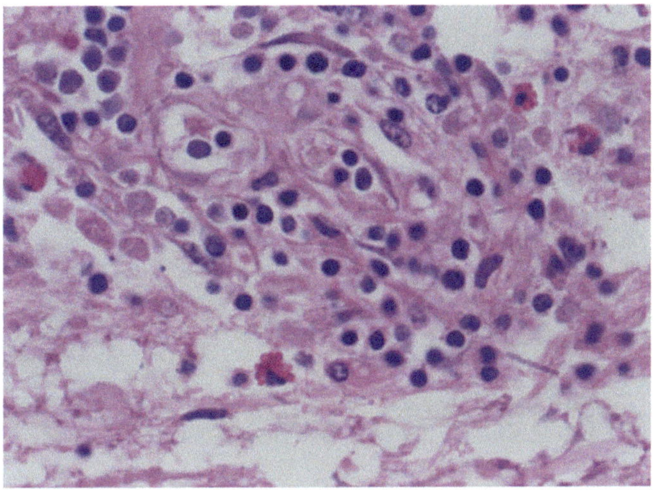

**Figure 3.48.** Horse. Spinal Cord. EPM. The inflammatory infiltrate may contain eosinophils and occasional multinucleate giant cells. (H&E)

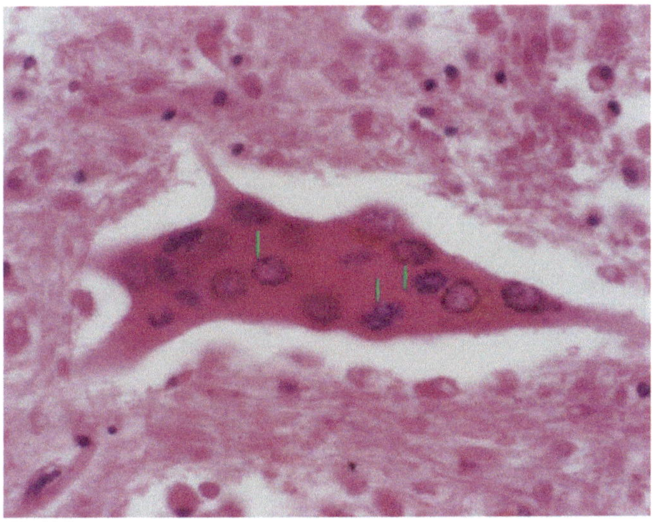

**Figure 3.49.** Horse. Spinal Cord. EPM. Schizonts (arrow) with merozoites of *S. neurona* are contained within the neuronal cell cytoplasm. (H&E)

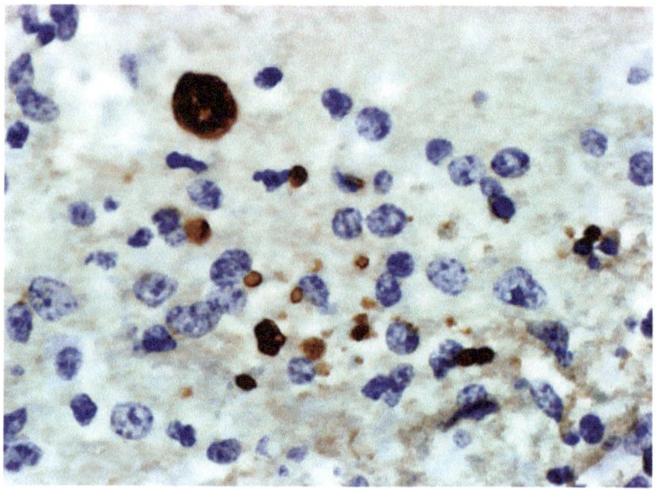

**Figure 3.50.** Horse. Spinal cord. EPM. *S. neurona* antigen within cyst and zooites. (IHC)

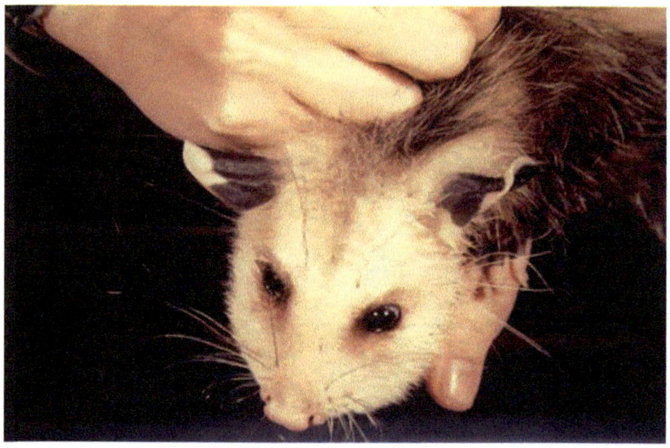

**Figure 3.51.** Opossum (*Didelphis virginiana* or *albiventris*). Considered the definitve host in the life cycle of *S. neurona*.

*Neospora hughesi* has been reported as another protozoal agent in similar mixed inflammatory cases of protozoal encephalomyelitis.

*c. Bacterial*

Bacteria to be considered for meningoencephalitis or cerebral abscesses are *Streptococci equi* subsp. *equi* or *zooepidemicus*), *Listeria monocytogenes, Klebsiella pneumoniae, Borrelia burgdorferi, and Rhodococcus equi. Clostridium tetani* and *Clostridium botulinum* cause clinical neurologic disease, but they do not induce pathologic changes.

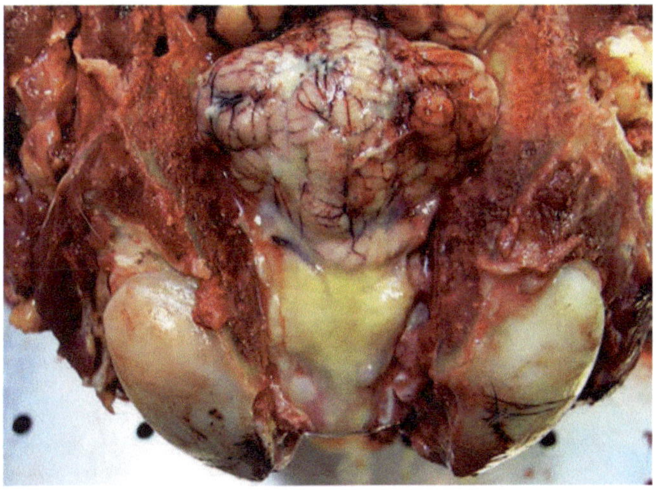

**Figure 3.52.** Horse. Brain. Purulent Meningoencephalitis. *S. equi* subsp. *zooepidemicus* was isolated.

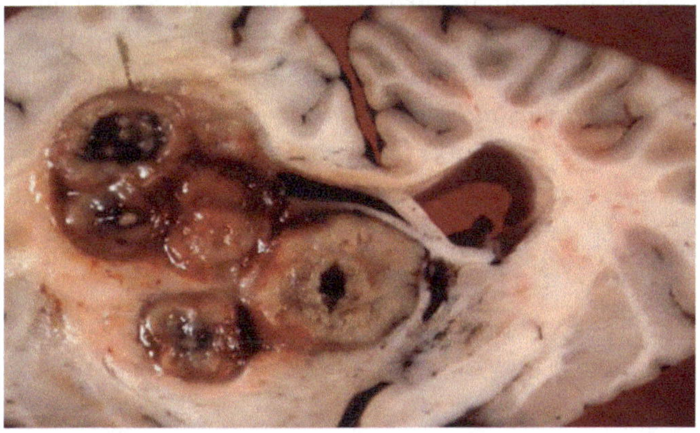

**Figure 3.53.** Horse. Brain. Cerebral Hemisphere. Abscesses. *S. equi* subsp. *equi* was cultured.

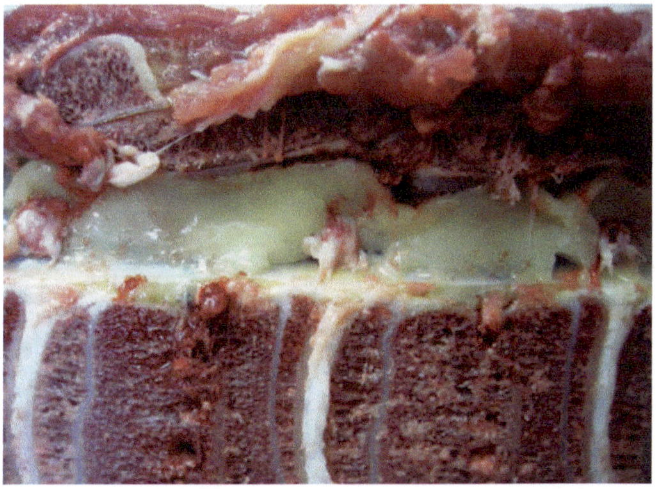

**Figure 3.54.** Horse. Spinal Cord. Epidura. Pyogranulomatous Inflammation. *Rhodococcus equi* was cultured.

*d. Mycotic*

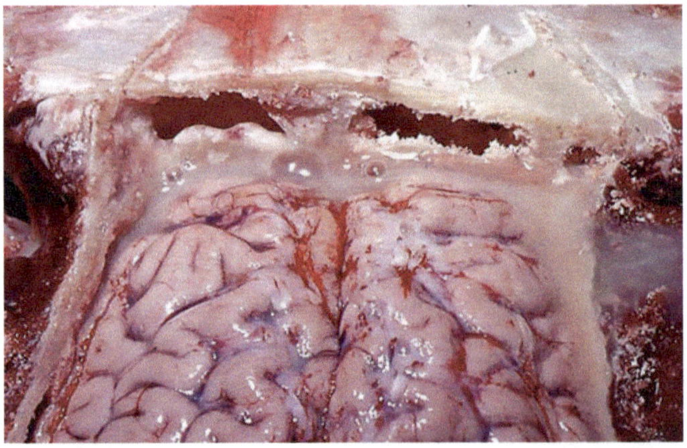

**Figure 3.55.** Horse. Brain. Rostral Brain. Cryptococcosis. A mucinous exudate has accumulated at the rostral brain typical for infection with *Cryptococcus neoformans*. The likely route of entry is aerogenous. (Courtesy Dr. J. King, Cornell University.)

*Aspergillus* sp. and *Mucor* sp. can also be involved in mycotic CNS disease. Very rarely, Amoeba such as *Acanthamoeba* sp. and *Balamuthia mandrillaris* are involved as causative agents for meningoencephalitis.

*e. Parasitic*

Aberrantly migrating larvae of certain equine endoparasites are quite destructive to the brain and spinal cord. Multifocal necrosis, hemorrhage, and inflammation may randomly develop at multiple levels of the CNS. Larvae can be demonstrated after multiple sectioning. Parasitic larvae under consideration include *Strongylus vulgaris*, *Setaria* sp. (Asia), *Hypoderma* sp., *Parelaphostrongylus tenuis* sp., and *Halicephalobus gingivalis*.

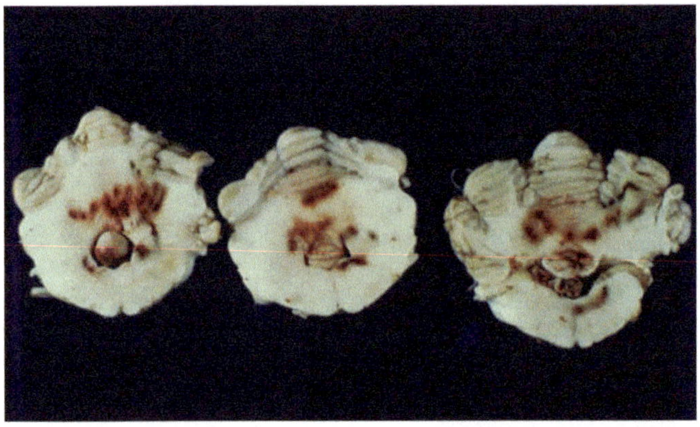

**Figure 3.56.** Horse. Cerebellum. *Halicephalobus gingivalis*. Larval migration tracts are present in multiple foci.

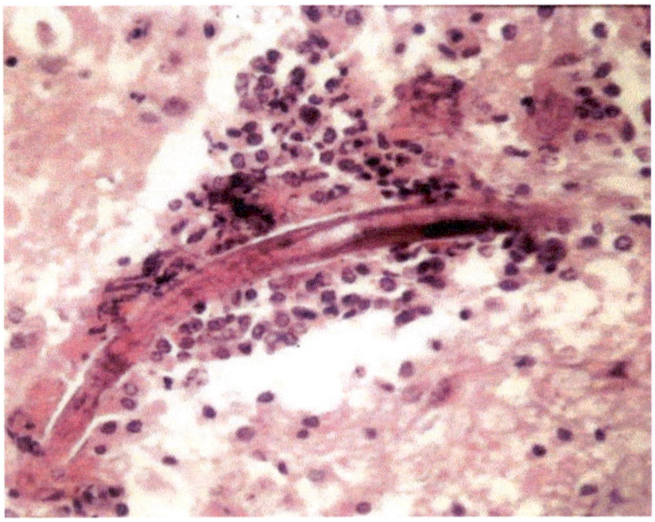

**Figure 3.57.** Horse. Cerebellum. *Halicephalobus gingivalis*. Rhabditiform larvae are surrounded by inflammatory cells. There is evidence of malacia. The parasite is one of the many causes of ataxia in the horse. (H&E)

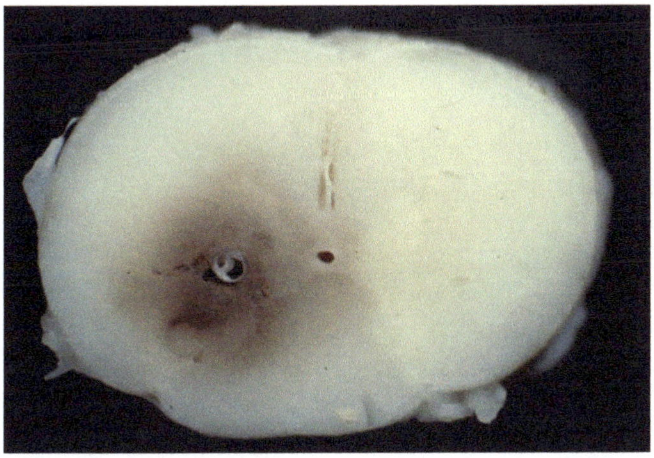

**Figure 3.58.** Horse. Spinal Cord. Donkey. *Strongylus vulgaris*. Cross section of parasite is present in the center of focal hemorrhage and malacia.

### *5. Traumatic injuries*

The injuries and consequences to the brain and spinal cord depend on three factors: severity, speed, and duration. Trauma to the skull may result in fractures of basilar bones resulting in hemorrhage and laceration of the adjacent brain tissue. Penetrating foreign bodies need to be considered as a cause also. Trauma to the spinal column may lead to vertebral fractures, spinal cord contusion, or laceration.

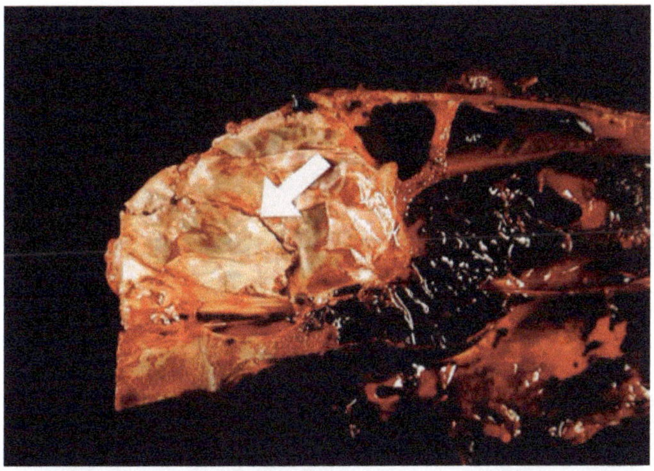

**Figure 3.59.** Horse. Skull. Fracture of Baso-Sphenoid Bone. The arrow denotes the sharp fracture line with subsequent hemorrhage of the basilar brain. The horse fell on the head after rearing. Rupture of cervical muscles may also be present in these cases.

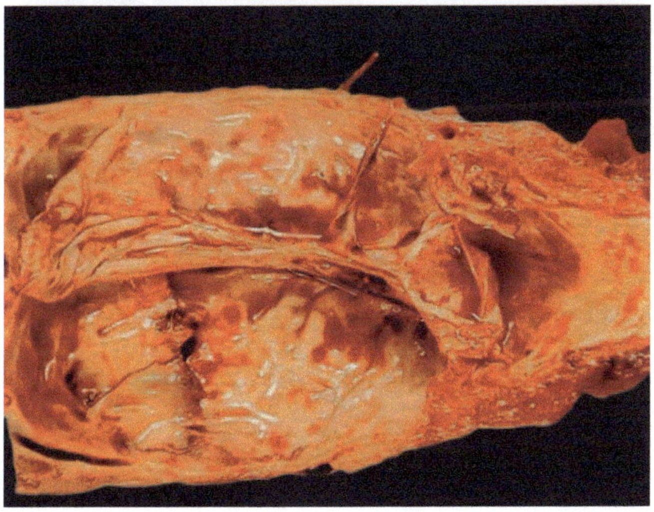

**Figure 3.60.** Horse. Skull. Fracture of Parietal Bone.

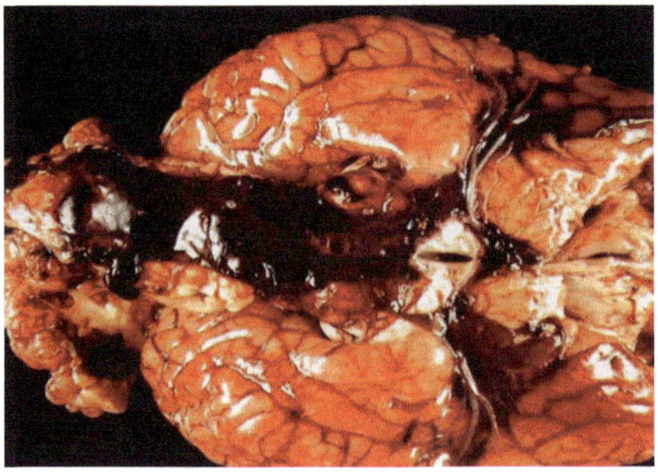

**Figure 3.61.** Horse. Base of Brain. Contrecoup Hematoma.

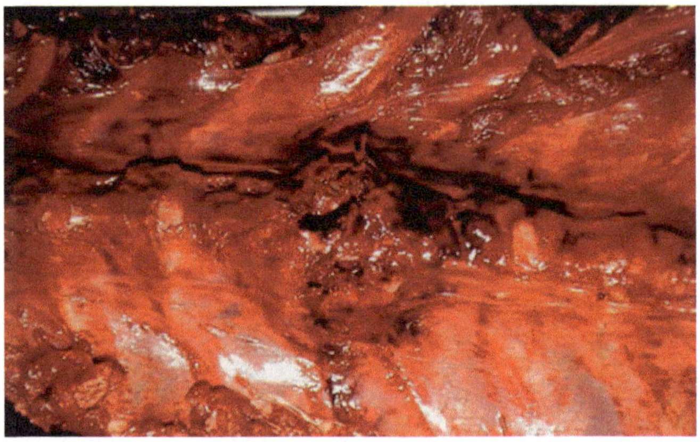

**Figure 3.62.** Horse. Spinal Cord. Fractures. The compound fracture of a vertebral body occurred at T5 with resulting compression of the overriding spinal cord. Lightning may be considered as cause of unexpected fractures of well-protected vertebrae in otherwise healthy horses. Also malicious electrocution needs to be considered as a cause.

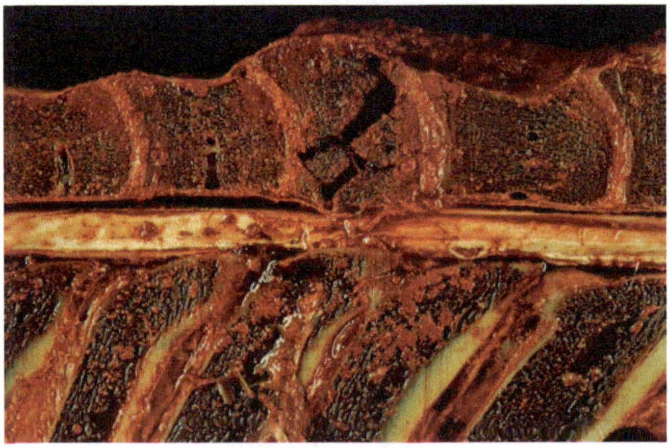

**Figure 3.63.** Horse. Fracture of the thoracic segment, especially T10 T12, is more typical as to location.

## 6. *Neoplastic*

Primary cerebral tumors are extremely rare in horses. Occasional ependymomas, choroid plexus tumors, and meningiomas have been described. Metastasizing tumors include malignant melanomas and hemangiosarcomas. Tumors within the epidural space of the spinal cord may be schwannomas, lymphomas, hemangiomas, hemangiosarcomas, or plasma cell tumors with a compressing effect on the overriding spinal cord. Peripheral nerve sheath tumors may have similar compressive effects. Pituitary tumors are discussed in Chapter 11, "Disease of the Endocrine System."

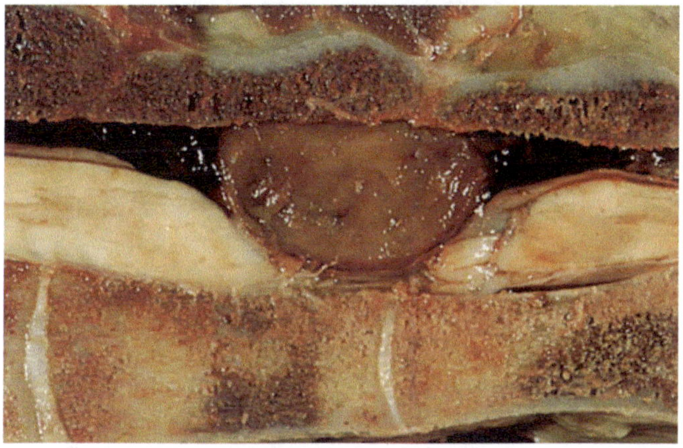

**Figure 3.64.** Horse. Epidural Space. The focal space-occupying tan mass was diagnosed as a schwannoma. Differential diagnosis: lymphoma, paraganglioma, plamacytoma. (Courtesy Dr. P. Habecker, University of Pennsylvania.)

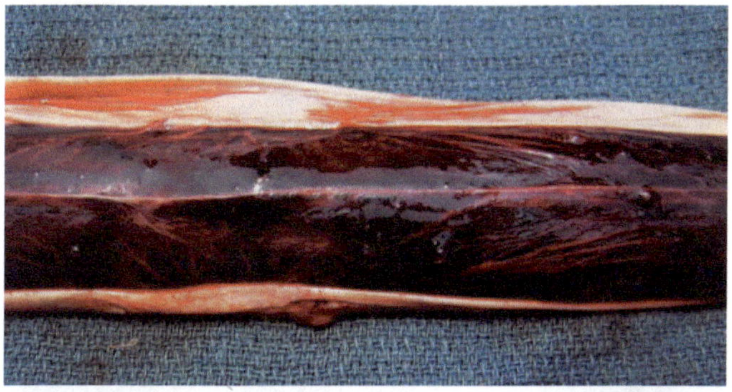

**Figure 3.65.** Horse. Cervical Cord. Hemorrhage from lymphoma.

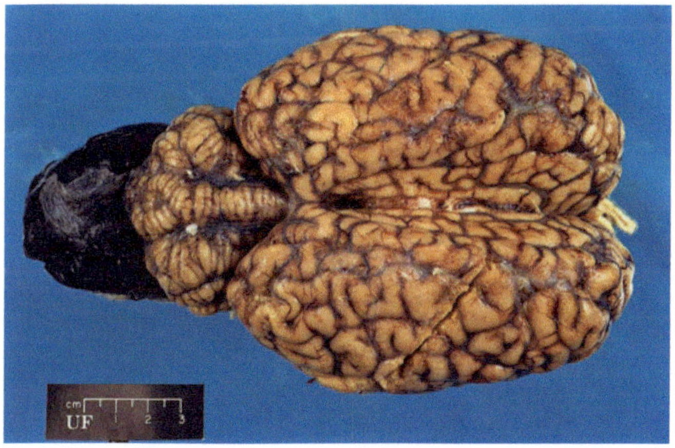


**Figure 3.66.** Horse. Medulla Oblongata. A malignant melanoma has invaded the medulla oblongata.

## 7. *Miscellaneous*

### *a. Choroid plexus cholesteatoma*

These granular growths commonly occur at the site of the lateral or fourth ventricles. They are incidental findings with no neurologic impact.

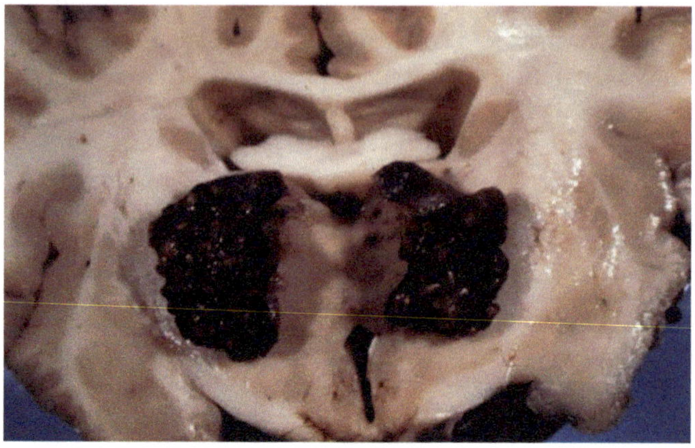

**Figure 3.67.** Horse. Brain. Cholesteatoma. A granular mass is present in the lateral ventricles on sagittal section.

### *b. Epidural synovial cyst*

Considered the result of synovial membrane detachment from degenerative facet joint disease, the proliferating tissue may compress spinal nerves.

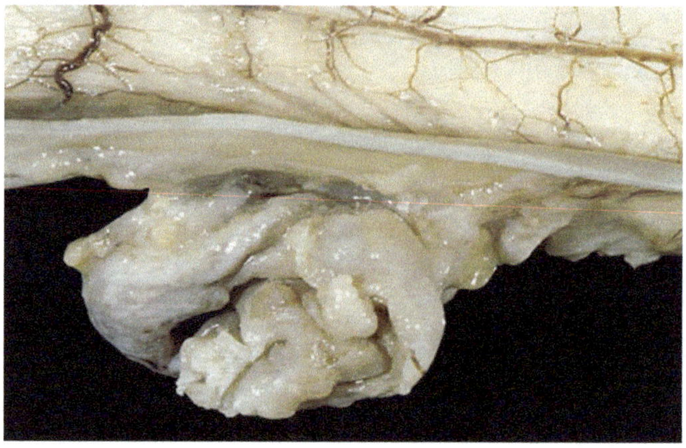

**Figure 3.68.** Horse. Epidural Synovial Cyst. A gelatinous gray folded tissue compresses the spinal cord in a collar-like fashion next to the spinal nerves at the level of C6. (Courtesy Dr. P. Habecker, University of Pennsylvania.)

## II. Peripheral nervous system

### 1. *Polyneuritis equi (polyradiculitis, cauda equina neuritis)*

The disease of adult horses progressively involves the sacrocaudal nerves to produce clinical signs of hind leg paresis and urinary bladder paralysis with secondary rupture and uroperitoneum. The exact cause is unknown. An immune-mediated antimyelin basic protein disorder is postulated.

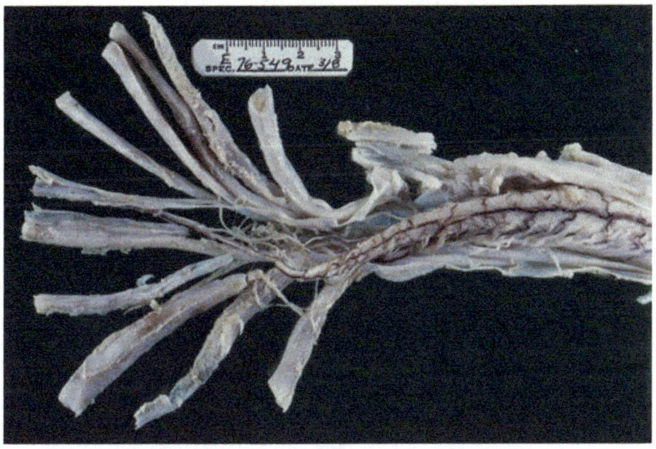


**Figure 3.69.** Horse. Cauda Equina. Neuritis. The filum terminale is markedly thickened due to an extensive inflammation.

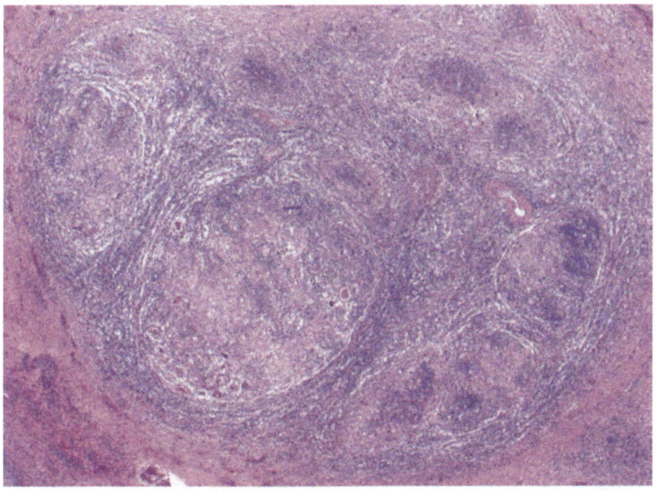

**Figure 3.70.** Horse. Cauda Equina. Neuritis. There is microscopic evidence of severe mononuclear cell infiltration of the nerve roots, almost completely obliterating them. In chronic cases the inflammation may become granulomatous to include giant cells and collagen. (H&E)

### 2. *Grass sickness*

This seasonal disease has been mainly reported to occur in Great Britain with some cases seen on the European continent. Very rare cases of grass sickness have been reported from the United States. The disorder apparently affects young horses grazing on pastures in the springtime. It is thought to be the result of a neurotoxic agent affecting the autonomic function of neurons in sympathetic paravertebral ganglia. But also structural enteric neuronal damage contributes to intestinal dysautonomia leading to alimentary smooth muscle atonia and intestinal ileus, enhanced intestinal secretions and changes in fluid gradient exchange.

As to the cause, type C (group 3) toxins produced by *Clostridium botulinum* have been incriminated.

Clinical signs of grass sickness include colic, gastric reflux tympany, excessive salivation, and sweating. Muscle weakness and tremors, slow chewing, dysphagia, and drooping eyelids (ptosis) are additional signs.

Differential diagnosis should include pasture myodystrophy.

Gross findings include a fluid-filled gastrointestinal tract and splenomegaly. Microscopic features include dropout of neurons, chromatolysis with some inflammation of neurons of the paraganglia, and ganglia of the myenteric plexus.

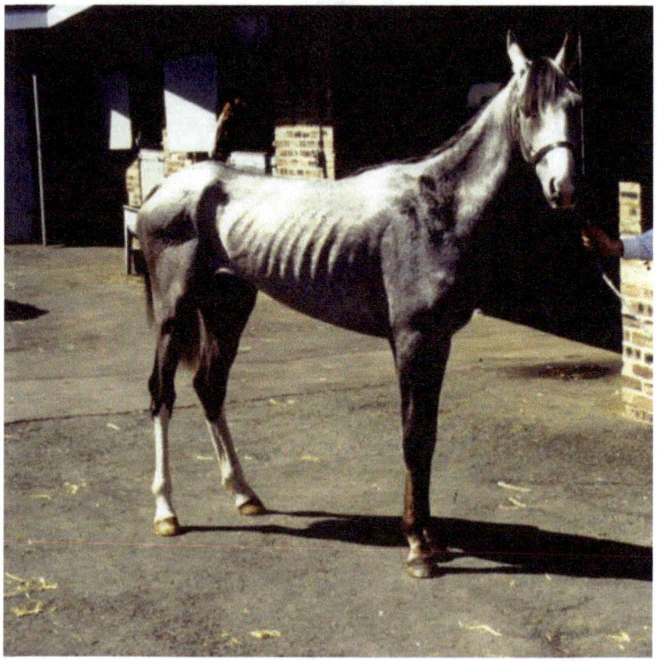

**Figure 3.71.** Horse. Whole Body. Grass Sickness. Severe emaciation from intestinal dysautonomia. (Courtesy Dr. E. Milne, Biobest Laboratories Ltd, UK.)

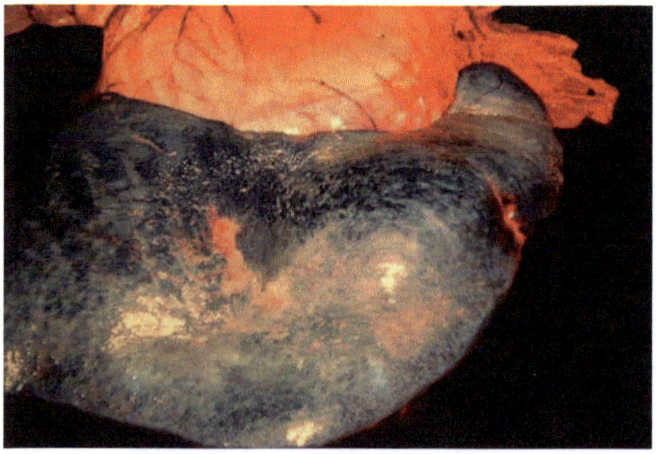

**Figure 3.72.** Horse. Spleen and Stomach. Grass Sickness. Both organs are markedly distended: the spleen by blood; the stomach by fluid.

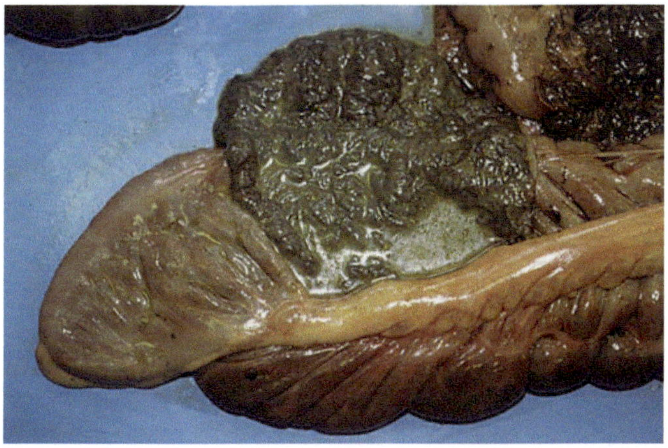

**Figure 3.73.** Horse. Cecum. Grass Sickness. The lumen is markedly distended by viscous fluid and digesta.

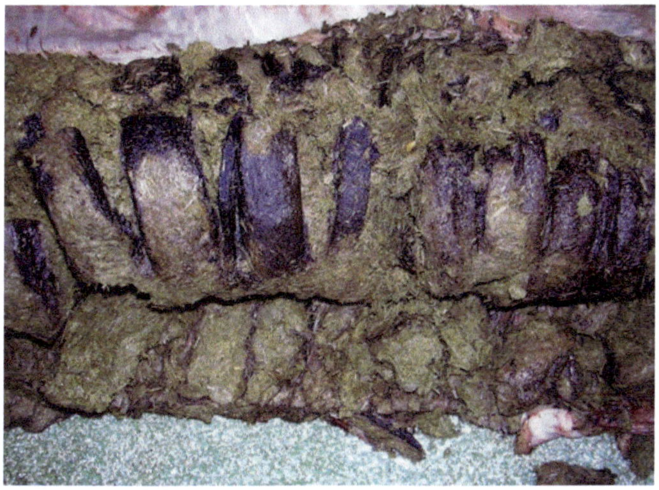

**Figure 3.74.** Horse. Colon. Grass Sickness. Black coating of the mucosa is hypothesized to be produced by *Clostridium botulinum* type C associated with the disease. The digesta often firmly adhere to the colonic mucosa. (Courtesy Dr. E. Milne, Biobest Laboratories Ltd, UK.)

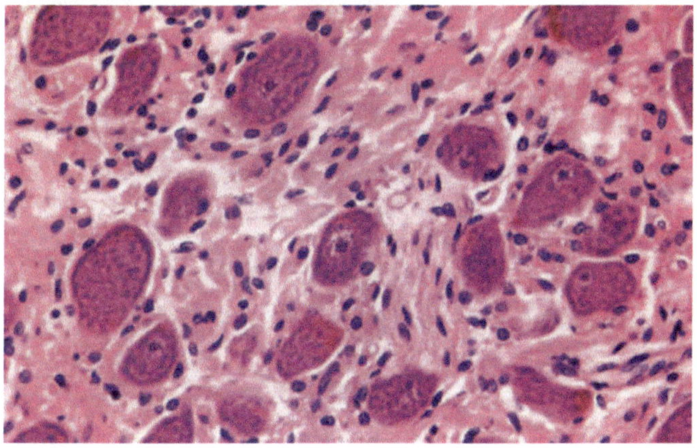

**Figure 3.75.** Horse. Mesenteric Ganglion. Normal histologic appearance for comparison. (H&E) (Courtesy Dr. E. Milne, Biobest Laboratories Ltd, UK.)

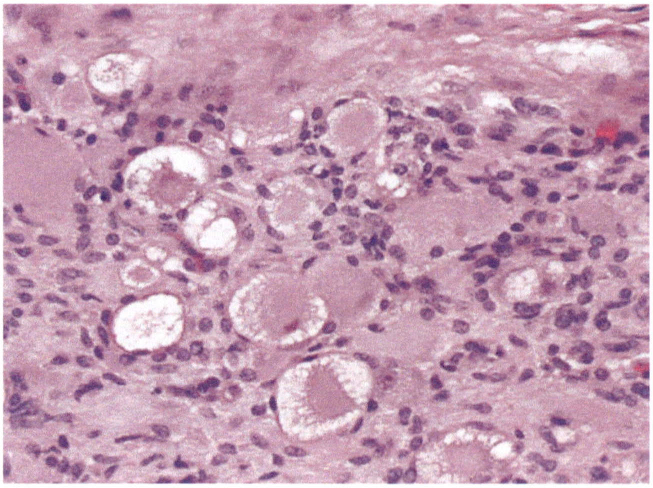

**Figure 3.76.** Horse. Myenteric Plexus. Grass Sickness. The celiac mesenteric ganglion is the target. Neurons are characterized by chromatolysis and vacuolation. (H&E) (Courtesy Dr. E. Milne, Biobest Laboratories Ltd, UK.)

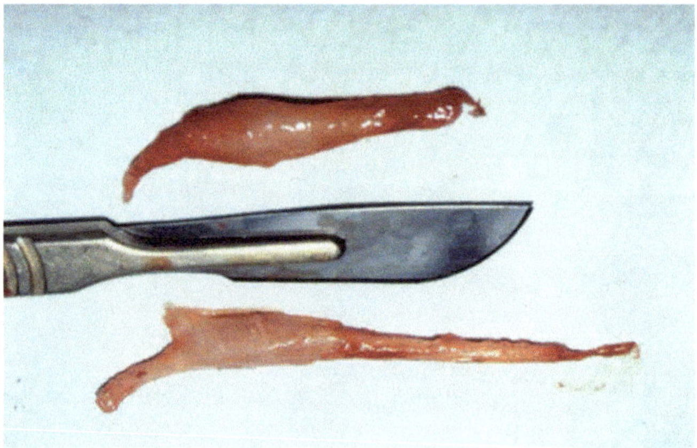

**Figure 3.77.** Horse. Superior Cervical Ganglion. Removed and displayed. (Courtesy Dr. E. Milne, Biobest Laboratories Ltd, UK.)

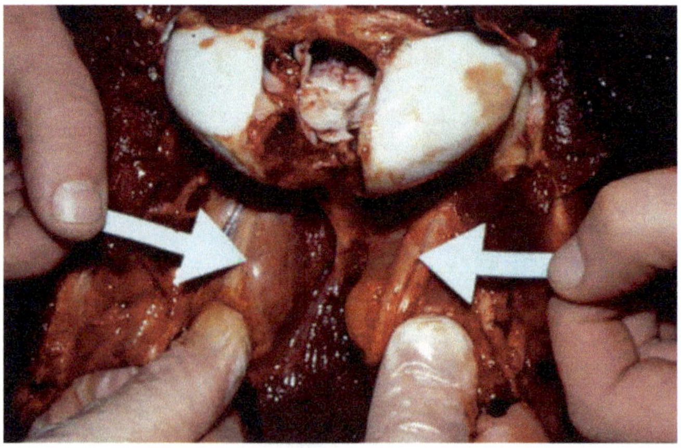

**Figure 3.78.** Horse. Superior Cervical Ganglion. Arrow denotes in situ location. (Courtesy Dr. E. Milne, Biobest Laboratories Ltd, UK.)

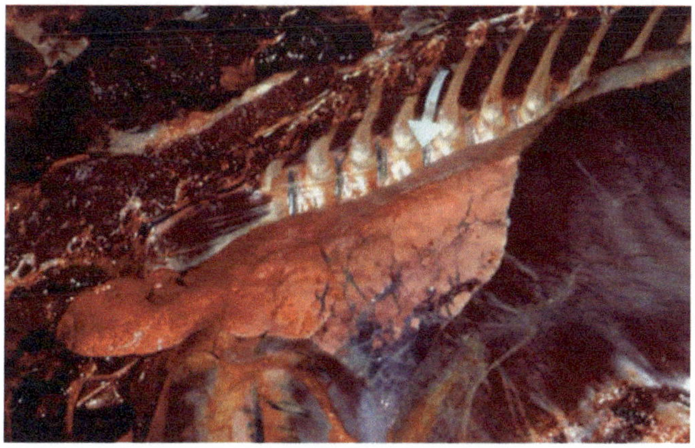

**Figure 3.79.** Horse. Thoracic Ganglionic Chain. Topographic location indicated by arrow. (Courtesy Dr. E. Milne, Biobest Laboratories Ltd, UK.)

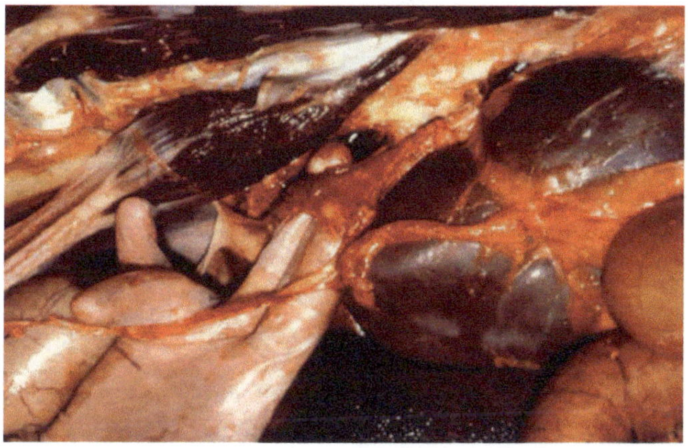

**Figure 3.80.** Horse. Celiac-Mesenteric Ganglion. Topographic location in abdomen indicated by palm of gloved hand. (Courtesy Dr. E. Milne, Biobest Laboratories Ltd, UK.)

### *3. Peripheral neuropathies*

Peripheral neuropathies are rare in horses. Recurrent laryngeal hemiphlegia neuropathy is mentioned in Chapter 9, "Diseases of the Muscular System." True stringhalt and Australian stringhalt are disorders with clinical signs of abnormal gait due to distal axonopathy with Wallerian degeneration of peripheral, largely myelinated hindlimb and forelimb nerves. A peripheral polyneuropathy with demyelination and inflammation of Schwann cells is made responsible for the knuckling syndrome in Scandinavian riding horses.

Other examples of peripheral neuropathies are femoral nerve paresis, entrapment of scapular nerve, lead poisoning, and amputation neuroma.

Peripheral nerve sheath tumors arise from Schwann cells. They need to be differentiated from neurofibromas and sarcoids in cases of cutaneous location. Other single tumors may be infiltrating squamous cell carcinoma or lymphoma.

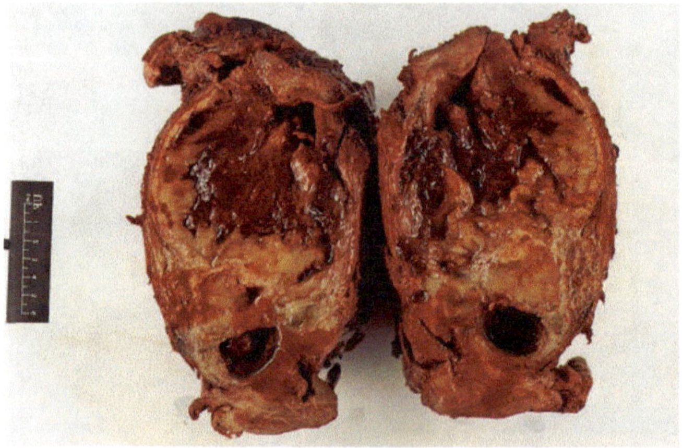

**Figure 3.81.** Horse. Hindlimb. Malignant Peripheral Nerve Sheath Tumor. A multilobulated mass with large areas of hemorrhage and necrosis.

## Selected references


Bogaert L, Heerden MV, Ceck HE, Chiers K. 2011. Molecular and immunohistochemical distinction of equine sarcoid from schwannoma. *Vet Pathol* 48(3): 737–741.

Cantile C, Del Piero F, Di Guardo G, Arispici M. 2001. Pathologic and immunohistochemical findings in naturally occurring West Nile virus infection in horses. *Vet Pathol* 38:414–421.

Castillo-Olivaris J, Wood J. 2004. WNV infection in horses. A review. *Vet Res* 35:467–483.

Cottrell DF, McGorum BC, Pearson GT. 1999. The neurology and enterology of equine grass sickness: a review of basic mechanisms. *Neurogastroenterol Motil* 11(2):79–92.

Hudson N, Mayhew I, Pearson G. 2001. A reduction in intestinal cells of Cajal in horses with equine dysautonomia (grass sickness). *Auton Neurosci* 92(1–2): 37–44.

James FM, Engiles JB, Beech J. 2010. Meningitis, cranial neuritis, and radiculitis associated with *Borrellia burgdorferi* infection in a horse. *J Am Vet Med Assoc* 237(10):1180–1185.

Locombe RF, Huntington PJ, Friend SC, Jeffcott LB, Luff AR, Finkelstein DK. 1992. Pathological aspects of Australian stringhalt. *Equine Vet J* 24(3):174–183.

Newton JR, Wylie CE, Proudman CJ, McGorum BC, Poxton IR. 2010. Equine grass sickness: are we any nearer to answers on cause and prevention after a century of research? *Equine Vet J* 42(6):477–481.

Porter MB, Long MT, Getman LM, et al. 2003. West Nile virus encephalomyelitis in horses: 46 cases (2001). *J Am Vet Med Assoc* 222:1241–1247.

Schuler LA, Khaitsa ML, Dyer RW, Steltenow CL. 2004. Evaluation of an outbreak of West Nile virus infection in horses: 569 cases. *J Am Vet Med Assoc* 225:1084–1089.

Shotton HR, Lincoln J, McGorum BC. 2011. Effects of equine grass sickness on sympathetic neurons in prevertebral and paravertebral ganglia. *J Comp Pathol* 145(1):35–44.

# 4 Diseases of the Respiratory System

I. Upper respiratory tract
   1. Structures of normal nose
   2. Sinonasal disorders
      a. Paranasal sinus cyst
      b. Ethmoid hematoma
      c. Nasal polyp
      d. Sinonasal inflammation
   3. Guttural pouch diseases
   4. Pharynx/larynx/epiglottis disorders
   5. Sinonasal neoplasia
II. Lower respiratory tract
   1. Trachea
   2. Lung
      a. Recurrent airway obstruction
      b. Exercise-induced pulmonary hemorrhage
      c. Pneumonias
      d. Pulmonary neoplasia
      e. Pleuritis
   3. Diaphragmatic hernia
   4. Pleural mesothelioma

*Color Atlas of Equine Pathology*, First Edition. Claus D. Buergelt and Fabio Del Piero.

# I. Upper respiratory tract

## *1. Structures of normal nose*

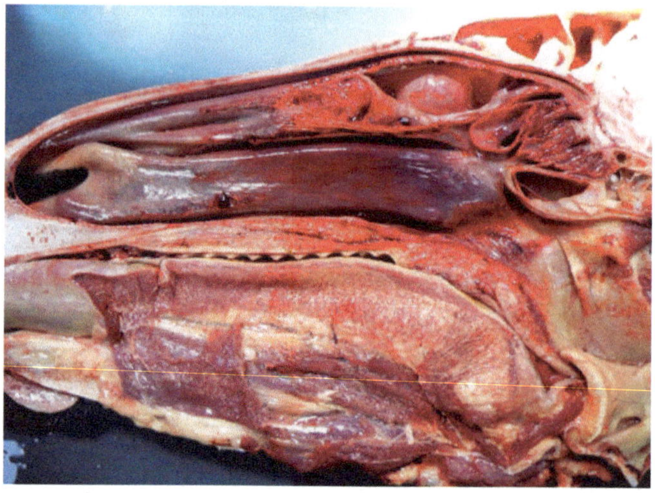

**Figure 4.1.** Horse. Nose. Midsaggital Section. Normal structures of the nasal passages are exposed.

## *2. Sinonasal disorders*

### *a. Paranasal sinus cyst*

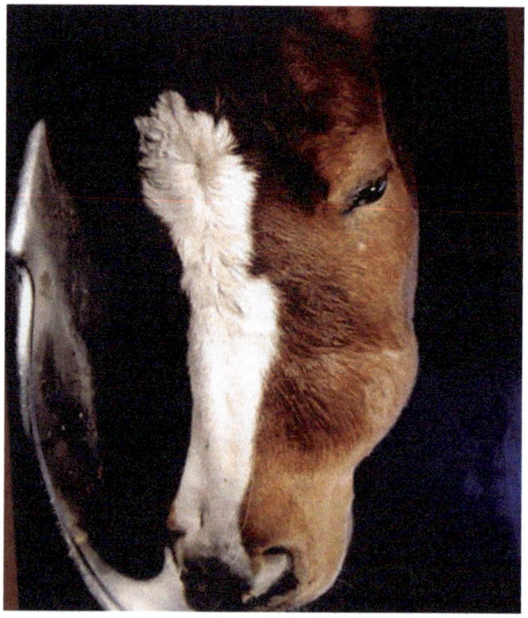

**Figure 4.2.** Horse. Head. Nasal Deviation. A unilateral facial deformity is associated with nasal septum deviation. Differential diagnoses include branchial cyst, paranasal cyst, ossifying fibroma, congenital dental deformities, abscessation, nutritional osteodystrophy, and nasal neoplasia.

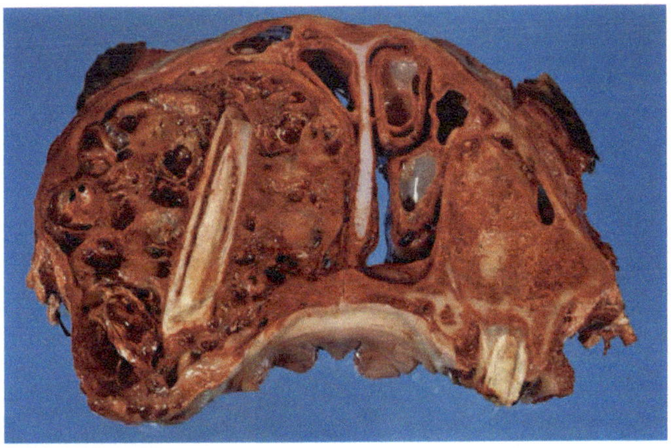

**Figure 4.3.** Horse. Nasal Cavity. Paranasal Cyst. A multiloculated cystic growth has occupied and expanded into half of the nasal cavity thus slightly deviating the septum. The surrounding molar tooth has been dislodged. The paranasal sinuses of the opposite nasal cavity are filled with mucin. The cyst mainly arises from the caudal maxillary sinus.

*b. Ethmoid hematoma*

This slowly growing tissue proliferation arises from the mucosa of the caudal nasal cavity or ethmoid labyrinth. The pathogenesis is not understood because this tissue proliferation acts like a locally invasive neoplasm but morphologically is not. It clinically leads to small volume epistaxis.

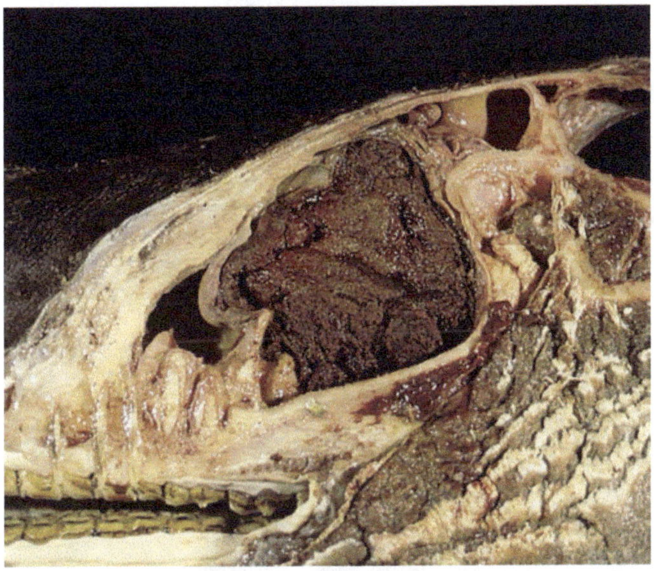

**Figure 4.4.** Horse. Sinus. Ethmoid Hematoma. A reddish granular tissue mass expands cranially from the ethmoid plate and is evident after fenestration of the sinus.

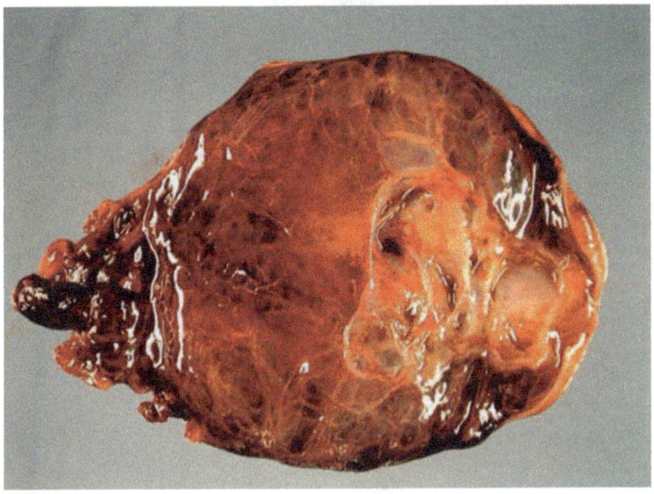

**Figure 4.5.** Horse. Caudal Nasal Cavity. Ethmoid Hematoma. An amorphous, soft, jelly, grapelike growth has been surgically removed from the ethmoid plate of a horse with repetitive nose bleeding.

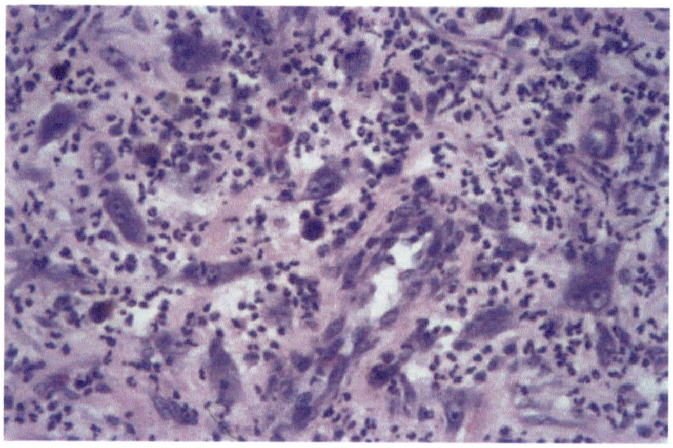

**Figure 4.6.** Horse. Ethmoid Hematoma. Mixed cellular inflammation that includes histiocytes and giant cells is one microscopic feature of ethmoid hematoma. (H&E)

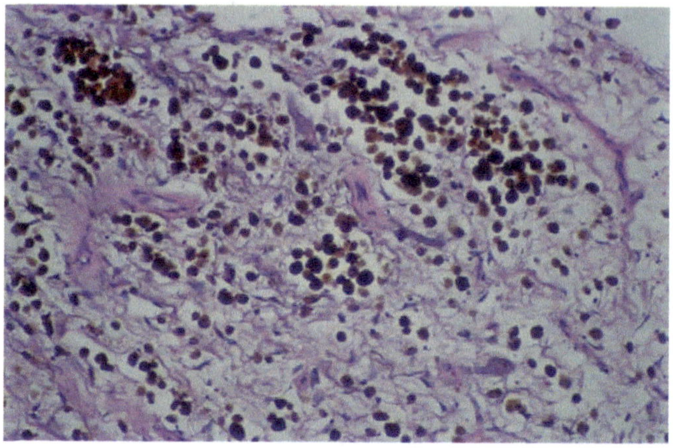

**Figure 4.7.** Horse. Ethmoid Hematoma. Mineralized collagen and hemosiderin-laden macrophages are additional microscopic features. (H&E)

### *c. Nasal polyp*

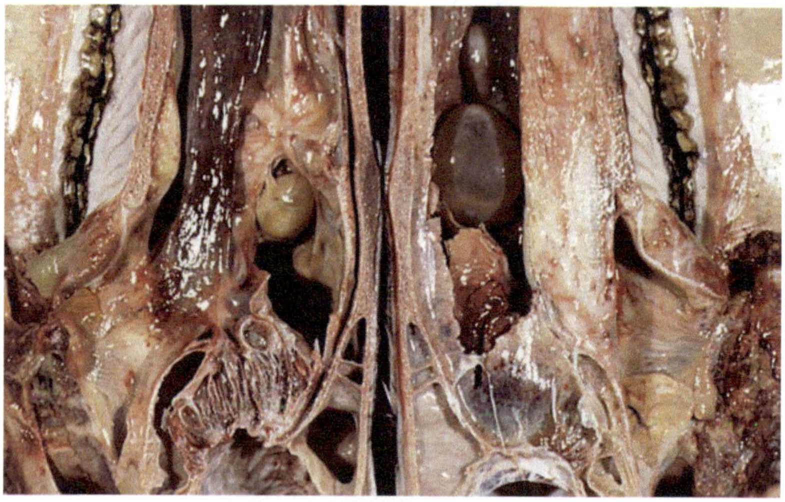

**Figure 4.8.** Horse. Nasal Cavity. Polyps. Oval, partially cystic growths are deep in the caudal nasal passages. Nasal polyps originate from the ethnoturbinates. (Courtesy Dr. P. Habecker, University of Pennsylvania.)

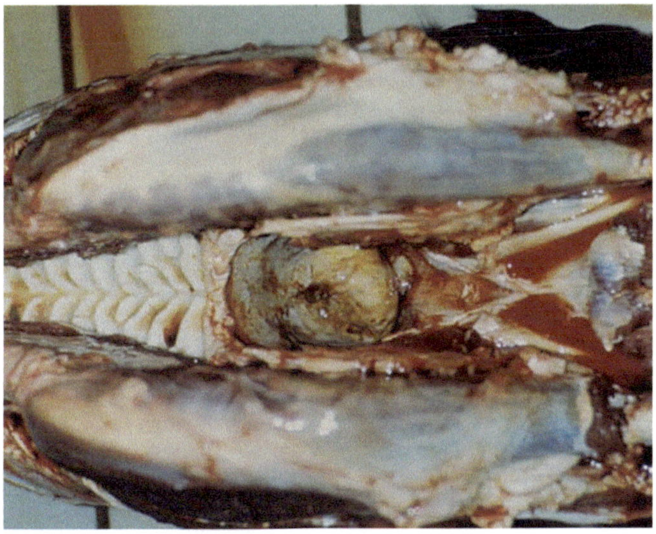

**Figure 4.9.** Horse. Nasopharynx. Polyp. A single round mass has obliterated the pharynx. Nasopharyngeal polyps originate from the middle ear. (Courtesy Dr. P. Habecker, University of Pennsylvania.)

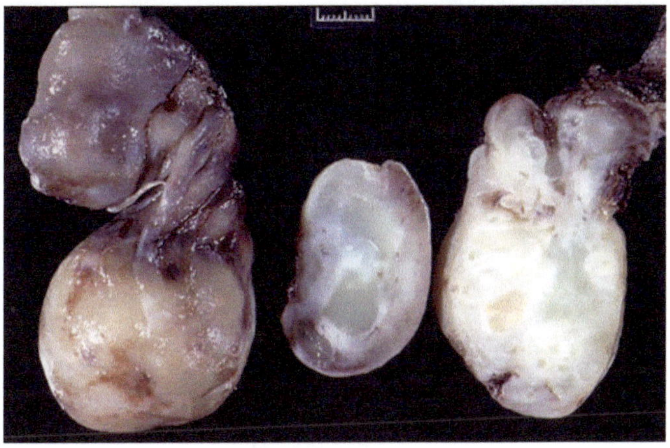

**Figure 4.10.** Horse. Nasal Polyps. Pedunculated, gelatinous tissue surgically removed from the nose. (Courtesy Dr. J. King, Cornell University.)

*d. Sinonasal inflammation*

Viruses, bacteria, and fungi have to be considered as etiologic agents. If bacteria are involved, these usually are *Streptococci* sp. or *Fusobacterium* sp. Noninfectious causes may be environmental, irritants, or trauma. The inflammatory response can be classified depending on the nature of the exudate as catarrhal, mucinous, hemorrhagic, purulent, and granulomatous.

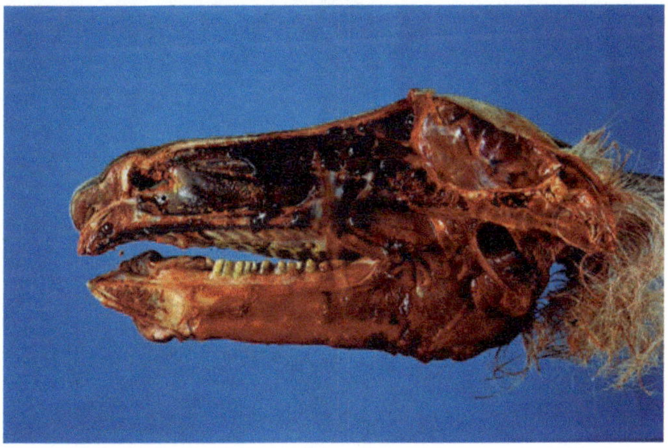

**Figure 4.11.** Horse. Nose. Midsaggital Section. Fibrinohemorrhagic Rhinitis. *Fusobacterium* sp. Destruction of nasal conchae. Trauma. Differential diagnosis should be nasal neoplasia or ethmoid hematoma.

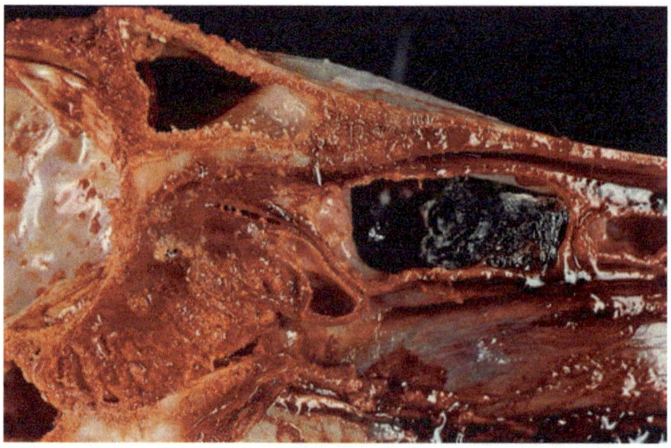

**Figure 4.12.** Horse. Nose. Midsaggital Section. Fungal Hemorrhagic Sinusitis. Aspergillosis. Differential diagnosis should be trauma or hemangiosarcoma.

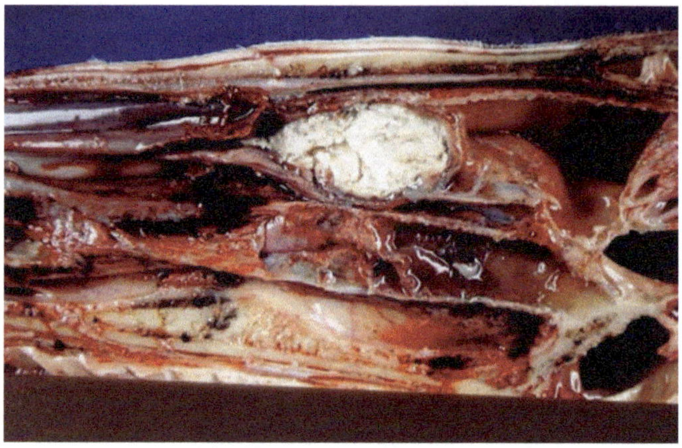

**Figure 4.13.** Horse. Nose. Midsaggital Section. Caseous Rhinitis Aspergillosis (Aspergilloma). A fibrinonecrotic inflammation is considered more common with fungal infections.

Other fungi to affect the nasal cavity are *Coccidioides immitis* and *Cryptococcus neoformans*.

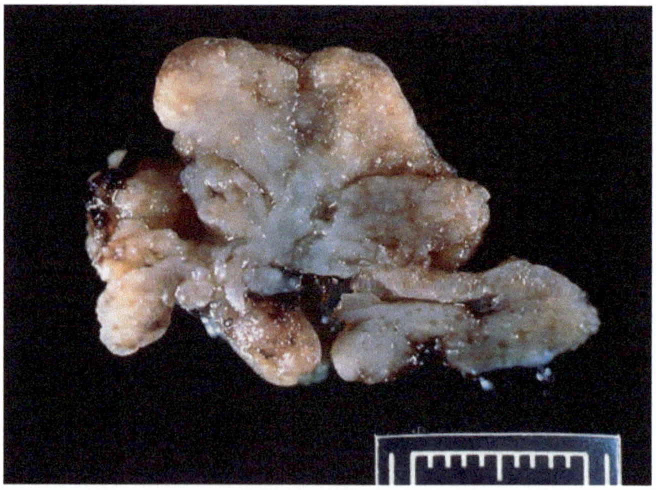

**Figure 4.14.** Horse. Nose. Rhinosporidiosis. This granulomatous disease typically affects the nasal septum and sinuses. Tumorlike, soft, polypoid, glistening nodules are grossly visible. (Courtesy Dr. D. Meuten, North Carolina State University.)

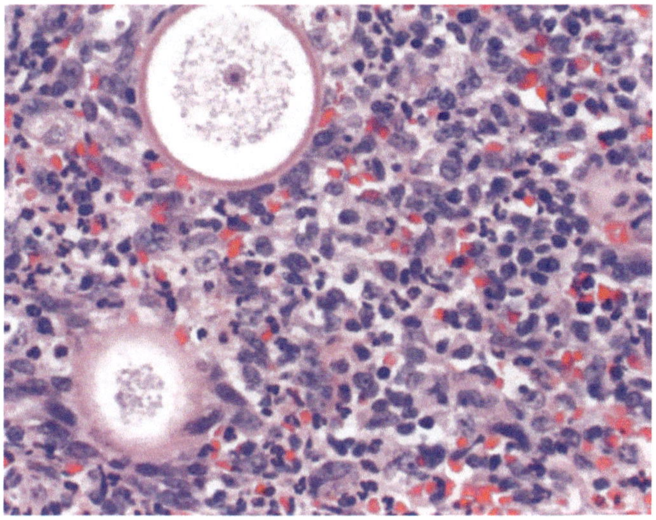

**Figure 4.15.** Horse. Rhinosporidiosis. The pyogranuloma histologically is characterized by large oval sporangia containing numerous endospores. *Rhinosporidium seeberi*, the causative organism, is now considered an aquatic protistan parasite. (H&E)

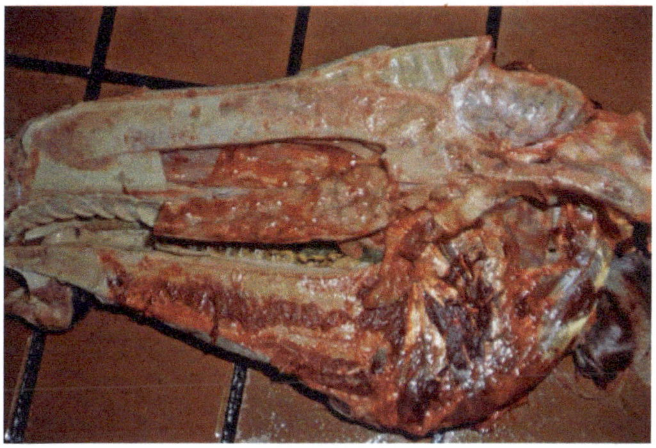

**Figure 4.16.** Horse. Nose. Midsaggital Section. Granulomatous Rhinitis. Pythiosis. Differential diagnosis: nasal amyloidosis. (See Chapter 13, "Diseases of the Skin (Integument).")

The nasal form of glanders is an example of infection with an exotic, zoonotic bacillus. The agent (*Burkholderia mallei*) causes granulomas and ulcers in the nasal septum.

### *3. Guttural pouch diseases*

Also known as eustachian tube diverticula, the guttural pouches in the horse are large pockets on either side of the caudoventral head, lined by a thin, smooth, shiny mucosa. Each guttural pouch is partially divided by the stylohyoid bone, connected with the pharynx and traversed by the internal carotid artery as well as by cranial nerves and cranial ganglia. Because of this close anatomic relationship of blood vessels, nerves, and pharyngeal opening, the guttural pouches are susceptible to pathogens of the upper respiratory tract with a sometimes serious outcome such as severe fatal epistaxis. Dysphagia and Horner's syndrome are other clinical signs of guttural pouch diseases resulting from damage of the adjacent cranial nerves and ganglia.

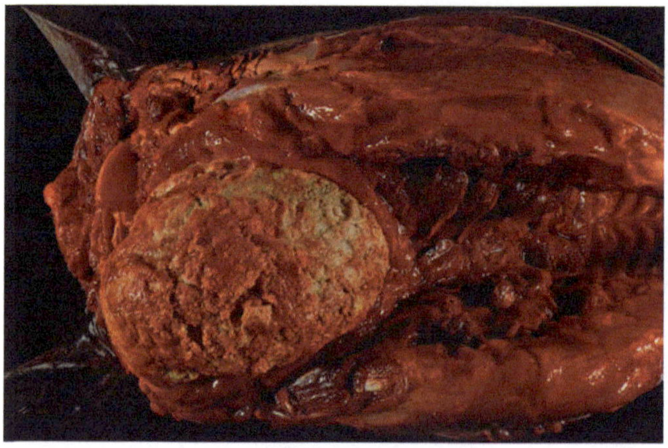

**Figure 4.17.** Horse. Guttural Pouch. Empyema. The pouch is unilaterally distended and filled by abundant thick, fibrinopurulent exudate. Infectious organisms that may be recovered are *Streptococcus equi* subsp. *equi* or *Streptococcus equi* subsp. *zooepidemicus*. Intermittent, unilateral mucopurulent nasal discharge is a common clinical sign, often increasing when the horse lowers the head. Epistaxis is uncommon.

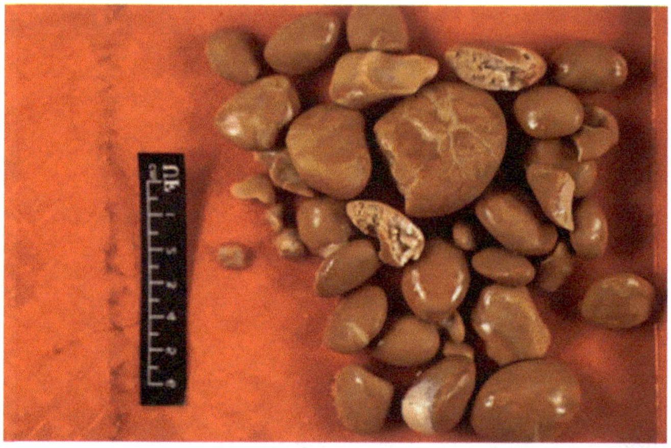

**Figure 4.18.** Horse. Guttural Pouch. Chondroids. Inspissated concretions can form with chronic infection.

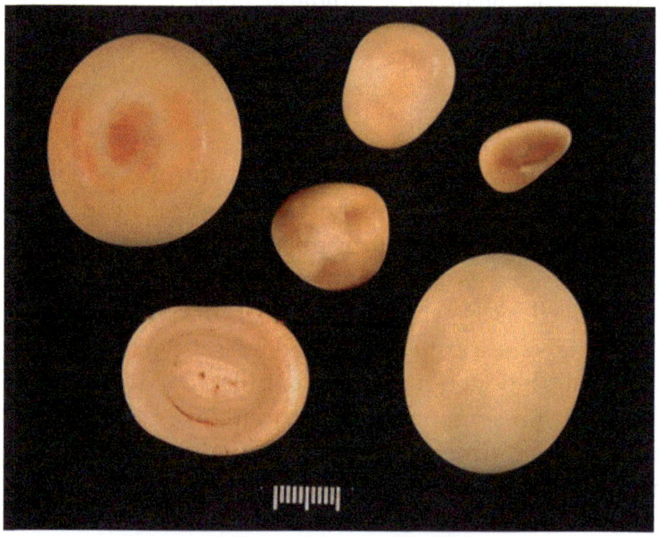

**Figure 4.19.** Horse. Guttural Pouch. Chondroids. Cross sections.

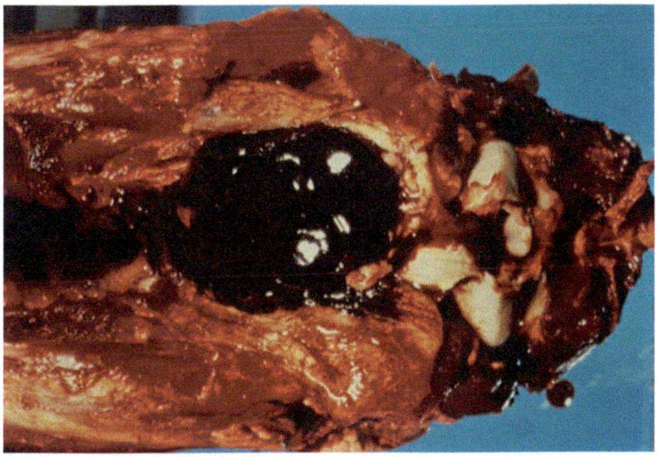

**Figure 4.20.** Horse. Guttural Pouch. Hematoma Due to Mycosis or Pythiosis. Usually unilateral, it is the result of aspergillosis or in the Southeast of the United States due to pythiosis.

*Aspergillus nidulans* is a common resident of the guttural pouch. The mycotic infection can spread through the wall of the pouch, with fungi invading the nearby internal carotid artery to induce thrombosis and dissection aneurysm with massive bleeding, sometimes leading to exsanguination. The pathogenesis of the aneurysm may be partially due to fracture of the stylohyoidal apparatus or joint instability due to chronic joint degeneration.

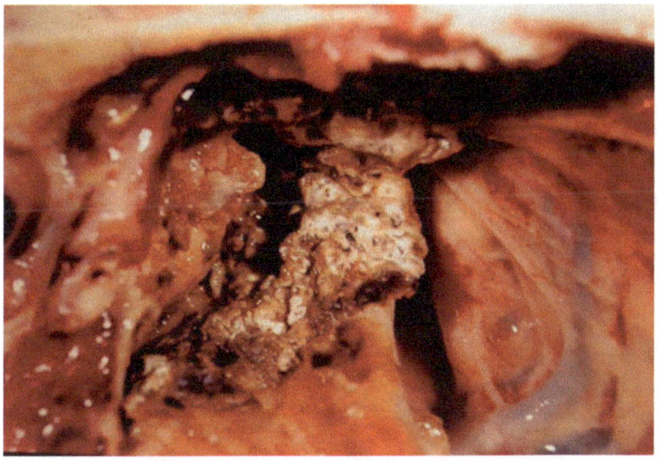

**Figure 4.21.** Horse. Guttural Pouch. Mycosis. Once the blood is removed, there is evidence of a friable, cauliflower-like dry exudate covering the pouch wall.

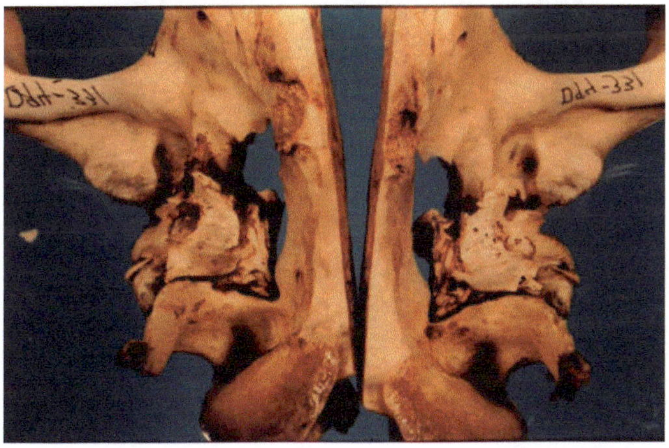

**Figure 4.22.** Horse. Stylohyoidal Bone Apparatus. Guttural Pouch. There is evidence of chronic arthritis with exostoses and fractures in a horse with guttural pouch mycosis. The bone changes might be partially responsible for traumatic damage to the adjacent internal carotid artery and might aid the angioinvasion of resident fungi.

## 4. Pharynx/Larynx/Epiglottis disorders

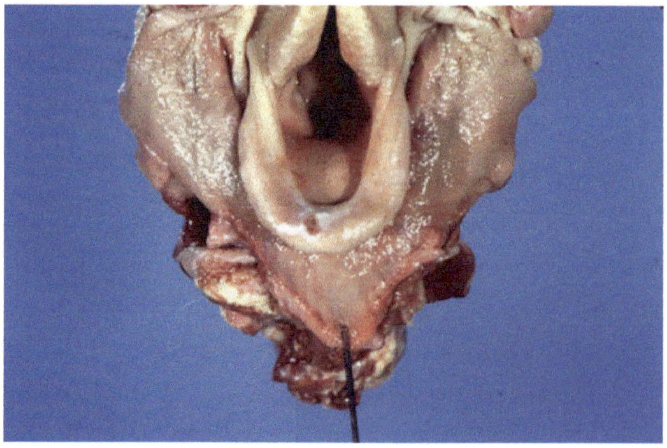

**Figure 4.23.** Horse. Larynx. Epiglottal (Laryngeal) Entrapment. This is the result of redundant mucosa and the cause of upper airway obstruction with exercise intolerance and respiratory noise noticed in racehorses, but also seen in non-racehorses, and is followed by subepiglottic granuloma and subepiglottic cyst formation. Entrapped membranes become thickened. (Courtesy Dr. J. King, Cornell University.)

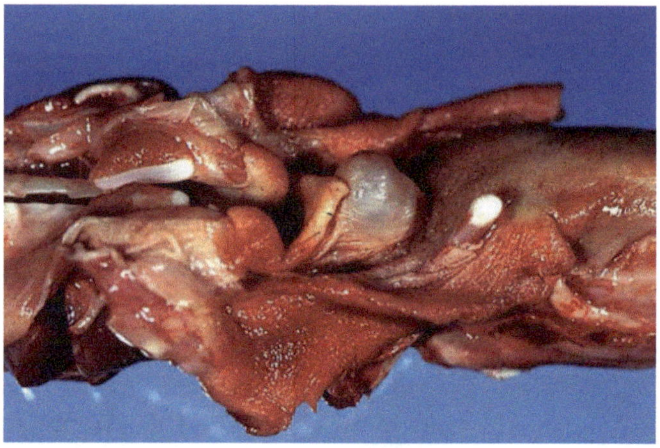

**Figure 4.24.** Horse. Epiglottis. Congenital Subepiglottal Cyst. A small cyst surrounds the epiglottis. (Courtesy Dr. J. King, Cornell University.)

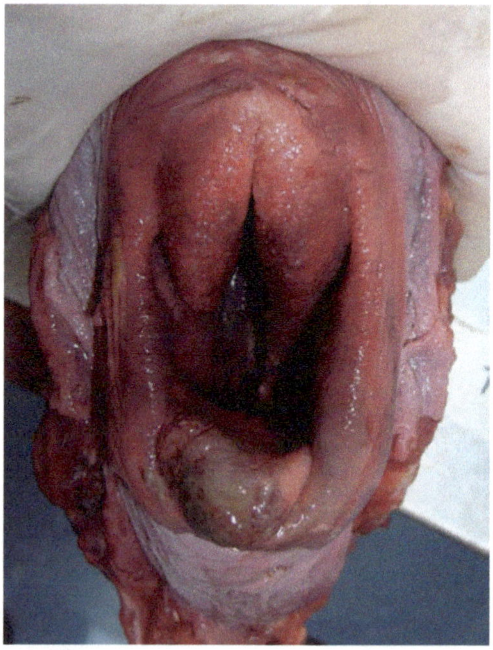

**Figure 4.25.** Horse. Epiglottis. Hypoplasia and Granuloma. (Courtesy Dr. P. Habecker, University of Pennsylvania.)

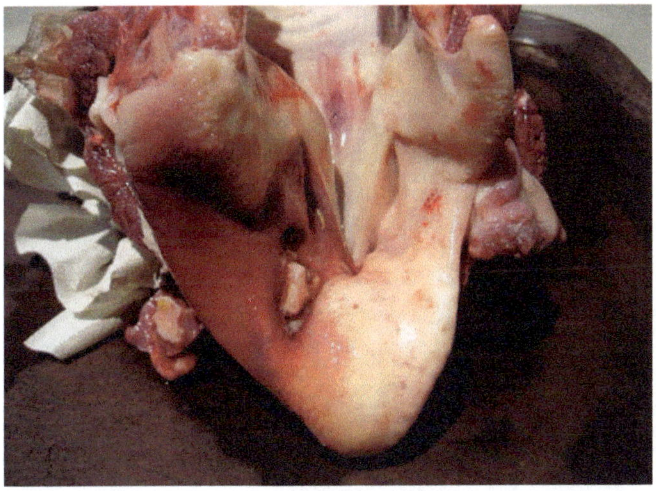

**Figure 4.26.** Horse. Aryepiglottic Fold. Anaerobic bacterial infection. Necrosuppurative, locally extensive, chronic, moderate laryngitis.

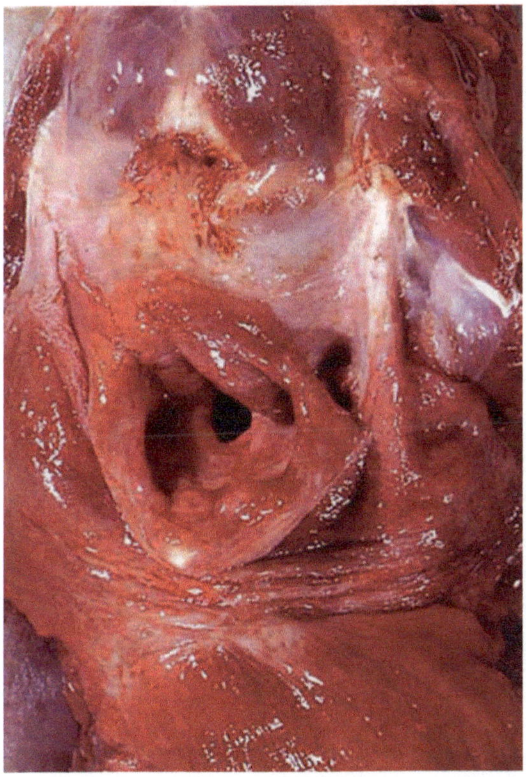

**Figure 4.27.** Horse. Larynx. Cicatrix Syndrome. The nasopharyngeal cicatrix syndrome occurs in two forms. The acute phase is characterized by inflammation and the presence of a diphtheritic membrane, whereas the chronic condition is characterized by scar tissue in the pharynx rostral to the epiglottis. Also included are deformity of the epiglottis, inflammation of the arytenoid cartilage, scarring and thickening of the vocal cords. The condition has been reported from Texas. Detection is made by endoscopic examination. (Courtesy Dr. J. King, Cornell University.)

Other abnormalities associated with the epiglottis are dorsal abscesses.

### *5. Sinonasal neoplasia*

Nasal neoplasms occur more often than thought and mainly arise from the caudal maxillary sinuses. The common tumor types include squamous cell carcinomas, adenocarcinomas, fibro-chondro-osseous and dental tumors, and hemangiosarcomas. On occasion lymphosarcomas, meningiomas, and carcinoids have been reported. Most of the sinonasal tumors are malignant, destroying nasal structures by local invasion and frequently causing facial deformity, loss of teeth, and breathing difficulty. Spread to regional draining lymph nodes may occur, but distant metastases are very rare. Grossly, the sinonasal tumors are indistinguishable as to histogenesis, and microscopic examination is mandatory for morphologic classification. Figure 4.28, Figure 4.29, Figure 4.30, Figure 4.31, Figure 4.32, and Figure 4.33 are representative of the various tumor lineages.

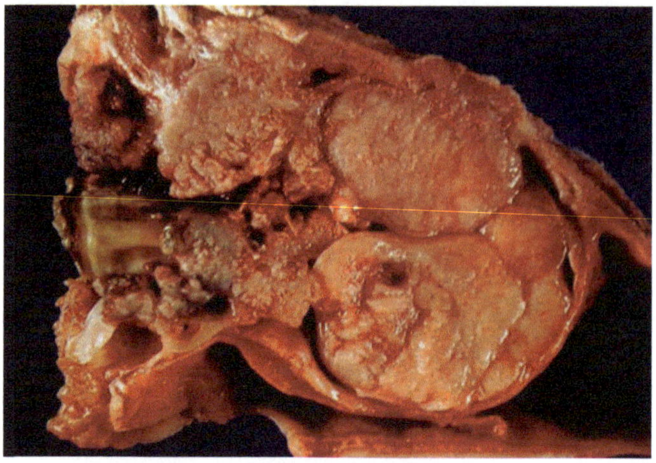

**Figure 4.28.** Horse. Nasal Cavity. Squamous Cell Carcinoma.

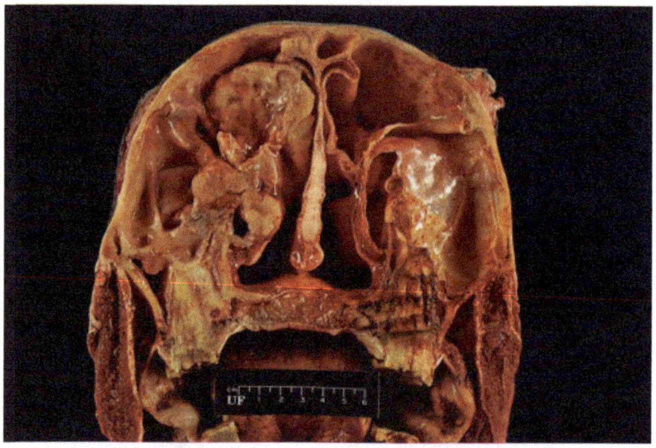

**Figure 4.29.** Horse. Nasal Cavity. Adenocarcinoma.

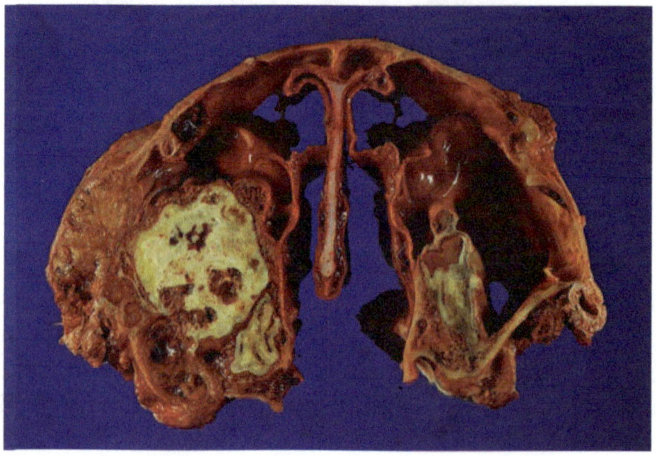

**Figure 4.30.** Horse. Nasal Cavity. Osteosarcoma.

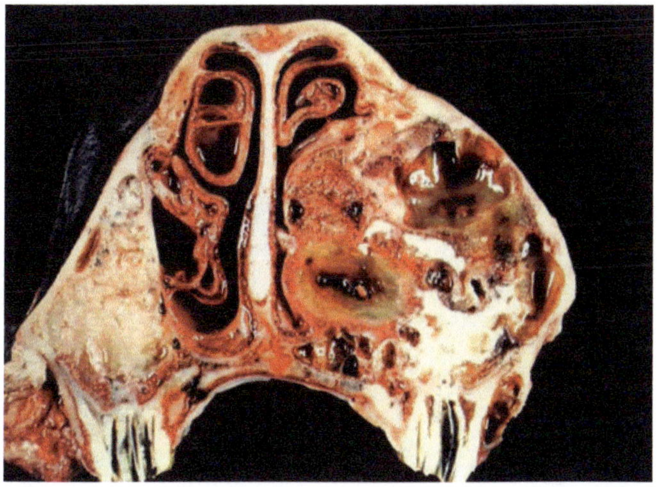

**Figure 4.31.** Horse. Nasal Cavity. Odontocementoma.

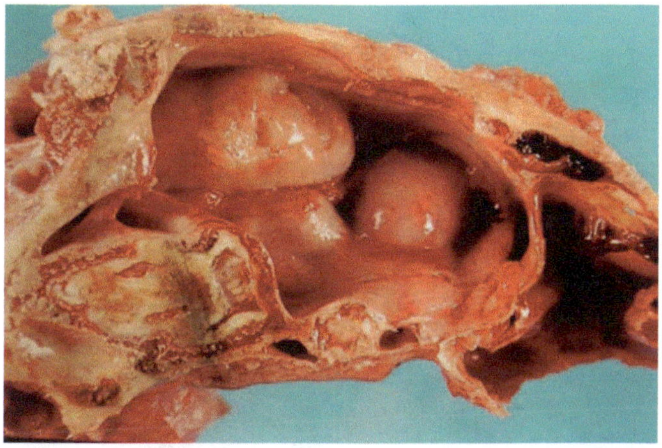

**Figure 4.32.** Horse. Nasal Cavity. Carcinoma.

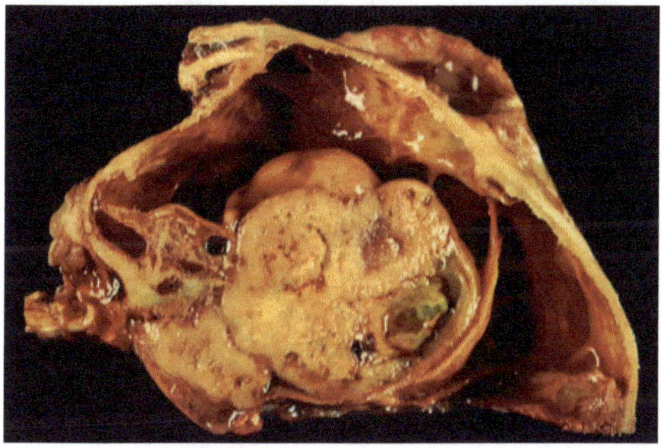

**Figure 4.33.** Horse. Nasal Cavity. Lymphoma.

All of these growths are destructive while invading various tissues of the nose. Their histologic makeup has to be identified by microscopy.

# II. Lower respiratory tract

## 1. Trachea

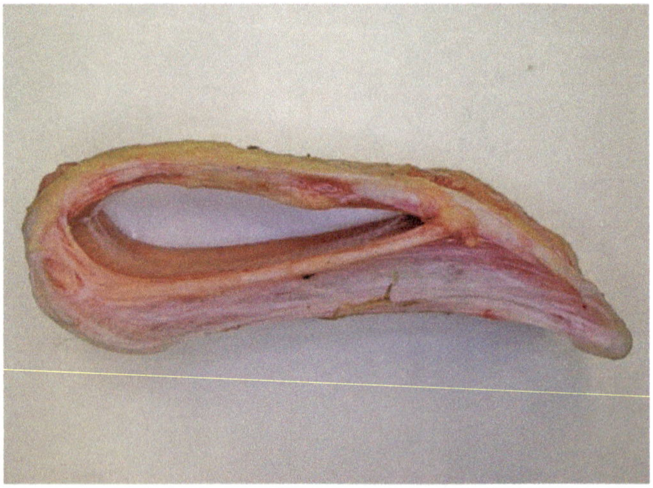

**Figure 4.34.** Horse. Trachea. Tracheal Collapse. The tracheal lumen is narrow due to widening of the dorsal tracheal ligament in an older horse. Occurs with some frequency in Miniature horses. It is the result of chondrodysplasia of the cartilaginous rings. (Courtesy Dr. J. Roberts, National Zoo, Washington DC.)

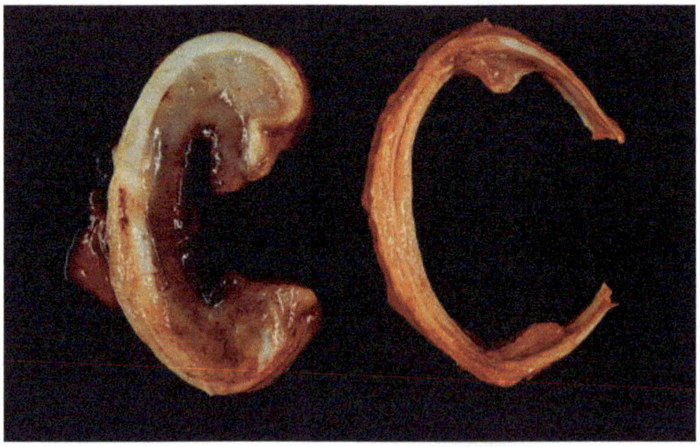

**Figure 4.35.** Horse. Trachea. Inflammation. The mucosal lining of the ring on the left is thickened by edema and inflammatory reaction from repeated intubation. The tracheal ring on the right is unremarkable.

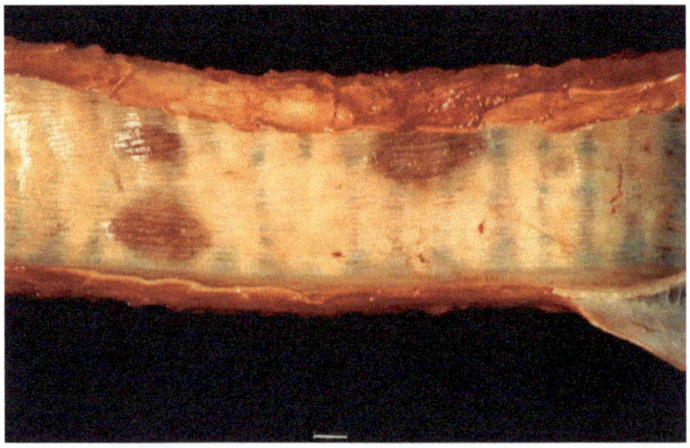

**Figure 4.36.** Horse. Trachea. Lymphoma. As part of the multicentric distribution, several raised nodules are present in the mucosa resulting from neoplastic lymphocytes. The gross differential diagnosis is mycotic tracheitis.

## 2. Lung

### *a. Recurrent airway obstruction*

This condition, formerly known as chronic obstructive pulmonary disease (COPD), is seen in middle-age horses that are stabled for a long period of time and surrounded by and fed damp hay over a lengthy period of time. It is the result of a delayed hypersensitivity response to antigens that are persistently inhaled. It leads to bronchospasm and the accumulation of mucus and exudate in bronchioles with eosinophils and lymphocytes around bronchioles. Pulmonary emphysema and lack of pulmonary collapse are common gross changes. Inflammatory mediators and histamine are stimuli involved in the pathogenesis. Increased respiratory efforts, particularly after exercise, and dry cough are clinical signs of recurrent airway obstruction (RAC).

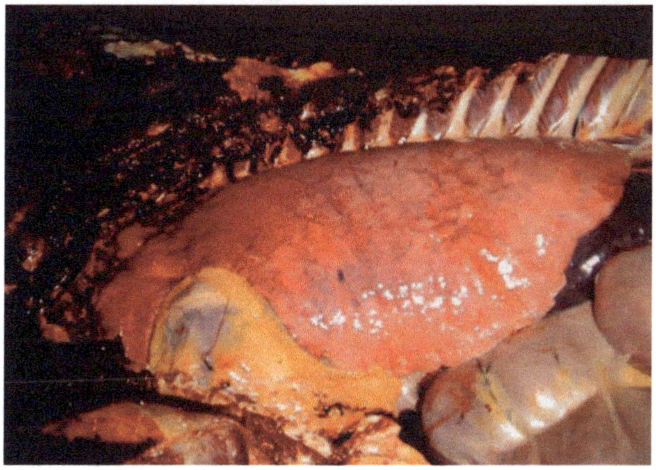

**Figure 4.37.** Horse. Lung. RAC. The lungs are not collapsed and have rib impressions.

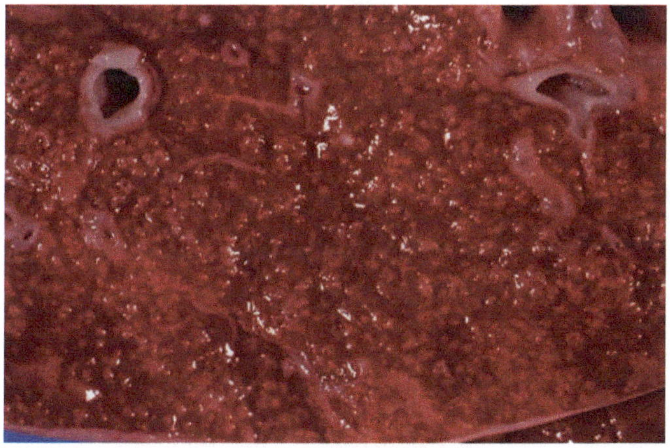

**Figure 4.38.** Horse. Lung. RAC. On cross section, the lungs show bubble-like elevations, suggesting peribronchiolitis, bronchiolitis, and accumulation of intrabronchiolar mucus and inflammatory cells.

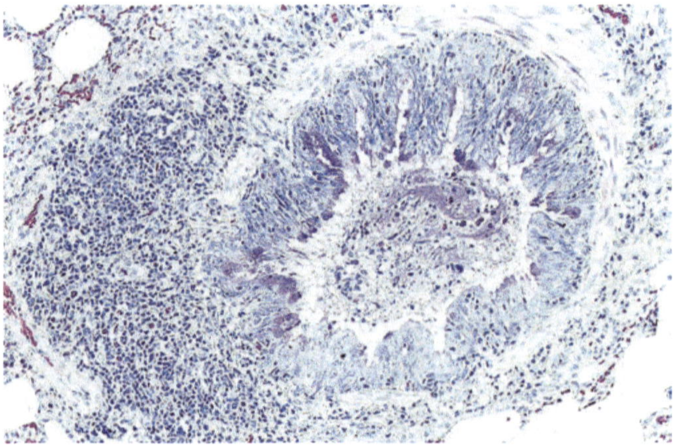

**Figure 4.39.** Horse. Lung. Mucoid Bronchiolitis. Intraluminal bronchiolar mucus with neutrophils and eosinophils. Severe peribronchiolar lymphocytic, plasmacytic, and eosinophilic infiltrations. (Giemsa)

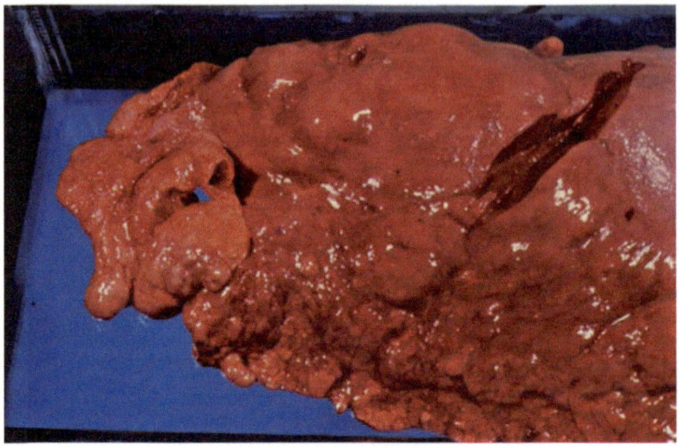

**Figure 4.40.** Horse. Lung. RAC. Rarely, the lung is excessively aerated representing marked, diffuse parenchymal emphysematous bulging (heaves).

*b. Exercise-induced pulmonary hemorrhage*

Commonly seen in horses under exercise and during racing, its pathogenesis is not fully understood. It has been proposed that veno-occlusive remodeling, particularly in the caudo-dorsal lung fields, leading to hemorrhage, fibrosis, and angiogenesis is a contributory factor. Mitral valve regurgitation leading to pulmonary venous hypertension is considered an alternative mechanism in exercise-induced pulmonary hemorrhage (EIPH). EIPH is one of the three major factors in acute epistaxis. The other two are ethmoid hematoma and guttural pouch mycosis.

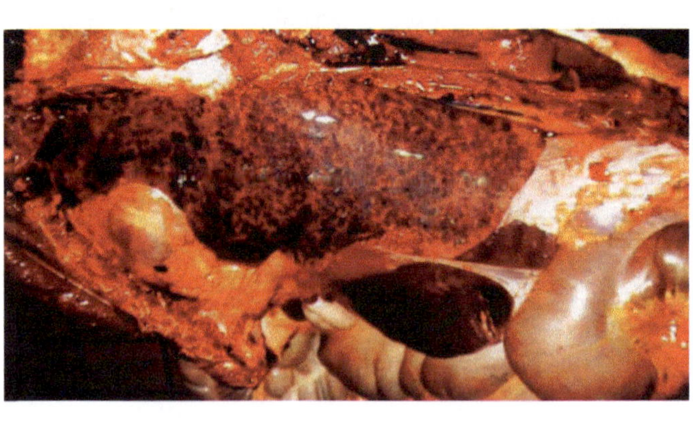

**Figure 4.41.** Horse. Thorax. EIPH. The lungs are uncollapsed and the caudodorsal lung areas are deeply reddened.

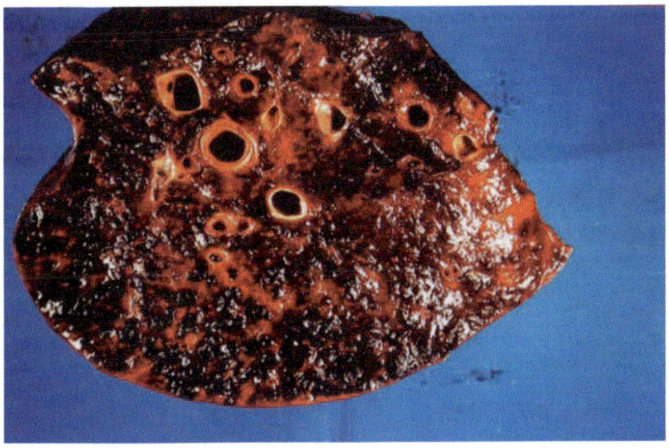

**Figure 4.42.** Horse. Lung. EIPH. The cross section of the lung field is red. Disseminated intravascular coagulopathy should be considered as a differential diagnosis.

*c. Pneumonias*

i. Aspiration

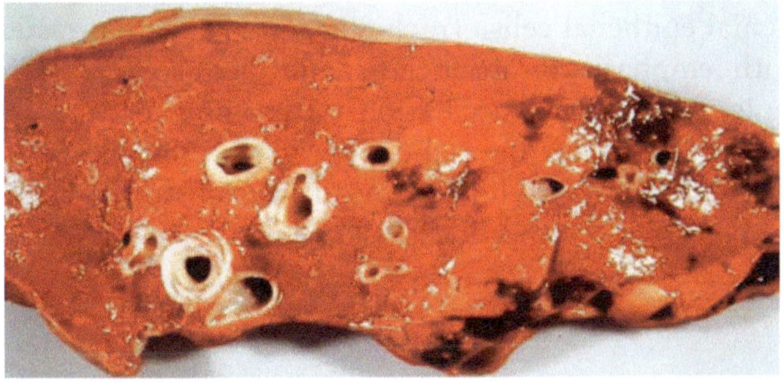

**Figure 4.43.** Horse. Lung. Aspiration Pneumonia. This horse was treated with mineral oil via gastric tube and aspirated some of the fluid. Discrete dark brown discoloration of several of the cranial lobules is present.

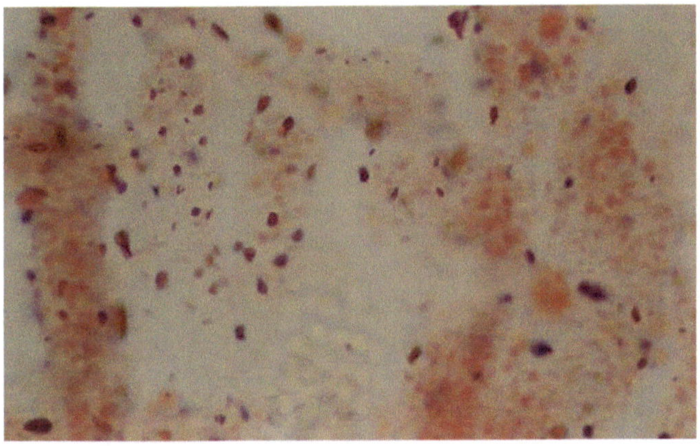

**Figure 4.44.** Horse. Lung. Mineral Oil Aspiration. Fat droplets can be demonstrated within alveoli. (Oil red O)

ii. Viral pneumonia. Disease examples are equine adenovirus infection, equine viral rhinopneumonitis (EVR), equine viral arteritis (EVA), equine influenza, African horse sickness, and equine morbillivirus (Hendra virus). EVR, EVA, and adenovirus infection are covered in Chapter 2, "Diseases of Foals and Juveniles." African horse sickness and Hendra virus are mentioned as exotic diseases in Appendix C.

## Equine influenza

Two subtypes of influenza virus are recognized in the horse: orthomyxovirus A/Equi-1 and orthomyxovirus A/Equi-2. The disease is a threat to the racing horse and breeding industries and generally associated with high morbidity and low mortality in adult horses and complicated by secondary bacterial infection. Foals and pregnant mares are particularly susceptible to the influenza virus. Neonatal loss and dystocia are complications in term pregnant mares. Influenza virus replicates within the respiratory epithelial cells causing necrosis of tracheal and bronchial epithelial cells. Tracheitis and broncho-interstitial pneumonia with emphasis on bronchitis and peribronchitis are typical histopathologic changes. Vaccination is recommended as prevention. Equine strain H3N8 has been shown to have jumped species with a current distribution in greyhounds and in various other canine breeds clustered in shelters or other locations.

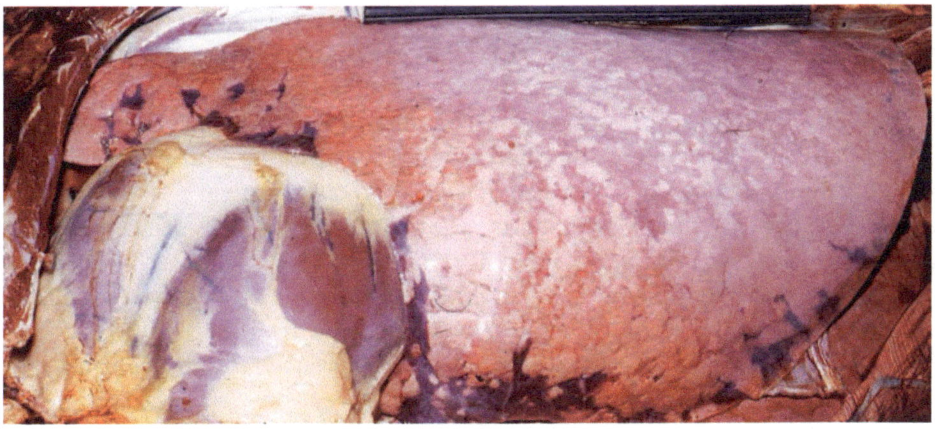

**Figure 4.45.** Horse. Lung. Influenza. There is evidence of several plum-colored foci in lobules concentrated in the cranioventral lung. (Courtesy Dr. T. Blunden, Animal Health Trust, UK.)

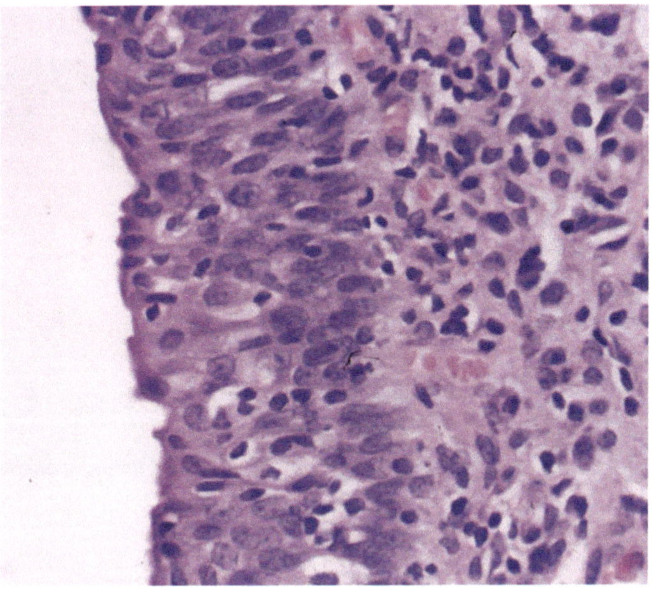

**Figure 4.46.** Horse. Trachea. Influenza. Microscopic changes include a moderate infiltration of lymphocytes and occasional plasma cells in the epithelium and submucosa. (H&E) (Courtesy Dr. T. Blunden, Animal Health Trust, UK.)

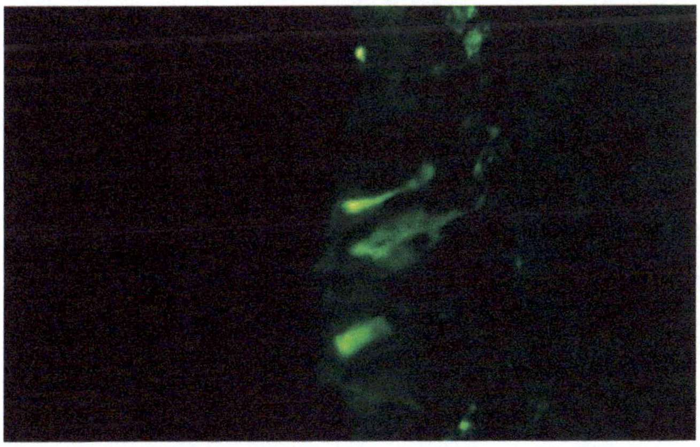

**Figure 4.47.** Horse. Trachea. Influenza. Distribution of viral antigen via fluorescence microscopy is demonstrated within the cytoplasm of the respiratory mucosa. (FA) (Courtesy Dr. T. Blunden, Animal Health Trust, UK.)

iii. Bacterial pneumonia. These are the most commonly occurring pneumonias in the adult horse. The causative bacteria are usually gram-positive, although gram-negative bacteria can be seen. Predisposing factors are transport (greater than 500 miles) and training and grouped together (aggregation) in restricted areas (racetrack barns; boarding barns). Surveys of larger numbers of horses with bacterial pneumonia identified *Streptococcus equi* subsp *zooepidemicus*, *Actinobacillus suis*-like bacteria, *Actinobacillus equuli*, Pasteurellaceae, and anaerobic cocci as common isolates. Most of the bacteria colonize the pharynx/tonsil as saprophytes. *Rhodococcus equi* is covered as an important pulmonary pathogen in Chapter 2, "Diseases of Foals and Juveniles." Gross patterns of pneumonias are diffuse, multifocal, locally extensive, cranioventral, and embolic. Portal of entry usually is aerogenous.

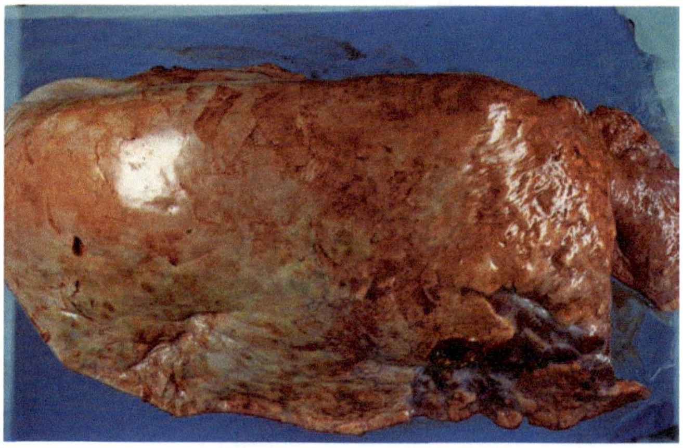

**Figure 4.48.** Horse. Lung. Cranioventral Pneumonia. There is evidence of brown consolidation of the cranial lung. *Aeromonas* sp. was isolated.

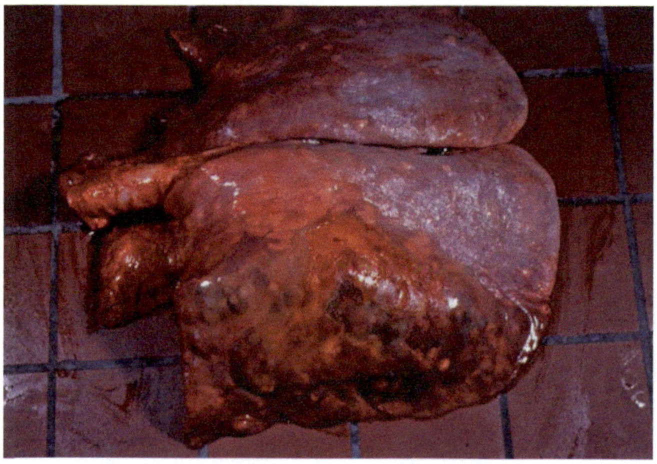

**Figure 4.49.** Horse. Lung. Multinodular Pneumonia. Multiple confluent nodules, fluctuating on touch, bulge the pleura. The pneumonia is representative of *Rhodococcus equi* infection.

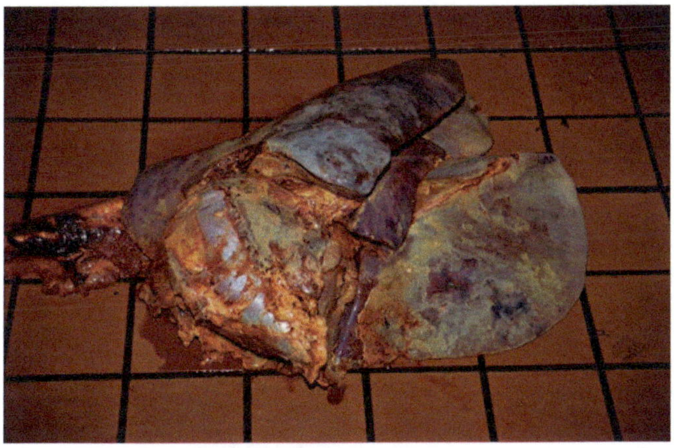

**Figure 4.50.** Horse. Lung. Cranioventral Pneumonia. This locally extensive, almost diffuse pneumonia resulted from *Steptococcus equi* subsp. *zooepidemicus*.

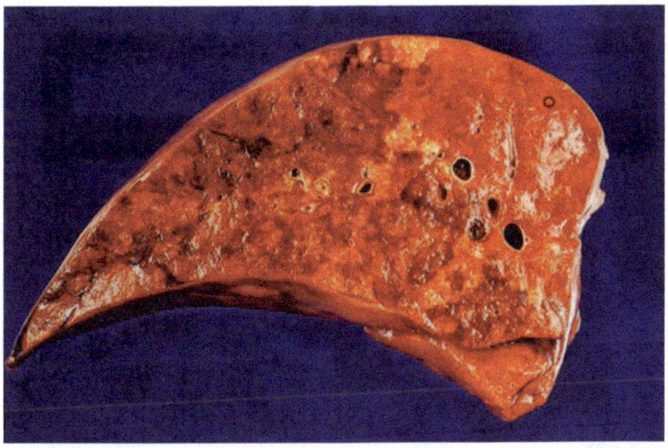

**Figure 4.51.** Horse. Lung. Necrohemorrhagic Pneumonia. Shipping Fever. The lung has a mottled, necrotizing, hemorrhagic pattern on cross section. *Pasteurella multocida* was isolated from the lung of this horse shipped over a long distance.

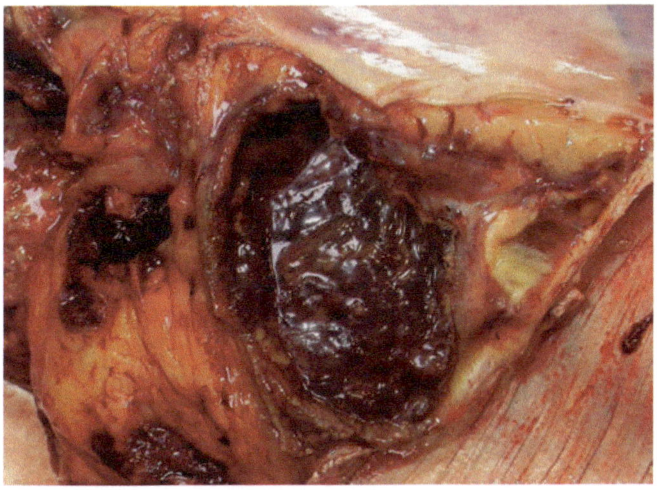

**Figure 4.52.** Horse. Lung. Cranioventral Necrosuppurative Pneumonia. On cross section a sequestrum is featured by a brown red exudate. *Pseudomonas aeruginosa*, *Streptococcus equi* subsp. *zooepidemicus*, and *Prevotella* sp. were identified.

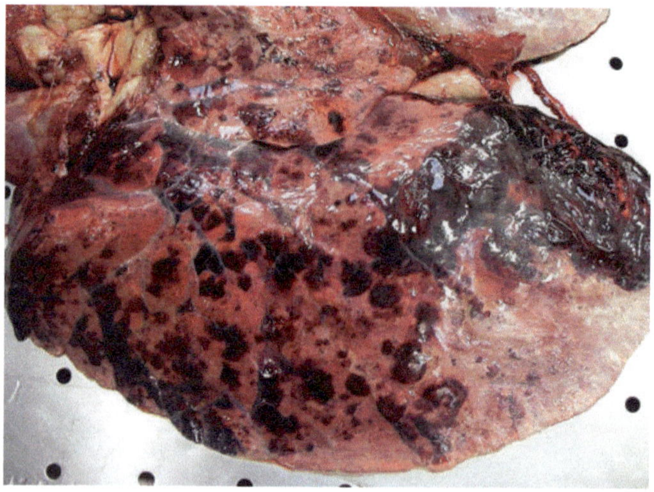

**Figure 4.53.** Horse. Lung. Multifocal Necrohemorrhagic Pneumonia and Diffuse Edema. *Salmonella enteric serovar Newport MDR-ampC* was isolated in this case.

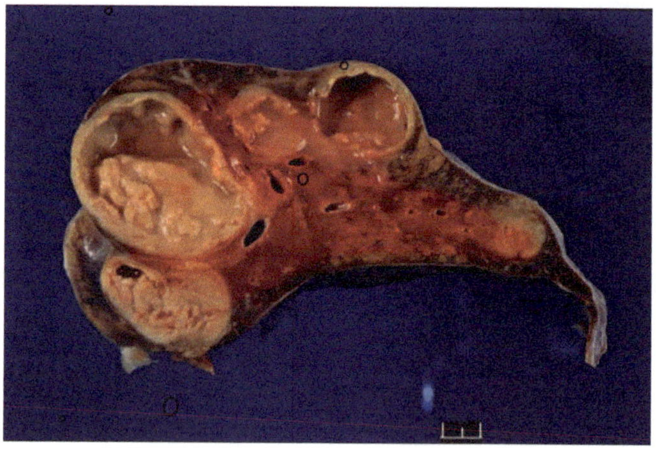

**Figure 4.54.** Horse. Lung. Multiple Abscesses. *Coccobacilli* sp. were cultured.

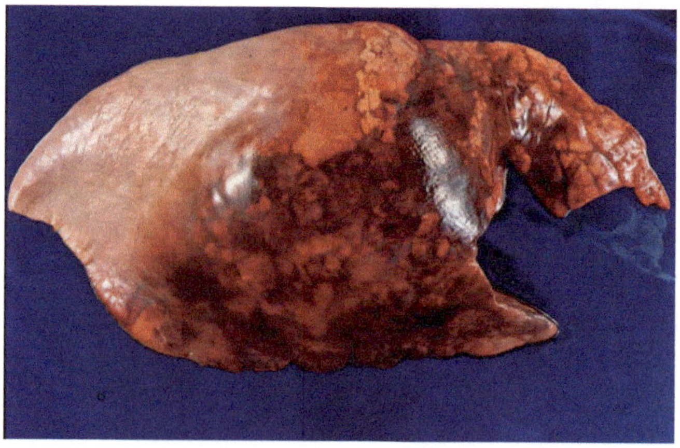

**Figure 4.55.** Horse. Lung. Cranioventral Necrohemorrhagic Pneumonia. Cause: hemolytic *Streptococci* sp.

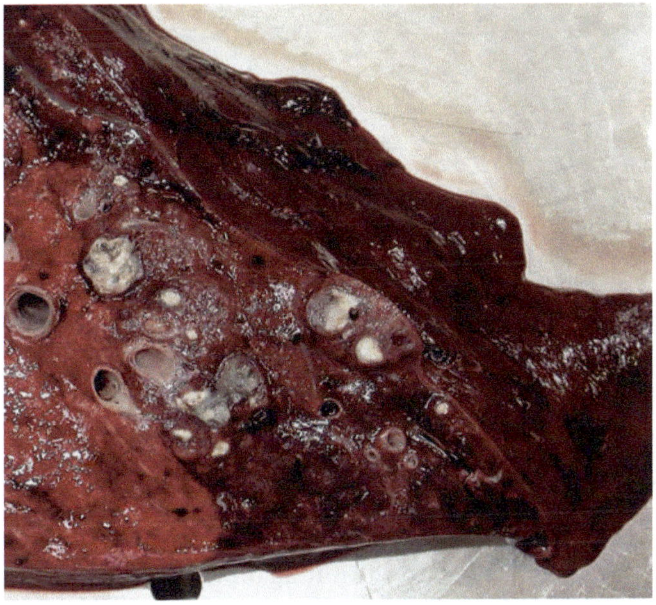

**Figure 4.56.** Lung. Cross section. Cranioventral Suppurative Bronchopneumonia. *Streptococcus equi* subsp. *zooepidemicus* was isolated.

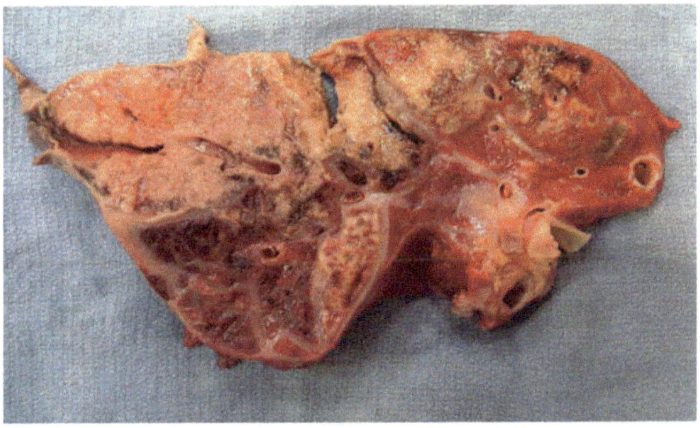

**Figure 4.57.** Horse. Lung. Locally Extensive Pneumonia. Marbled cross section. *Staphylococcus aureus* was isolated. (Courtesy Dr. J. Engiles, University of Pennsylvania.)

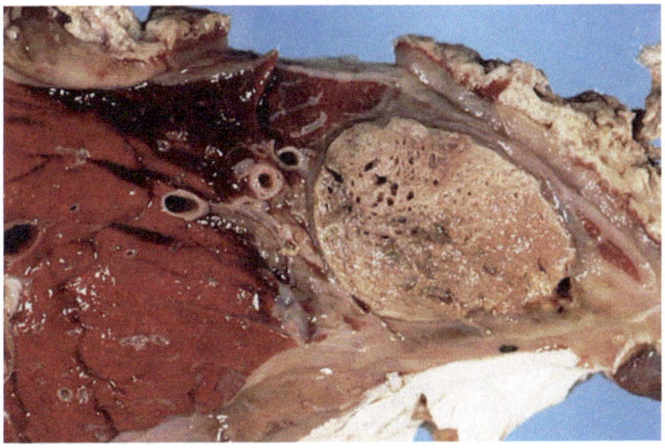

**Figure 4.58.** Horse. Lung. Pneumonia. Cross Section. Cranioventral Necrosuppurative Bronchopneumonia with Sequestrum and Fibrionous Pleuritis. *Streptococcus equi* subsp. *zooepidemicus* was identified.

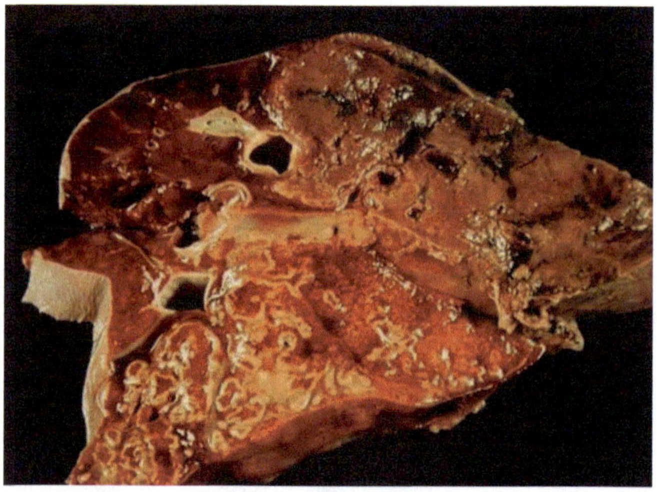

**Figure 4.59.** Horse. Lung. Locally Extensive Pneumonia. Multiple confluent areas of necrosuppurative bronchopneumonia occupy most of the lung. *Klebsiella pneumoniae* was isolated.

iv. Mycotic pneumonia. The pattern of fungal pneumonia by virtue of hematogenous spread is embolic. The most frequent recognized cause of mycotic pneumonia is pulmonary aspergillosis. Pulmonary histoplasmosis and cryptococcosis are rarer pathogens.

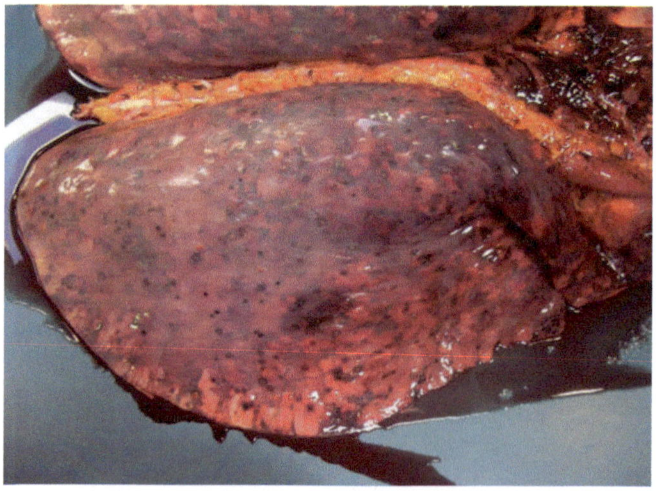

**Figure 4.60.** Horse. Lung. Multifocal Embolic Necrohemorrhagic Pneumonia. Angioinvasive *Aspergillus* fungi secondary to *Salmonella* typholocolitis. (Courtesy Dr. P. Habecker, University of Pennsylvania.)

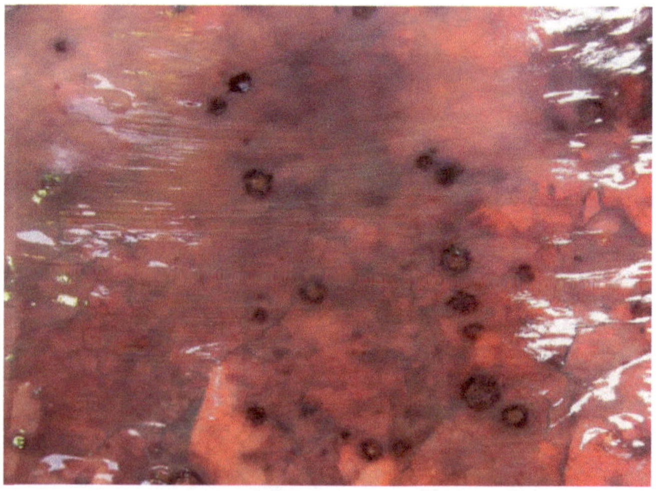

**Figure 4.61.** Horse. Lung. Surface. Necrohemorrhagic Embolic Mycotic Pneumonia. Small discrete red-gray foci suggest the presence of angioinvasive fungi. (Courtesy Dr. P. Habecker, University of Pennsylvania.)

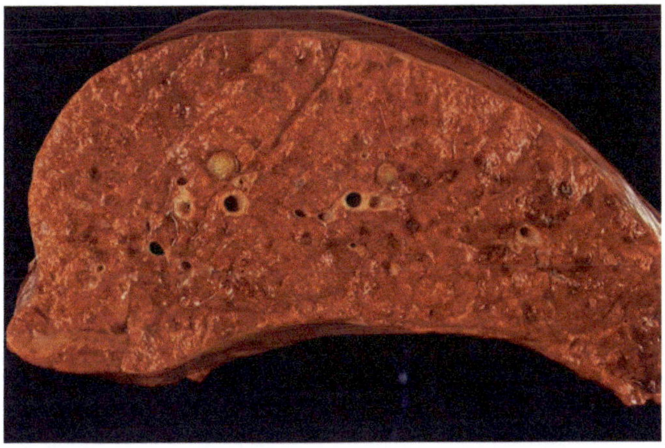

**Figure 4.62.** Horse. Lung. Angioinvasive Necrohemorrhagic Mycotic Pneumonia. Discrete yellow and red foci are disseminated on cross section.

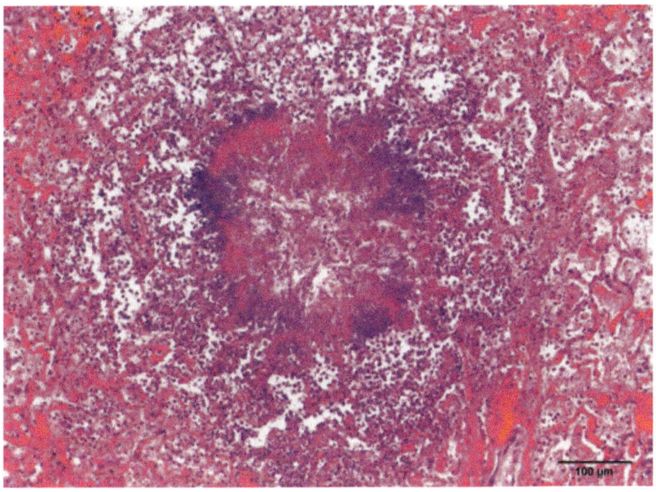

**Figure 4.63.** Horse. Lung. Mycotic Pneumonia. Angiocentric necrotizing and hemorrhagic pneumonia with *Aspergillus* sp. hyphae and capillary thrombosis. (H&E)

v. Parasitic pneumonia. The equine lungworm *Dictyocaulus arnfieldi* has a direct life cycle. Other forms of verminous pneumonia are due to migrating larvae of *Draschia* sp. or *Parascaris equorum*. *Halicephalobus gingivalis* larvae may also migrate through the lung.

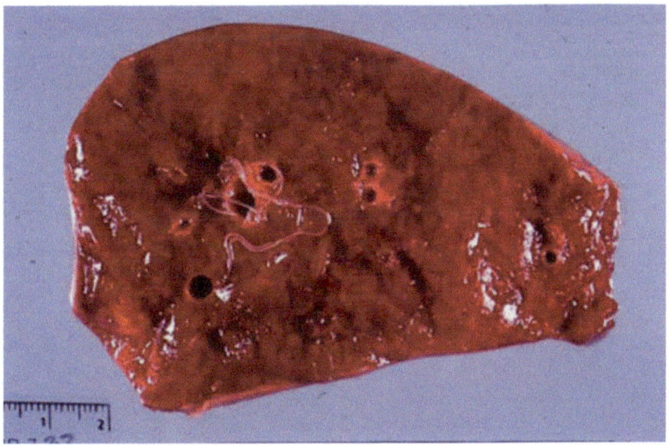

**Figure 4.64.** Horse. Lung. Verminous Pneumonia. *D. arnfieldi* adults are present in airways. (Courtesy Dr. J. Roberts, National Zoo, Washington, DC.)

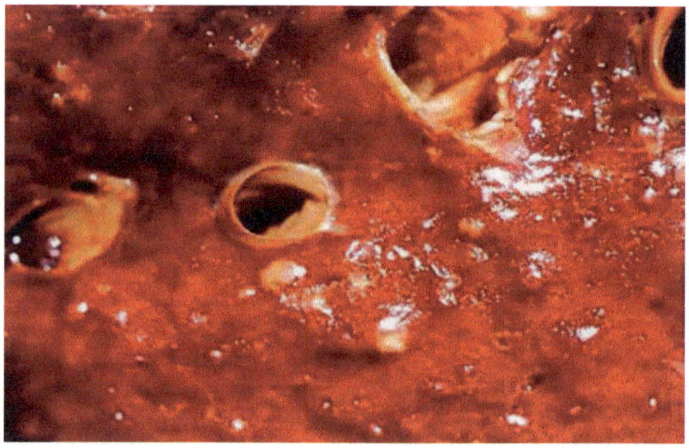

**Figure 4.65.** Horse. Lung. Verminous Pneumonia. The small yellow bulging nodules on cross section are the result of migrating endoparasitic larvae, in this case *Ascarid* larvae. Result of migrating *Ascarid* larvae.

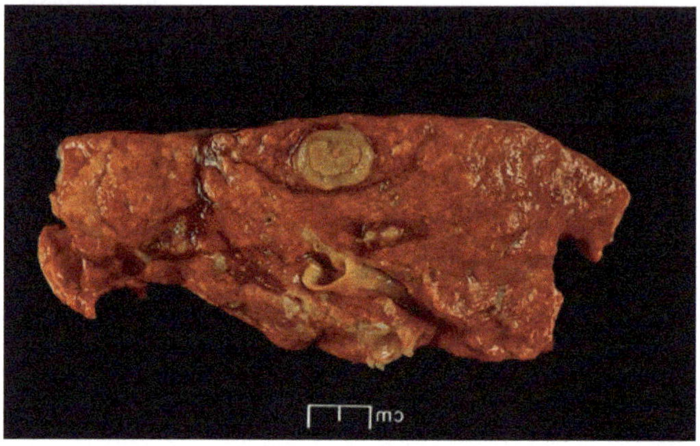

**Figure 4.66.** Horse. Lung. Verminous Pneumonia. Initiating migrating larvae may be *Ascarids, Habronema* sp., or *Halicephalobus gingivalis. Habronema* sp. was identified in this case.

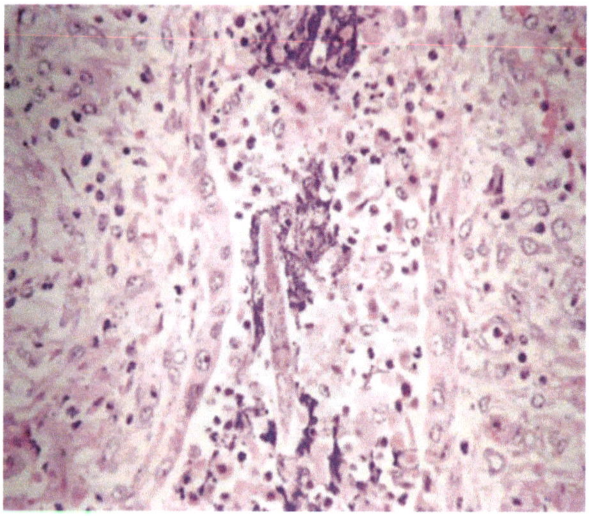

**Figure 4.67.** Horse. Lung. Verminous Pneumonia. *Halicephalobus gingivalis* larva is surrounded by epithelioid macrophages intermingled with lymphocytes. (H&E)

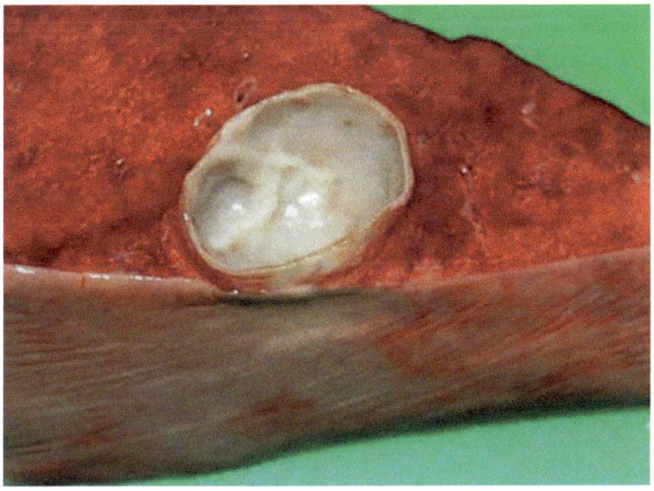

**Figure 4.68.** Horse. Lung. Hydatid Cyst. *Echinococcous granulosus*. These cysts can also be encountered in the liver.

## vi. Miscellaneous

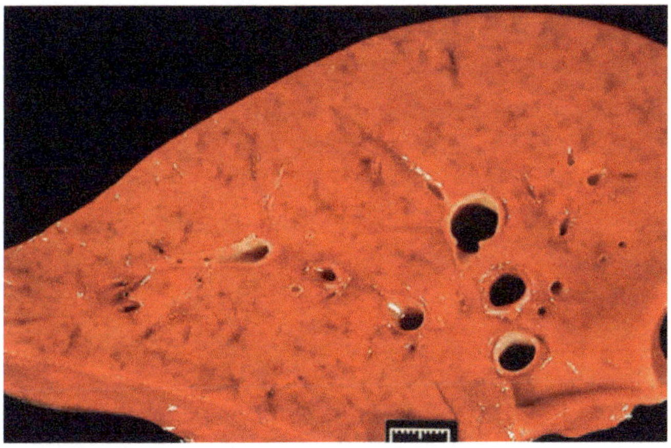

**Figure 4.69.** Horse. Lung. Pneumonia. *Pneumocystis jiroveci* formerly *carinii*. The lung on cross section is consolidated. The acute phase of this infection is characterized as a protein-rich exudative pneumonia. Differential diagnosis: pulmonary edema from vasculotropic EHV-1 infection (young adults), endotoxic shock, influenza. (Courtesy Dr. J. Edwards, Texas A&M University.)

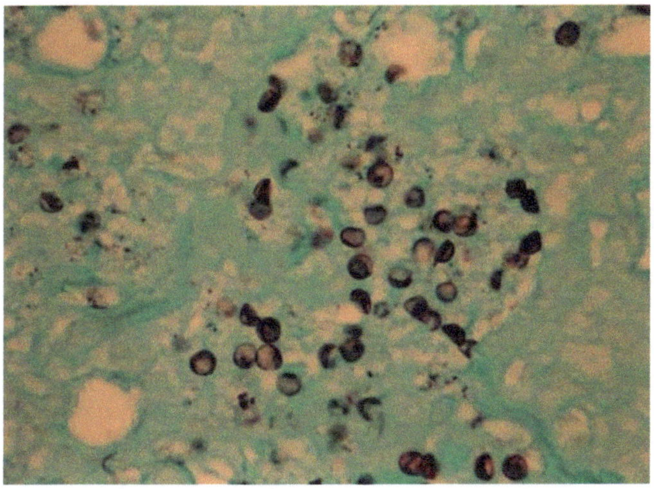

**Figure 4.70.** Horse. Lung. *Pneumocystis jiroveci* formerly *carinii*. A silver stain microscopically demonstrates small black oval structures within alveoli. (GMS)

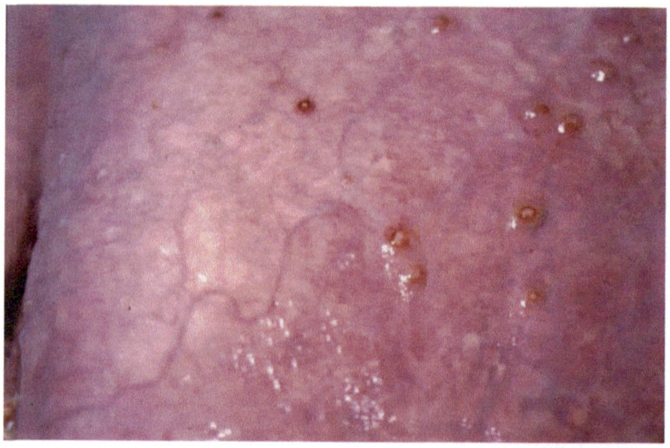

**Figure 4.71.** Horse. Lung. Sterile Granulomatosis. Also known as equine sarcoidosis, this granulomatous reaction on the visceral pleura is of uncertain etiology and should be considered as a differential diagnosis for mycotic pneumonia. Mycobacterial DNA has been sporadically identified by PCR in these lesions.

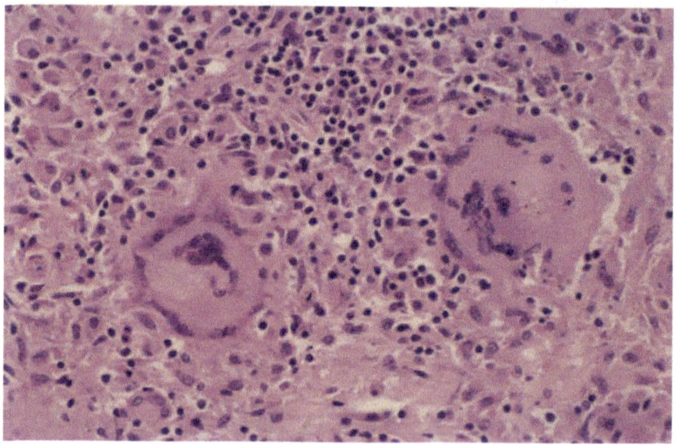

**Figure 4.72.** Horse. Lung. Sterile Granulomatosis. Microscopically, it is composed of epithelioid macrophages and multinucleate, inflammatory giant cells. (H&E)

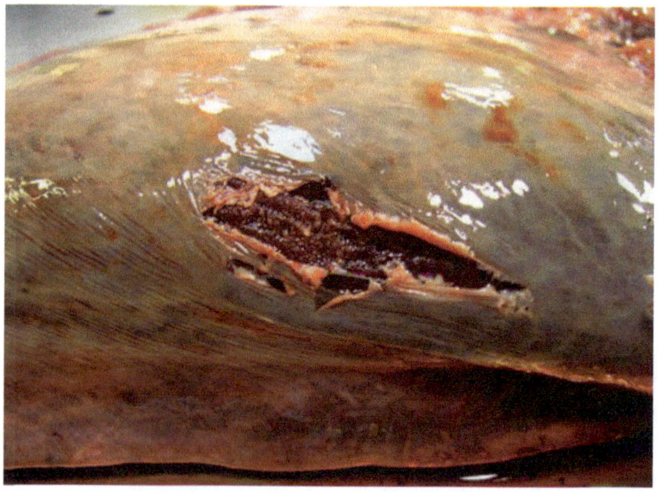

**Figure 4.73.** Horse. Lung. Puncture. Trauma. Superficial parenchymal laceration resulted in hemothorax.

## Equine multinodular pulmonary fibrosis

### Pathologic features

Equine multinodular pulmonary fibrosis (EMPF) is a newly recognized entity of interstitial pneumonia in horses thought to be associated with equine herpesvirus type 5 (EHV-5). The disorder when clinically diagnosed is mainly present in its chronic form. Chronic interstitial pneumonia is the end result of injury to the alveolar-interstitial unit of the lung with repair attempts by type II pneumocytes and alveolar fibrosis. The disease typically shows up in older horses.

### Gross findings

The entire lung fails to collapse upon removal from the thorax due to lack of air. The lung is diffusely firm, meaty, and liver-like on touch. It has a mottled tan to brown discoloration from loss of airspace. In the more advanced cases, the lungs reveal randomly interspersed distinct pale white-tan firm, bulging nodules of various dimension ranging from 1 to 10 cm in diameter. Typically the airways are not involved. There is very little normal lung parenchyma left in this disease process. Tracheobronchial lymph nodes are markedly enlarged.

### Microscopic findings

The terminal form is characterized by diffuse proliferation of type II pneumocytes rendering an adenomatoid pattern to the alveolar lining. Alveolar spaces are infiltrated by neutrophils. Alveolar macrophages are interspersed among the neutrophilic exudate and on occasion reveal distinct amphophilic intranuclear viral inclusion bodies (EHV-5). Alveoli are commonly replaced by collagen and increased elastic fibers. This connective tissue is the constituent of the grossly distinct bulging white firm nodules.

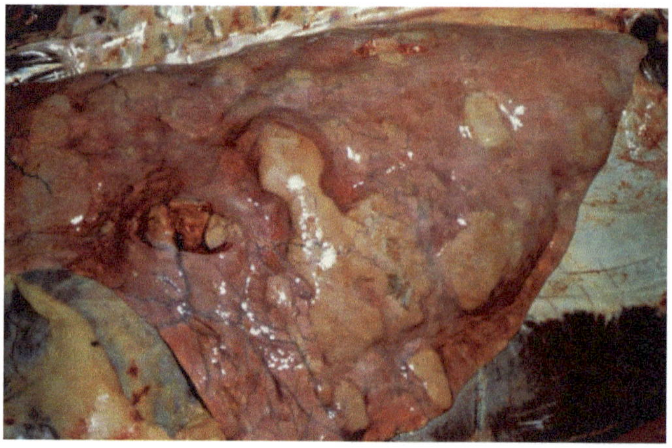

**Figure 4.74.** Horse. Lung. Equine Multinodular Pulmonary Fibrosis (EMPF). The lung has a mottled pattern; pink to tan foci alternate with nonaerated raised pale nodules.

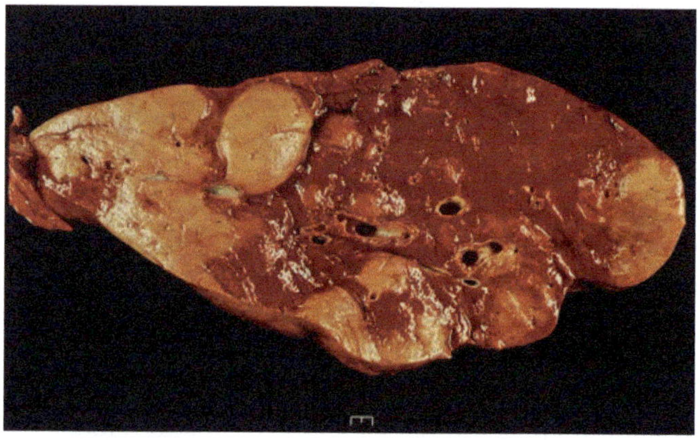

**Figure 4.75.** Horse. Lung. EMPF. On cross section the pulmonary parenchyma contains distinct tan bulging nodules and dark meaty zones, all nonaerated.

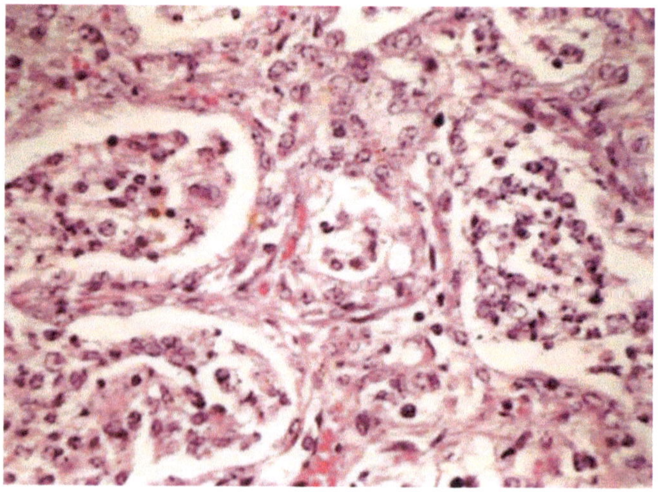

**Figure 4.76.** Horse. Lung. EMPF. Epithelization of alveolar lining characterizes the early chronic phase of interstitial pneumonia. The alveolar lumen contains neutrophils and macrophages. The interstitium contains lymphocytes, plasma cells, and some fibroblasts. (H&E)

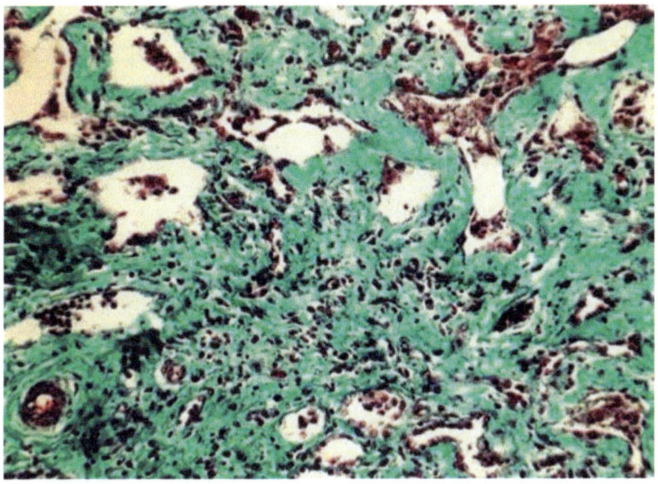

**Figure 4.77.** Horse. Lung. EMPF. Collagen has accumulated within the interstitial space to induce fibrosis. (Masson's trichrome)

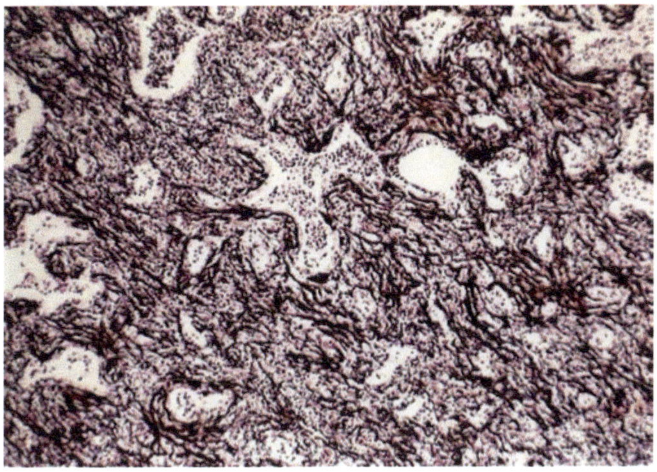

**Figure 4.78.** Horse. Lung. EMPF. Dense foci of elastic fibrils are within widened interstitial spaces. (Manuel's reticulin)

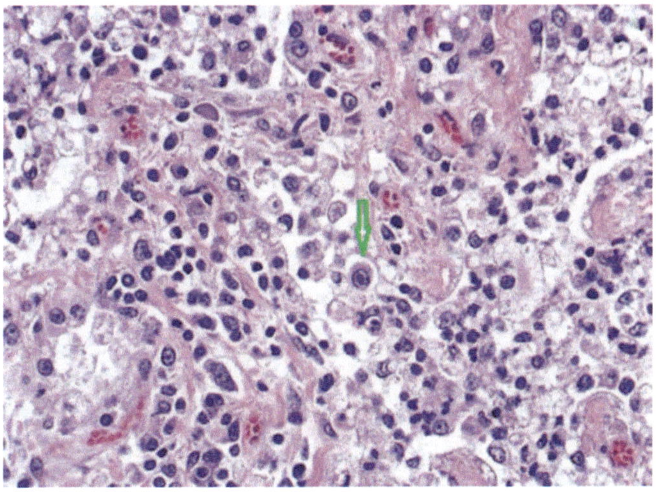

**Figure 4.79.** Horse. Lung. EMPF. The alveolar-interstitial unit has been replaced by type II pneumocytes, alveolar macrophages, plasma cells, and lymphocytes. Arrow denotes amphophilic intranuclear herpes viral inclusion body in alveolar macrophage (Fig.4.80). (H&E)

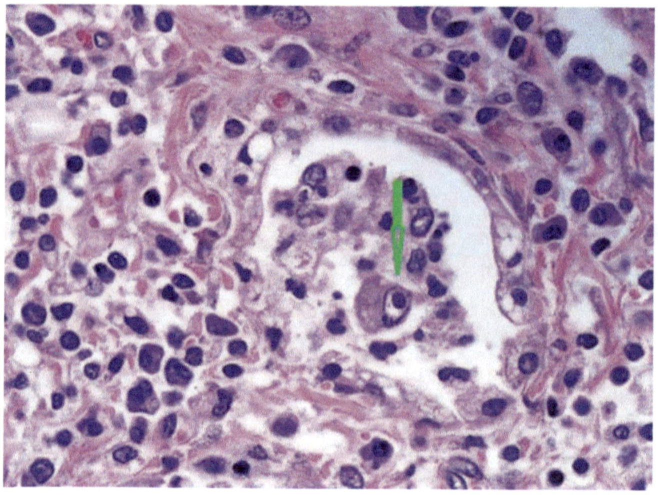

**Figure 4.80.** Horse. Lung. EMPF. Arrow denotes amphophilic intranuclear herpes viral inclusion body in alveolar macrophage. (H&E)

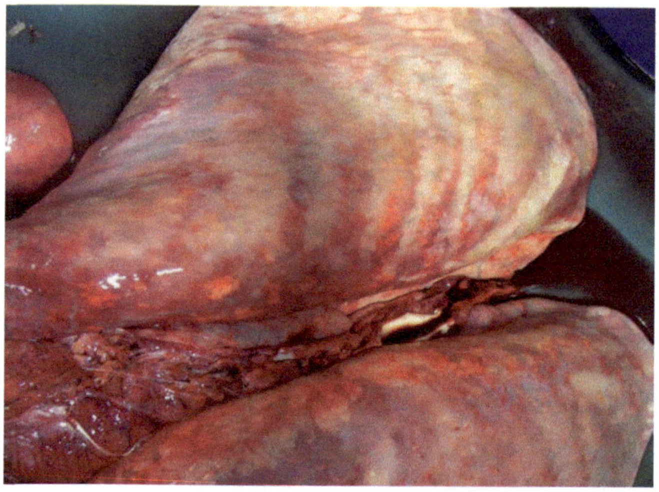

**Figure 4.81.** Horse. Lung. EMPF. In some cases of the disease, bulging nodules are absent and the gross pattern of consolidation is homogeneously diffuse.

## Equine multinodular pulmonary fibrosis – Fact sheet

**Definition:** Diffuse interstitial pneumonia of adult horses associated with equine herpesvirus type 5, a gamma herpesvirus

**Incidence:** Diagnosed in individual hoses in the United States, Canada, and Europe

### Gross findings

- Severe pneumonia with diffuse pattern or bulging fibrous nodules
- Enlarged tracheobronchial lymph nodes

### Microscopic findings

- Severe chronic interstitial pneumonia with fibrosing alveolitis and sporadic amphophilic intranuclear inclusion bodies in alveolar macrophages
- Reactive tracheobronchial lymphadenitis

### Differential diagnosis

- *Rhodococcus equi* interstitial pneumonia
- Silicate pneumoconiosis
- *Perilla mint* and *Crofton weed* pneumotoxicosis
- *Crotalaria* toxicosis (generally seen also as hepatic fibrosis)
- Exposure to high concentrations of oxygen (oxygen toxicosis)
- Primary and secondary pulmonary neoplasia

*d. Pulmonary neoplasia*

Primary lung tumors are rare in horses. If there is evidence of pulmonary neoplasia, metastases should be taken into consideration first and other primary sites looked for. Metastasizing hemangiosarcomas to the lung and pleura have been reported with some frequency. Other metastasizing tumors include carcinomas and lymphomas. Of primary pulmonary neoplasia two types have been described: adenocarcinoma and granular cell tumors.

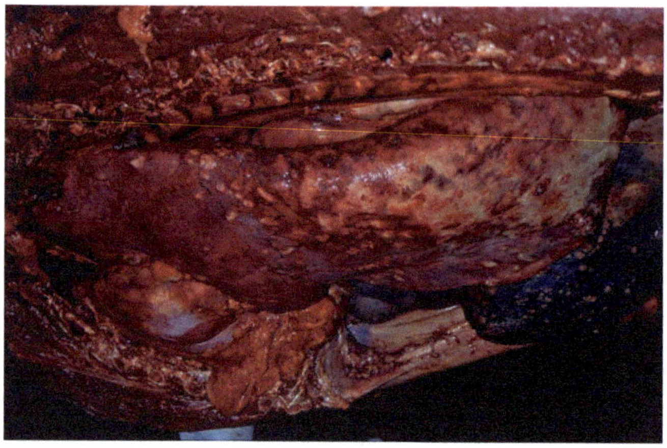

**Figure 4.82.** Horse. Lung. Primary Adenocarcinoma. A sharply delineated homogeneous tissue has replaced the marginal parts of the dorsal lung lobes. The tumor metastasized to the liver.

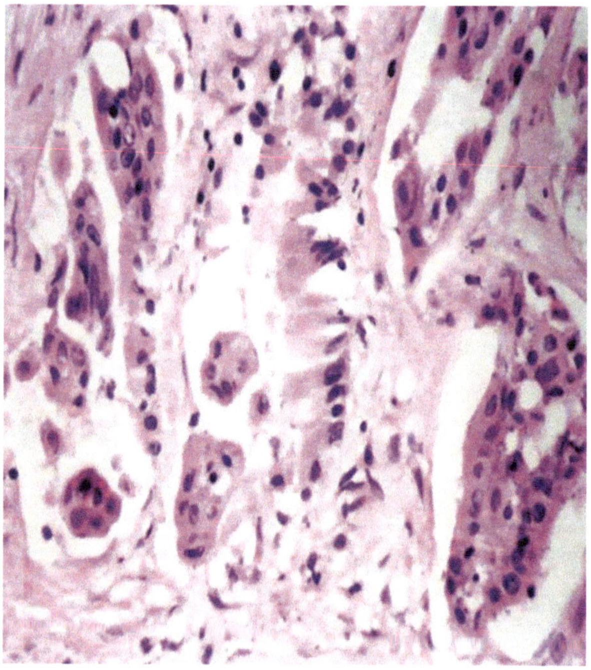

**Figure 4.83.** Horse. Lung. Primary Adenocarcinoma. Microscopic examination identified an adenocarcinoma with desmoplasia. Differential diagnosis: squamous cell carcinoma (mules). (H&E)

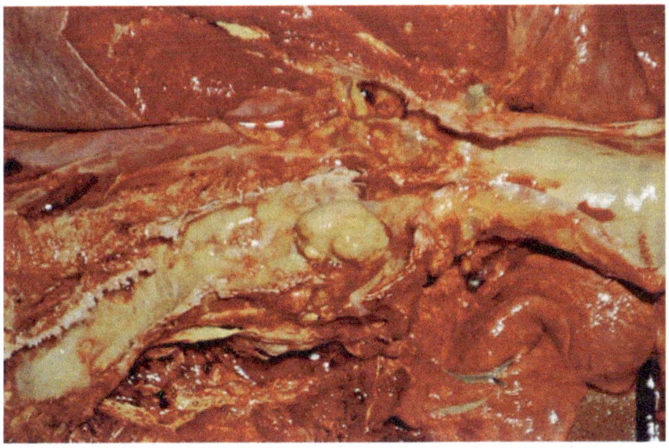

**Figure 4.84.** Horse. Lung. Granular Cell Tumor. A small yellow nodule is present close to the tracheal bifurcation, the typical location for this tumor in the horse. The tumor is of neural differentiation.

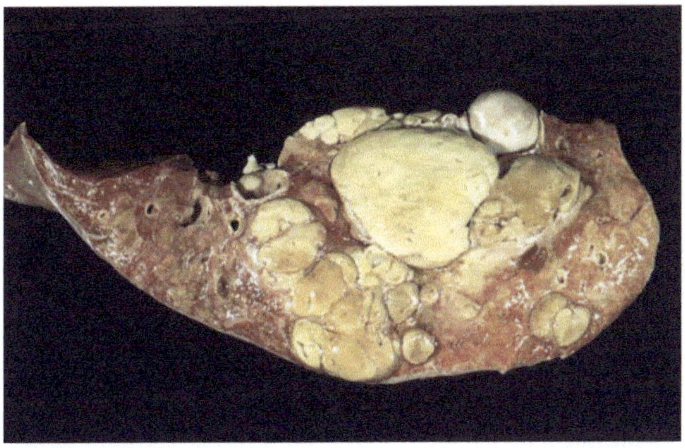

**Figure 4.85.** Horse. Lung. Granular Cell Tumor. Large, yellow nodules are present on cross section. (Courtesy Dr. P. Habecker, University of Pennsylvania.)

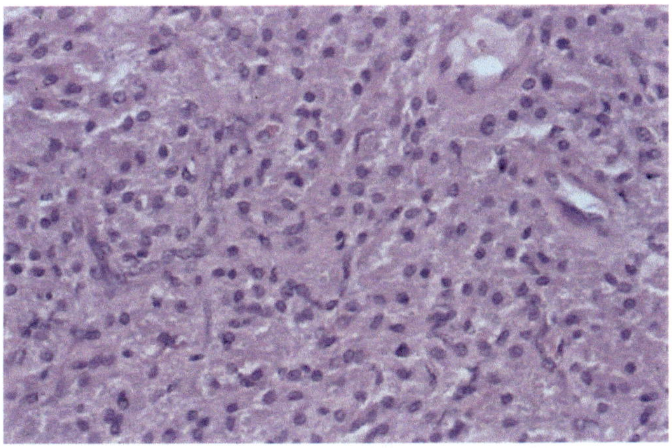

**Figure 4.86.** Horse. Lung. Granular Cell Tumor. Microscopic features of the neoplastic cells are a prominent eosinophilic, granular cytoplasm with peripheral hyperchromatic round nuclei. (H&E)

The cytoplasm of granular cell tumors stains positive with periodic acid-Schiff and is immunohistochemically positive for vimentin and S-100 suggesting neural crest, possibly Schwann cell origin.

### *e. Pleuritis*

Most cases are of bacterial etiology and may be secondary to a pneumonia or to a ruptured lung abscess. Pleuritis may be acute or chronic and unilateral or bilateral. Risk factors for pleuritis are strenuous exercise or long-distance transportation. It can also be associated with head restraint and lowering of the head interfering with the horse's capability to clear the trachea. Opportunistic oropharyngeal microbes contaminate the lower respiratory tract in these instances. Fibrinopurulent exudate accumulates in the thorax; with time, adhesions of the lung to the chest wall ensue. Among various bacterial isolates, *Mycoplasma felis* has been reported as a cause of pleuritis in the horse.

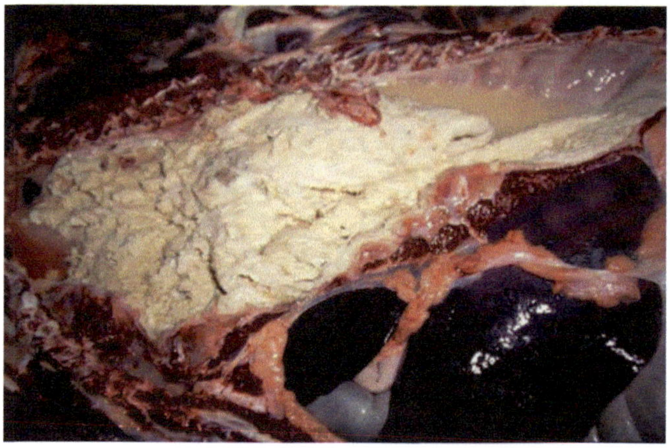

**Figure 4.87.** Horse. Thorax. Empyema from Ruptured Abscess. A diffuse, partially inspissated exudate accumulated in the thorax.

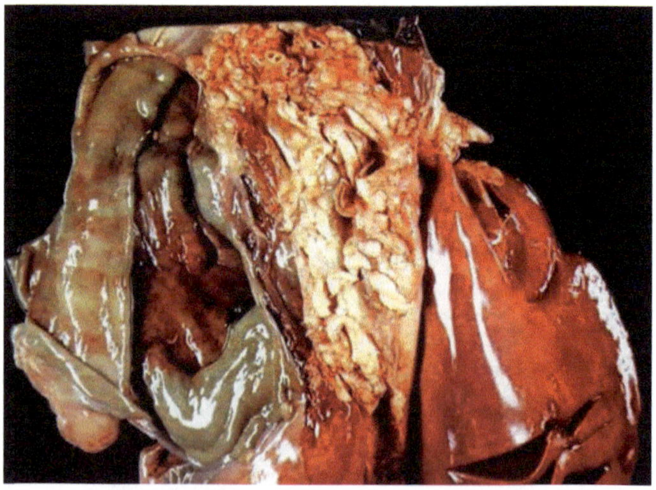

**Figure 4.88.** Horse. Thorax. Pleuropneumonia and Empyema. An underlying pulmonary abscess that ruptured can be responsible for thoracic empyema.

Pleural effusions of noninflammatory origin may result in hydrothorax or hemothorax.

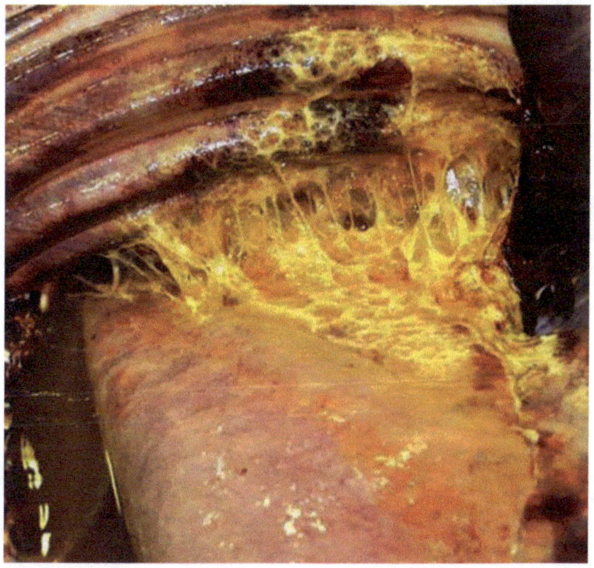

**Figure 4.89.** Horse. Thorax. Fibrinous Pleuritis. Sheets of thick fibrin adhere to the lung and parietal pleura. A large volume of straw-colored fluid poured from the thorax.

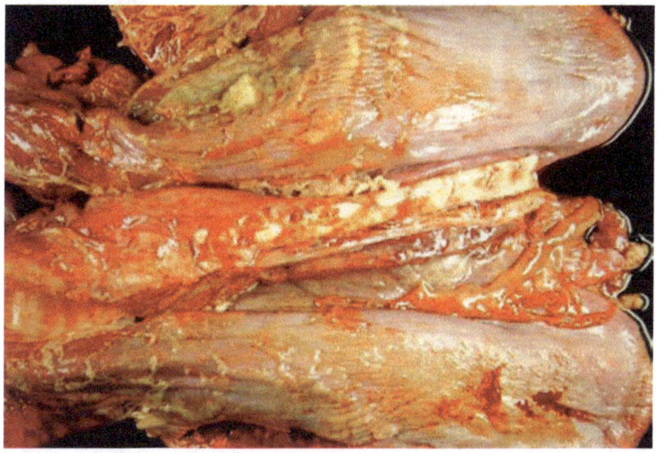

**Figure 4.90.** Horse. Thorax. Chronic Fibrous Pleuritis. The cranial portions of the lung are covered by fibrous tissue likely resulting in adhesions to the parietal pleura.

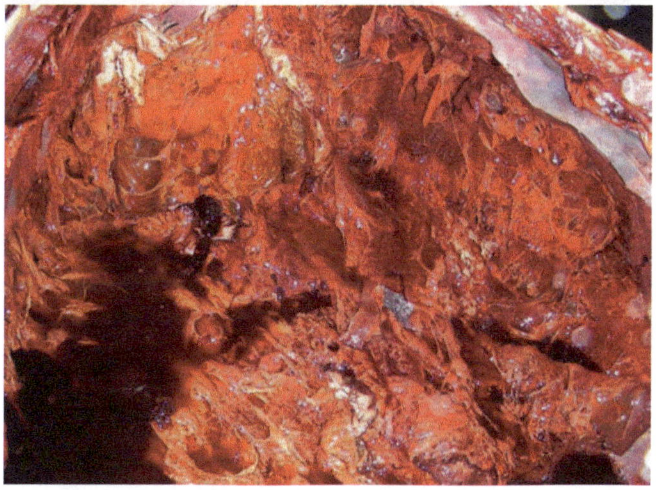

**Figure 4.91.** Horse. Thorax. Fibrinonecrotic Septic Pleuritis. Fractured ribs were the cause.

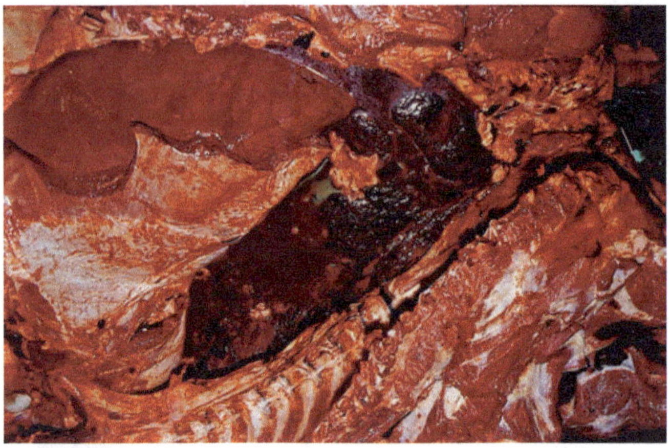

**Figure 4.92.** Horse. Thorax. Hemothorax. Ruptured major blood vessels (aortic aneurysms) are usual causes for hemothorax.

### *3. Diaphragmatic hernia*

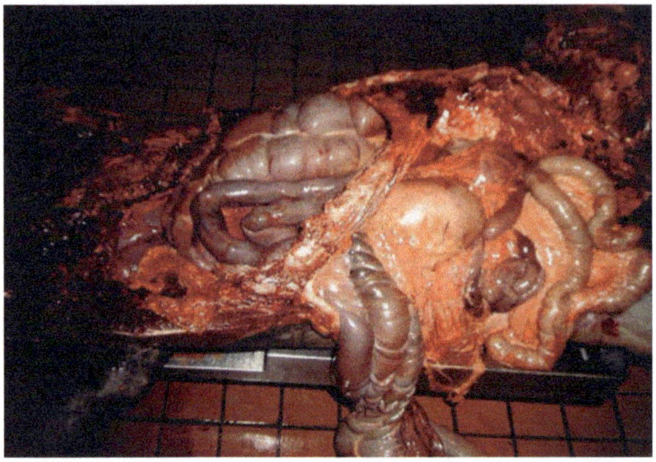

**Figure 4.93.** Horse. Thorax. Diaphragmatic Hernia. Loops of large colon and small intestine are found within the chest. Strenuous exercise, hard fall, or trauma from heavy objects may be preceding events. Postmortem diaphragmatic hernias may also occur in horses.

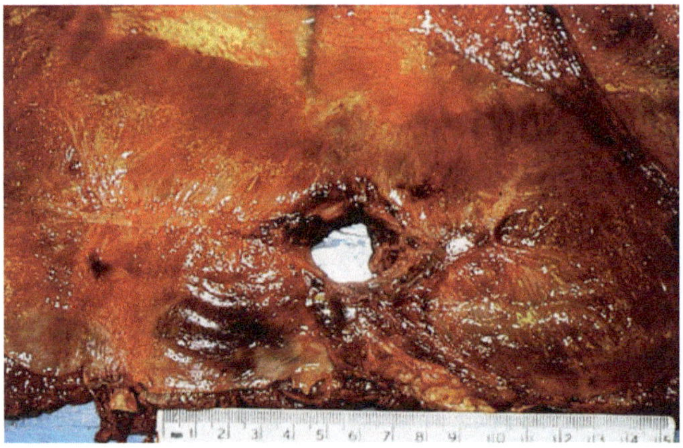

**Figure 4.94.** Horse. Diaphragmatic Hernia. An open ring in the diaphragm allows loops of intestine to penetrate the chest.

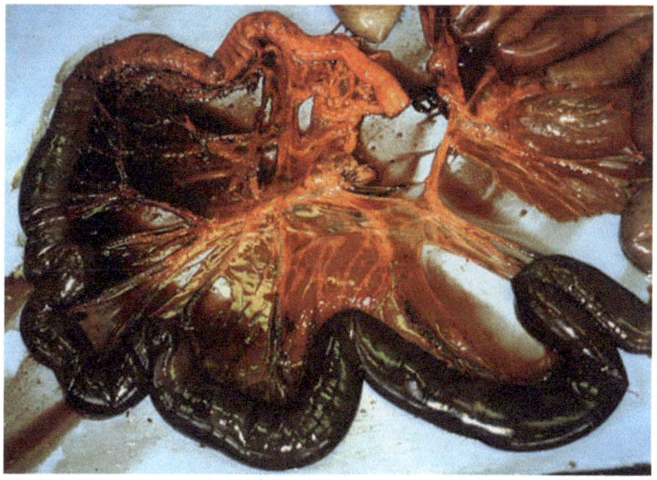

**Figure 4.95.** Horse. Diaphragmatic Hernia. Ischemic necrosis of the small intestinal loops after herniation.

### *4. Pleural mesothelioma*

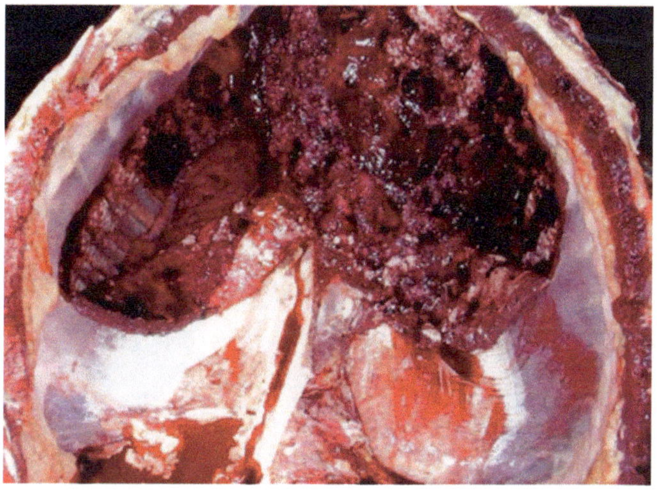

**Figure 4.96.** Horse. Thorax. Mesothelioma. A red confluent cauliflower-like growth is coating the parietal pleura.

## Selected references

Aitken MA, Parente EJA. 2011. Epiglottal abnormalities in mature nonracehorses: 23 cases (1990–2009). *J Am Vet Med Assoc* 238(12):1634–1638.

Barclay AJ, Paton DJ. 2000. Hendra (equine morbillivirus). *Vet J* 160(3):169–176.

Begg AP, Reece RJ, Hum S, Townsend W, Gordon A, Carrick J. 2011. Pathological changes in horses dying with equine influenza in Australia, 2007. *Aust Vet J* 89(Suppl 1):19–22.

Buergelt CD, Hines SA, Cantor G, et al. 1986. A retrospective study of proliferative interstitial lung disease of horses in Florida. *Vet Pathol* 23:750–756.

Hooper PT, Ketterer PJ, Hyatt AD, Russel GM. 1997. Lesions of experimental equine morbillivirus pneumonia in horses. *Vet Pathol* 34(4):312–322.

Niedermaier G, Poth T, Gehlen H. 2010. Clinical aspects of multinodular pulmonary fibrosis in two warmblood horses. *Vet Rec* 166:426–430.

Nobre D, Dagli ML, Haraguchi M. 1994. *Crotalaria junco* intoxication in horses. *Vet Hum Toxicol* 36:445–448.

Norman TE, Chaffin MK, Bisset WT, Thompson JA. 2012. Association of clinical signs with endoscopic findings in horses with nasopharyngeal cicatrix syndrome: 118 cases (2003–2008). *J Am Vet Med Assoc* 240(6):734–739.

Williams KJ, Maes R, Del Piero F, et al. 2007. Equine multinodular pulmonary fibrosis: a newly recognized herpesvirus-associated fibrotic lung disease. *Vet Pathol* 44:849–862.

Wong DM, Belgrave R, Williams KJ, et al. 2008. Equine multinodular fibrosis in five horses. *J Am Vet Med Assoc* 232:898–905.

# 5 Diseases of the Cardiovascular System

I. Heart
  1. Congenital cardiovascular anomalies
    a. Ventricular septal defect
    b. Common truncus arteriosus
    c. Patent ductus arteriosus
    d. Vascular ring anomaly and megaesophagus
  2. Pericardial diseases
  3. Myocardial diseases
    a. Necrosis/degeneration
    b. Myocarditis
  4. Endocardial disorders
    a. Fibrosis and mineralization
    b. Valvular fibrosis (endocardiosis)
    c. Valvular endocarditis
  5. Cardiomyopathy

II. Vessels
  1. Vasculitis
    a. Equine viral arteritis
    b. Purpura hemorrhagica
    c. Verminous endarteritis
    d. Parasitic nodules in ascending aorta
  2. Vascular thrombosis and injuries
    a. Aortic-iliac thrombosis
    b. Jugular vein thrombosis
    c. Carotid artery injection
    d. Aortic rupture
    e. Rupture of middle uterine artery
    f. Hemomelasma ilei
  3. Vascular neoplasia

*Color Atlas of Equine Pathology*, First Edition. Claus D. Buergelt and Fabio Del Piero.

The equine heart occupying the ventral middle mediastinal space extends between ribs 2 and 6. It is surrounded by a pericardium attached to the sternum. The weight of the heart depends on breed, sex, and age. Generally, it averages 0.6% of the total body weight (3.45 kg average heart weight) in horses without exercise training. It can reach 1.04% of body weight in horses under training and exercise. Small horses have relatively heavier hearts than large horses. The shape of the equine heart is that of a cone with the sharp apex formed by the left ventricle.

The equine heart, as in all mammals, has three physiologic features: (1) it is a pump supplying oxygenated blood to the dependent organs of the body and returning venous blood to the lungs for oxygenation; (2) it contains a conduction system associated with specialized cardiocytes receiving and supplying electrical stimuli; and (3) as an endocrine organ it contains hormone-producing cardiocytes to secrete a peptide hormone defined as atrial natriuretic factor.

A healthy heart is especially important for the equine athlete. Cardiac markers such a troponins are used for the clinical diagnosis of myocardial disease in the horse.

An orderly dissection of the heart is necessary to avoid mutilation of anatomic structures for the assessment of pathologic processes. Several techniques have been proposed. The method used at the University of Florida is described in Chapter 1.

## I. Heart

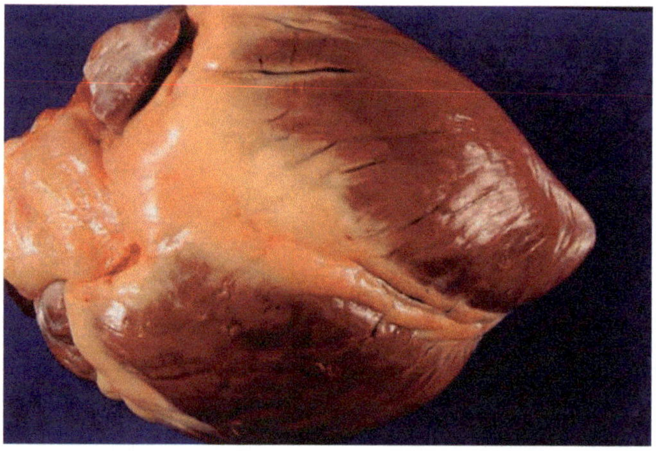

**Figure 5.1.** Horse. Normal Heart. The apex is exclusively formed by the left ventricle in the healthy equine heart.

### *1. Congenital cardiovascular anomalies*

In the horse, these anomalies have been reported as ventricular septal defect (VSD) and less frequently as atrial septal defect (ASD), patent ductus arteriosus (PDA), common truncus arteriosus, tetralogy of Fallot, vascular ring anomaly, complete transposition of greater vessels, and double-outlet right ventricle and tricuspid valve atresia.

*a. Ventricular septal defect*

VSD is the most frequently occurring single defect in the horse. It is usually a membranous defect high in the ventricle, but apical muscular defects can be encountered. A small VSD often remains unnoticed clinically, but in larger ones there may be evidence of pulmonary edema in the case of a left-to-right blood shunt due to overflooding of the lungs, or there may be cyanosis in the case of a shunt reversal from right to left. The right ventricle undergoes hypertrophy in the latter case. Animals with VSD range in age from neonates to 2 years.

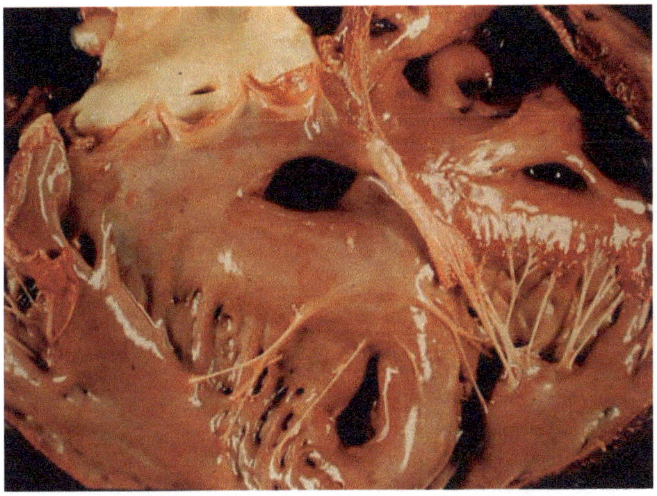

**Figure 5.2.** Horse. Heart. Ventricular Septal Defect. There is evidence of both a high ventricular and apical septal defect in this 2-month-old thoroughbred colt. (Reprinted with permission from Cambridge University Press.)

*b. Common truncus arteriosus*

This anomaly is defined as one major vessel leaving the ventricular part of the heart. The single vessel receives unoxygenated blood through a high ventricular ventricular defect. The condition leads to cyanosis.

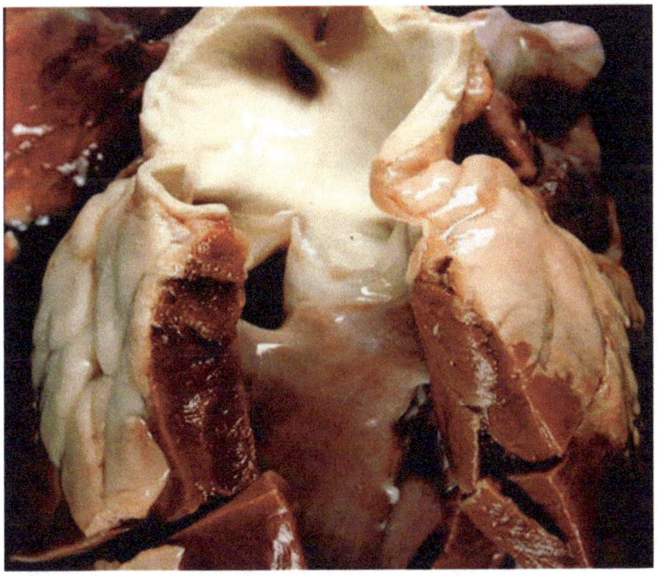

**Figure 5.3.** Horse. Heart. Common Truncus Arteriosus. One large vessel overriding a ventricular septal defect exits the heart. A high VSD is present.

*c. Patent ductus arteriosus*

The ductus arteriosus is a tubular muscular structure of the fetal circulation that connects the pulmonary trunk with the ascending aorta and allows blood to bypass the lungs. In the horse it closes physiologically within 3 days after birth to obliterate and to become the ligamentum arteriosum. There is usually a left-to-right shunting of blood with pulmonary circulatory overload. Pulmonary hypertension in long-standing cases may lead to shunt reversal, cyanosis, and aneurysm of the pulmonary artery as in this case.

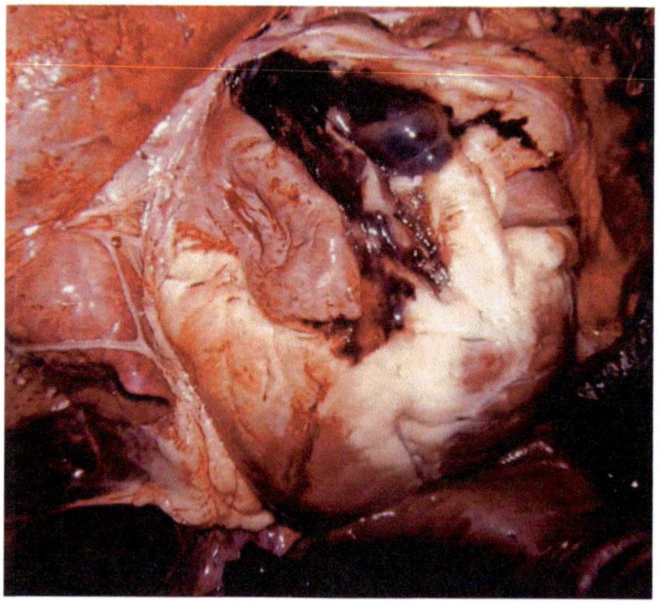

**Figure 5.4.** Horse. Heart. Major Vessels. Patent Ductus Arteriosus. An aneurysm of the pulmonary artery is indicated by the red discoloration of the wall.

*d. Vascular ring anomaly and megaesophagus*

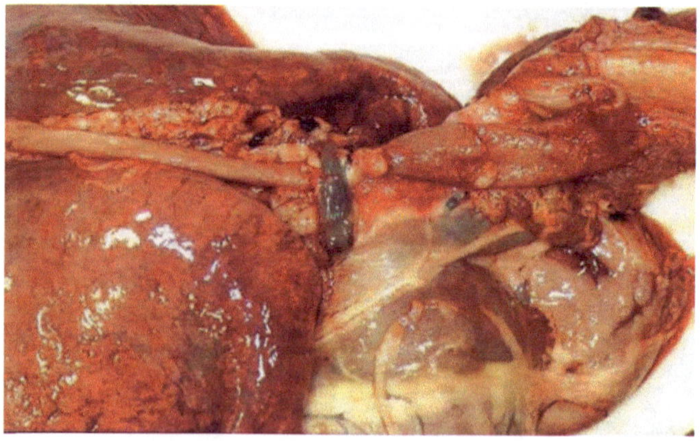

**Figure 5.5.** Horse. Vessel. Persistent Right Fourth Aortic Arch. A vascular ring over the esophagus has created a compression of the esophagus at that site with cranial distension of the esophagus creating a megaesophagus. (Courtesy Dr. J. Roberts, National Zoo, Washington, DC.)

## 2. Pericardial diseases

Two types of pericardial inflammatory processes are distinguished: effusive, often nonseptic, and fibrinous septic pericarditis. The cause of the effusive form is unknown; bacteria are frequently isolated from the fibrinous form. The principal bacterial isolates are *Actinobacillus* sp., *Streptococcus* sp., *Enterococcus* sp., and *Klebsiella pneumoniae*. Bacterial inflammation of the pericardium usually is hematogenous in origin as to the portal of entry. A special form of fibrinous pericarditis has been reported in adult horses in conjunction with the mare reproductive loss syndrome since its occurrence in 2001 (see Chapter 12, "Diseases of the Reproductive System").

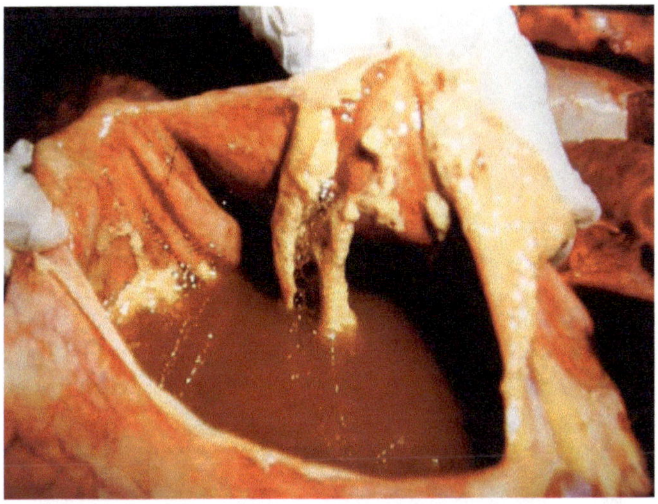

**Figure 5.6.** Horse. Heart. Septic Pericarditis. The severely distended pericardium is the result of the accumulation of a brown septic exudate. *Arcanobacterium pyogenes* was isolated in this case.

Hydropericardium and hemopericardium from cardiac tamponade or cardiac hemangiosarcoma are other types of fluid accumulation in the pericardium.

## 3. Myocardial diseases

Diseases of the myocardium can be divided into primarily degenerative and primarily inflammatory entities.

### a. Necrosis/degeneration

Nutritional or toxic factors need to be taken under consideration as etiology. Vitamin E/selenium deficiency is an example of a nutritional disorder. Ionophore antimicrobials (e.g., monensin, lasalocid), *Cassia occidentalis*, blister beetle cantharidin, oleander cardenolides (*Nerium oleander*), adonis cardenolides (*Adonis aestivalis*), and mycotoxins are etiologic examples for toxic cardiomyopathies.

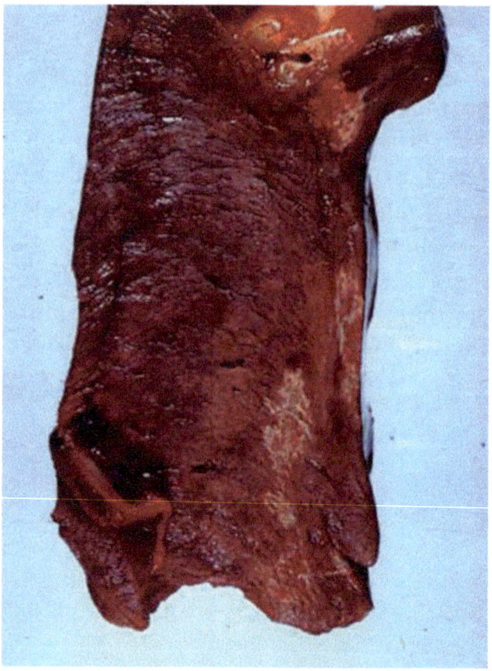

**Figure 5.7.** Horse. Heart. Myocardium. Necrosis. Blister Beetle. The gray foci in the myocardium represent myocyte necrosis. (Courtesy J. Roberts, National Zoo, Washington, DC.)

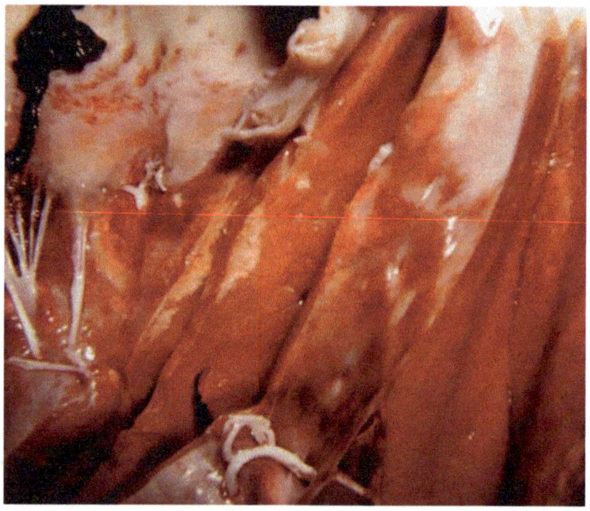

**Figure 5.8.** Horse. Heart. Myocardium. Vitamin E/Selenium Deficiency. This nutritional myopathy is rare in horses and usually affects foals. Patches of white foci are present in the myocardium of the left ventricle. (Reprinted with permission from Cambridge University Press.)

*b. Myocarditis*

Myocarditis is relatively rare in horses. Viruses such as the alphavirus of eastern equine encephalitis or equine infectious anemia, bacteria such as Streptococci, fungi such as *Aspergillus* sp. or nematodes such as *Halicephalobus gingivalis* are recognized etiologic causes for myocarditis.

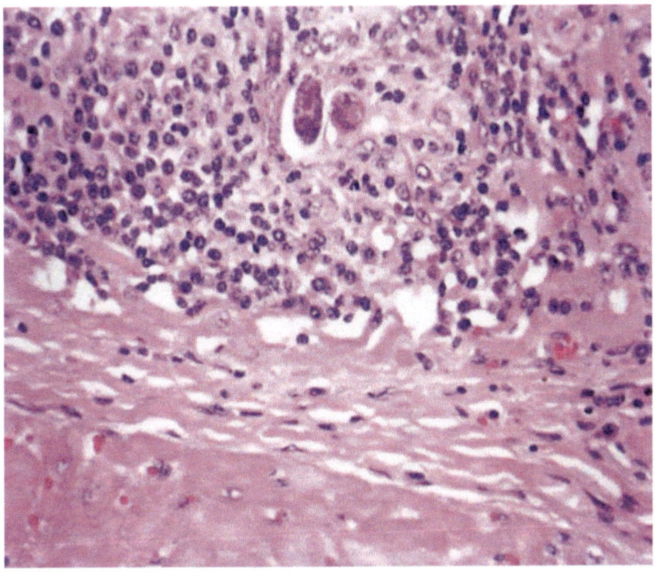

**Figure 5.9.** Horse. Heart. Parasitic Myocarditis. This horse had a granulomatous parasitic myocarditis due to *Halicephalobus gingivalis* as an incidental finding at necropsy. A few larvae are embedded within granulomatous inflammation. (H&E)

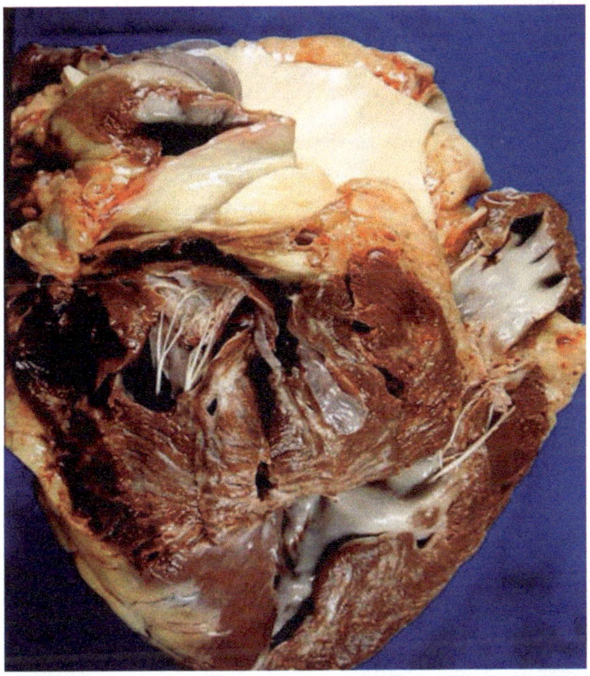

**Figure 5.10.** Horse. Heart. Myocardial Fibrosis. Very old horses develop myocardial fibrosis as end-stage lesions of previous inflammation or degeneration, replacing myocardium with collagen (myocardial scar). In this heart major areas of the myocardium have been replaced by gray streaks of collagen tissue.

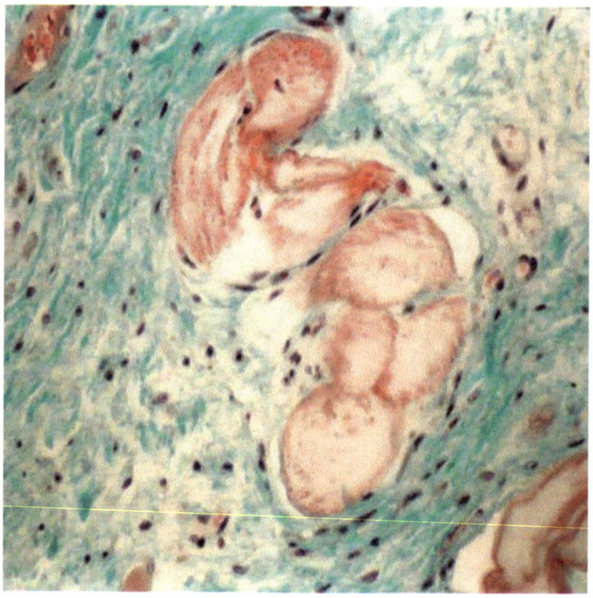

**Figure 5.11.** Horse. Heart. Myocardial Fibrosis. Dense layers of collagen have encircled Purkinje myocytes potentially interfering with the function of the conduction system. Such a change may result in sudden death of the animal. (Trichrome)

### *4. Endocardial disorders*

The endocardium as a thin membrane lines the ventricles, atria, and valves. It is susceptible to degenerative and inflammatory changes.

#### *a. Fibrosis and mineralization*

Focal endocardial fibrosis may be the result of blood regurgitation and circulatory disturbance due to valvular insufficiency. Endocardial fibroelastosis denotes diffuse thickening of the entire endocardium along ventricles. This may lead to congestive heart failure due to interfering with ventricular myocardial contraction. A few such cases have been reported in the horse.

Endocardial mineralization is metastatic as the result of pseudohypervitaminosis D from consumption of toxic plants such as *Cestrum diurnum*. Similar mineralization occurs in the intima of the aorta and in tendons and ligaments. It has to be differentiated from hypercalcemia as a paraneoplastic syndrome secondary to lymphoma.

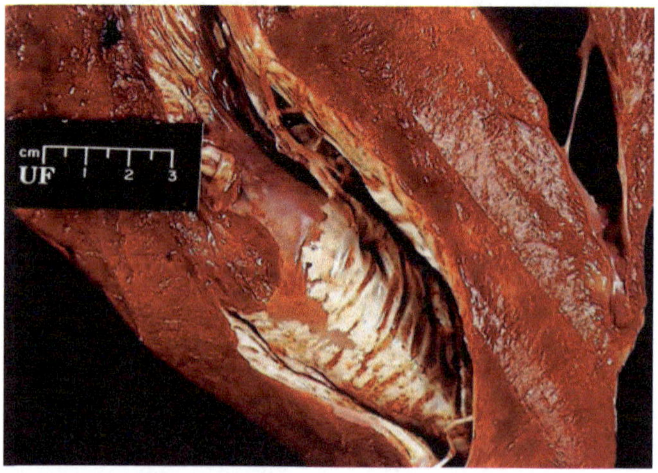


**Figure 5.12.** Horse. Heart. Endocardial Mineralization. White gritty streaks cover the apical endocardium in this case of *Cestrum diurnum* toxicity.

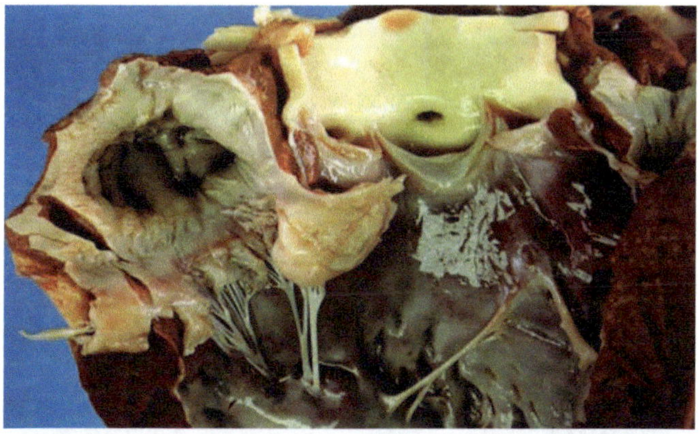

**Figure 5.13.** Horse. Heart. Endocardial Mineralization. Gritty plaques cover the endocardium of the left atrium in this case of *Cestrum diurnum* toxicity. Jet lesions from valvular fibrosis (endocardiosis) are another finding in this heart.

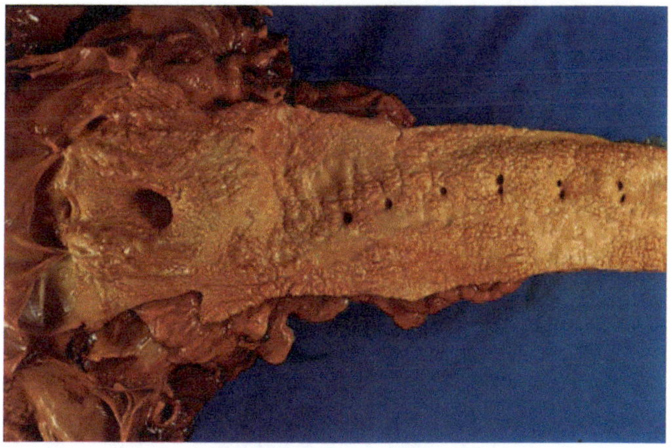

**Figure 5.14.** Horse. Aorta. Intimal Mineralization. The two segments have a streaky roughening of the intima. *Cestrum diurnum* toxicity.

*b. Valvular fibrosis (endocardiosis)*

The condition is characterized by thickening of the leaflets of the valves due to fibroblast proliferation and collagen deposition within the valvular matrix. The mitral valves are most commonly affected with the thickening being either diffuse or involving the free edge of the leaflet. The covering endothelium is spared by this process and remains smooth. Fibrous thickening of the chordae tendineae may occur simultaneously. It has been suggested that the valvular changes are the result of wear and tear, increased blood pressure, or both. Hemodynamic changes due to failure of valvular compliance rarely lead to congestive heart failure.

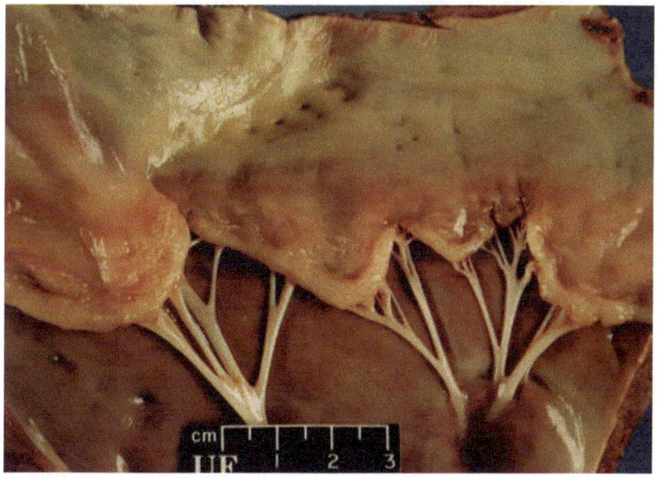


**Figure 5.15.** Horse. Heart. Mitral Valve Fibrosis (Endocardiosis). The thickening in this 25-year-old horse is diffuse with rounded edges of the opaque leaflets.

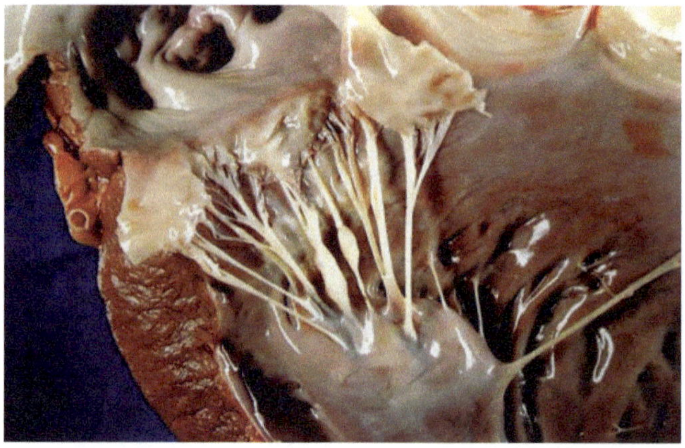

**Figure 5.16.** Horse. Heart. Mitral Valve Fibrosis (Endocardiosis).The valvular opaqueness is diffuse; chordae tendineae are nodularly thickened also. These may rupture from weakening at the insertion site to the papillary muscle. Chordal rupture is frequently overlooked at routine dissection of the heart.

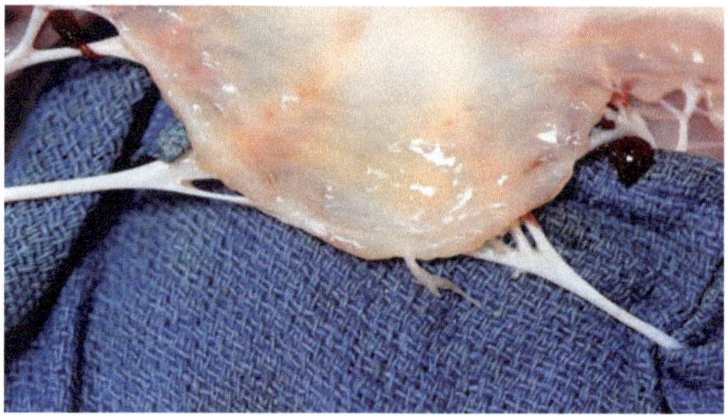

**Figure 5.17.** Horse. Heart. Mitral Valve. Rupture of Chorda Tendinea. Valvular fibrosis and edema are also present. Pulmonary edema is a fatal complication.

### *c. Valvular endocarditis*

Inflammation of the endocardium is either mural or valvular. Generally, valvular endocarditis is more frequent than mural endocarditis. The aortic valves are involved most frequently followed by the mitral valves. Bacteria isolated from valvular vegetations are both gram-positive and gram-negative.

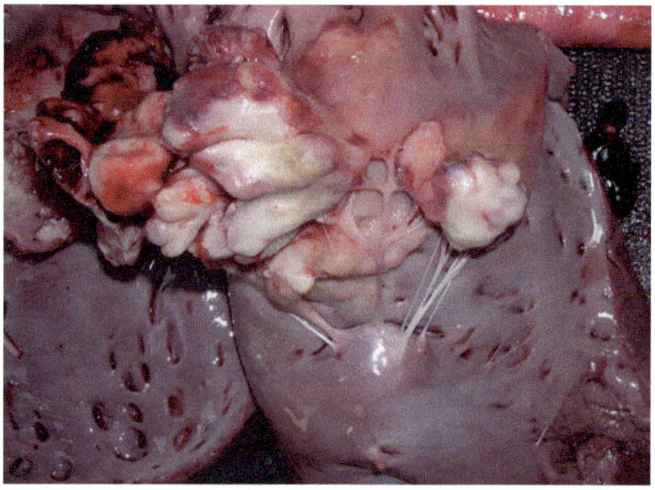

**Figure 5.18.** Horse. Heart. Tricuspid Valve. Valvular Endocarditis. Chronic. Differential diagnosis: neoplasia.

In earlier stages of the disease, the valvular lesions are cauliflower-like and of friable texture. Because of the friable texture of the vegetation, emboli may shower from the left heart valves to the kidneys or spleen where infarcts may develop. Septic emboli rarely shower through the coronary arterial ostia into the myocardium where small infarcts or myocarditis may occur. Emboli from the right heart valves would reach the lung and usually do not cause infarcts in the lung.

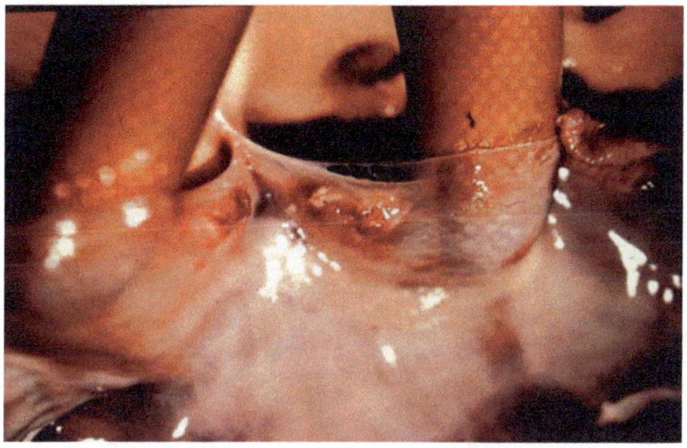

**Figure 5.19.** Horse. Heart. Aortic Semilunar Valves. Friction Rubs (Arantius, Bianchi, Morgagni nodules). Small nodules on the lateral edge of the cusps develop as a mirror image from rubbing against each other. They should not be confused with vegetations.

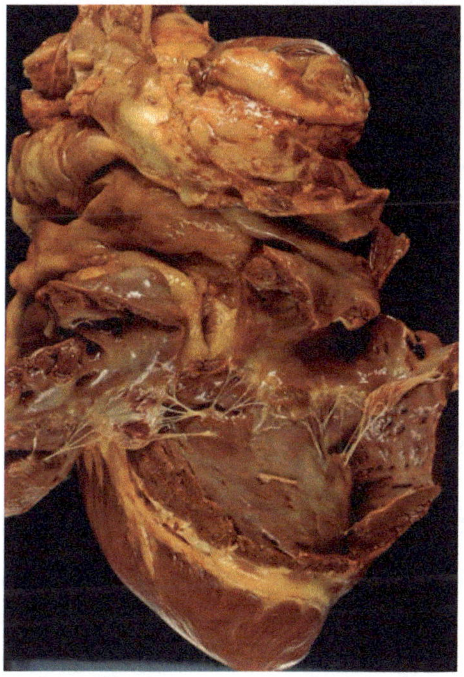

**Figure 5.20.** Horse. Heart. Lymphoma. Enlarged lymph nodes at the base of the heart are embedded in adipose tissue. The atrium is also involved.

### *5. Cardiomyopathy*

Cardiomyopathy is defined as heart muscle disease of unknown etiology. The condition results in cardiomegaly and heart failure. Three forms are distinguished: dilated (dilatative), hypertrophic, and restrictive. Cardiomyopathies have been well characterized in humans, dogs, and cats. The condition is rare in horses, and only individual equine cases have been described.

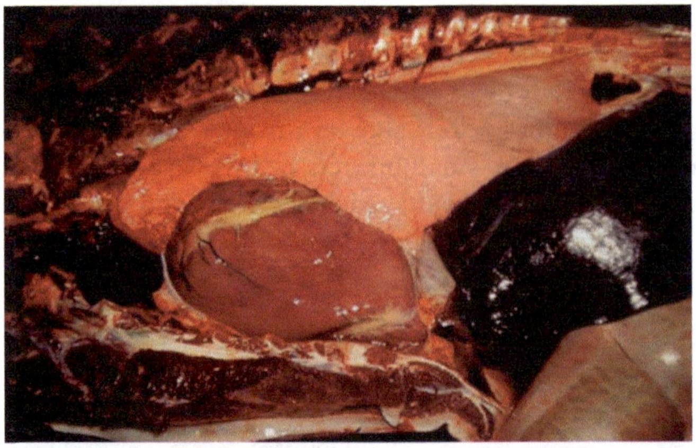

**Figure 5.21.** Horse. Thorax and Abdomen. Cardiomyopathy in Situ. The heart is enlarged and shows a thin-wall profile. The liver is enlarged and deep blue indicating venous congestion.

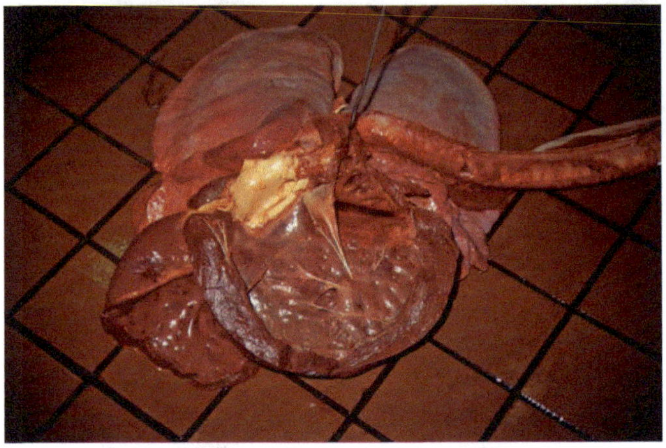

**Figure 5.22.** Horse. Heart. Dilated Cardiomyopathy. The opened left heart shows a thin wall and a flattened papillary muscle profile. Attached lungs show rib impressions suggesting pulmonary edema. (Reprinted with permission from Cambridge University Press.)

## II. Vessels

### *1. Vasculitis*

Vasculitis in horses is frequently associated with infectious agents such as viruses, bacteria, rickettsia, and endoparasites.

#### *a. Equine viral arteritis*

The disease is caused by an RNA virus belonging to the genus *Arterivirus* (family Arteriviridae). The virus is inhaled or transmitted during mating and colonizes leukocytes, some epithelia (lung, vesicular glands, adrenal cortex, renal tubular epithelium), vascular endothelium, and myocytes. It clinically results in widespread edema, especially of the subcutis. Pregnant mares may abort. Aborted fetuses usually do not harbor the virus or may not have serum antibodies. The virus causes fibrinoid necrosis and panvasculitis of small arteries, veins, and lymphatics. Interstitial pneumonia, renal tubular necrosis, inflammation of the male accessory sex glands, serositis with excess fluid accumulation in the subcutis, thorax, abdomen, and pericardium, and a papular sometimes ulcerative dermatitis are pathologic findings. Virus isolation, indirect immunohistochemistry, and polymerase chain reaction are used to diagnose the disease. Differential diagnoses include African horse sickness, equine infectious anemia, equine ehrlichiosis, purpura hemorrhagica, and pulmonary vasculotropic equine herpesvirus-1 infection in yearling horses.

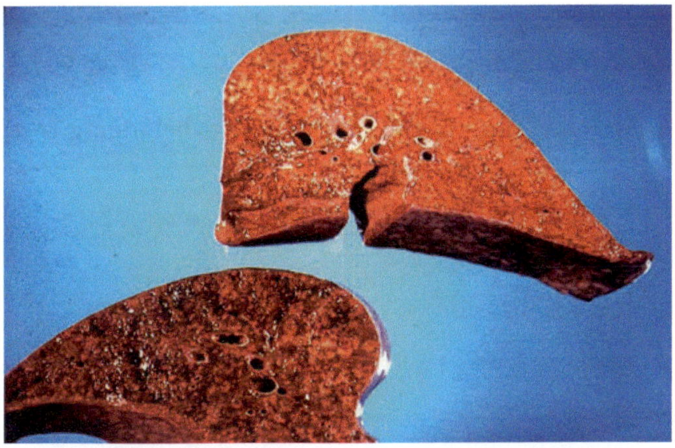

**Figure 5.23.** Horse. Lung. Viral Arteritis. Interstitial pneumonia. The cross section is firm and marbled.

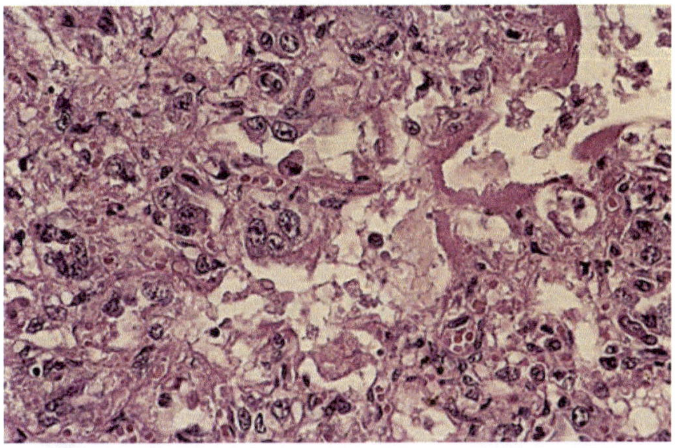

**Figure 5.24.** Horse. Lung. Viral Arteritis. Interstitial pneumonia. Type 2 pneumocyte proliferation and hyaline membranes are histologic features. (H&E)

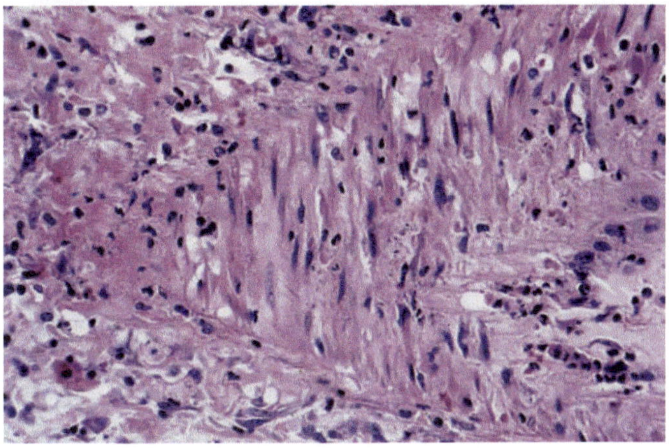

**Figure 5.25.** Horse. Lung. Viral Arteritis. Vasculitis. Lymphocytic vasculitis with lymphocyte and myocyte necrosis (tangential section). (H&E)

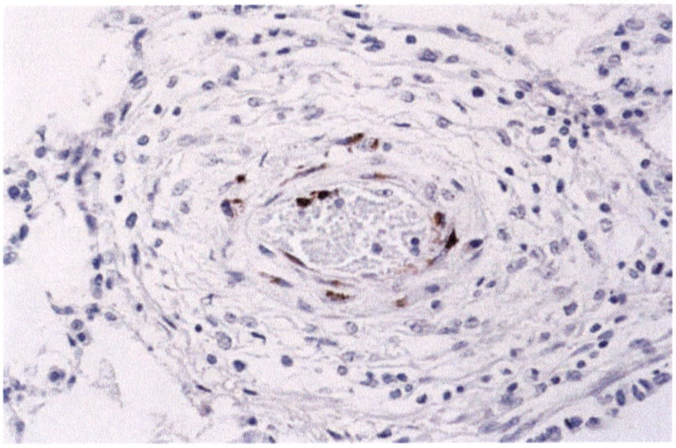

**Figure 5.26.** Horse. Lung. Viral Arteritis. Vasculitis and edema with intracytoplasmic EAV antigen within endothelium and tunical myocytes. (IHC)

## Equine viral arteritis – Fact sheet

Definition: Systemic disease caused by a virus belonging to the family of Arteriviridae.

### Transmission

- Inhalation/Aerosolization
- Sexual contact

### Pathogenesis

- Virus seeds to lung and bronchial lymph nodes
- Dissemination via infected monocytes

### Gross findings

- Diffuse subcutaneous edema
- Pleural and pericardial effusion
- Petechiae and ecchymoses in small intestine
- Interstitial pneumonia

### Microscopic findings

- Tunica media fibrinoid necrosis of small arteries, veins, lymphatics, and panvasculitis
- Pulmonary edema and interstitial pneumonia
- Edema and hemorrhage in intestine and lymphoid organs
- Renal tubular necrosis

### Diagnosis

- Virus isolation
- Serology via virus microneutralization
- Indirect immunohistochemistry (antemortem skin test and postmortem tissues)

### Differential diagnosis

- African Horse Sickness
- Purpura Hemorrhagica
- Equine Ehrlichiosis and Anaplasmosis, Equine Piroplasmosis, and Equine Infectious Anemia

### *b. Purpura hemorrhagica*

Equine purpura hemorrhagica is the result of an acute necrotizing vasculitis that causes subcutaneous edema in the distal limbs, ventrum, and head as well as subcutaneous and muscular petechiae. Details and images of the condition are presented in Chapter 15, "Diseases of the Hemolymphatic System."

### *c. Verminous endarteritis*

Resulting from migrating fourth-stage larvae of *Strongylus vulgaris,* severe obstructive thrombosis may occur associated with the wall of the cranial mesenteric root. Additional endarteritis and aneurysmal dilation of the vessel may ensue. Horses as young as 3 months may be affected. On occasion, larvae can be identified within the thrombi. Emboli from the nidus of thrombosis may shower through the ileocolic, cecal, and colonic arterial tributary to induce intestinal infarcts. Such events clinically lead to recurrent colic. The examination of the cranial mesenteric root was an integral part and mandatory procedure of the equine necropsy to rule out the presence of parasitic endarteritis during times when horses carried endoparasites.

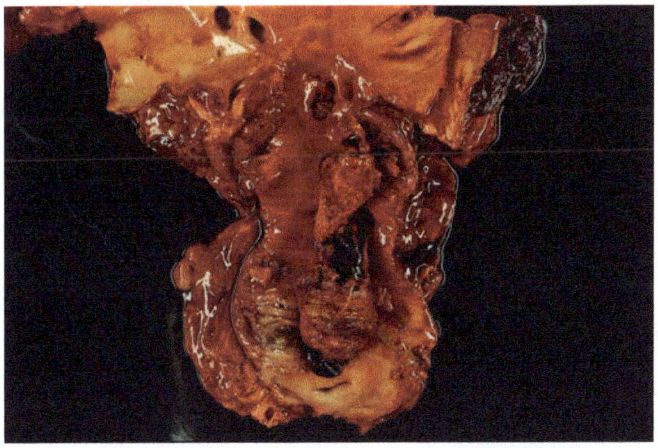

**Figure 5.27.** Horse. Cranial Mesenteric Root. Verminous Endarteritis. A large friable clot of fibrin and blood built up and occluded the mesenteric root. A *Strongylus vulgaris* larvae can be visible extending from clot into the lumen. On occasion, the inflamed, weakened, and dilated vascular wall may rupture to cause a fatal hemoabdomen.

### *d. Parasitic nodules in ascending aorta*

These typically are present as incidental findings in the intima of the ascending aorta usually above the semilunar valve cusps but sometimes within the cusp. The nodules are discrete, smooth, firm, and white as end-stage encapsulation to the presence of *Strongylus vulgaris* larvae that migrated up the abdominal and thoracic aorta into the ascending aorta where they died. The nodules have to be differentiated from chronic valvulitis.

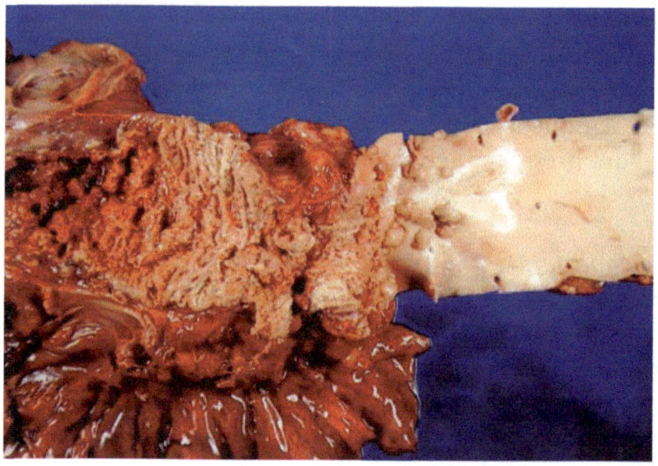

**Figure 5.28.** Horse. Aorta. Parasitic Nodules. The intima is seeded by several smooth nodules and by fibrin thrombi intermixed with hemorrhagic foci indicating a more active reaction to the presence of *Strongylus vulgaris* larvae. Larval migration beyond the ascending aorta is rare and rupture of granulomas may cause thrombosis of the carotid artery and brain infarcts.

## 2. Vascular thrombosis and injuries

### a. Aortic-iliac thrombosis

Sporadically seen in racing standardbred and thoroughbred horses, massive thrombi occlude the terminal aorta at the iliac bifurcation. Coldness of hind limbs and intermittent lameness may be associated clinical signs. It has been hypothesized that this condition may be a sequel to preceding *Strongylus vulgaris*–induced endarteritis of the cranial mesenteric root.

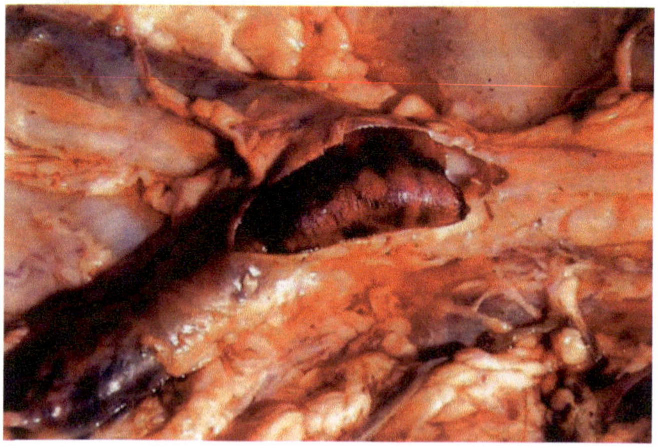

**Figure 5.29.** Horse. Terminal Aorta. Saddle Thromboembolus. A single large thrombus has occluded the lumen of the terminal aorta and the iliac arteries. (Reprinted with permission from Cambridge University Press.)

### b. Jugular vein thrombosis

Thrombophlebitis can develop in the jugular veins from repeated short-interval intravenous injection. Venous distension in such a condition may be obvious. The thrombus may be septic with bacteria or fungi colonizing. Emboli may shower into the lungs with usually no clinical consequences.

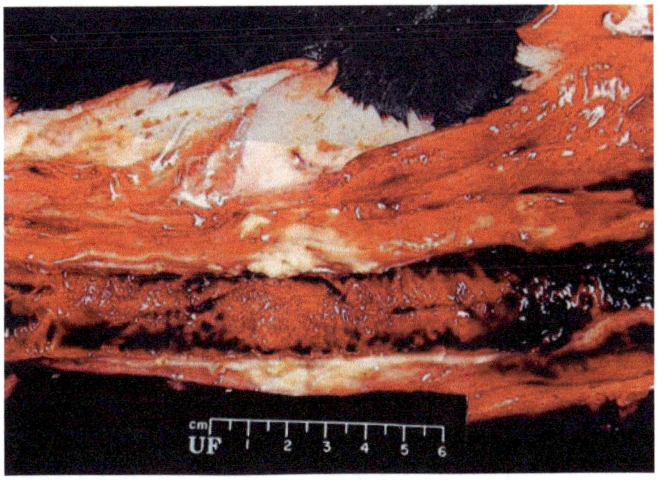


**Figure 5.30.** Horse. Jugular Vein Thrombosis. A large long thrombus occludes the vessel. It may develop after venipuncture in septic animals or in association with disseminated intravascular coagulopathy (DIC).

### *c. Carotid artery injection*

An attempt to inject medication into the jugular vein may mistakenly reach the carotid artery with fatal consequences. In this event it is mandatory to search for the injection site or needle puncture via a thorough inspection. Perivascular hemorrhage associated with the injection site may be a helpful indicator for faulty puncture.

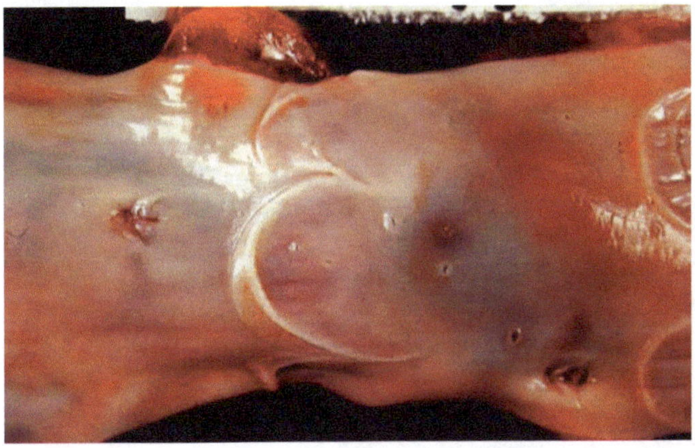

**Figure 5.31.** Horse. Carotid Artery. Two small needle punctures are evident in the intima.

### *d. Aortic rupture*

They may occur after sudden movement of the whole body toward the ground (fall, mating) causing blood vessel traction.

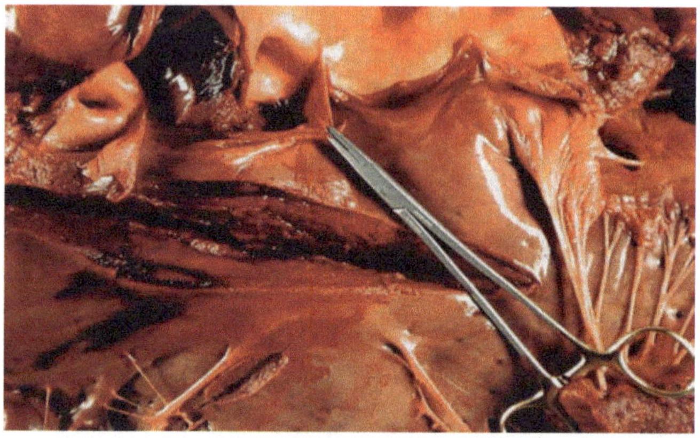

**Figure 5.32.** Horse. Aorta. Rupture. Acute intramyocardial hemorrhage.

Older stallions are reported to rupture the ascending aorta spontaneously. The event is the result of a weakening of the vessel wall due to age and a sudden increase of blood pressure when stressed. The rupture typically occurs in the ascending segment of the aorta with fatal hemothorax as the outcome. On occasion the rupture happens immediate to the aortic ring (opening), and in this case the rupture needs to be verified by inspecting the inside of the aortic semilunar valve cusps.

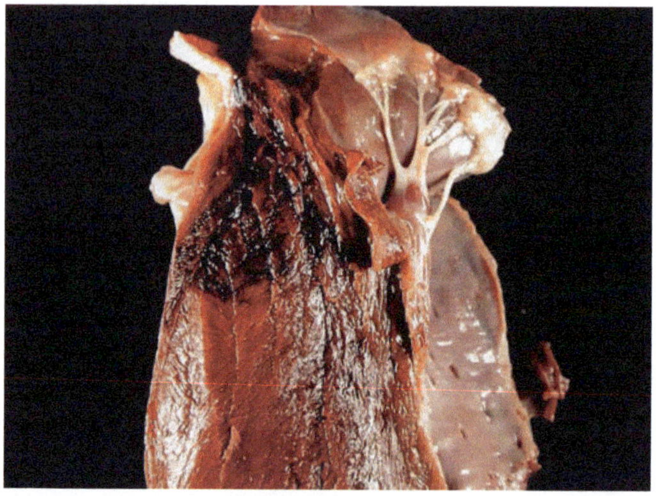

**Figure 5.33.** Horse. Myocardium. Aortic Rupture. A large focus of intramyocardial hemorrhage is present beneath the aortic semilunar cusp. It is the result of aortic rupture in an older stallion.

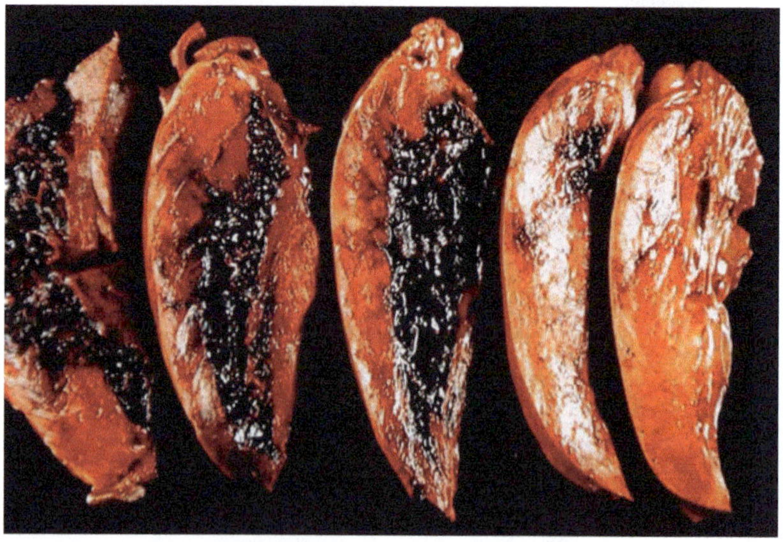

**Figure 5.34.** Horse. Myocardium. Aortic Rupture. Major portions of the myocardium are dissected by blood after a rupture of the aortic ring had occurred in an older stallion. No blood was present in the thorax.

*e. Rupture of middle uterine artery*

In older mares after repeated pregnancy in late term gestation, the middle uterine artery may develop a dissecting aneurysm due to structural weakening of the vessel wall. Hemoabdomen is a fatal outcome.

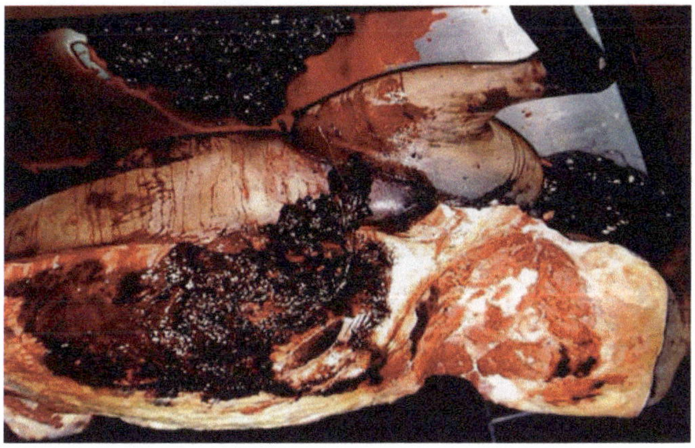

**Figure 5.35.** Horse. Hemoabdomen. An older mare in late term pregnancy had ruptured the middle uterine artery.

Other larger vessels can rupture also due to odd traumas or during horse races, but these events are very sporadic.

*f. Hemomelasma ilei*

An incidental finding at necropsy, the discovery has challenged the opinion as to etiology. Hemomelasma ilei typically appears at the antimesenteric serosal surface of the ileum as black (red) pea-size to walnut-size plaques. Originally thought to be the result of aberrant migrating larvae of *Strongylus vulgaris*, hemomelasma ilei nonetheless is seen in horses when endoparasitism is no longer an issue. One present hypothesis is that they are tears of weak serosal blood vessels particularly susceptible to hyperperistalsis of a muscular ileum. Another present hypothesis is that they are serosal vascular injuries from intestinal kinking.

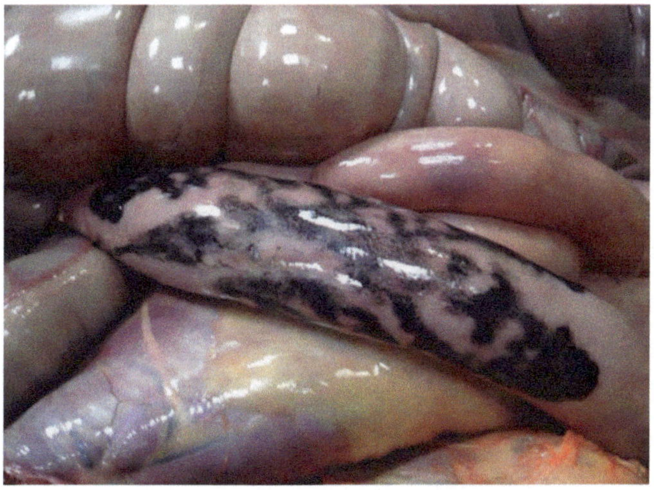

**Figure 5.36.** Horse. Ileum. Black Hemomelasma Ilei. Elevated black and serpiginous plaques are present on the serosa at the antimesenteric site. The black discoloration is the result of hemosiderosis from previous hemorrhage and postmortem pseudomelanosis.

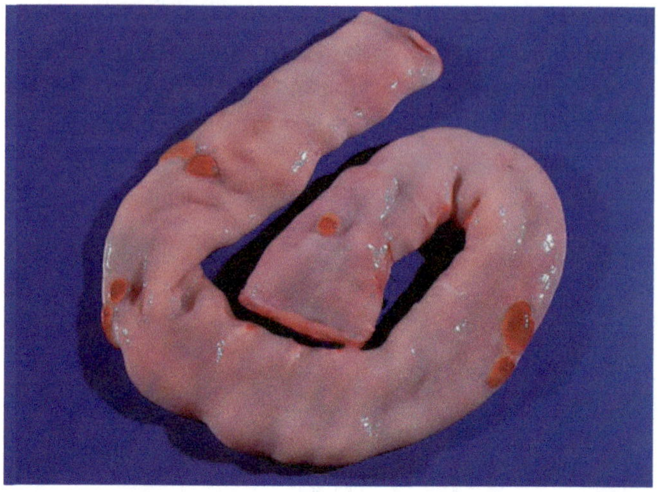

**Figure 5.37.** Horse. Ileum. Serosa. Red Hemomelasma Ilei. The nodules are comprised of fibrous tissue and hemosiderosis.

### *3. Vascular neoplasia*

Tumors of endothelial origin are either hemangiomas or hemangiosarcomas depending on their histologic features and biologic behavior. Such tumors can occur at any site where there are blood vessels. Preferential organs in the horse are the respiratory or musculoskeletal systems. Other sites are the skin, eye, and central nervous system. Thoroughbreds are overrepresented in reported neoplastic collections. The differential diagnoses include tumors arising from lymphatic vessels defined as lymphangioma or lymphangiosarcoma, tumor-like proliferation of mature vascular tissue, defined as hamartoma, or vascular proliferations in the skin of young horses diagnosed as angiomatosis or angiectasia. Factor VIII-related antigen can be applied as an immunohistochemical marker for vascular endothelium demonstration.

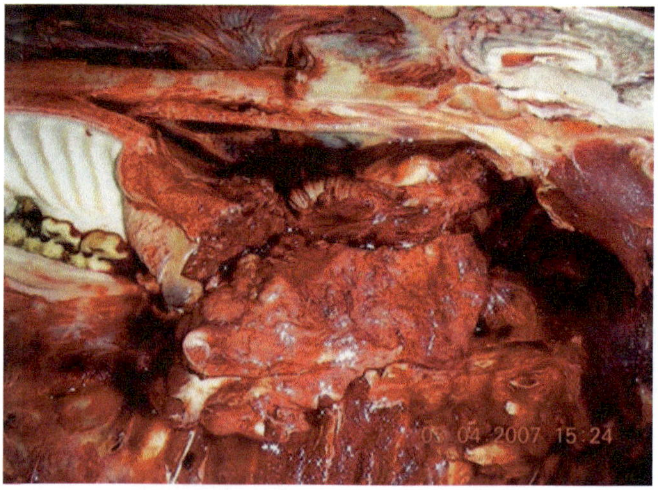

**Figure 5.38.** Horse. Oropharynx. Hemangiosarcoma. A multilobulated, fleshy red-tan growth occupies the site of the oropharynx. Epistaxis was one of the clinical signs noticed in this draft horse.

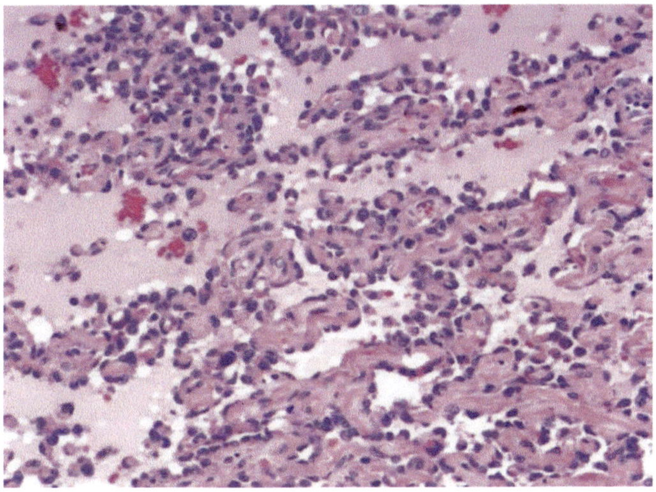

**Figure 5.39.** Horse. Oropharynx. Hemangiosarcoma. Microscopically, streams of endothelial-like neoplastic cells are resting on collagen to form vascular canals filled with serum and some red blood cells. (H&E)

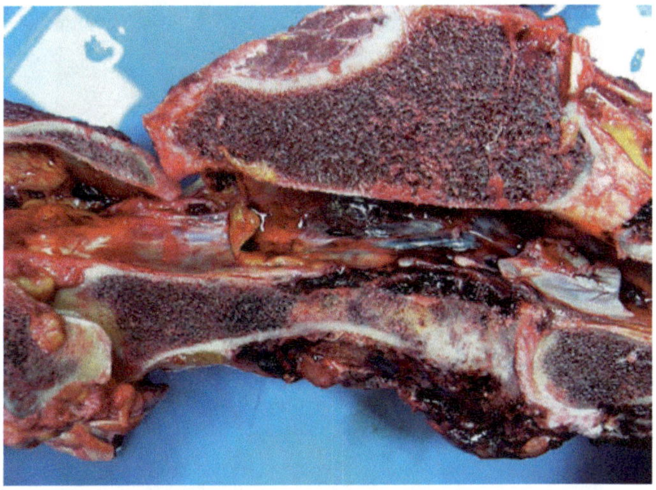

**Figure 5.40.** Horse. Vertebra at C-2. Hemangiosarcoma. A fleshy circumscribed growth is located at the ventral part of the vertebra and within the epidural space. The tumor arose from the vasculature of the bone. Differential diagnosis: malignant melanoma. (Courtesy Dr. P. Habecker, University of Pennsylvania.)

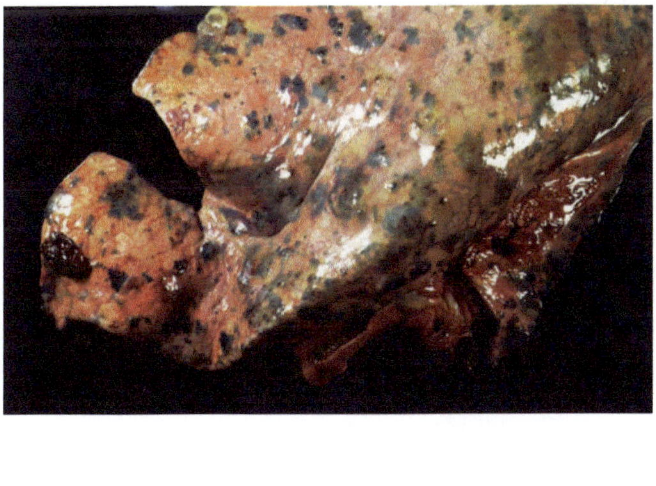

**Figure 5.41.** Horse. Lung. Hemangiosarcoma. Metastasis occurred to the lungs. The tumor also disseminated to the brain and kidney. (Courtesy Dr. P. Habecker, University of Pennsylvania.)

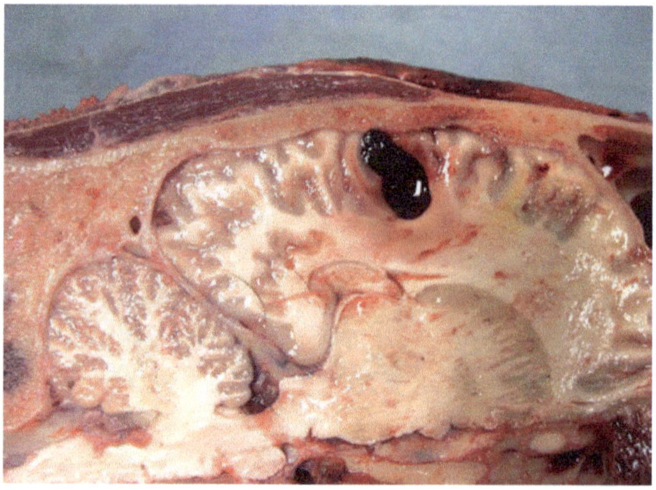

**Figure 5.42.** Horse. Brain. Hemangiosarcoma. Site of metastasis. (Courtesy Dr. P. Habecker, University of Pennsylvania.)

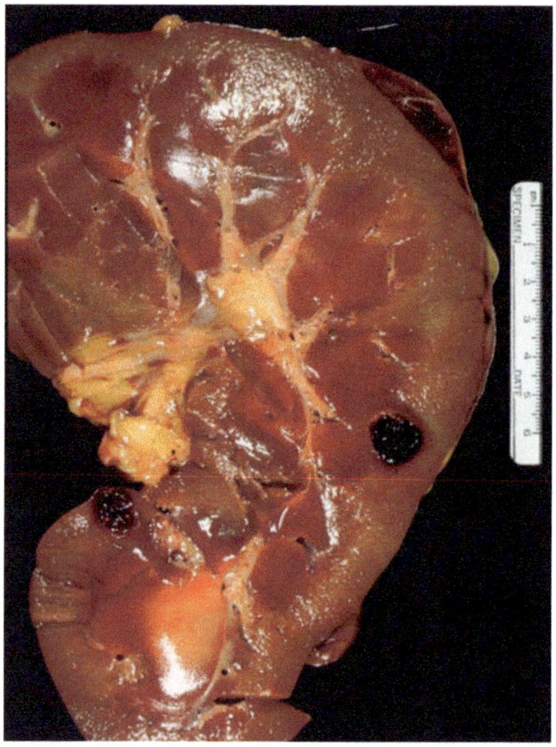

**Figure 5.43.** Horse. Kidney. Hemangiosarcoma. Site of metastasis of the same tumor. (Courtesy Dr. P. Habecker, University of Pennsylvania.)

## Selected references



Bolin DC, Donahue JM, Vickers ML, et al. 2005. Microbiologic and pathologic findings in an epidemic of equine pericarditis. *J Vet Diagn Invest* 17(1):38–44.

Buergelt CD. 2003. Equine cardiovascular pathology: an overview. *Anim Health Res Rev* 4(2):109–129.

Decloedt A, Verleyer T, DeClercq G, et al. 2012. Acute and long term cardiomyopathy and delayed neurotoxicity after accidental lasalocid poisoning in horses. *J Vet Intern Med* 26(4):1005–1011.

Del Piero F. 2000. Equine viral arteritis. *Vet Pathol* 37:287–296.

Else RW, Holmes JR. 1972. Cardiac pathology in the horse. 1. Gross pathology. *Equine Vet J* 4:1–8.

Sage AM. 2002. Cardiac disease in the geriatric horse. *Vet Clin North Am Equine Pract* 18(3):575–589.

Seahorn JL, Slovis NM, Reimer JM, Carey VJ, Donahue JG, Cohen ND. 2003. Case-control study of factors associated with fibrinous pericarditis among horses in central Kentucky during spring 2001. *J Am Vet Med Assoc* 223(6):832–838.

Woods LW, Filigenzi MS, Booth MC, Rodger LD, Arnold JS, Puschner B. 2004. Summer pheasant's eye (*Adonis aestivalis*) poisoning in three horses. *Vet Pathol* 41(3):215–220.

Worth LT, Reef VB. 1998. Pericarditis in horses: 18 cases (1986–1995. *J Am Vet Med Assoc* 212(2):248–253.

# 6 Diseases of the Gastrointestinal System

**With contributions by Julie B. Engiles**

I. Diseases of the oral cavity
   1. Anomalies
   2. Dental diseases
   3. Dental tumors
   4. Diseases of the buccae and tongue
II. Diseases of the esophagus
   1. Obstruction of the lumen
   2. Inflammation
   3. Idiopathic hypertrophy of the distal esophagus
   4. Neoplasia
III. Diseases of the stomach
   1. Gastric rupture
   2. Gastric ulcers
   3. Gastric parasites
   4. Gastric neoplasia
IV. Noninfectious diseases of the intestinal tract
   1. Anomalies
      a. Atresia
      b. Aganglionosis
      c. Meckel's diverticulum
      d. Ileal hypertrophy
   2. Displacements and strangulation
      a. Volvulus
      b. Torsion
      c. Strangulation lipomas
      d. Intussusception
      e. Foramen epiploicum herniation
      f. Nephrosplenic ligament entrapment
      g. Mesodiverticular band
      h. Mesenteric rent
      i. Diaphragmatic hernia
      j. Intestinal infarcts

*Color Atlas of Equine Pathology*, First Edition. Claus D. Buergelt and Fabio Del Piero.

3. Intraluminal foreign bodies
   a. Sand impaction
   b. Enteroliths
4. Rectal (colonic) perforation
5. Intestinal diverticulum
6. Large intestinal tympany

V. Infectious diseases of the intestinal tract
1. Inflammation
   a. Catarrhal enteritis
   b. Hemorrhagic enteritis
   c. Fibrinonecrotic enteritis
   d. Ulcerative enteritis
   e. Granulomatous enteritis
   f. Hyperplastic enteritis
   g. Inflammatory bowel diseases
2. Drug-induced enteropathy
3. Endoparasites
   a. Nematodes
   b. Cestodes
   c. Trematodes
   d. Enteric coccidiosis
4. Intestinal neoplasia
5. Miscellaneous

VI. Diseases of the peritoneum
1. Inflammation
2. Neoplasia
3. Miscellaneous

In frequency, diseases of the gastrointestinal tract rank number one in large animals. Great economic losses may arise from disorders of the gastrointestinal tract. Although many gastrointestinal tract diseases are preventable due to available protective medication or vaccines, and improved management and feeding practices, others continue to occur in the horse, simply as the result of anatomic and genetic peculiarities of this species.

Due to the anatomic length of the gastrointestinal tract, an orderly investigation is recommended and to separate the tract into four segments: stomach, small intestine, colon-cecum, and transverse colon-rectum.

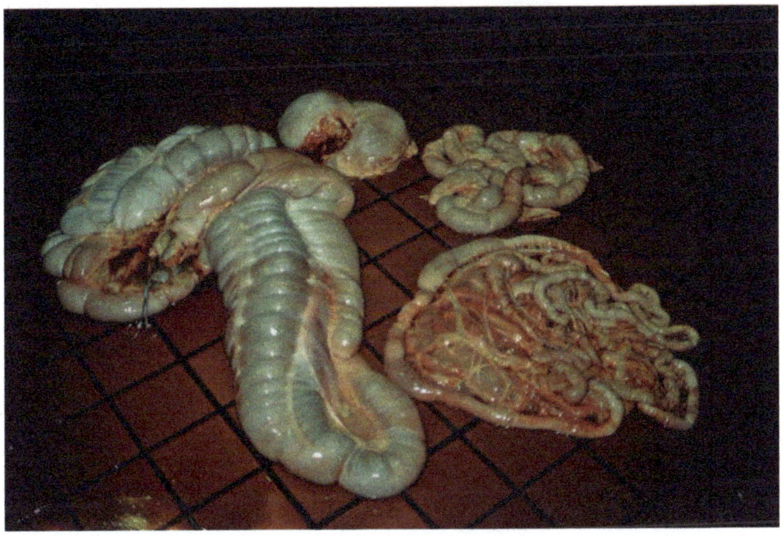

**Figure 6.1.** Horse. Gastrointestinal Tract. Normal. For more detailed inspection, the gastrointestinal tract has been divided into four segments. (Reprinted from Equine Medicine and Surgery, Colahan et al., Figure 3-55, Page 122, Copyright Elsevier, 1999.)

## I. Diseases of the oral cavity

Careful examination of the oral cavity structures is mandatory for both clinicians and pathologists.

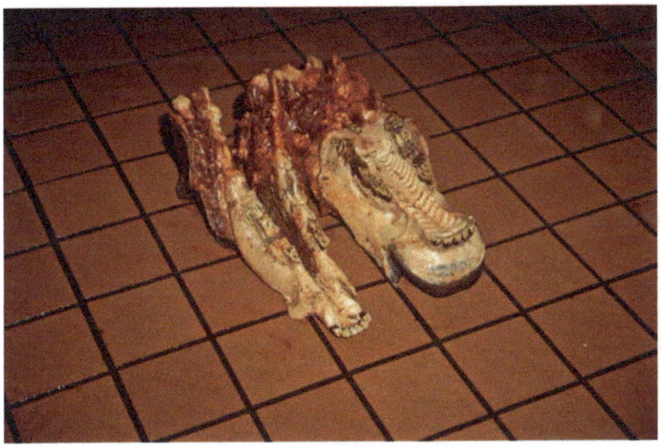

**Figure 6.2.** Horse. Jaws. Examination for Dental Wear. Separation of the mandible from the maxilla facilitates examination of molar teeth.

## 1. Anomalies

The normal development of the oral cavity depends largely on the organized growth of a synchronized embryologic process. Failure of tissue integration and of tissue fusion may lead to a variety of malformations, the most frequent of which are facial fissures, brachygnathia, and cleft palate (palatoschisis).

## 2. Dental diseases

Dental diseases are frequently overlooked as the single cause of cachexia. Equine dentistry is a regular service of practitioners to the equine industry. Pathologists have a relaxed attitude toward careful inspection of teeth during the equine necropsy. The few dental disorders presented here do not do justice to equine dentistry as a clinical specialty and are simply individual occurrences to share with practitioners and pathologists.

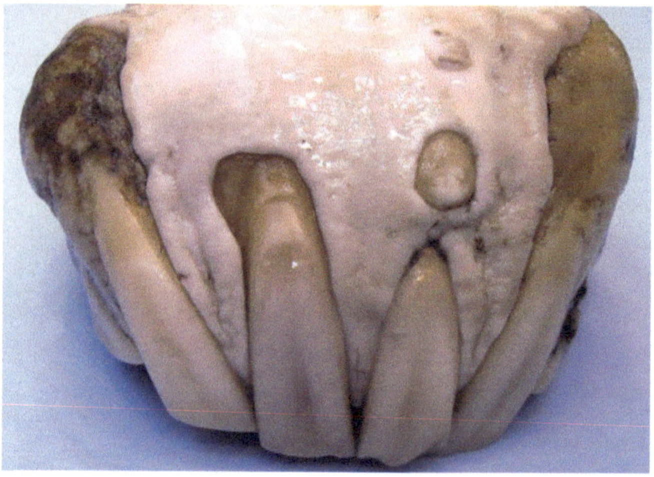

**Figure 6.3.** Horse. Incisors. Equine Odontoclastic Tooth Resorption and Hypercementosis (EOTRH). A painful disorder of mainly the incisor teeth, it is thus far of unknown etiology in horses older than 15 years. Macroscopic examination reveals bulbous enlargement by a rough cemental surface at the apical aspect. (Courtesy Dr. R. Smedley, Michigan State University.)

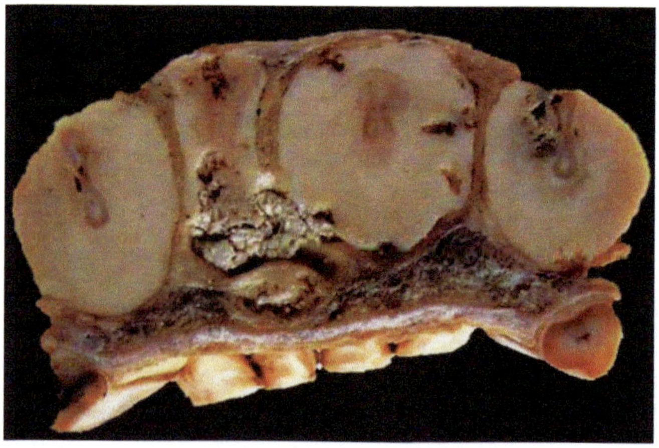

**Figure 6.4.** Horse. Incisors. Equine Odontoclastic Tooth Resorption and Hypercementosis Syndrome (EOTRH). The enlargement observed on the surface is best seen as thickening on cross section. The dental changes should not be confused with cementoma. (Courtesy Dr. R. Smedley, Michigan State University.)

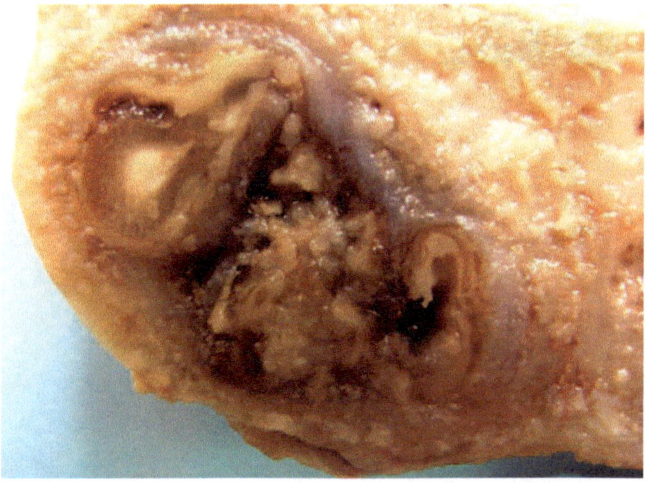

**Figure 6.5.** Horse. Incisors. Equine Odontoclastic Tooth Resorption and Hypercementosis (EOTRH). In some incisors depressions, perforations and focal lytic changes with necrotic tissue and focal remnants of the periodontal ligament can be found. Inflammatory lesions in the pulp cavity and alveolar bone can be present in some cases. (Courtesy Dr. R. Smedley, Michigan State University.)

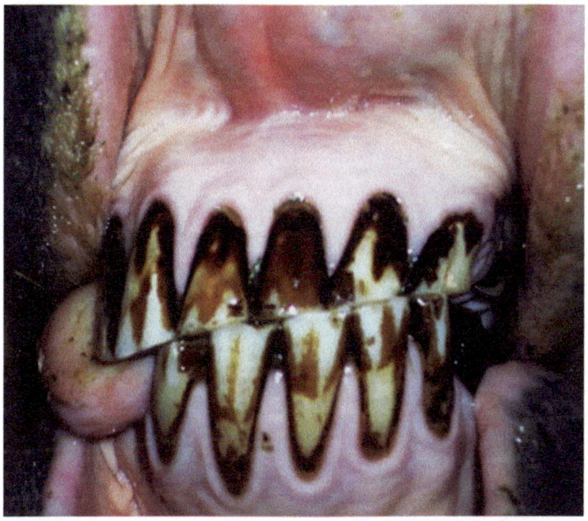

**Figure 6.6.** Horse. Teeth. Incisors. Diagonal Incisors. The condition leads to malocclusion. (Courtesy Dr. T. Banner, Gainesville, FL.)

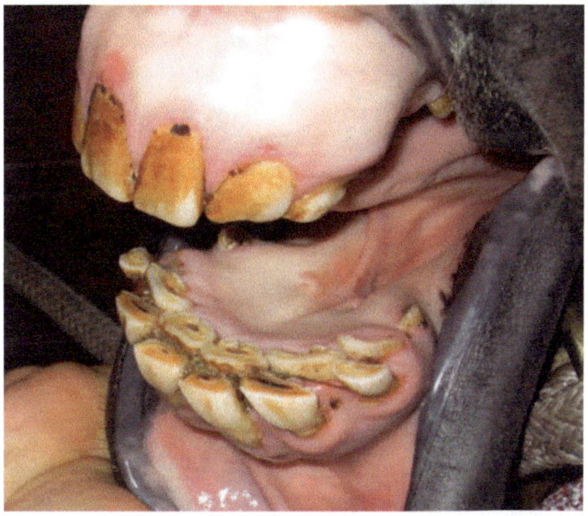

**Figure 6.7.** Horse. Teeth. Incisors. Double Incisors. The condition may lead to periodontal disease. (Courtesy Dr. Toots Banner, Gainesville, FL.)

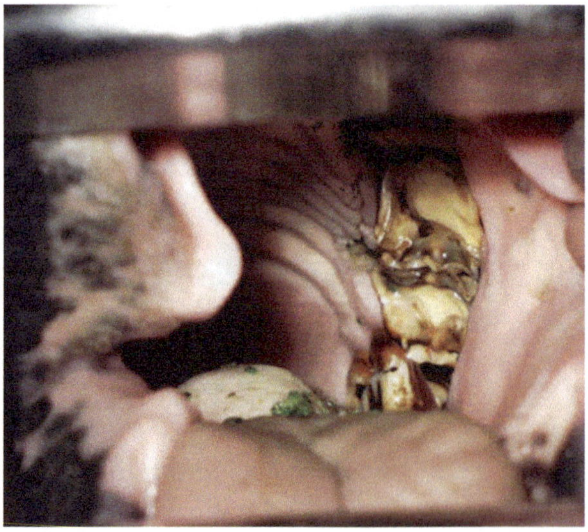

**Figure 6.8.** Horse. Teeth. Geriatric Teeth. Much of the enamel is gone, leaving dentin and cementum exposed. The worn occlusal surfaces have reduced grinding functions. (Courtesy Dr. T. Banner, Gainesville, FL.)

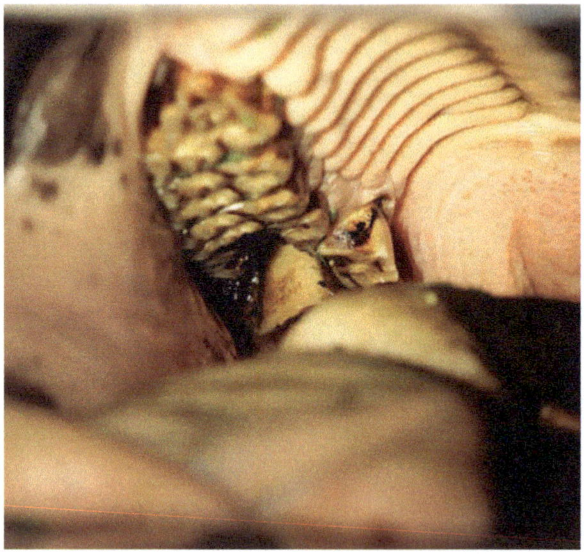

**Figure 6.9.** Horse. Teeth. Molar. Split Molar. Acts like a fractured tooth. (Courtesy Dr. T. Banner, Gainesville, FL.)

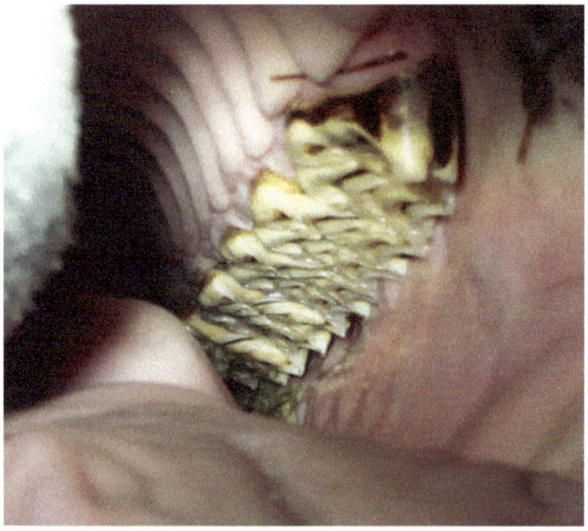

**Figure 6.10.** Horse. Teeth. Molar. Points and Hooks. Can injure soft tissue and predispose to abnormal masticatory motion. (Courtesy Dr. T. Banner, Gainesville, FL.)

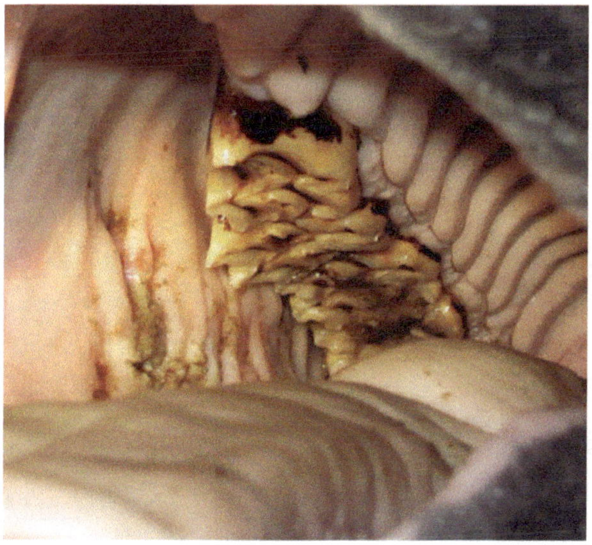

**Figure 6.11.** Horse. Teeth. Molar. Wave. Leads to malocclusion and gingival margin displacement, usually involving fourth premolar and first molar teeth. (Courtesy Dr. T. Banner, Gainesville, FL.)

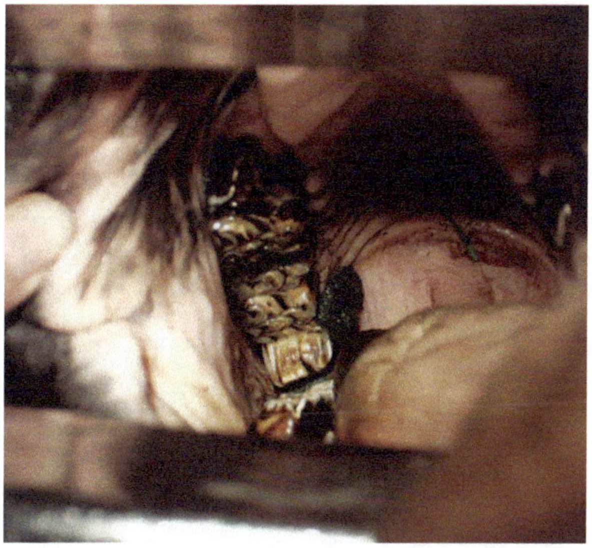

**Figure 6.12.** Horse. Teeth. Step Mouth and Molar Step. Abrupt changes in crown height along the arcade are known as "step mouth." Excessive length is due to lack of an opposing tooth. (Courtesy Dr. T Banner, Gainesville, FL.)

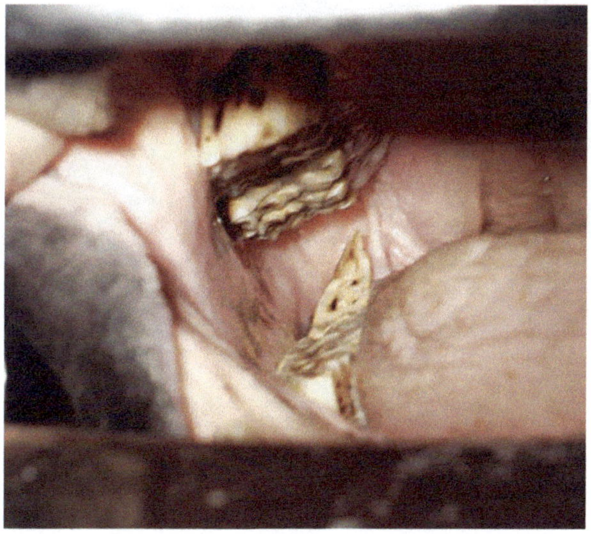

**Figure 6.13.** Horse. Teeth. Caudal Hook. (Courtesy Dr. T. Banner, Gainesville, FL.)

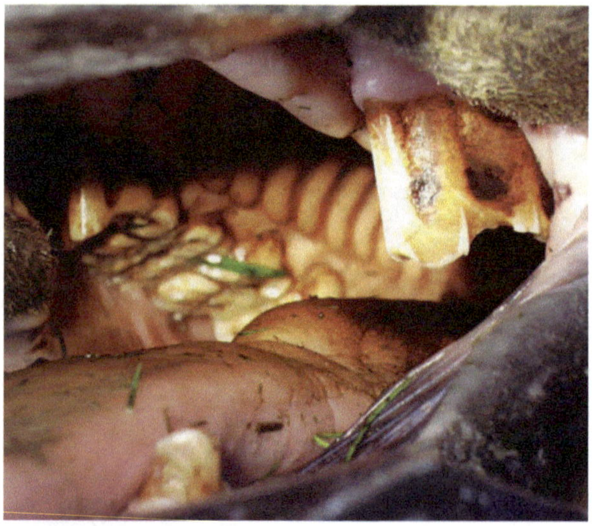

**Figure 6.14.** Horse. Teeth. Rostral Hook. (Courtesy Dr. T. Banner, Gainesville, FL.)

### *3. Dental tumors*

*Contributed by Dr. Julie B. Engiles, University of Pennsylvania*

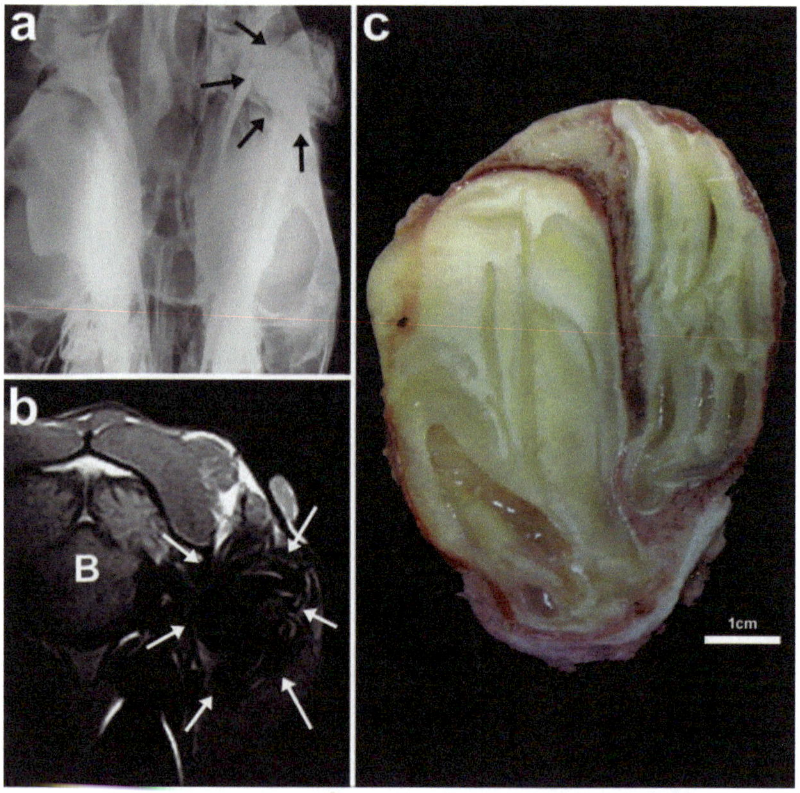


**Figure 6.15.** Horse. Head. Peripheral Compound Odontoma ("ear tooth") in a 2-year-old warmblood gelding with a hard swelling caudal to the right ear. (a) Ventral-dorsal digital radiographic projection of the skull shows a discrete radiopaque mass just caudal to the zygomatic arch (arrows) that protrudes laterally. (b) Transverse T1-weighted short tau inversion recovery. Magnetic resonance imaging (MRI) shows a well-defined mass of low signal intensity, consistent with dense mineralized material, containing curvilinear arrays of high signal intensity, consistent with fluid (arrows). The brain (B) is labeled for orientation. (c) Gross photograph of a sagittal section from the surgically excised mass shows two dysplastic but well-formed mineralized odontogenic structures that contain curvilinear fluid-filled cysts as seen in the MRI.

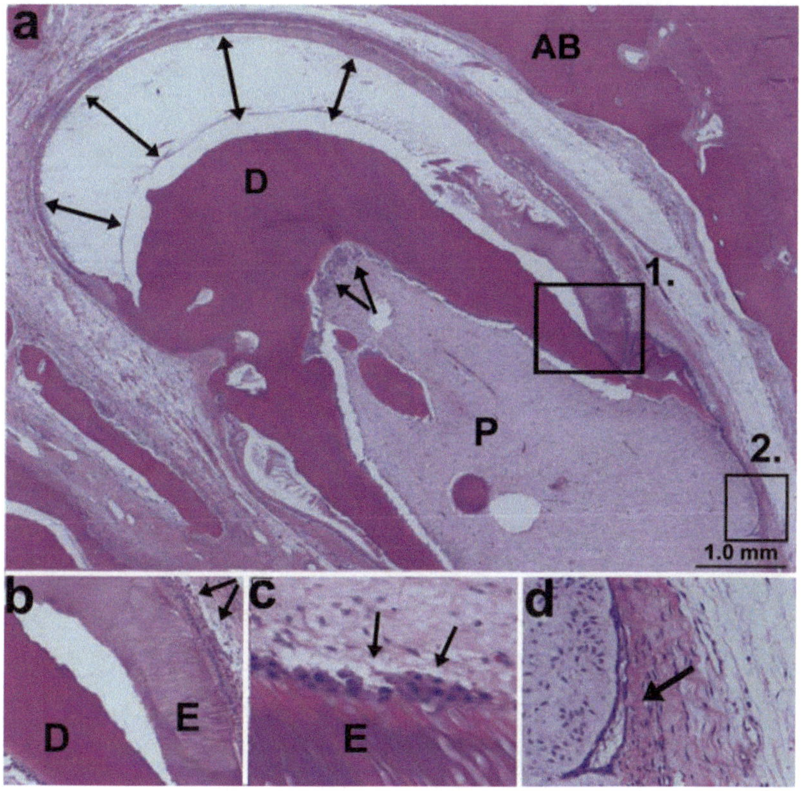


**Figure 6.16.** Horse. Head. Peripheral Compound Odontoma of decalcified H&E-stained sections of the mass in Fig. 6.15. (a) There is a well-organized odontogenic structure that includes an outer margin of alveolar bone (AB), a cystic cavity formed by the enamel organ (double-headed arrows), underlying dentin (a and b; D) subtended by odontoblasts (arrows), and an inner core of pulp (P). Higher magnification photomicrograph of the framed region 1. shows arrays of dentin tubules (D in b) that abut enamel tubules (E in b and c), which are lined by ameloblasts (arrows in b and c). Higher magnification photomicrograph of the framed region 2. shows Hertwig sheath composed of inner and outer enamel epithelium responsible for induction of root dentin. Remnants of Hertwig sheath become cell rests of Malassez, which are thought to be the origin of fibromatous/ossifying epulis, most common in dogs.

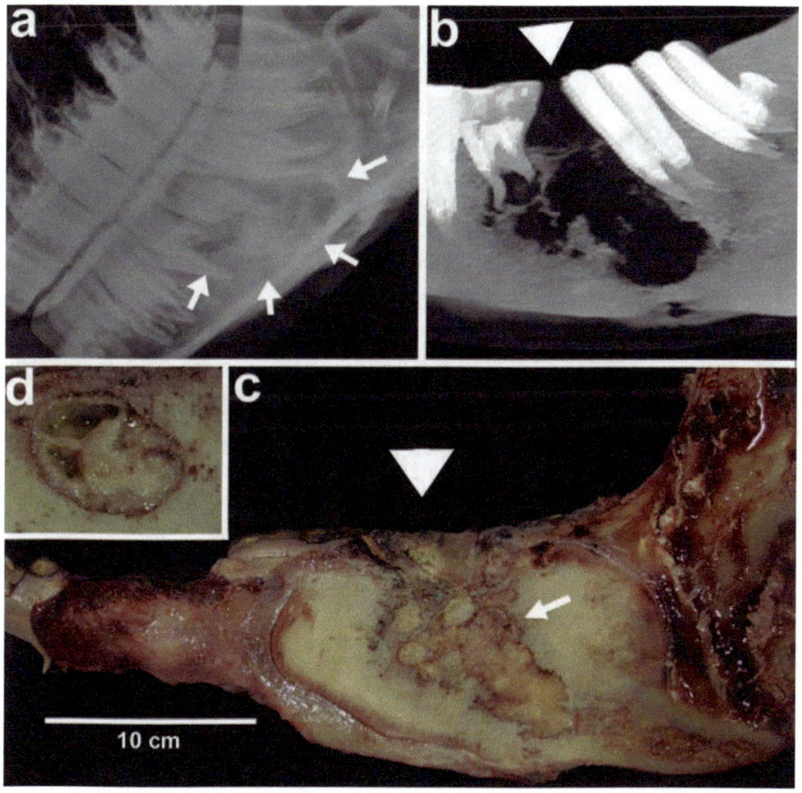


**Figure 6.17.** Horse. Mandible. Ameloblastic Fibro-Odontoma. Digital radiographic projections and gross photos of a juvenile horse that presented with a rapidly enlarging rostral mandibular mass. Although the mass effaced the entire right and part of the left mandibular rami, and displaced the incisors and canine teeth, the mass had well-defined caudal margins (a, b). Gross photos taken prior to partial mandibulectomy show severe enlargement of the mandible with focal ulceration of the lingual mucosa (c). A sagittal section of the surgically excised mass shows irregular nodules of hard to gritty gray-white mineralized foci admixed with firm red-tan tissue (d).

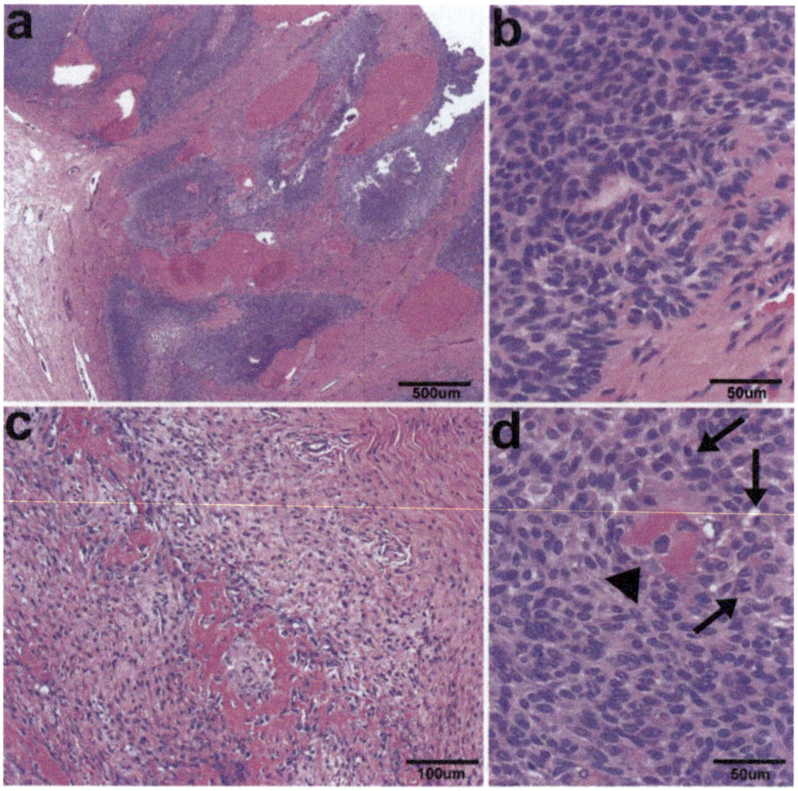


**Figure 6.18.** Horse. Mandible. Ameloblastic Fibro-Odontoma. H&E-stained decalcified sections of the mass show lobules of basophilic cells interspersed by eosinophilic islands of mineralized bone/cementum/dentin and spindle-shaped cells embedded in a collagenous matrix (a, c). Higher magnification of the basophilic lobules show primitive hyperchromatic blunt spindle-shaped cells that palisade along the external margin and also form rosettes, resembling ameloblastic epithelium (b). In other regions, the spindle cells have slightly different morphology with frequent mitoses (d, arrows), and surround small islands of unmineralized osteoid/dentin/cementum (d, arrowhead).

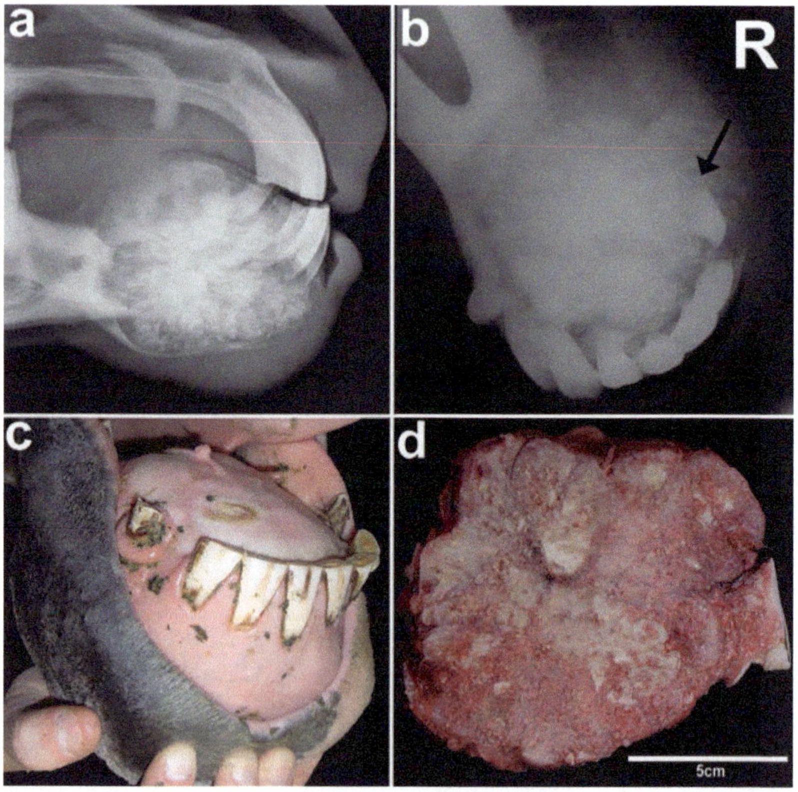


**Figure 6.19.** Horse. Mandible. Primary intraosseous odontogenic squamous cell carcinoma in an adult horse that presented with weight loss and mandibular swelling. Lateral digital radiographic projection (a) that shows multiloculated radiolucencies infiltrating the mandibular ramus. Computed tomography of the same region shows loss of the first molar (b, arrowhead) lysis of the fourth premolar tooth roots and similar radiolucent cavities. Gross photo shows a multinodular proliferation of firm tan tissue that infiltrates the mandibular ramus and extends to the gingival surface (c). Some nodules contain fluid-filled centers (d). The remaining structures in the oral cavity and draining lymph nodes were unaffected.

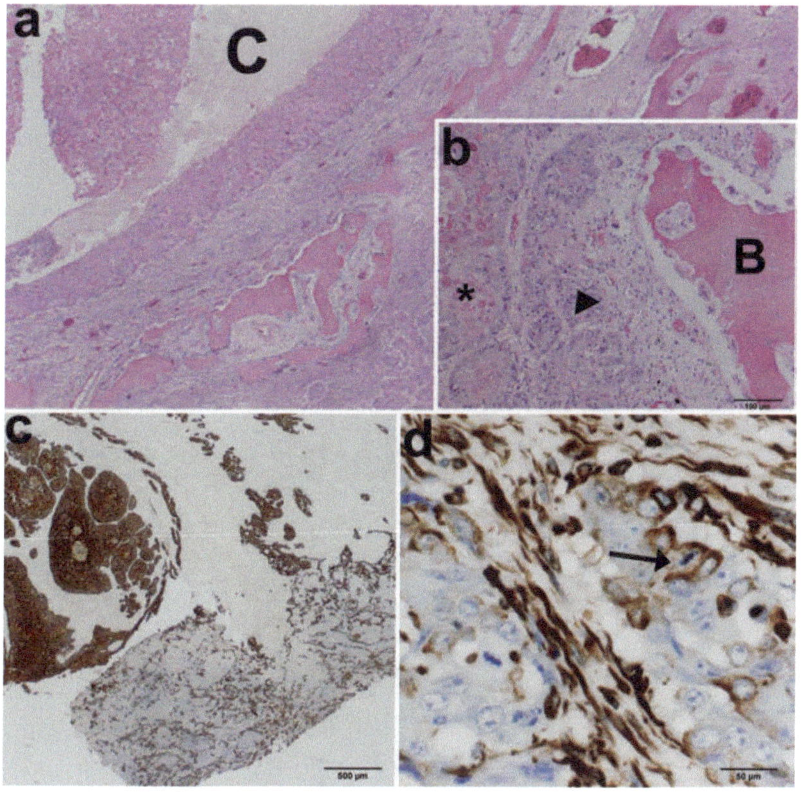


**Figure 6.20.** Horse. Mandible. Primary intraosseous odontogenic squamous cell carcinoma: H&E-stained nondecalcified sections from the cystic nodules. Neoplastic stratified squamous epithelium surrounds cystic cavities filled with pale eosinophilic fluid and sloughed cells (a, "**C**"). Islands of neoplastic cells show prominent keratinization (b, asterisk) or little keratinization, resembling basal cells (b, asterisk). Immunohistochemistry for AE1/AE3 cytokeratin shows abundant antigen expression by neoplastic cells that form large discrete lobules as well as infiltrative thin cords/trabeculae (c). Neoplastic squamous epithelium also demonstrates vimentin expression (d), which can be seen in a squamous cell undergoing mitosis (d, arrow).

### *4. Diseases of the buccae and tongue*

Color changes associated with the normal pink of the visible oral mucous membrane may include pallor, cyanosis, petechiae, ecchymoses, congestion, and icterus, all important clues for the identification of disease entities affecting different internal organ systems.

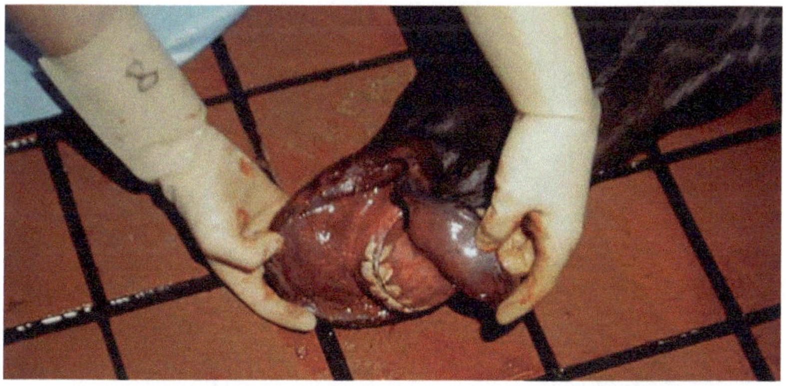

**Figure 6.21.** Horse. Oral Mucosa. Muddy Red. Color change in shock or cyanosis.

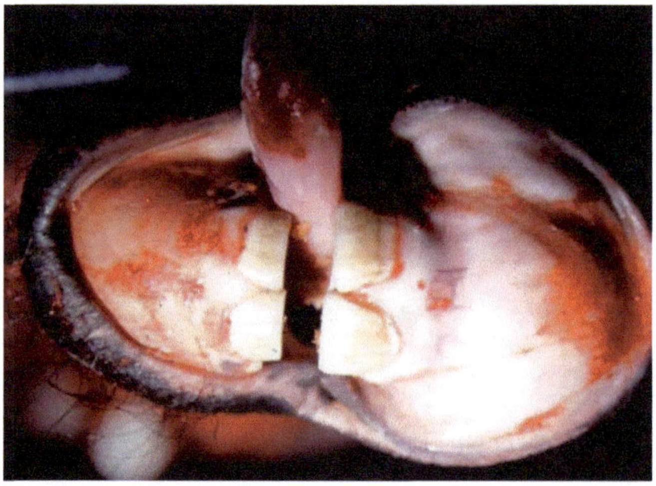

**Figure 6.22.** Horse. Oral Mucosa. Multifocal Red. Color change after drug reaction to nonsteroidal anti-inflammatory drugs (NSAIDs), infection such as infectious equine anemia, or immune dyscrasia such as pemphigus or purpura hemorrhagica. (Reprinted with permission from the Animal Technology Institute of Taiwan, Republic of China)

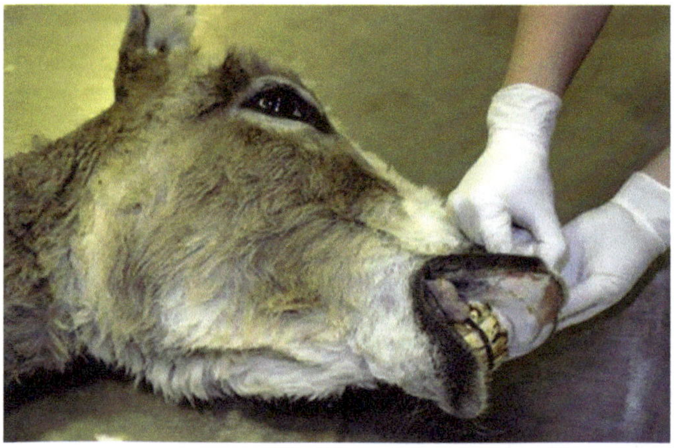

**Figure 6.23.** Donkey. Oral Mucosa. White. Color change from anemia. (Courtesy Dr. J. Roberts, National Zoo, Washington, DC.)

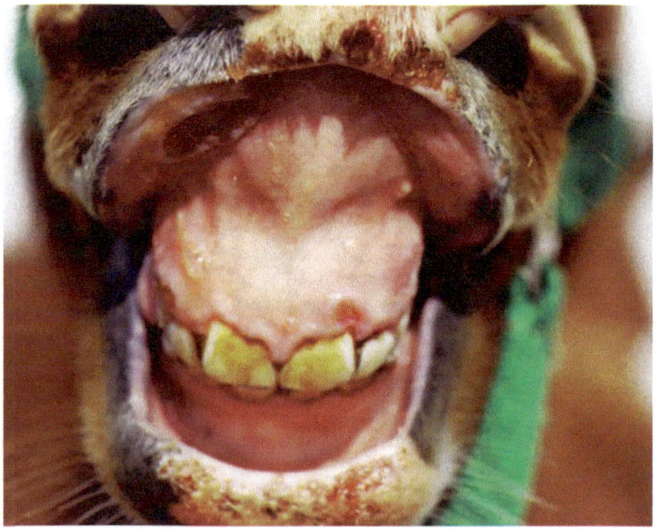

**Figure 6.24.** Horse. Mouth. Plant-induced Ulcerative Stomatitis and Cheilitis. Fleshy ulcers are present in the mucosa of the upper lips and in the gingiva above the incisors. The skin of the lips is ulcerative and eczematous. These lesions have developed from consumption of yellow foxtail (*Setaria lutescens*) grass barbs. (Courtesy Dr. P. Habecker, University of Pennsylvania.)

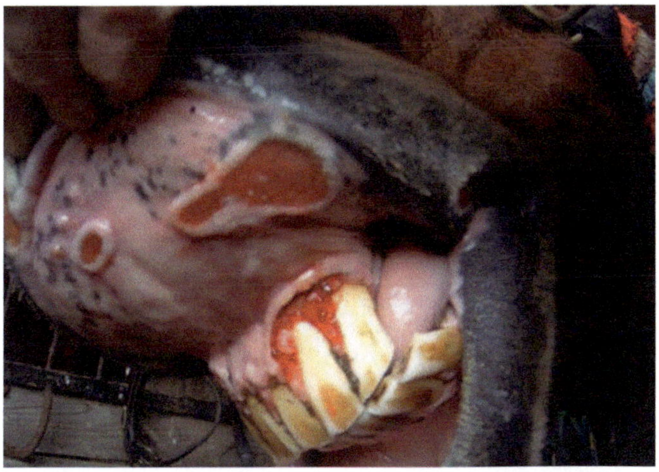

**Figure 6.25.** Horse. Mouth. Plant-induced Ulcerative Stomatitis and Cheilitis. After consumption of the grass, spikelets of seed heads burrow into the equine oral gingiva to cause an ulcerative, granulomatous, fibrous foreign body inflammation. (Courtesy Dr. P. Habecker, University of Pennsylvania.)

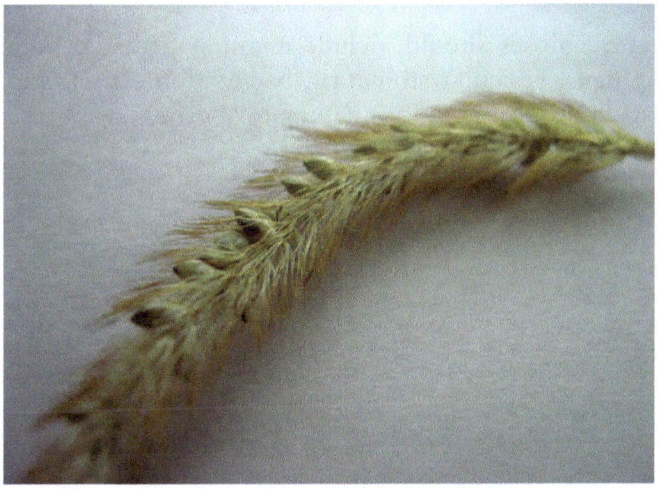

**Figure 6.26.** *Setaria lutescens*. (Courtesy Dr. P. Habecker, University of Pennsylvania.)

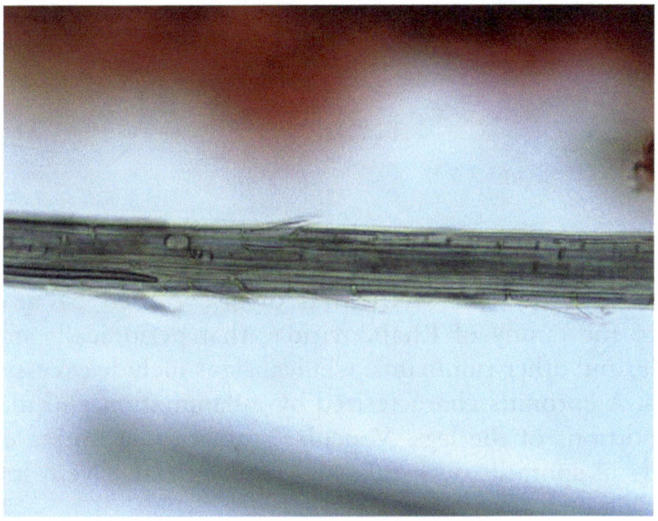

**Figure 6.27.** Barbs of *Setaria lutescens*. These are penetrating the gingiva or lips. (Courtesy Dr. P. Habecker, University of Pennsylvania.)

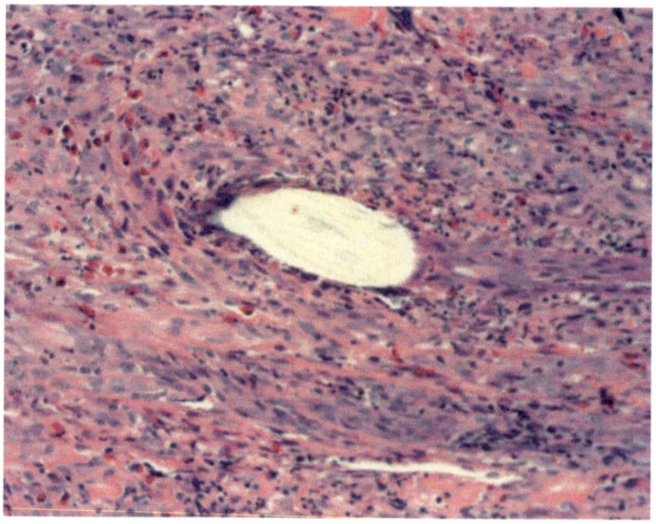

**Figure 6.28.** Horse. Mouth. Plant-induced Ulcerative Stomatitis and Cheilitis. Microscopically, a plant barb is embedded within a dense foreign body pyogranulomatous reaction with eosinophils. (H&E) (Courtesy Dr. P. Habecker, University of Pennsylvania.)

Differential diagnoses should include immune-mediated bullous diseases such as pemphigus, vesicular stomatitis, bacterial infection, and reaction to treatment with nonsteroidal anti-inflammatory drugs.

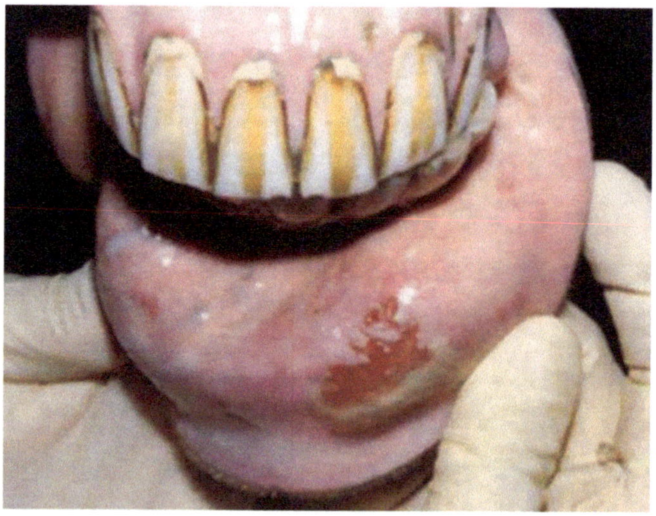

**Figure 6.29.** Horse. Lips. Vesicular Stomatitis. Muzzle. Some focal erosive changes are present in the mucosa.

Vesicular stomatitis is a RNA viral disease caused by a vesiculovirus belonging to the family of Rhabdoviridae that periodically infects horses, swine, cattle, and other ruminants. Clinical signs include excessive salivation and blisters. A coronitis characterized by inflammation and ulcers involves the lower portions of the legs. Vesicular stomatitis in horses occurs in the United States as sporadic outbreaks and requires extensive restriction in the trade including quarantine.

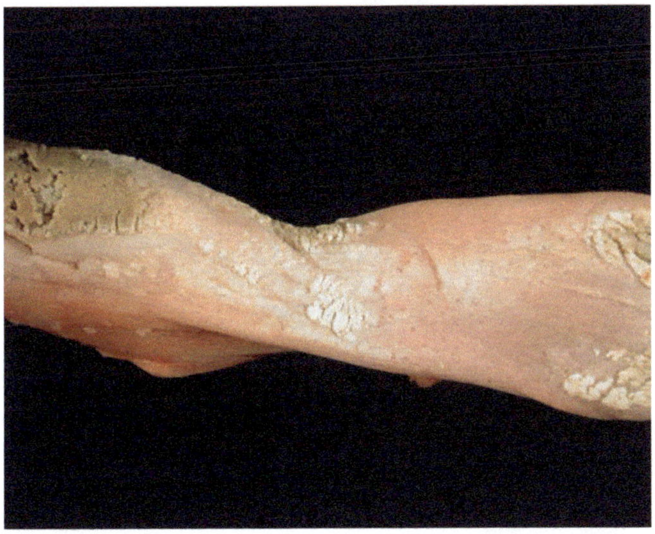

**Figure 6.30.** Horse. Tongue. Glossitis and Parakeratosis. Multifocal dry exudate on the surface from bacterial infection. Differential diagnosis is candidiasis (thrush).

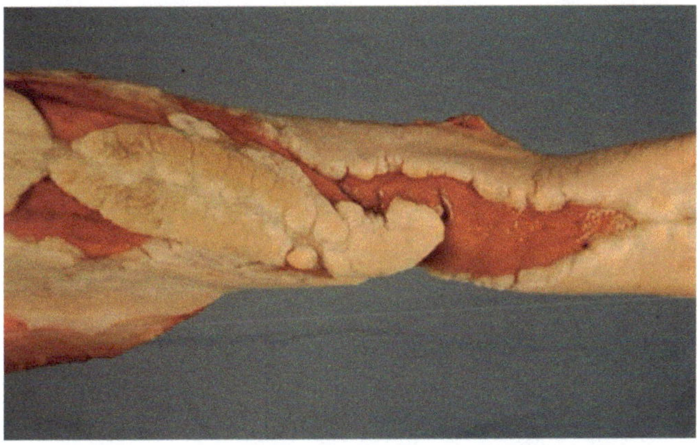

**Figure 6.31.** Horse. Tongue. Ulcers. Multifocal chronic ulcerative glossitis from dental attrition. Differential diagnosis: nerve paralysis from intraglossal neoplasia (squamous cell carcinoma).

## II. Diseases of the esophagus

As a tubular organ, the esophagus provides the route of passage for masticated food to the stomach. It is divided into three anatomic segments: cervical, thoracic, and abdominal. There are four anatomic narrowings: at the caudal larynx, thoracic inlet, base of the heart and diaphragmatic hiatus. Esophageal diseases in the horse are relatively rare compared with diseases in other compartments of the gastrointestinal tract.

### *1. Obstruction of the lumen*

This can be the result of impaction, choke, and strictures. Narrowing of the lumen also occurs from compressive changes due to disease processes outside the esophagus (soft tissue inflammation from trauma). Of additional critical clinical importance are perforations because they induce severe cellulitis.

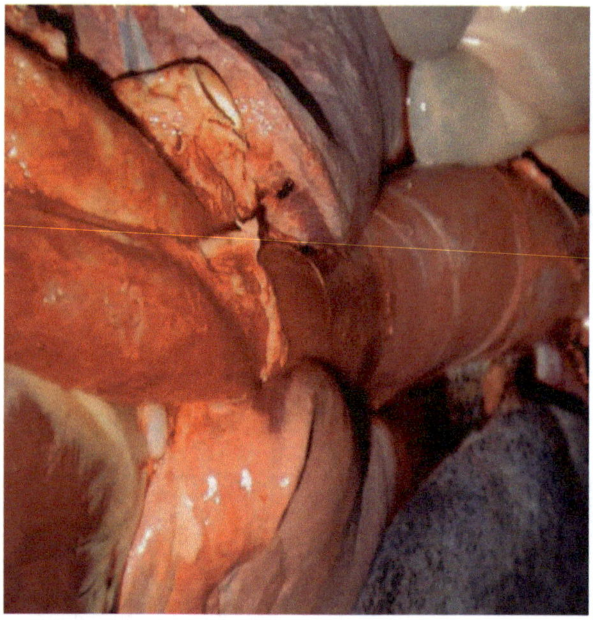

**Figure 6.32.** Horse. Megaesophagus. Impaction. The esophagus is diffusely distended.

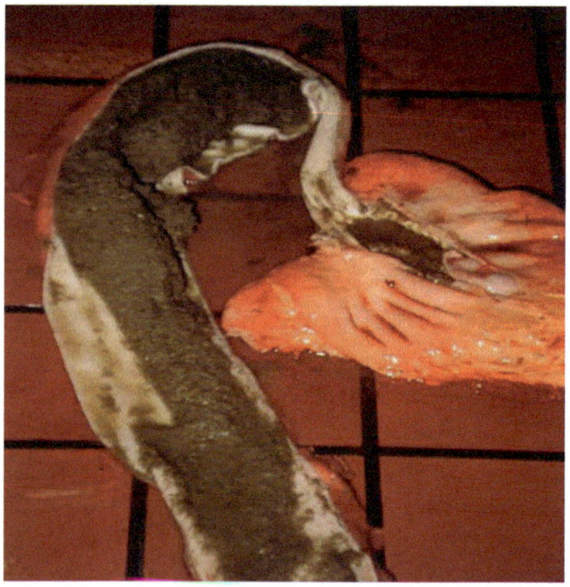

**Figure 6.33.** Horse. Megaesophagus. Ingesta as the result of gastric functional stricture or impaction occupy the lumen. Aspiration pneumonia may occur as a complication. Differential diagnosis: diffuse idiopathic megaesophagus, megaesophagus from vascular ring anomaly.

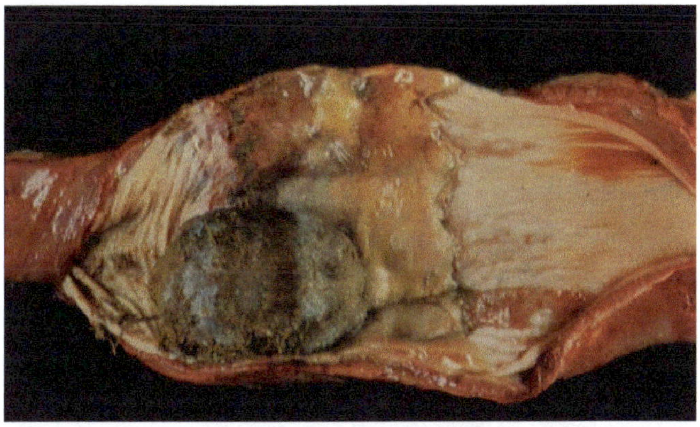

**Figure 6.34.** Horse. Esophagus. Foreign Body (Choke). Foreign object entrapment occurs at the site of the esophageal narrowings. The entrapped object causes pressure necrosis of the adjacent mucosa. (Reprinted with permission from the Animal Technology Institute of Taiwan, Republic of China)

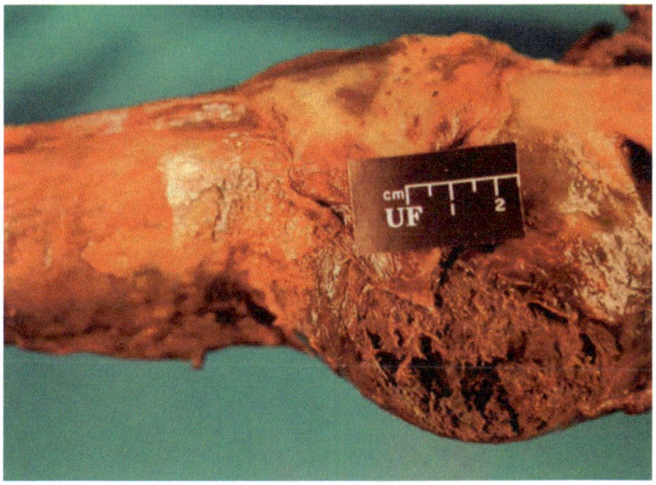


**Figure 6.35.** Horse. Esophagus. Foreign Body (Choke). When prolonged, the entrapment may lead to weakening of the wall to cause an inflammatory pseudo-diverticulum and cellulitis of the periesophageal soft tissue. (Reprinted with permission from the Animal Technology Institute of Taiwan, Republic of China)

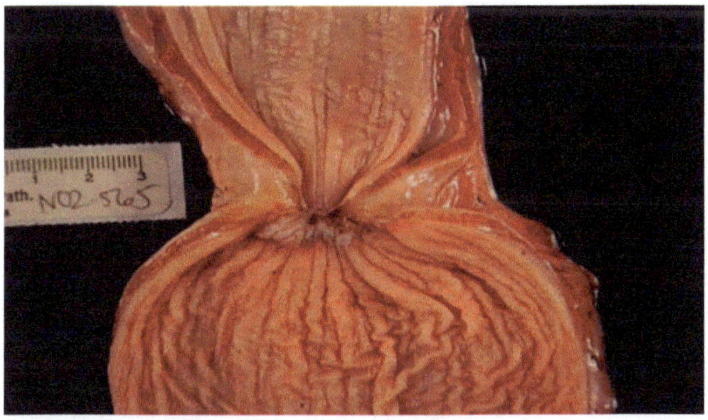

**Figure 6.36.** Horse. Esophagus. Foreign Body (Choke). Stricture developed from the healing process of the necrotic mucosa after removal of the object. (Reprinted with permission from the Animal Technology Institute of Taiwan, Republic of China)

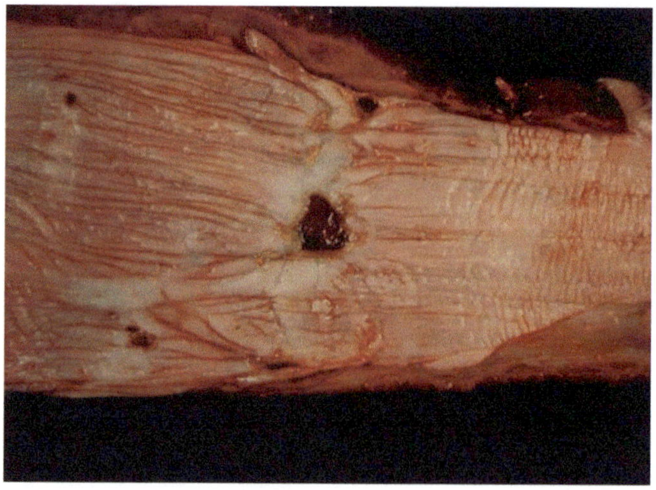

**Figure 6.37.** Horse. Esophagus. Perforation. Result of injury from passing a medical instrument (gastric tube). Erosion and ulceration of the esophagus are described in the section on gastroduodenal ulcer disease in Chapter 2, "Diseases of Foals and Juveniles."

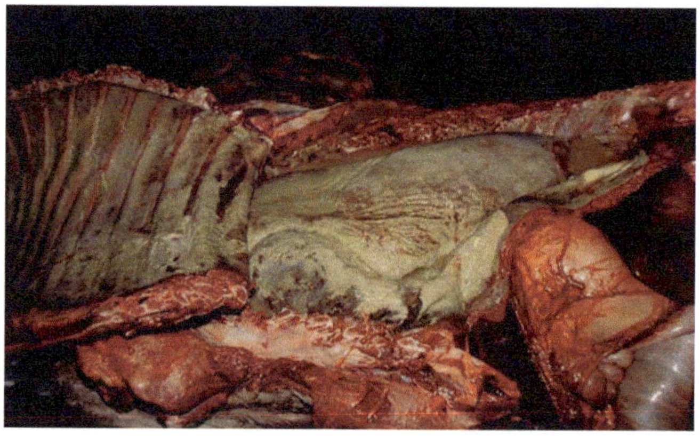

**Figure 6.38.** Horse. Esophagus. Stricture interfering with food passage resulted in perforation, septic fibrinous pleuritis, and empyema.

## *2. Inflammation*

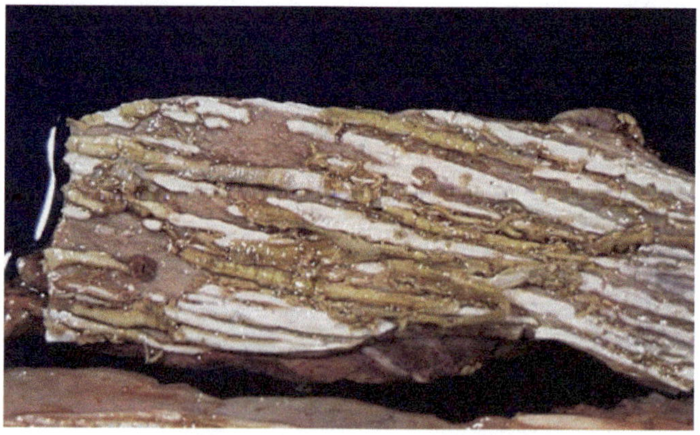

**Figure 6.39.** Horse. Esophagus. Reflux Esophagitis. Ascending linear erosive and ulcerative changes are present in the mucosa that also exhibits hyperkeratosis. Differential diagnosis: corrosive and chemical burns.

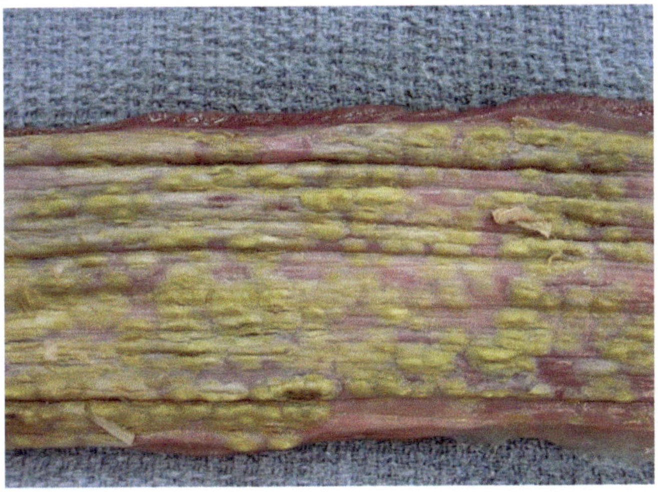

**Figure 6.40.** Horse. Esophagus. Parakeratosis due to *Candida* sp. Opportunistic infection in a leukopenic horse infected with *Salmonella* sp. and treated with antimicrobials.

### *3. Idiopathic hypertrophy of the distal esophagus*

Older horses (12.5 ± 5.6 years) frequently develop along the caudal 20 cm of the distal esophagus a thickening of the wall without exhibiting clinical signs of dysfunction, an incidental finding at necropsy. This is due to hypertrophy of the smooth muscle cells involving the circular layer of the tunica muscularis without fibrosis or inflammation. The cause remains elusive. The condition does not develop in the proximal portions of the esophagus that is composed of skeletal musculature or in the middle 20 cm that is skeletal muscle intermixed with smooth muscle cells.

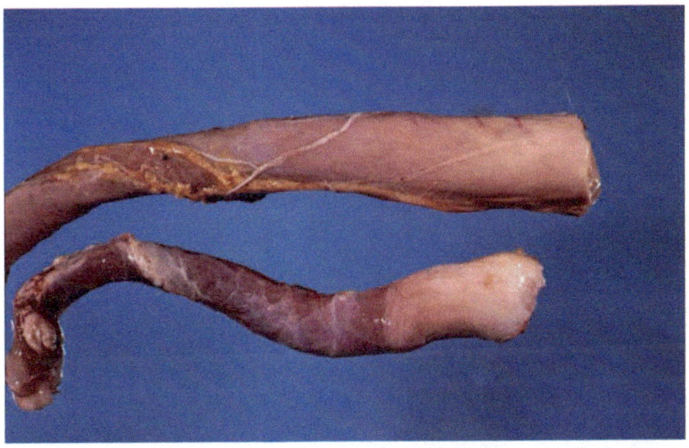

**Figure 6.41.** Horse. Distal Esophagus. Muscular Segmental Distal Hypertrophy.

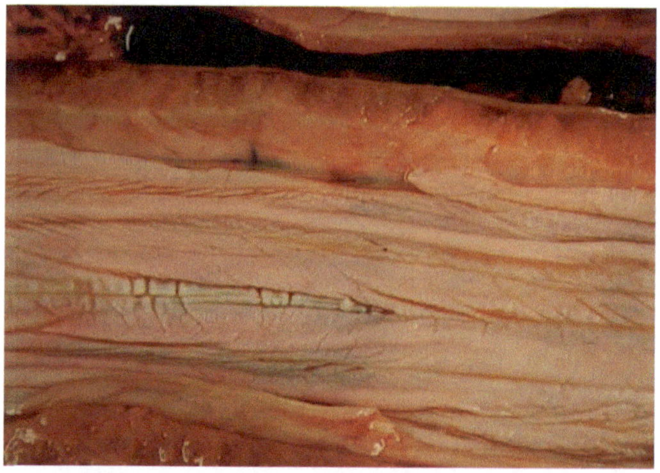

**Figure 6.42.** Horse. Distal Esophagus. Muscular Hypertrophy (Courtesy Dr. P. Habecker, University of Pennsylvania.)

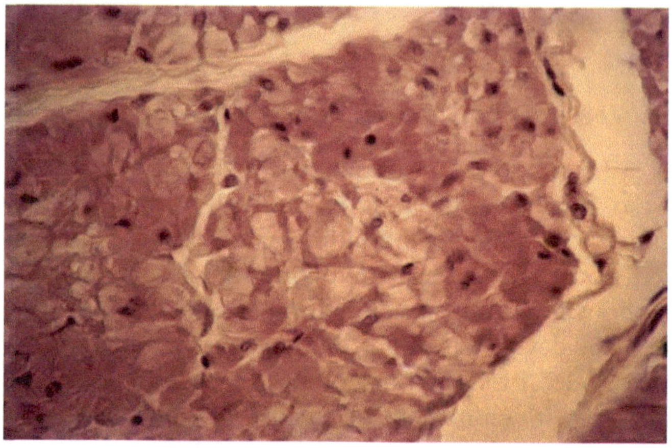

**Figure 6.43.** Horse. Distal Esophagus. Muscular Hypertrophy. Several smooth muscle myocytes exhibit hydropic changes in sarcoplasm. (H&E)

### *4. Neoplasia*

Primary tumors arising from the esophageal mucosa are rare and generally squamous cell carcinomas.

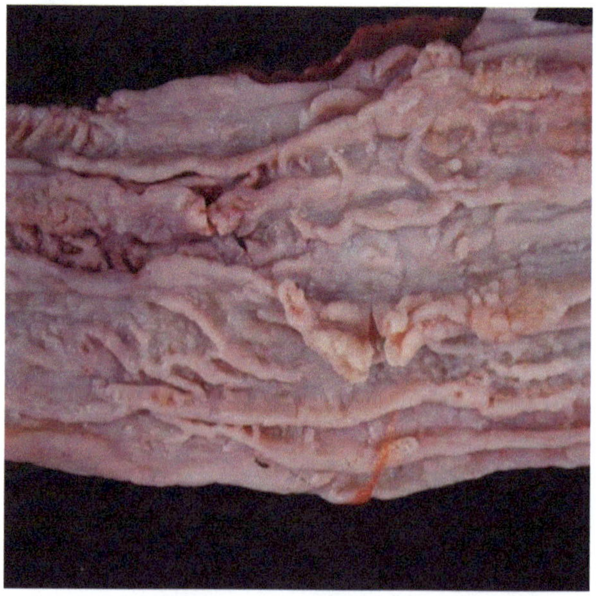

**Figure 6.44.** Horse. Esophagus. Squamous Cell Carcinoma. The mucosa is characterized by small discrete elevations distorting the longitudinal mucosal folds.

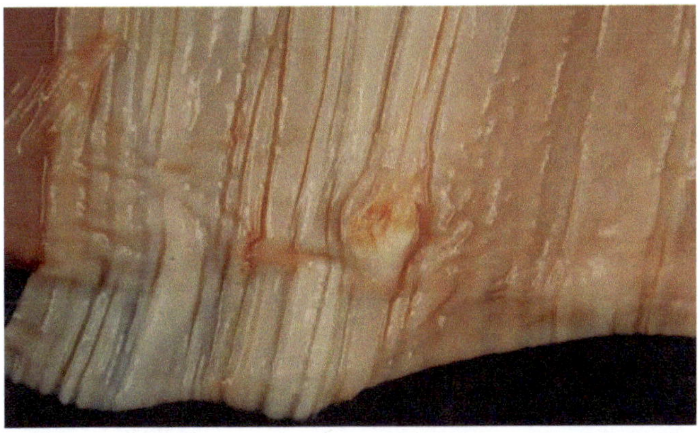

**Figure 6.45.** Horse. Distal Esophagus. Papilloma. This small, cauliflower-like, single elevation of the mucosa of the distal esophagus represents equine papillomavirus-induced papilloma.

## III. Diseases of the stomach

### *1. Gastric rupture*

Most of the cases are the result of overeating, impaction, ileus, or intestinal obstruction; some of the cases are simply idiopathic. Horses with histories of both acute and chronic colic are susceptible to gastric ruptures. Death occurs before there is time for peritonitis to develop. Gastric rupture is one of the causes of sudden death in the horse. Gastric rupture typically occurs at the greater curvature. Rupture sequence is: (1) muscularis, (2) serosa, (3) mucosa.

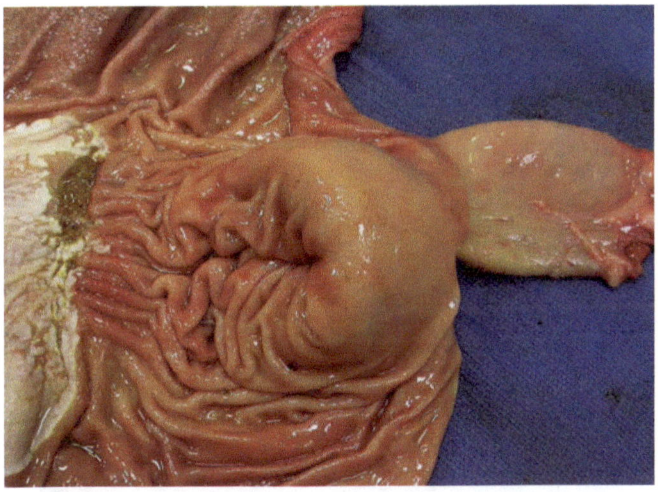

**Figure 6.46.** Horse. Stomach. Pyloric Sphincter Hypertrophy. A distinct bulge of the mucosa at the pylorus is the result of marked hypertrophy of the sphincter muscle. This might be a cause for gastric rupture. Other causes of gastric rupture are impaction or intestinal obstructions such as strangulating lipoma, ileus.

Events of gastric rupture are shown in Figure 6.47, Figure 6.48, Figure 6.49, and Figure 6.50.

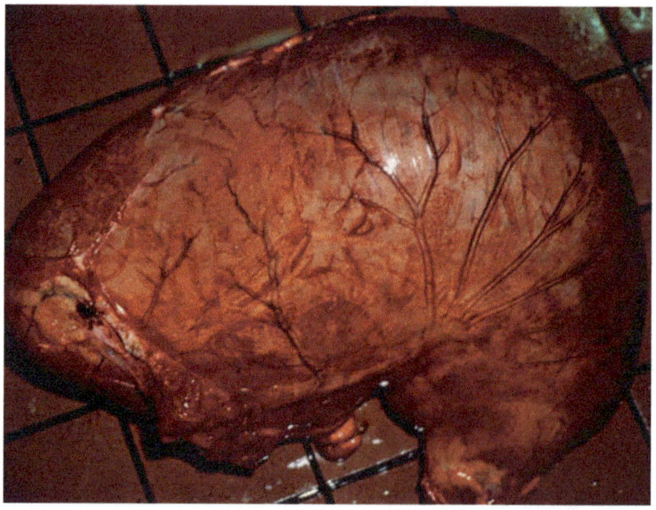

**Figure 6.47.** Horse. Stomach. Distension. The stomach is markedly distended but not ruptured. Overeating with grass/alfalfa hay induces risk for rupture; grain may reduce risk. Gastric distension also occurs in grass sickness. (Reprinted with permission from the Animal Technology Institute of Taiwan, Republic of China.)

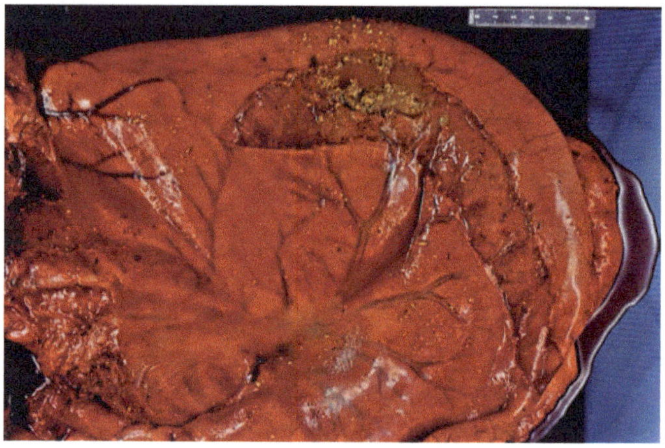

**Figure 6.48.** Horse. Stomach. Incomplete Rupture. The stretched serosa has dissected from the muscularis. The rent in the serosa usually is the longest; it is less in the tunica muscularis, and the smallest in the mucosa. The tunica muscularis apparently is the weakest of the stomach layers. (Reprinted with permission from the Animal Technology Institute of Taiwan, Republic of China.)

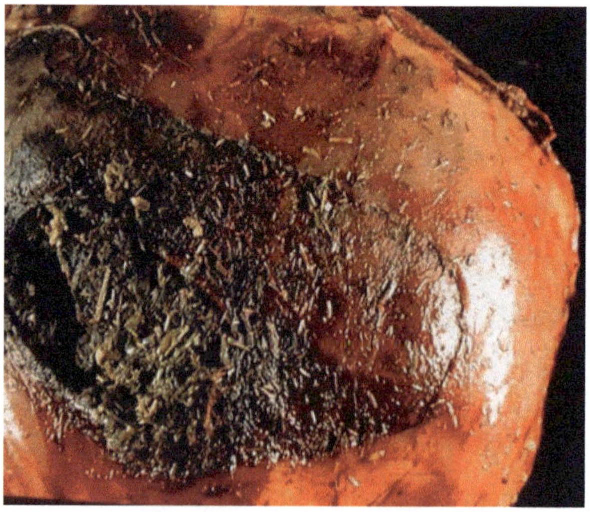

**Figure 6.49.** Horse. Stomach. Full-Wall Rupture. Feed has spilled to the serosal surface. (Reprinted with permission from the Animal Technology Institute of Taiwan, Republic of China.)

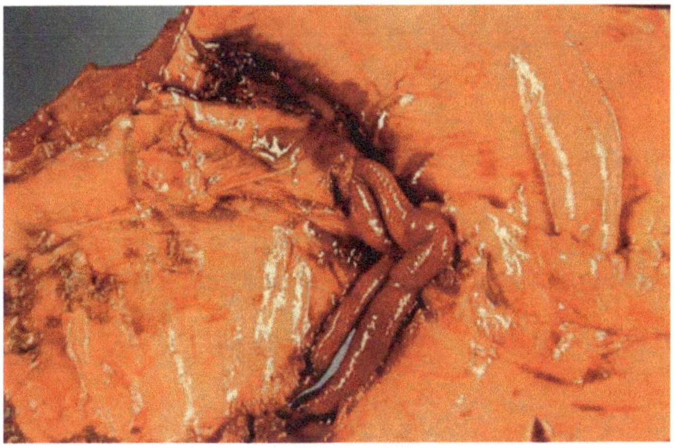

**Figure 6.50.** Horse. Stomach. Mucosa. The torn mucosa has swollen, ragged, hemorrhagic edges differentiating it as an antemortem rupture from a postmortem rupture. (Reprinted with permission from the Animal Technology Institute of Taiwan, Republic of China.)

### *2. Gastric ulcers*

Gastroduodenal ulcer disease in foals is presented in Chapter 2, "Diseases of Foals and Juveniles." Mucosal tears at the plicate margin are normal findings due to incomplete keratinization. In the literature they mistakenly have been diagnosed as erosions/ulcers.

Gastric ulcers are largely recognized in performance horses. Ulcers may affect both compartments of the equine stomach. They have to be differentiated from erosions, which are shallow, not extending beyond the basal membrane of the mucosa. There are several causes for gastric erosions and ulcers: dietary, parasitic, trauma (stomach tube), neoplasia, and drugs. Interestingly, an association with *Helicobacter* sp. has not been convincingly verified with gastric ulcers in the horse. On rare occasions, *Salmonella enterica* can be isolated from the glandular mucosa ulcers in conjunction with intestinal salmonellosis. Antemortem diagnosis of ulceration is achieved by endoscopy. Scoring systems as to severity and location have been developed. Clinical signs include recurrent colic, poor appetite, and weight loss.

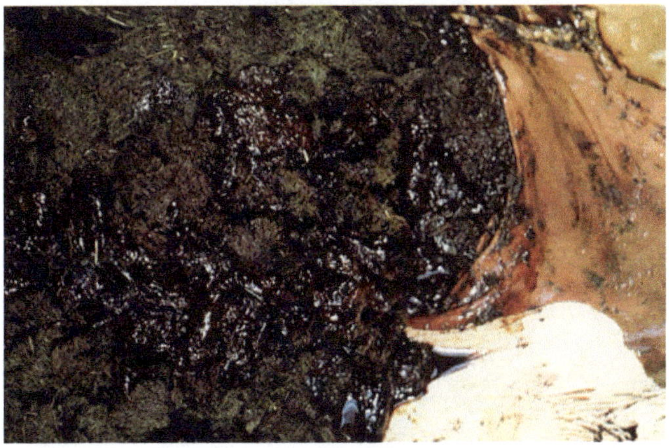

**Figure 6.51.** Horse. Stomach. Bleeds. Clotted blood is intermingled with ingesta. The blood was ingested and digested from a bleeding guttural pouch mycosis and had an apple cider odor. Differential diagnosis: bleeding ulcer.

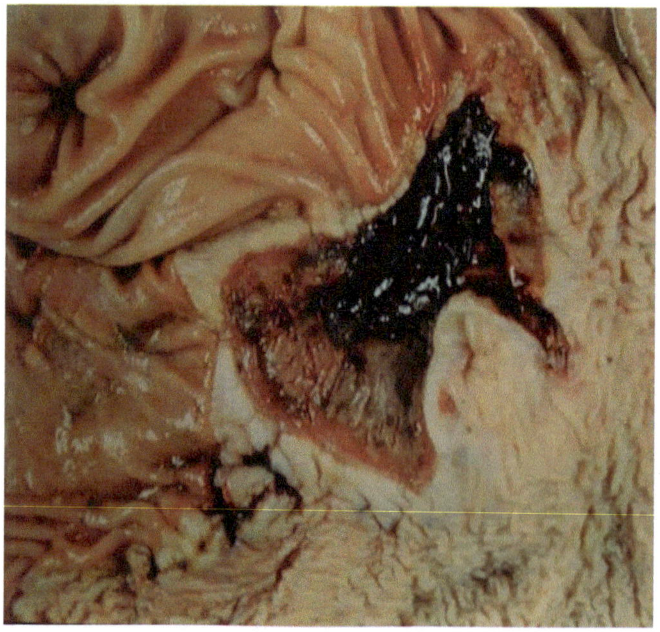

**Figure 6.52.** Horse. Stomach. Bleeding Ulcer. A crater in the nonglandular compartment of the stomach is covered by blood. The mucosal defect was deep enough to involve submucosal blood vessels to cause bleeding into the intestinal tract. This adult horse had a history of being repeatedly treated with NSAIDs. (Reprinted with permission from the Animal Technology Institute of Taiwan, Republic of China.)

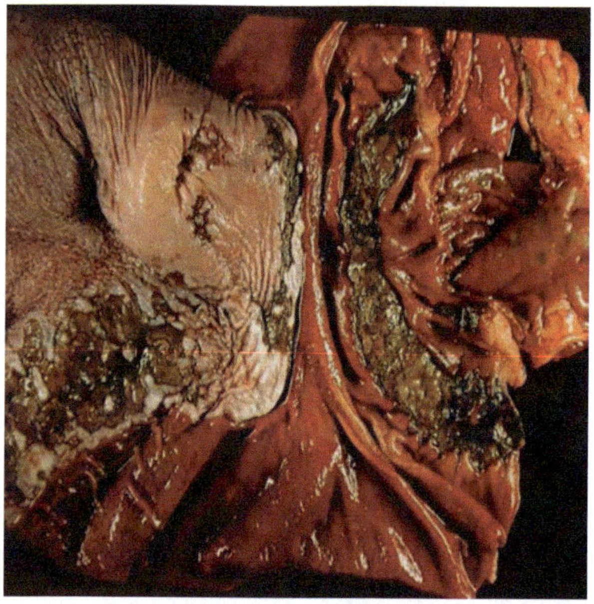

**Figure 6.53.** Horse. Stomach. Chronic Ulcers. These frequently occur in racehorses.

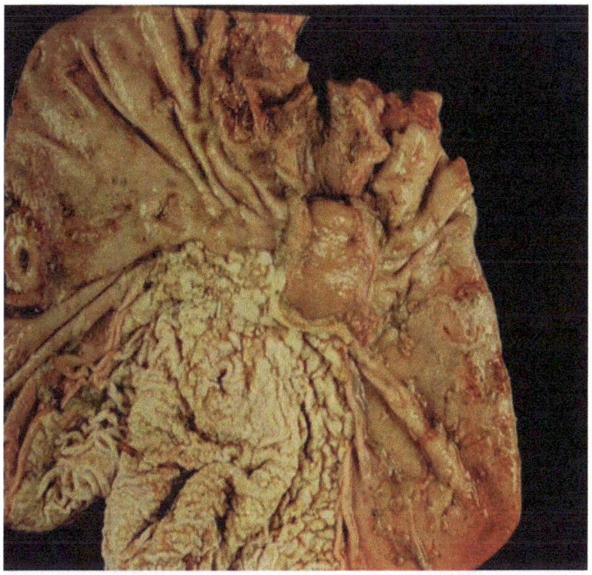

**Figure 6.54.** Horse. Stomach. Mucosal Breaks and Elevations. Hyperkeratosis of nonglandular stomach. Erosions and shallow ulcers of glandular mucosa are present. (Reprinted with permission from the Animal Technology Institute of Taiwan, Republic of China.)

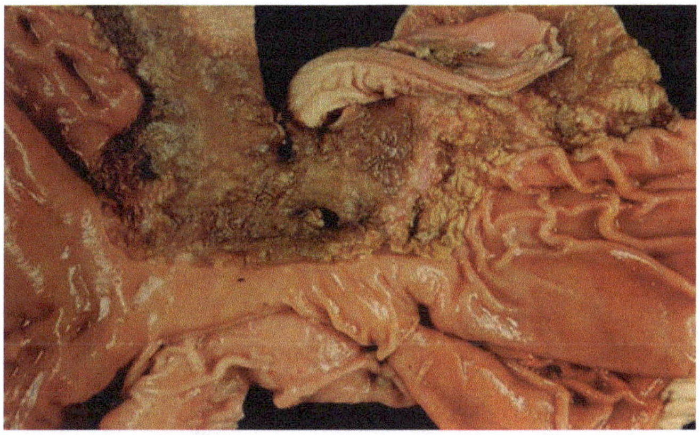

**Figure 6.55.** Horse. Stomach. Perforation. This event may be a fatal complication leading to peritonitis. (Reprinted with permission from the Animal Technology Institute of Taiwan, Republic of China.)

In the Southwest of the United States, alfalfa hay when cropped and crimped to hay may be contaminated with entrapped three-striped blister beetles, belonging to the genus *Epicauta* sp. The beetles contain terpenoid cantharidin. As little as 4–6 mg of dried *Epicauta* beetles can kill a horse due to hypocalcemia, hypomagnesemia, or cardiac failure from necrosis of myocardial tissue. The mechanism for the metabolic changes is unknown.

### Cantharidin toxicosis – Gross findings

- Within the gastrointestinal tract und urothelium, cantharadin causes mucosal blisters, hemorrhage, and necrosis.
- The heart may exhibit myocardial necrosis

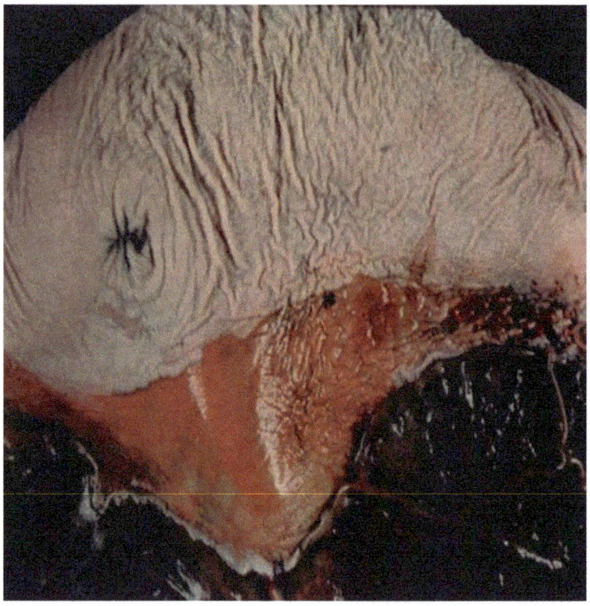

**Figure 6.56.** Horse. Stomach. Hyperemia. Focal reddening in the glandular mucosa is caused by *Epicauta* sp. Small erosions are present.

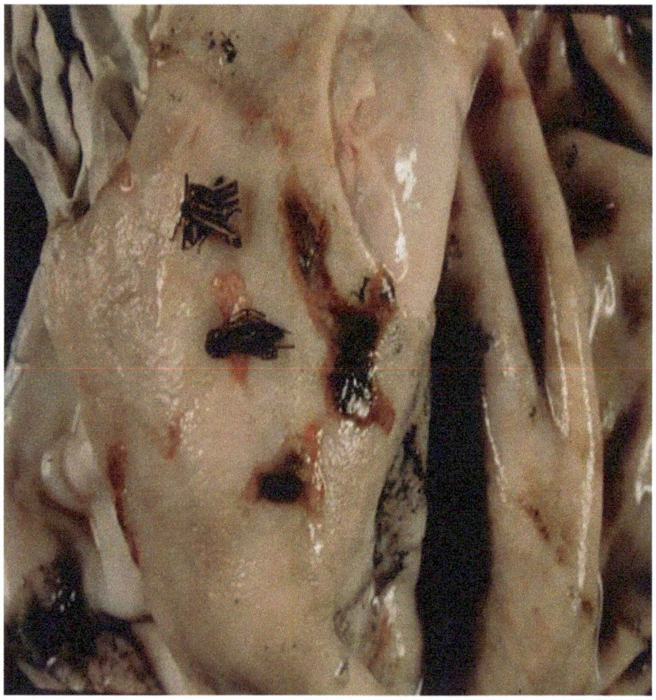

**Figure 6.57.** Horse. Stomach. *Epicauta* sp. Detection of parts of blister beetles in stomach contents screened via funnel supports the suspicion of cantharides toxicity.

## Cantharidin toxicosis – Mechanism of action

- Inhibition of protein phosphatase 2A
- Change of permeability of mitochondrial membranes
- Mucosal acantholysis

## Cantharidin toxicosis – Differential diagnosis

- Ingestion of chemicals or corrosives
- Acute arsenic toxicosis

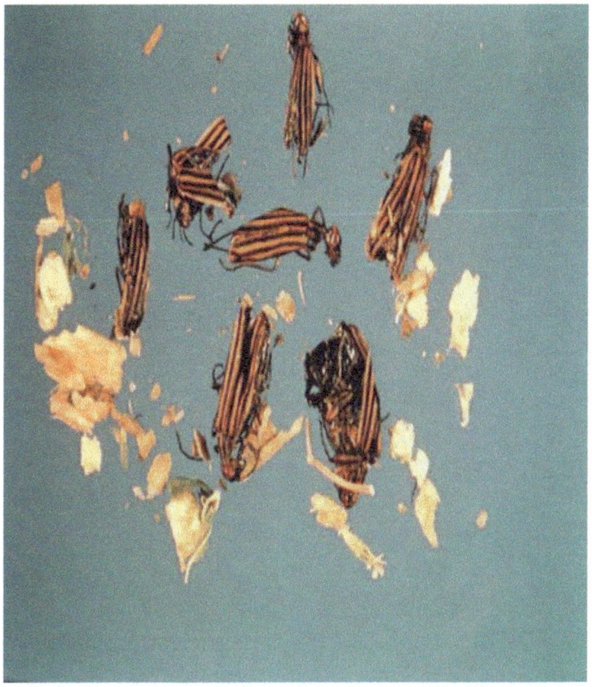

**Figure 6.58.** Wood Shavings. *Epicauta* sp. Hay shook from compressed bails releases blister beetles.

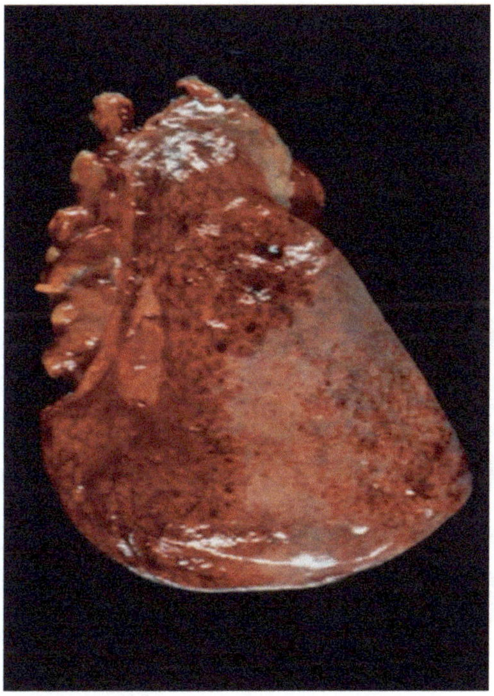

**Figure 6.59.** Horse. Urinary Bladder. Hyperemia. Reddening of the mucosa indicates hyperemia caused by *Epicauta* sp.

## Cantharidin toxicosis – Fact sheet

**Definition:** Toxicosis from cantharidin produced by blister beetles (Epicauta sp) entrapped in alfalfa hay

### Clinical features

- Abdominal pain
- Anorexia
- Hypocalcemia, hypomagnesemia

### Diagnosis

- Chemical analysis for cantharadin in urine or stomach contents by spectrophotometry
- Finding of blister beetles or their remnants in gastric contents

### *3. Gastric parasites*

In a 1998 study of 70 slaughtered horses in the Netherlands, *Trichostrongylus axei* was the most prevalent gastric parasite (51.4%), followed by *Gasterophilus intestinalis* (41.4%) and *Habronema* sp. (4.3%). Gastrointestinal parasites largely have disappeared since the introduction of effective anthelmintics such as ivermectin.

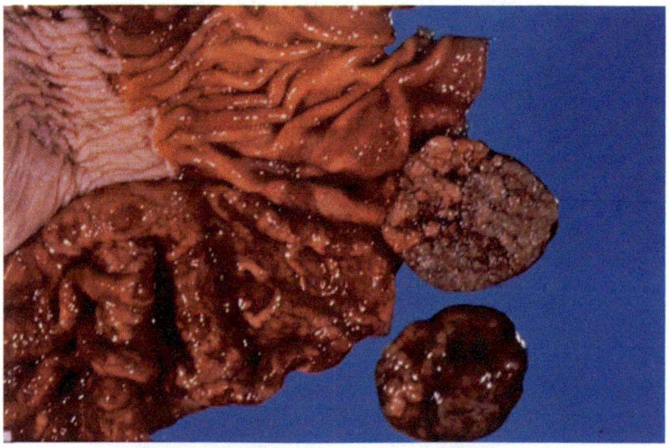

**Figure 6.60.** Horse. Glandular Mucosa. Fibrinous Hyperplastic Gastritis. Trichostrongylosis. The rugae are largely accentuated and covered by a fibrinous exudate. (Reprinted with permission from the Animal Technology Institute of Taiwan, Republic of China.)

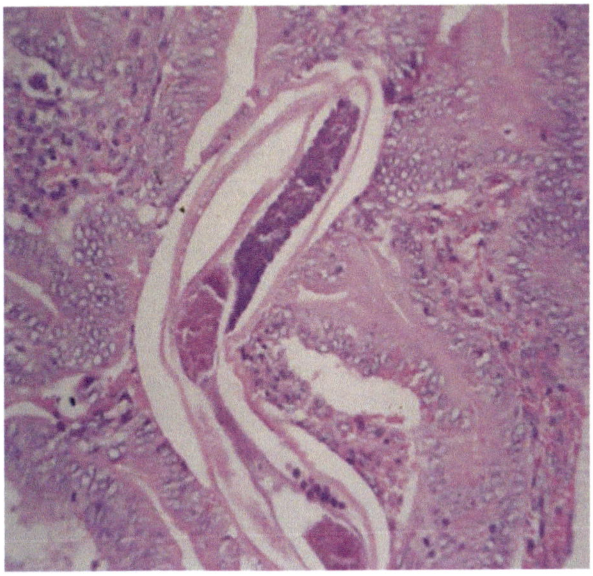

**Figure 6.61.** Horse. Stomach. Mucosa. Thickening is due to glandular hyperplasia and the presence of nematode larvae and/or adults within the gastric gland lumina with no inflammatory reaction. (H&E)

The adult worm of the nematode *Trichostrongylus axei* is tiny (0.5–0.8 cm long). The parasite enters the horse's stomach and intestine when the animal eats grass infected with eggs. The eggs hatch and the larvae move into the stomach and intestine where they mature. They induce a chronic gastroenteritis clinically. Affected horses typically graze with cattle or sheep also shedding eggs of the nematode.

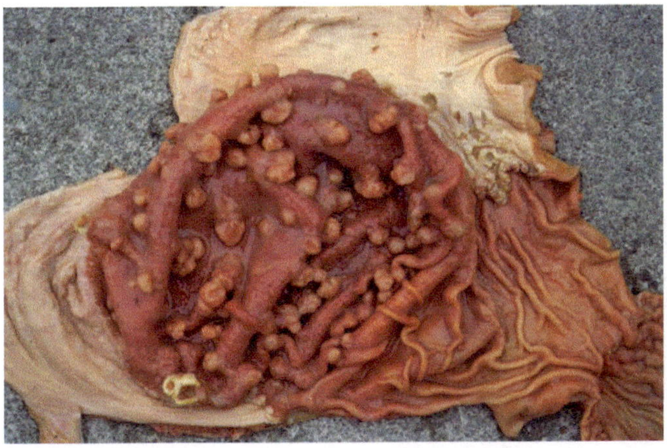

**Figure 6.62.** Horse. Glandular Stomach. Polypoid Rugal Hypertrophy. This condition is frequently encountered in ponies and should serve as differential diagnosis to trichostrongylosis (Courtesy Dr. L. Roth-Johnson, Eastham, MA.)

**Figure 6.63.** Horse. Stomach. Botfly. Larvae of botflies are loosely attached to the glandular mucosa just across the margo plicatus. Their location identifies them as *Gasterophilus intestinalis*. *G. nasalis* larvae are found embedded in the mucosa of the duodenum near the pylorus, whereas larvae of *G. hemorrhoidalis* attach to the tongue or mucosa of the mouth. When removed, larval attachment sites are associated with small, round, red ulcers.

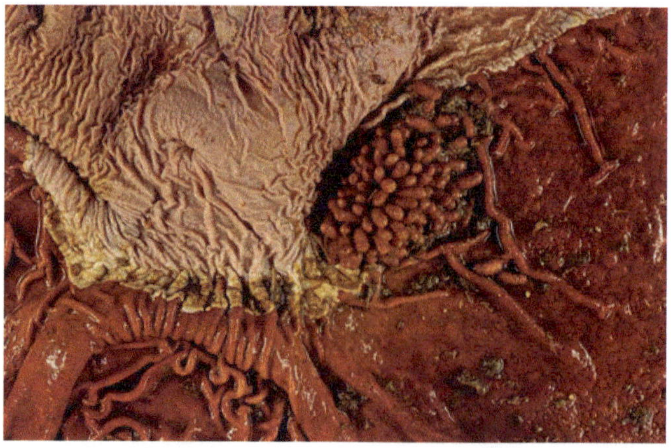

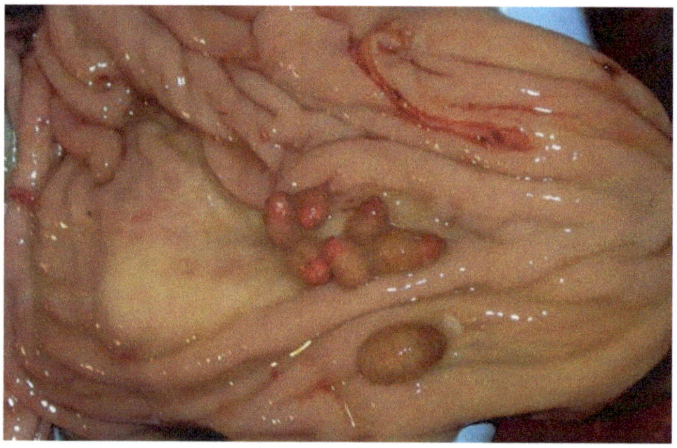

**Figure 6.64.** Horse. Pylorus. Botfly. Larvae of *Gasterophilus nasalis*.

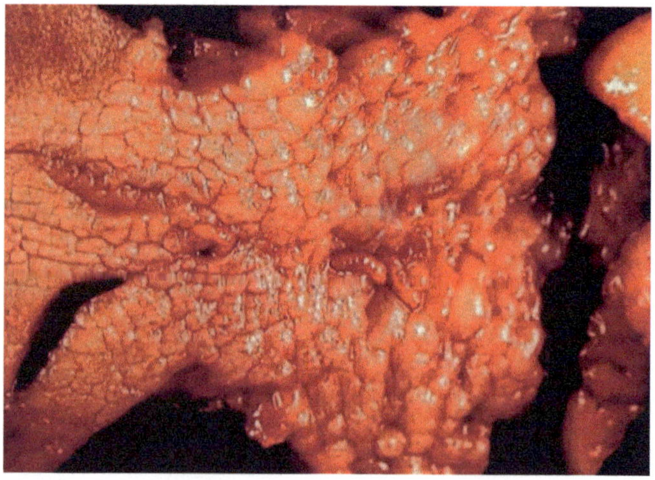

**Figure 6.65.** Horse. Tongue. Botfly. Eggs of *Gasterophilus hemorrhoidalis* attach to the hairs of the lips and larvae migrate into the mouth as seen here on the surface of the tongue. There is also evidence of grade 2 tonsillar lymphoid hyperplasia.

**Figure 6.66.** Horse. Skin. Botfly Eggs. The adult flies of the three species of horse bots have their eggs glued to the hair of various body parts of the horse, especially forelimbs and shoulder. Larvae hatch usually after the animal's licks the infested hair.

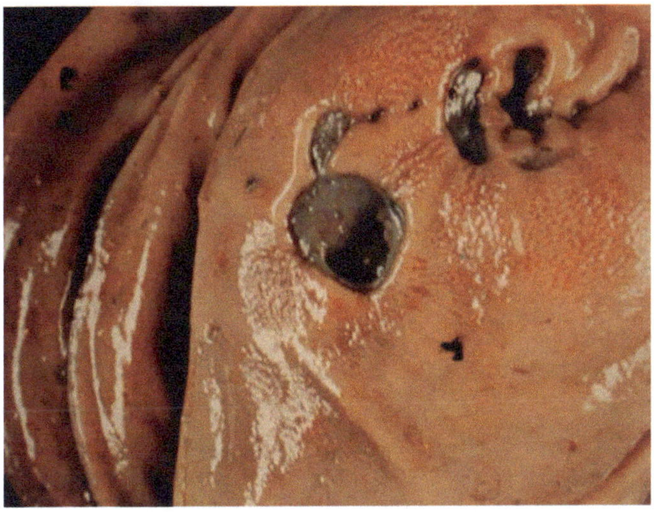

**Figure 6.67.** Horse. Stomach. Glandular Part. Parasitic Ulcerative Nodular Gastritis. A tumor-like swelling is present in the glandular mucosa compatible with infestation by *Habronema* sp. Several mucosal defects represent brood pouches of the adult stomach worms and a route for eggs to be passed into the lumen of the stomach. (Reprinted with permission from the Animal Technology Institute of Taiwan, Republic of China.)

The three species of stomach worms are *Habronema muscae*, *Habronema microstoma*, and *Draschia megastoma (insulae)*. Adults may measure 6–25 mm in size. Adults of *Draschia* burrow into the mucosa; the other species are free on the mucosa. The eggs or larvae are ingested by house flies (*Musca domestica*) or stable flies (*Stomoxys calcitrans*). Migrating larvae of *Draschia* may cause pulmonary nodules. Clinical signs are usually not observed.

## Gastric parasites – Fact sheet

### Types

- Nematodes: *Trichostrongylus axei*
  *Gasterophilus* sp.
  *Habronema* sp.; *Draschia* megastoma

### Location

- Glandular stomach, duodenum, tongue, pharynx

### Clinical signs

- Inconspicuous

### Gross findings

- Diffuse mucosal hypertrophy: *T. axei*
- Distinct focal shallow erosions: *G.intestinalis*
- Tumorlike mucosal elevations: *D. megastoma*

### 4. *Gastric neoplasia*

Squamous cell carcinoma is the most common primary gastric neoplasm in horses. It arises from the nonglandular compartment of the stomach. Affected horses ranged in age from 9 to 25 years in one study (median: 18 years). There apparently is no breed or sex predisposition. Inappetence, weight loss, lethargy, and tachypnea are consistent clinical findings. Hypercalcemia of malignancy occasionally is seen in some horses. Metastases occurred in most of the horses (18 of 23) in the study mentioned. Other rarer primary neoplasms encountered are gastrointestinal stromal tumor, leiomyoma, mesothelioma, adenocarcinoma, gastrinoma, fibropapilloma, and lymphoma.

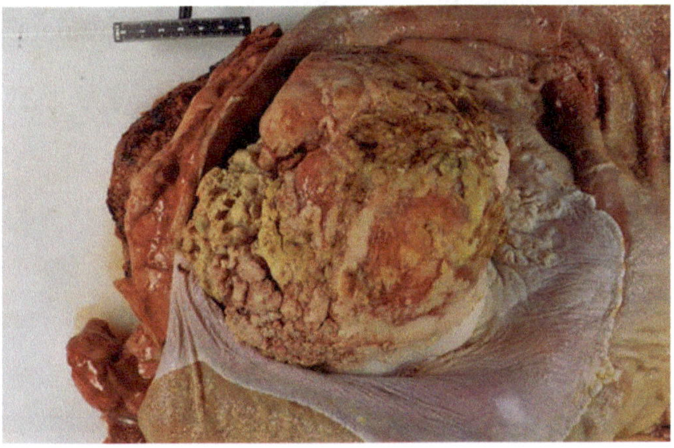

**Figure 6.68.** Horse. Stomach. Squamous Cell Carcinoma. A fleshy, ulcerative, cauliflower-like growth occupies the entire surface of the nonglandular stomach.

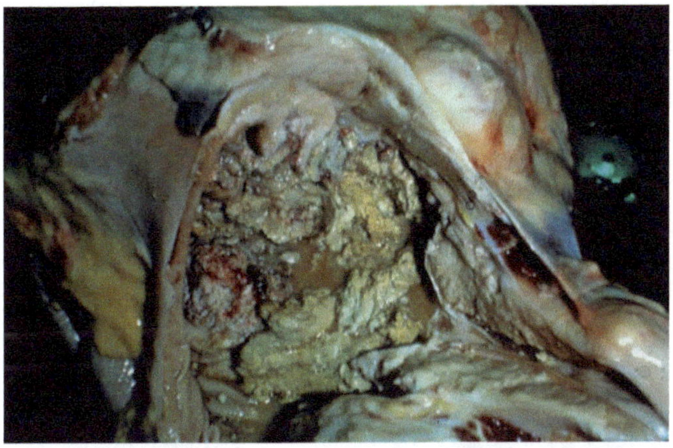

**Figure 6.69.** Horse. Stomach. Squamous Cell Carcinoma. A large crateriform moist mass has distended the entire stomach. Because there is marked necrosis of the keratinizing tumor, affected horses may exhibit malodorous breath clinically.

# IV. Noninfectious diseases of the intestinal tract

The intestinal mucosa is the most important stratum for digestion and absorption of nutrients and water. Nutrients, electrolytes, and water only become part of the body after they have crossed the lining of the intestine to enter the bloodstream. Digestion and protection from toxins and infectious agents are major functions of the intestine. The small intestinal tract is morphologically and functionally different from the large intestinal tract by the presence of villi that project from folds into the intestinal lumen. Most absorption and secretion occur in the small intestine. The principal function of the large intestine is absorption of sodium, chloride, and water as well as secretion of mucus.

The intestinal tract has its own specialized immune protection known as gut-associated lymphoid tissue (GALT). Both cellular and humoral immune responses represent defense mechanisms against pathogens and toxins.

## 1. Anomalies

### a. Atresia

Illustrated in Chapter 2, "Diseases of Foals and Juveniles."

### b. Aganglionosis

Described in Chapter 2, "Diseases of Foals and Juveniles."

### c. Meckel's diverticulum

This structure is considered to be a vestigial remnant of the omphalomesenteric duct and usually an incidental finding. It can become impacted with feces or give rise to intestinal strangulation. It is very rare in horses.

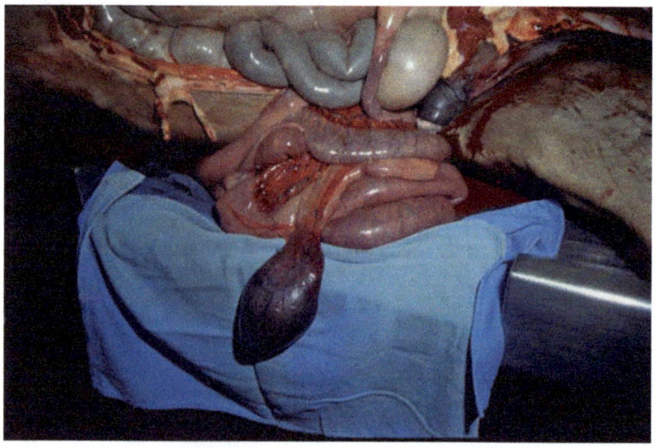

**Figure 6.70.** Horse. Small Intestine. Meckel's Diverticulum. A tubular structure is attached to and connected with the ileum at the antimesenteric surface. It can reach a length of 30 cm. Its mucosal lining is similar to that of the ileum.

### d. Ileal hypertrophy

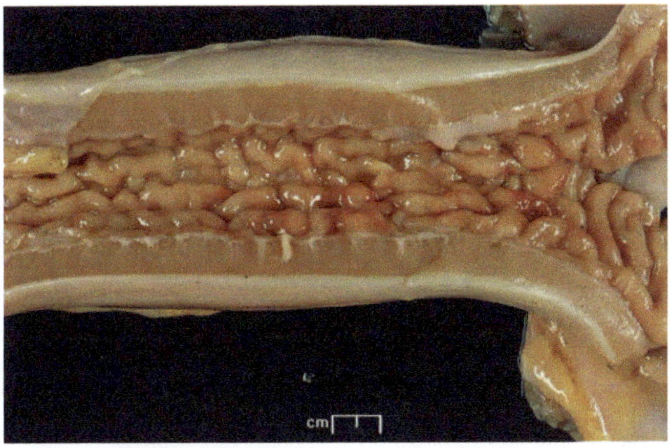


**Figure 6.71.** Horse. Ileum. Distal Hypertrophy. (Reprinted with permission from the Animal Technology Institute of Taiwan, Republic of China.)

The thickening is the result of muscular hypertrophy and hyperplasia, perhaps predisposed by ileocecal valve malfunction. Unlike in the distal esophagus, the thickening of the distal ileum can be associated with impaction and even perforation resulting in peritonitis. Despite increased muscle mass due to a lack of stroma in the wall, the impaction may predispose to the formation of a diverticulum characterized by a thin wall.

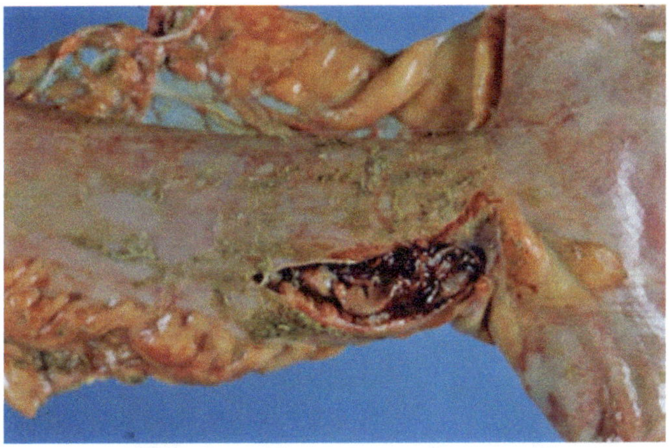

**Figure 6.72.** Horse. Ileum. Distal Hypertrophy and Rupture. (Reprinted with permission from the Animal Technology Institute of Taiwan, Republic of China.)

## 2. Displacements and strangulations

The vast majority of intestinal disorders are mechanical events related to anatomic peculiarities of the horse and are the main causes for equine colic. Other disturbances are primary vascular or neurogenic in etiology. All of them are responsible for obstruction to the passage of ingesta (strangulation) and venous stasis. Clinically they are associated with loss of water and electrolytes. Cardiovascular collapse or sepsis is the cause of death.

*a. Volvulus*

Volvulus is defined as a rotation of intestinal loops around the mesenteric attachment and occurs with frequency in species with a long small intestinal tract such as the horse.

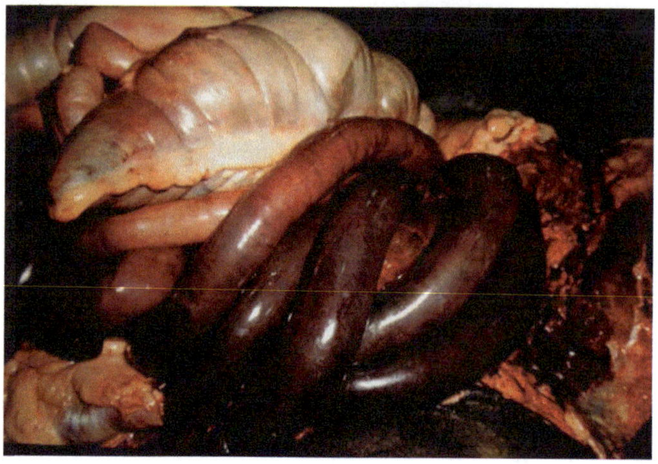

**Figure 6.73.** Horse. Small Intestine. Volvulus. Segments of the jejunum have rotated around the mesenteric attachment. The affected loops are red-blue due to venous engorgement from outflow obstruction. Devitalization of the intestinal wall leads to a breakdown of the intestinal barrier system.

*b. Torsion*

Torsion is defined as a rotation of intestinal segments around its longitudinal axis. This mainly occurs with segments of the large colon. Torsions can be up to 540 degrees. A different, rare variant of colon dislocation is a non-strangulating displacement of the right ventral colon causing compression of the major bile duct as the segments of the mesocolon come to rest close to the bile duct resulting in retention icterus as a clinical sign. There is no vascular compromise in this condition.

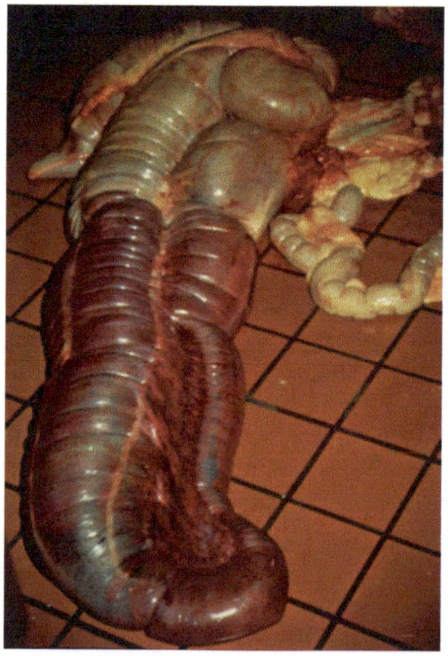

**Figure 6.74.** Horse. Colon. Torsion. Segments of the left colon have a deep reddish discoloration with sharp demarcation from the nonrotated, more fixed right colon segments.

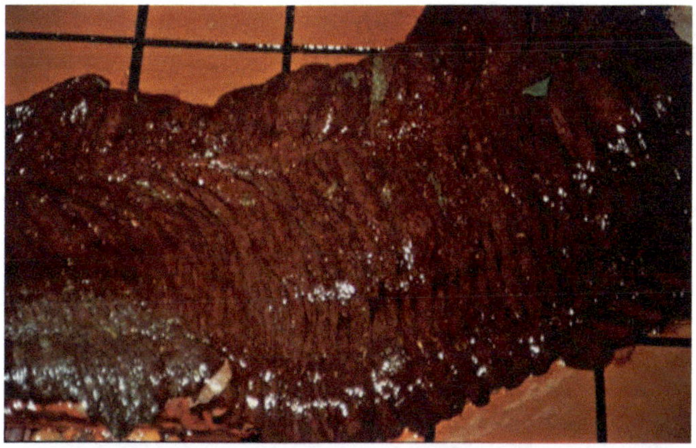

**Figure 6.75.** Horse. Colon. Torsion. When opened, the entire wall of the rotated colon is reddened and thickened by fluid (edema and some hemorrhage in wall). Unlike with enteric infections, the mucosa remains intact with intestinal displacements.

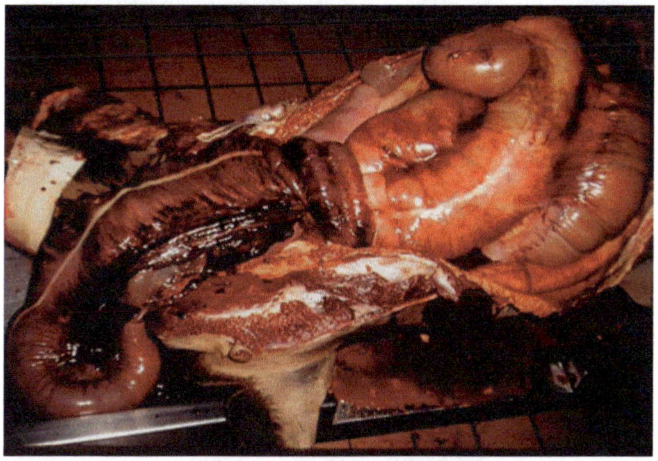

**Figure 6.76.** Horse. Colon. Torsion of 540 degrees.

*c. Strangulating lipomas*

Lipomas arise from the intestinal serosal or mesenteric surfaces of older horses. As they grow, lipomas change from sessile to pedunculated forms that may wrap around the adjacent intestinal loop to cause strangulation via intestinal knotting. Larger lipomas may outgrow their blood supply as they twist around their peduncle and as a consequence may undergo ischemic necrosis, color changes, and mineralization.

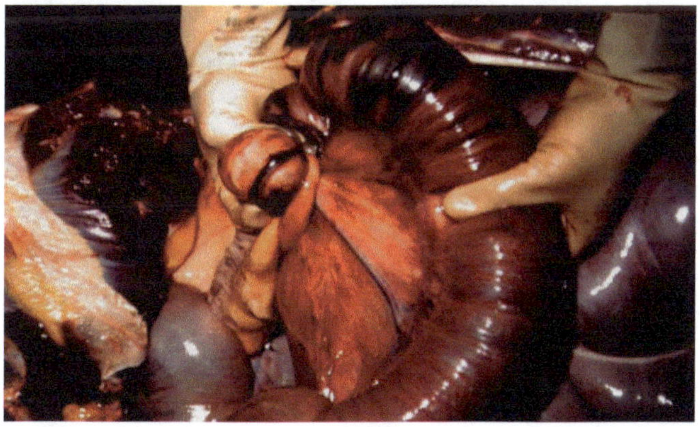

**Figure 6.77.** Horse. Small Intestine. Lipoma. A mass the size of a golf ball off the mesentery has knotted around the adjacent jejunum causing segmental hemorrhagic necrosis of the loop. (Reprinted with permission from the Animal Technology Institute of Taiwan, Republic of China.)

*d. Intussusception*

This condition is defined as telescoping of one intestinal segment into another. The slipping portion is the intussuscipiens; the receiving portion is the intussusceptum. Intestinal intussusceptions can be preceded by intestinal hypermotility or endoparasitism (ascarids and tapeworms). In the horse typical sites are ileocecum or cecocolon. Sporadic jejunal intussusception can occur.

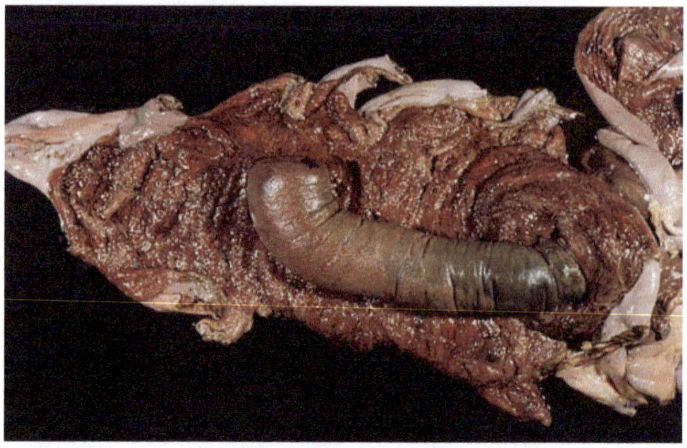

**Figure 6.78.** Horse. Ileocecal Intussusception. The terminal ileum has slipped into the cecum at the ileocecal junction. Ischemic necrosis is indicated by reddish, greenish discoloration. Postmortem intussusception has to be differentiated from antemortem telescoping. The difference is that the invaginating postmortem segment lacks adhesion and discoloration and can be easily removed.

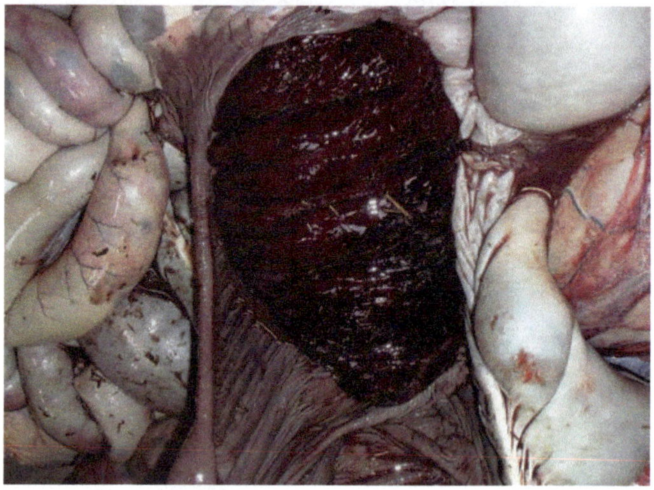

**Figure 6.79.** Horse. Cecocolic Intussusception.

*e. Foramen epiploicum herniation*

The foramen epiploicum constitutes an anatomic gap between the caudate lobe of the liver, stomach, and duodenum. This loose gap allows for invagination of portions of small intestine to occur resulting in strangulation of the displaced segment of the intestine.

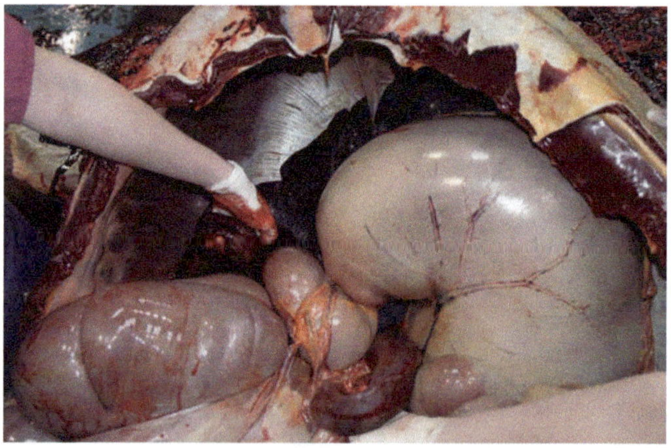

**Figure 6.80.** Horse. Cranial Abdomen. Foramen Epiploicum. Anatomic location (hand) of foramen epiploicum as gap between caudal liver, duodenum, and stomach.

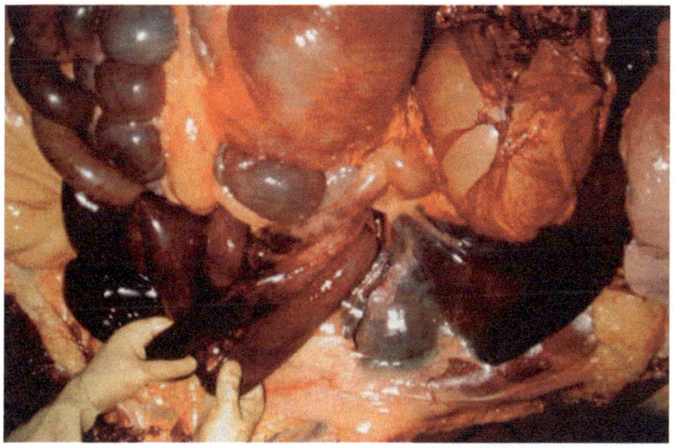

**Figure 6.81.** Horse. Small Intestine. Foramen Epiploicum Herniation. A loop of jejunum (hand) has slipped into the loose space between liver and duodenum. (Reprinted with permission from the Animal Technology Institute of Taiwan, Republic of China.)

*f. Nephrosplenic ligament entrapment*

The soft tissue site giving rise to intestinal entrapment acts like a fold between the spleen and left kidney.

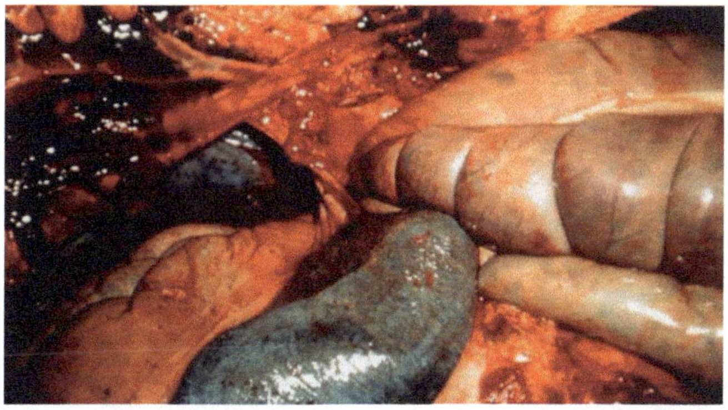

**Figure 6.82.** Horse. Spleen. Nephrosplenic Ligament Entrapment. This condition is defined as a form of left dorsal colon displacement where the ascending colon positioned dorsal to the spleen becomes entrapped in the space of the nephrosplenic ligament. (Reprinted with permission from the Animal Technology Institute of Taiwan, Republic of China.)

*g. Mesodiverticular band*

This structure is a vestigial remnant of the vitelline vessel.

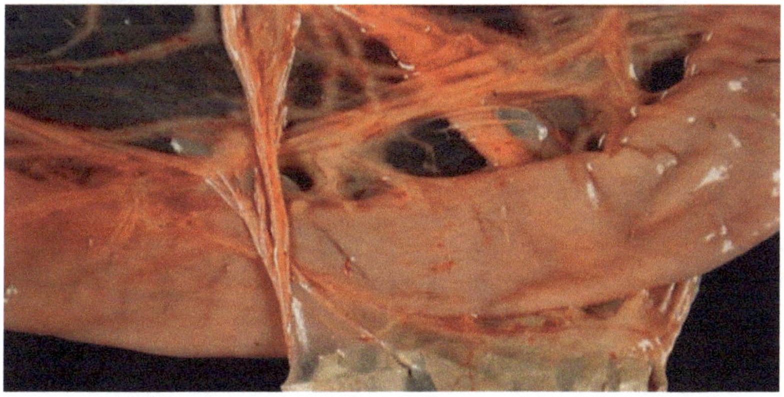

**Figure 6.83.** Horse. Small Intestine. Mesodiverticular Band. A stringlike structure has crossed the jejunum from one side of the mesenteric attachment to the other. Early surgical removal of the band is a cure preventing devitalization of the constricted loop. (Reprinted with permission from the Animal Technology Institute of Taiwan, Republic of China.)

*h. Mesentery rent*

Small intestinal loops can slip through tissue gaps within the mesentery.

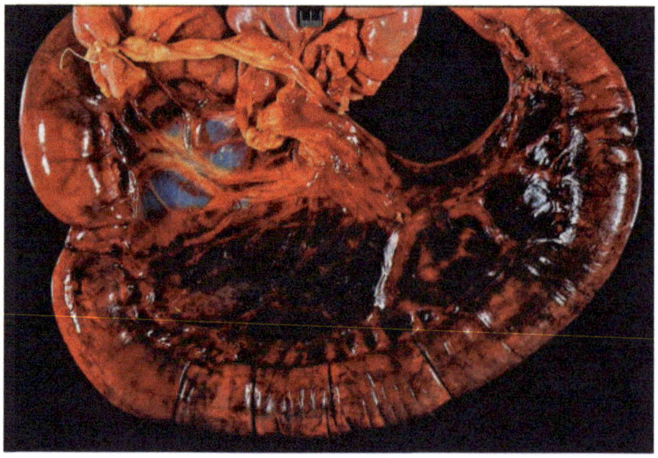

**Figure 6.84.** Horse. Mesentery. Rent. A congenital defect or tear has been the cause of jejunal invagination.

*i. Diaphragmatic hernia*

This condition is congenital or acquired via trauma. Gaps at the musculotendinous junction of the ventral diaphragm allow major portions of the intestinal tract and portions of the liver to slip into the thorax.

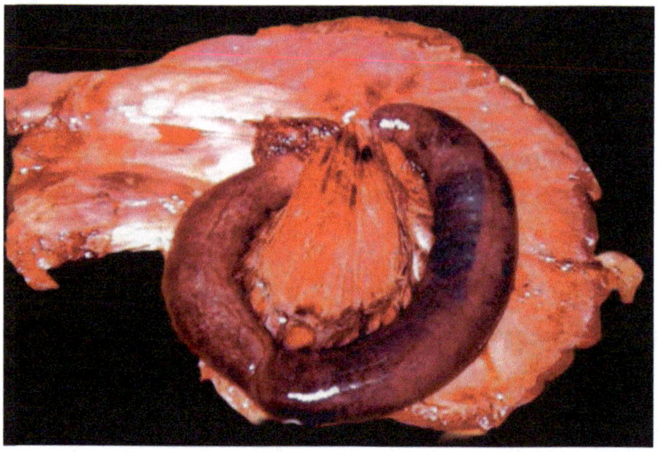

**Figure 6.85.** Horse. Diaphragm. Hernia. Portions of the intestinal tract telescope through the diaphragm into the thorax.

*j. Intestinal infarcts*

These are the result of vascular thrombosis blocking the blood supply of associated intestinal segments.

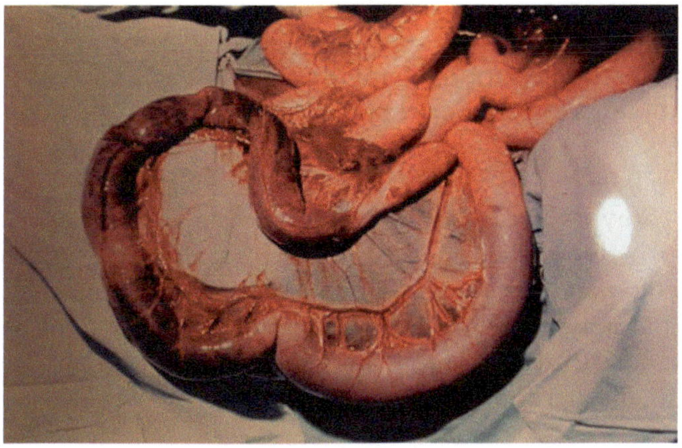

**Figure 6.86.** Horse. Small Intestine. Hemorrhagic Infarcts.

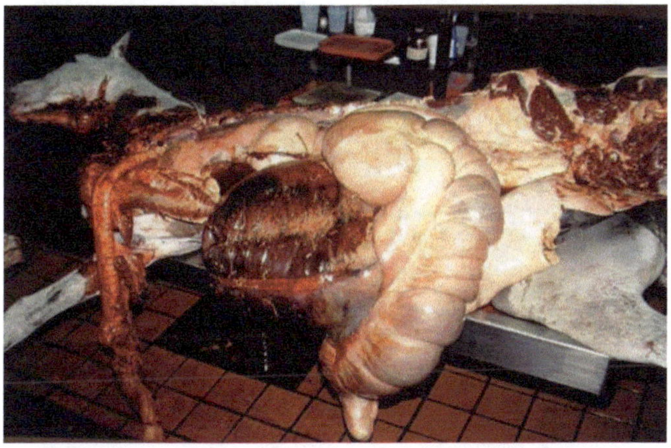

**Figure 6.87.** Horse. Colon. Hemorrhagic Infarcts. The cranial mesenteric root should be checked for evidence of fourth-stage larvae of *Strongylus vulgaris*.

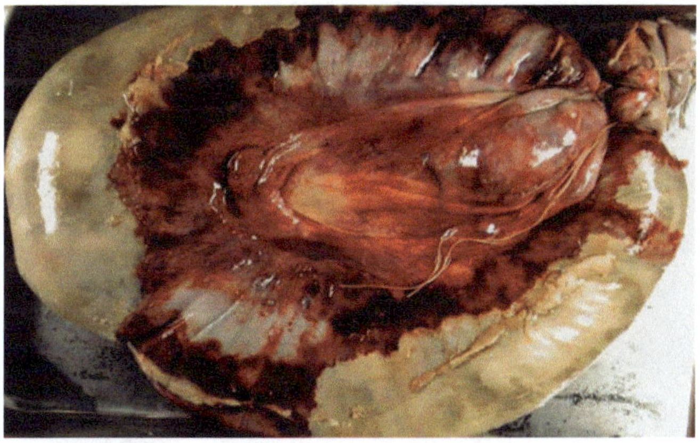

**Figure 6.88.** Horse. Pelvic Flexure of Colon. Hemorrhagic Infarct. Thromboembolic colitis from verminous cranial mesenteric root endarteritis clinically causing recurrent colitis.

### 3. *Intraluminal foreign bodies*

Intestinal foreign bodies not only are the cause for obstruction but may give rise to intestinal perforation or rupture leading to fatal peritonitis.

#### *a. Sand impaction*

Sand enteropathy in horses occurs when animals are kept on pastures with little grass growth and rich in sand. Ingested sand has a tendency to settle in the large colon and cecum rendering these organs extremely heavy. A large volume of sand may overwhelm the tract and the ability to clear itself. As it accumulates, sand causes irritation of the intestinal wall and weakening to cause rupture and peritonitis.

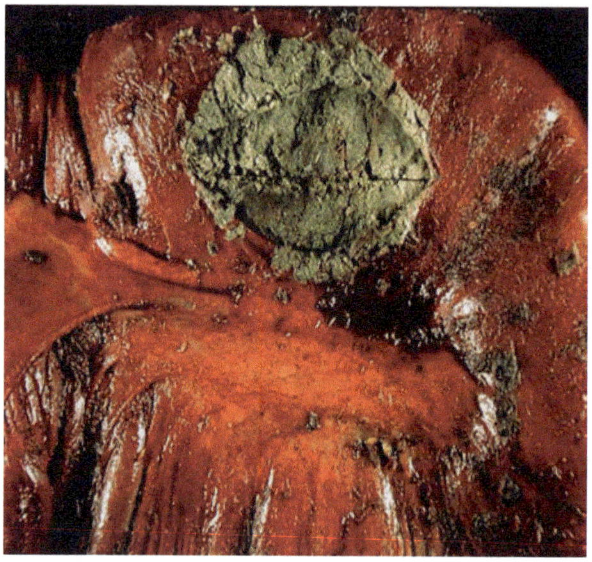

**Figure 6.89.** Horse. Colon. Rupture. The large colon has ruptured due to distension by sand and ingesta. An acute peritonitis is indicated by serosal reddening. (Reprinted with permission from the Animal Technology Institute of Taiwan, Republic of China.)

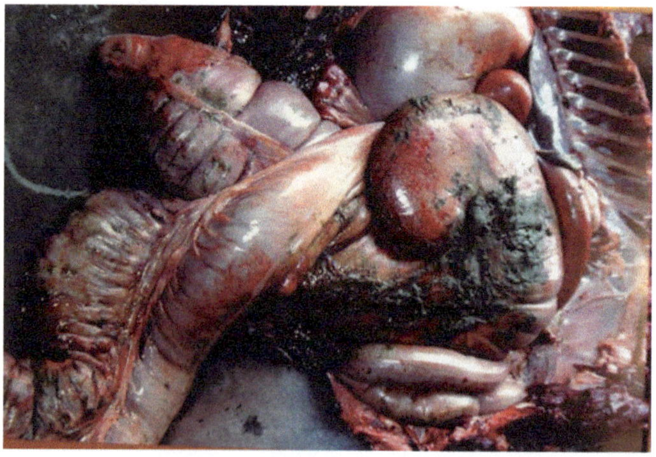

**Figure 6.90.** Horse. Cecum. Rupture. A distended cecum impacted by ingesta and sand has ruptured at the base.

*b. Enteroliths*

Mineral enteroliths typically form in horses fed on grain rich in phosphate and salts. Large amounts of unsplit salt escape into the colon to combine with ammonia-producing bacteria to form ammonium magnesium phosphate (triple phosphates). The growth of the enterolith depends on salts, a nidus for the precipitation of triple phosphates and some degree of intestinal hypomotility. The enteroliths grow like the rings of a tree. They may become heavy and large and then become entrapped at the transition into the transverse colon or the pelvic flexure. At these sites they may cause intestinal rupture. The nidus for mineral deposition may include nails, pebbles, brick fragments, or ropes.

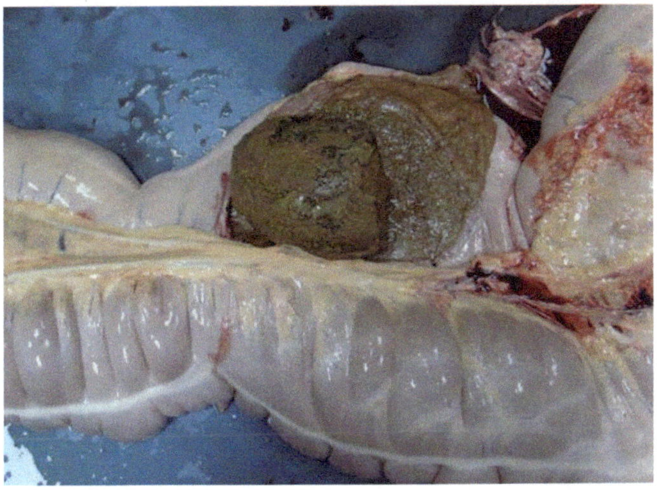

**Figure 6.91.** Horse. Colon. Rupture. An entrapped enterolith at this anatomically narrow site of the colon is the cause for the rupture.

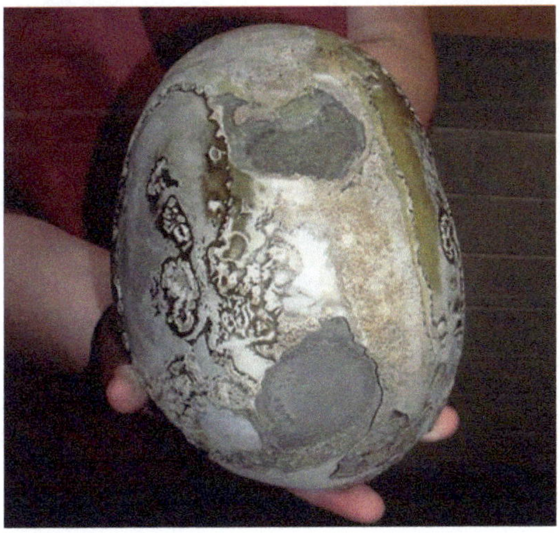

**Figure 6.92.** Horse. Colon. Enterolith. Surface profile.

### 4. Rectal (colonic) perforation

Obstetric intervention via the rectum, rectal palpation, or sadism may cause tearing of the rectum at its dorsal part with varying degrees of tissue destruction. Full-wall tearing is the most severe complication to cause cellulitis or peritonitis in the pelvic canal.

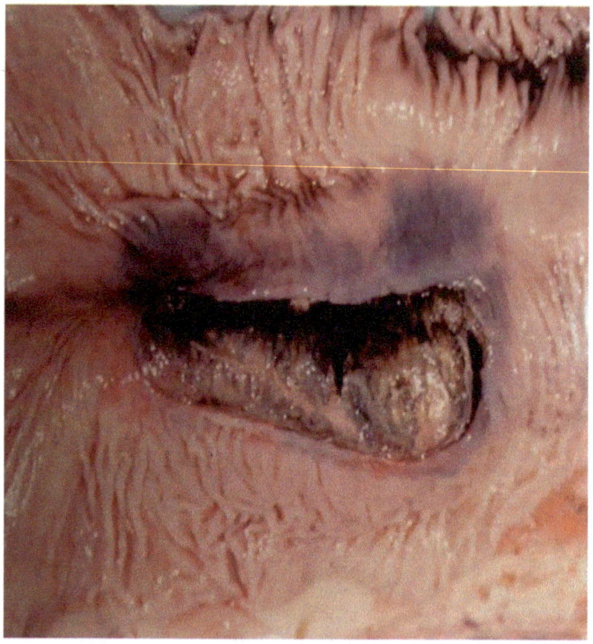

**Figure 6.93.** Horse. Dorsal Rectum. Perforation. A tear with rugged edges and hemorrhage occurred iatrogenically during rectal examination. A pathologic weakening of the wall due to preceding inflammation has to be ruled out via microscopic examination.

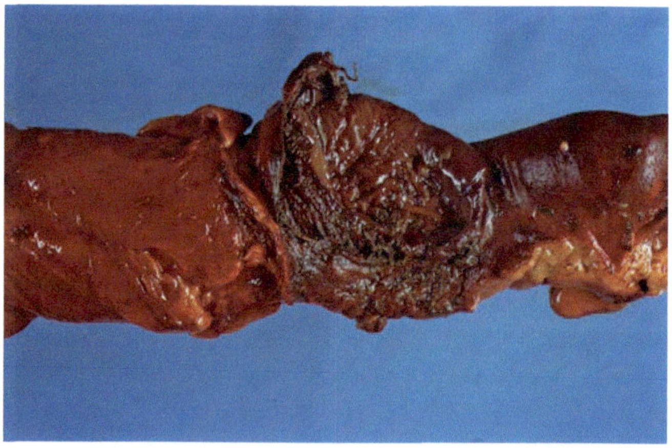

**Figure 6.94.** Horse. Small Colon. Rupture. May be associated with parturition or surgical straps.

### 5. *Intestinal diverticulum*

Intestinal diverticula are focal herniations of the mucosa into the serosa exhibiting focal external bulges. There is an opportunity to develop lodgings from entrapped ingesta and inflammation from pressure necrosis to cause intestinal rupture and peritonitis as the outcome. True or traction diverticula may be distinguished from false or propulsion diverticula. A true diverticulum includes mucosa and serosa; a false diverticulum involves herniation through the tunica muscularis.

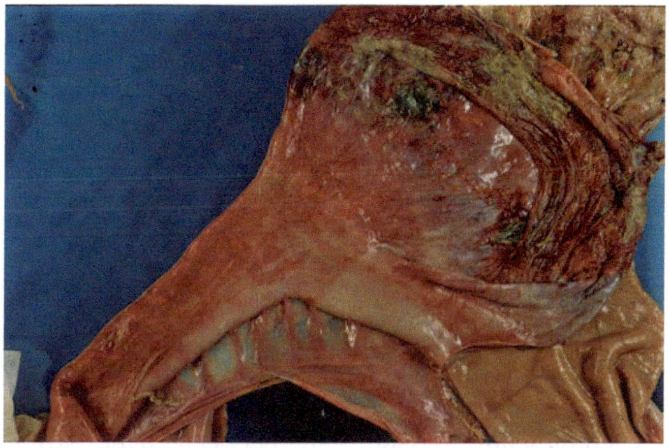

**Figure 6.95.** Horse. Small Intestine. Diverticulum. The opened diverticulum is composed of necrotic mucosa seen at the periphery; the center reflects serosa.

### 6. *Large intestinal tympany*

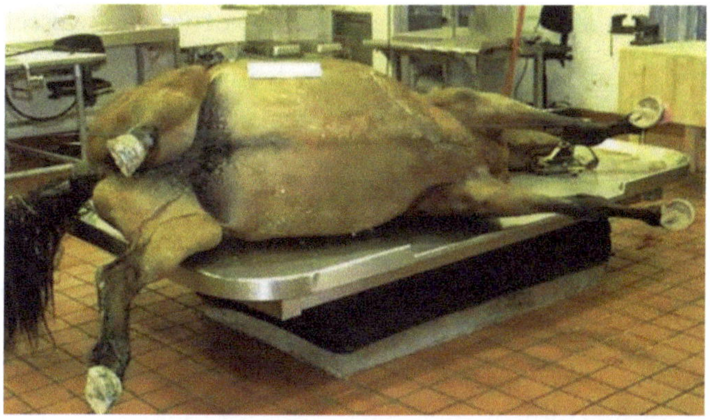

**Figure 6.96.** Horse. Whole Body. Young horse with distended abdomen submitted for a fresh necropsy. (Courtesy Dr. J. Roberts, National Zoo, Washington, DC.)

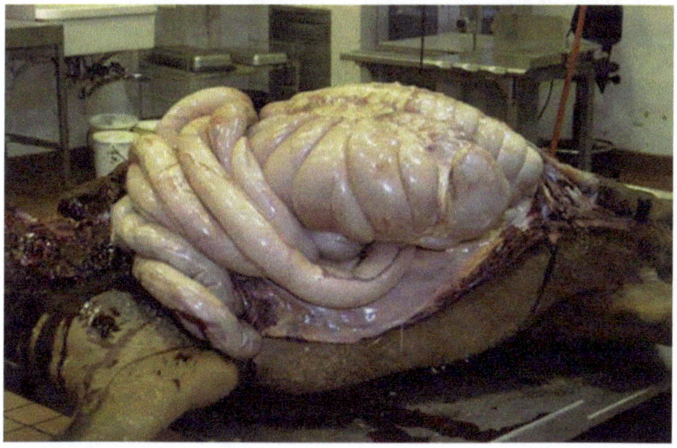

**Figure 6.97.** Horse. Opened Abdomen. Severe antemortem gaseous distension of the large intestine and also partially of the small intestine resulted from grain overload and will lead to metabolic derangements. Typically, this condition is seen in young, overconditioned, fast-growing horses. Intestinal contents exhibit brewer's yeast-like odor. Needs to be differentiated from postmortem condition. (Courtesy Dr. J. Roberts, National Zoo, Washington, DC.)

## Noninfectious disorders – Fact sheet

### I. Anomalies

- Atresia: Segmental interruption of intestinal lumen
- Aganglionosis: Neurogenic dysmotility
- Meckel's diverticulum: Vestigial omphalomesenteric duct remnant
- Ileal hypertrophy: Muscular layer thickening of the ileum

### II. Displacements and strangulations

- Volvulus: Rotation around mesenteric attachment
- Torsion: Rotation around longitudinal axis
- Strangulating lipoma: Pedunculated
- Intussusception: Telescoping of intestinal segments
- Foramen epiploicum: Tissue gap between liver, stomach, and duodenum
- Nephrosplenic ligament: Tissue fold between left kidney and spleen
- Mesodiverticular band: Vestigial remnant of vitelline vessel
- Mesenteric rent: Congenital defect or traumatic tear

### III. Intraluminal foreign bodies

- Sand impaction
- Enteroliths: Feed such as grain rich in ammonium magnesium phosphate

### IV. Rectal perforation

- Iatrogenic tear in dorsal rectum or colon

### V. Intestinal diverticulum

- Traction or true
- Propulsion or false

### VI. Grain overload

## V. Diseases of the intestinal tract: Infectious disorders

### Intestinal inflammation – Fact sheet

| Morphology | Etiology | Time |
|---|---|---|
| Catarrhal | Viral | Acute |
| Hemorrhagic | Bacterial | Chronic |
| Fibrinous | Parasitic | |
| Ulcerative | Mycotic | |
| Necrotic | Toxic | |
| Fibrinopurulent | Drug | |
| Granulomatous | Immune-mediated | |
| Hyperplastic | | |

### *1. Inflammation*

Intestinal inflammation can be classified according to site, depth, tissue response, time course, and etiology. Overlaps are frequent and limit clear-cut separation of its nature. Enteric inflammation is therefore most conveniently classified according to morphologic appearance, time course, and etiology.

#### *a. Catarrhal enteritis*

These are mainly viral in etiology and are most commonly caused by rotaviruses. Viral diagnosis is made by demonstrating negatively stained viral particles in feces with transmission electron microscopy, fecal enzyme-linked immunosorbent assay (ELISA), or polymerase chain reaction (PCR). Bacteria causing catarrhal (secretory) enteritis are *Escherichia coli* pathogens elaborating various enterotoxins of variable biologic properties and occasionally *Salmonella* sp. Diarrhea with water and electrolyte loss is a common clinical sign. In a recent clinical survey of foal diarrhea, 20% of the cases involved rotavirus, followed by *Clostridium perfringens* (18%), *Clostridium difficile* (13%), and *Salmonella enterica* (12%).

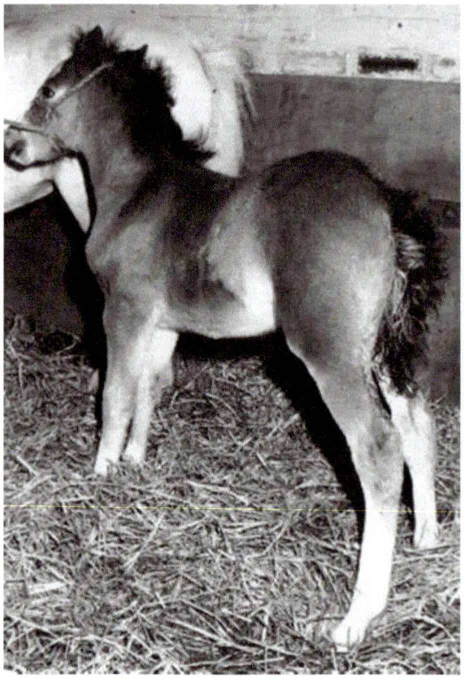

**Figure 6.98.** Foal. Rotavirus. Affected foals show evidence of watery diarrhea but minimal changes in the intestinal tract. Diagnosis can be made on fecal samples with commercial latex agglutination test kits, enzyme immunoassay, or PCR.

*b. Hemorrhagic enteritis*

Bacteria such as *Clostridium perfringens* and *Clostridium difficile* are examples as the cause for this type of enteritis, typically occurring in foals but also in adult horses. In adult horses, duodenitis/proximal jejunitis and colitis X (the term is abandoned these days) morphologically are other examples of hemorrhagic enterocolitis.

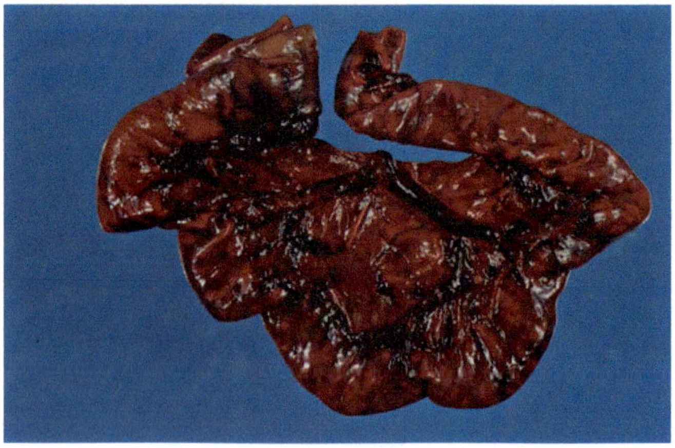

**Figure 6.99.** Horse. Small Intestine. Clostridial Disease. *C. perfringens* Type A Infection. Type C can also be involved. Diffuse hemorrhage affects the entire wall. The colon and cecum also may be involved.

This enteric microorganism is classified into five types (A–E) based on PCR detection of the genes encoding four major toxins (alpha, beta, epsilon, and iota). *C. perfringens* type A produces only alpha toxin. In addition, some strains of all the types may produce beta2 toxin and/or enterotoxin, which have been associated with diarrhea and enterocolitis in horses. It is noteworthy that *C. perfringens* type A is found in the intestine of normal horses.

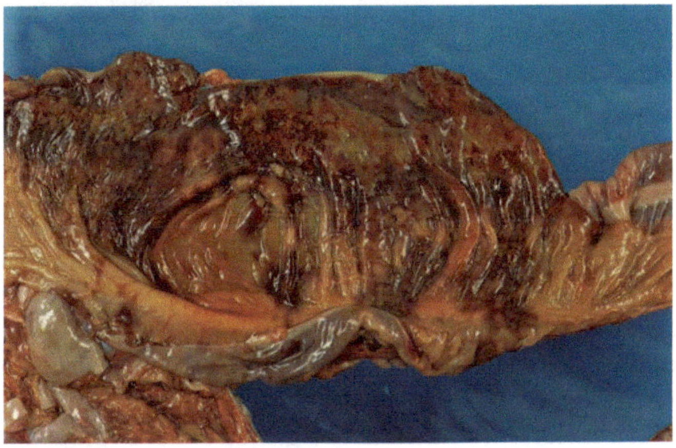

**Figure 6.100.** Horse. Colon. Clostridial Disease. *C. perfringens* type D infection. Hemorrhage and some edema are present. *C. perfringens* type D usually does not cause enteric disease in horses because it is rarely found in the intestine of normal horses. In this case it was thought to have been associated with colonic lesions.

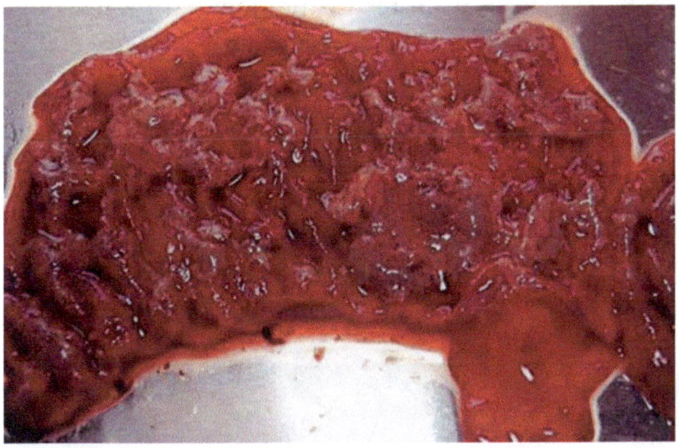

**Figure 6.101.** Horse. Colon. Clostridial Disease. Colon. Hyperemia and Edema. *Clostridium difficile* infection.

Abundant literature over the past years has identified *C. difficile* as an emerging enteric pathogen in horses with clinical signs of diarrhea. Diagnosis is usually based on detection of one or both of two major toxins, A and B, in intestinal content by commercial ELISA. Isolation of the microorganism from these specimens has some diagnostic value, but isolates need to be tested by PCR to demonstrate that they are toxigenic, as there are isolates that produce neither toxin A nor B. *C. difficile* may infect all ages of horses. In adults, the infection frequently is associated with typhlocolitis and to a lesser degree with small intestinal lesions. In foals, the opposite applies. The rate of carriers is low.

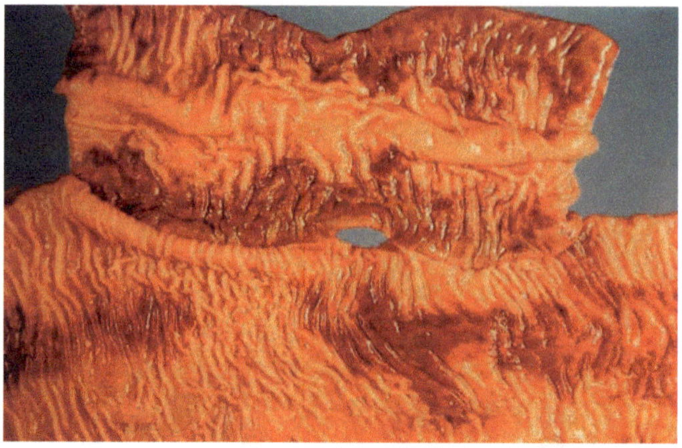

**Figure 6.102.** Horse. Duodenum. Anterior Enteritis. Acute Segmental Hemorrhage and Mucosal Necrosis. Severe reddening of the mucosa with some fibrin is present. (Reprinted with permission from the Animal Institute of Technology of Taiwan, Republic of China.)

The diagnosis was that of equine duodenitis/proximal jejunitis (EDPJ) or anterior enteritis based on the site of the changes, absence of significant enteric pathogen isolation, and clinical signs of colic, copious gastric reflux, and fluid accumulation in small intestine, endotoxemia, and the development of laminitis as clinical complications. The etiology of the syndrome is uncertain; some indications from the literature suggest a role of *C. difficile* toxins or fumonisin B1 toxicosis from feed contaminated by the fungus *Fusarium verticilloides (moniliforme)*. The involvement of *Salmonella* has been also suggested.

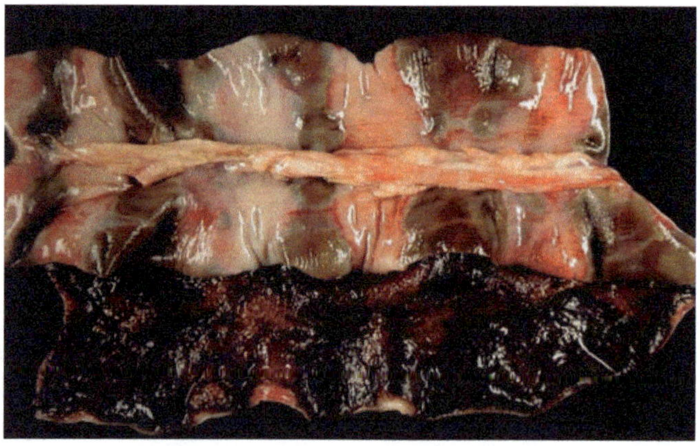

**Figure 6.103.** Horse. Duodenum. Anterior Enteritis. Hemorrhage and Necrosis. Abundant gastric reflux and intestinal distension are clinical complications. (Reprinted with permission from the Animal Institute of Technology of Taiwan, Republic of China.)

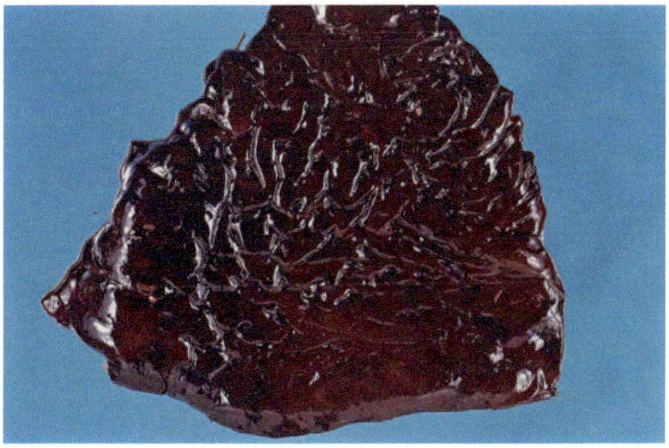

**Figure 6.104.** Horse. Colon. Colitis X. Venous Congestion. The wall of the colon is severely thickened by edema, and the mucosa suggests venous congestion. Largely enigmatic as to etiology in the past, the condition is now attributed to endotoxins released by *C. perfringens* type A or to certain genotypes of *C. difficile* toxins. The disease leads to endotoxemia and hypovolemic shock. The term *colitis X* is no longer used.

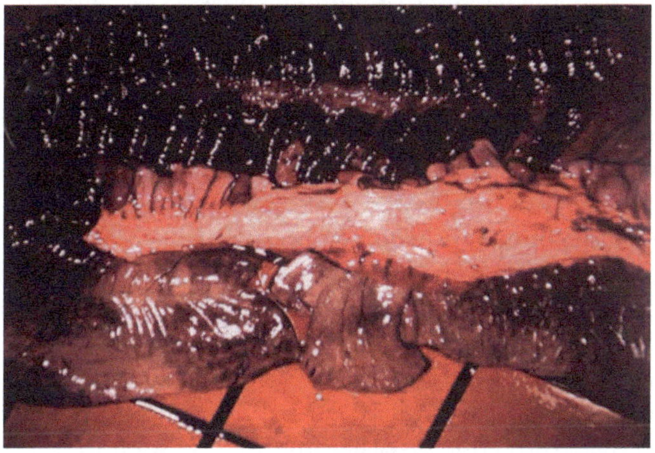

**Figure 6.105.** Horse. Colon. Acute Salmonellosis. Hyperemia, Hemorrhage, and Necrosis. Differential diagnosis: Clostridial disease or acute toxic right dorsal colitis.

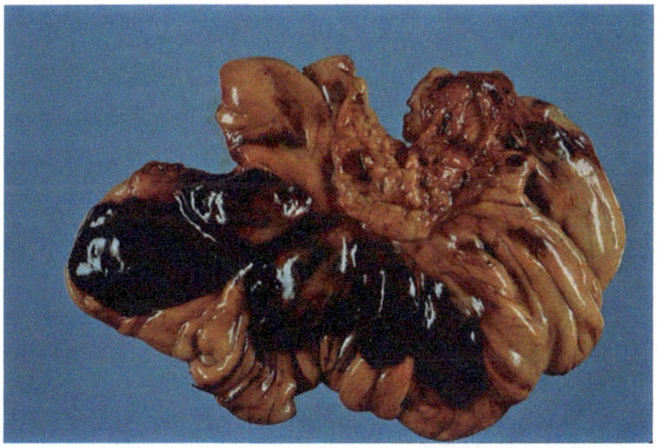

**Figure 6.106.** Horse. Colonic Lymph Node. Acute Salmonellosis. Hemorrhage. Lymphadenomegaly caused by edema, hemorrhage, and necrosis.

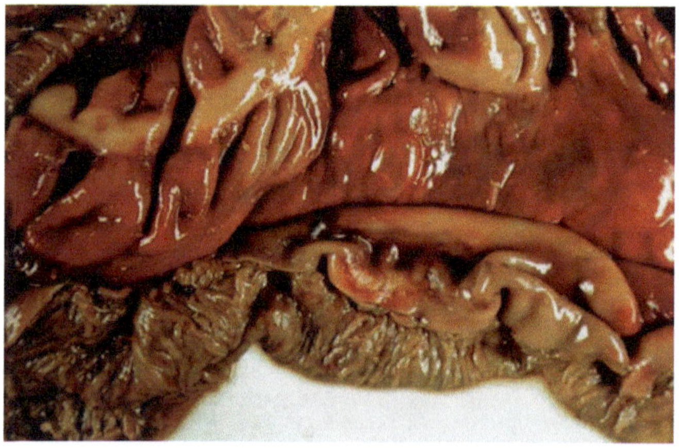

**Figure 6.107.** Horse. Colon. Transmural Salmonellosis. Fibrinous and Transmural Necrohemorrhagic Colitis.

*c. Fibrinonecrotic enteritis*

Salmonella is the prototype for this type of tissue reaction resulting from infection with *Salmonella enterica*. Salmonellosis is an important infectious disease of horses. It also is a zoonosis. Young animals are more susceptible to infection than adult animals that may be carriers. The bacilli produce an endotoxin. There are acute and chronic forms of salmonellosis. The acute disease phase produces intestinal edema, generalized ecchymoses, and hemorrhage inducing hemorrhagic enterocolitis. Later and more typical, the enteric mucosa of mainly the colon and cecum becomes fibrinous and necrotic to form casts in the lumen (pseudomembranes) defined as the subacute form of salmonellosis. The chronic form is characterized by a crusty mucosa. Draining mesenteric and colonic lymph nodes are enlarged due to lymphadenitis. Differential diagnosis is right dorsal colitis. Clinical complications include sepsis and laminitis. There are various nosocomial risk factors for salmonellosis including abdominal surgery. Certain *Salmonella* serotypes develop resistance to treatment with antibiotics. In addition to enterocolitis, the bacterium of the genus *Salmonella* are able to induce sepsis, hepatitis, gastritis, pneumonia, polyarthritis, osteomyelitis, meningitis, and chorionitis with abortion. Sporadic mycotic pneumonia may occur.

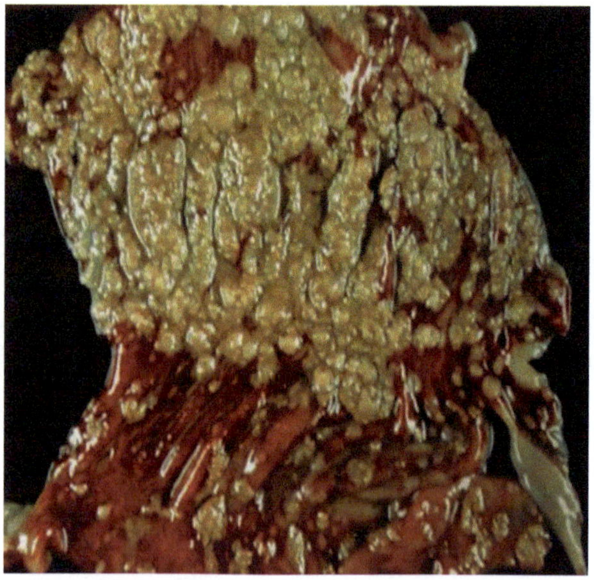

**Figure 6.108.** Horse. Colon. Subacute Salmonellosis. Fibrinonecrotic Colitis. Inspissated gray fibrin plaques are covering the mucosa.

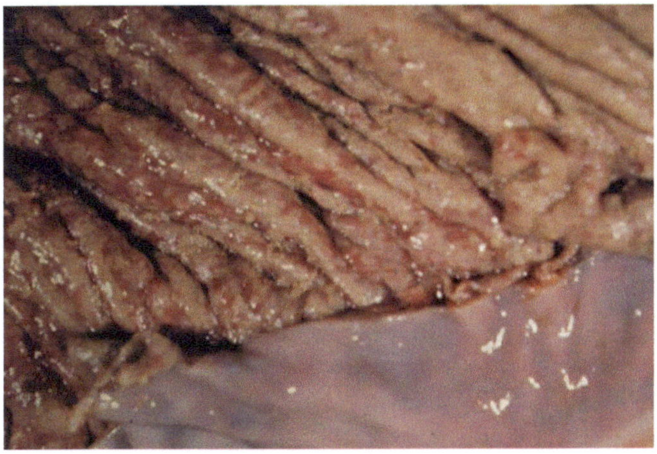

**Figure 6.109.** Horse. Colon. Chronic Salmonellosis. Fibrinonecrotic Colitis. A thick layer of exudate is diffusely covering the mucosa.

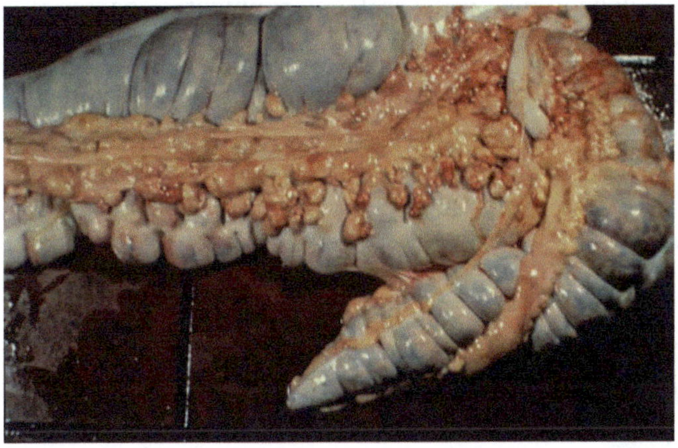

**Figure 6.110.** Horse. Colon, Cecum. Chronic Salmonellosis. Severe Lymphadenomegaly. Lymph node enlargement is caused by edema, lymphoid hyperplasia, sinus histiocytosis, and necrosis. Differential diagnoses should include rhodococcosis and lymphoma. (Reprinted with permission from the Animal Technology Institute of Taiwan, Republic of China.)

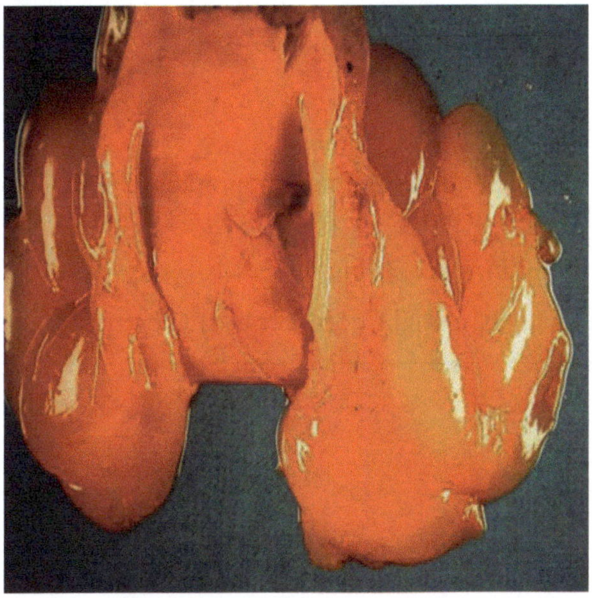

**Figure 6.111.** Horse. Colon. Salmonellosis. Edema. The submucosa is markedly edematous from hypoproteinemia and endotoxin-induced vascular permeability disturbance. Differential diagnoses include repositioning following displacement and Potomac horse fever.

## Equine salmonellosis – Fact sheet

### Definition

- Enteric or systemic infection with bacteria belonging to species *Salmonella enterica.*
- Zoonosis

### Incidence

- Variable depending on several environmental, bacterial, and host factors including carriers

**Range of Infection:** Inapparent, acute, subacute, chronic

### Complications

- Septicemia
- Laminitis
- Leukopenia

### Gross findings

- Diffuse hemorrhagic, fibrinonecrotic enterocolitis and typhlitis
- Intramural edema of colon and cecum
- Enlargement of mesenteric and cecocolonic lymph nodes
- Diffuse adrenocortical hemorrhage

### Microscopic findings

- Necrosis and mixed neutrophilic, mononuclear inflammation affecting mainly the mucosa
- Fibrin thrombi in mucosal blood vessels

**Differential Diagnosis:** Right dorsal colitis; Clostridial diseases *d. Ulcerative enteritis*

Potomac horse fever (PHF), also known as equine monocytic ehrlichiosis, is an example of this form of enteritis. PHF clinically is characterized by fever, dehydration, anorexia, leucopenia, and profuse diarrhea. Laminitis, subcutaneous edema of the ventral abdomen, and abortion may occur as clinical complications. The causative agent is *Neorickettsia ristic ii*. It may infect horses of all ages mostly during the summer months. *N. risticii* is a gram-negative obligate intracellular bacterium that infects monocytes and is transmitted often by helminthic trematodes and insects harboring flukes during the warmest period of the year. The infected monocytes have a predilection for the lamina propria and submucosa of the colon and cecum. Differential diagnoses include salmonella infection, drug toxicosis (antibiotics, NSAIDs), and endotoxic shock. Mortality of untreated cases range between 15% and 35%. Vaccination may be preventive.

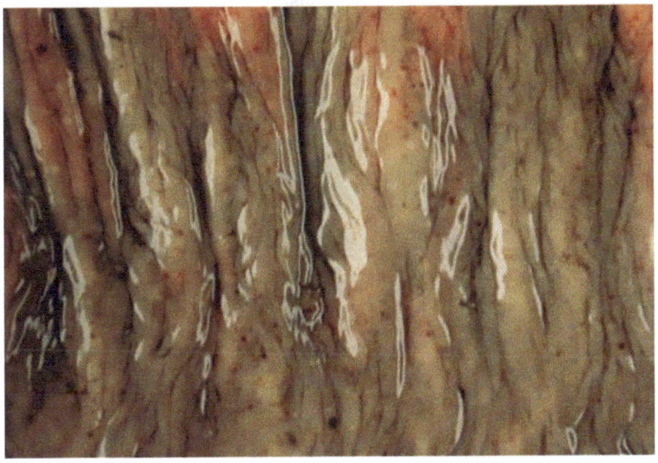

**Figure 6.112.** Horse. Colon. Potomac Horse Fever. Colitis. Multifocal mild erosive colitis with edema. The gross changes of PHF may be subtle and characterized by stellate round erosions in a mildly thickened mucosa. (Reprinted with permission from the Animal Technology Institute of Taiwan, Republic of China.)

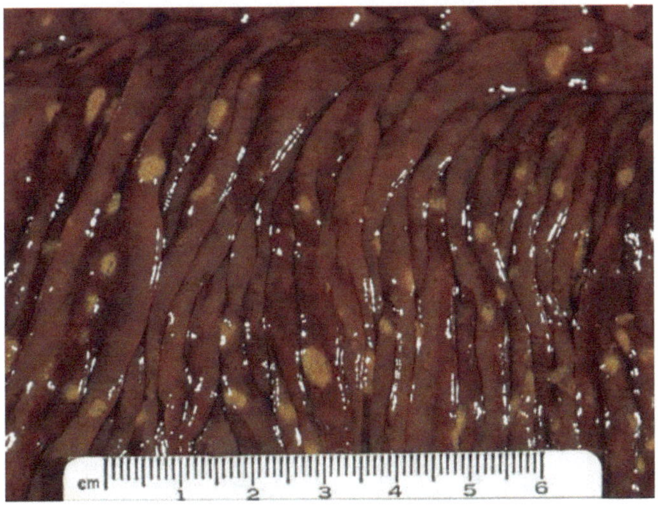


**Figure 6.113.** Horse. Colon. Potomac Horse Fever. Fibrinous and Ulcerative Colitis. Accentuated mucosal folds are characterized by white fibrin caps. (Courtesy Dr. P. Habecker, University of Pennsylvania.)

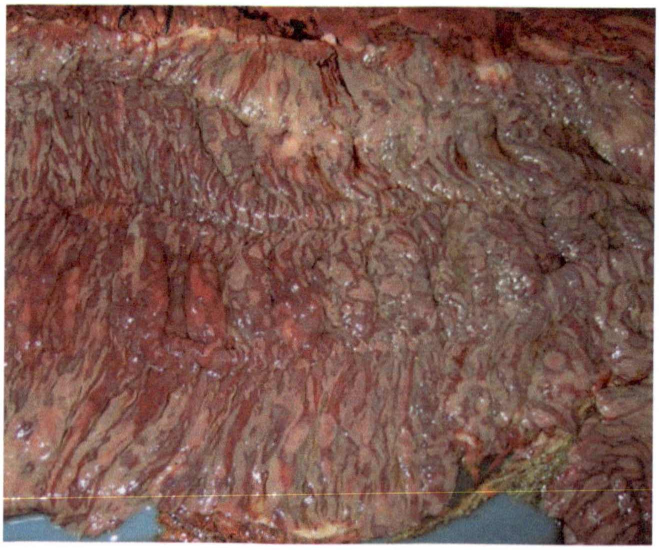

**Figure 6.114.** Horse. Colon. Potomac Horse Fever. Mucosal Infarcts.

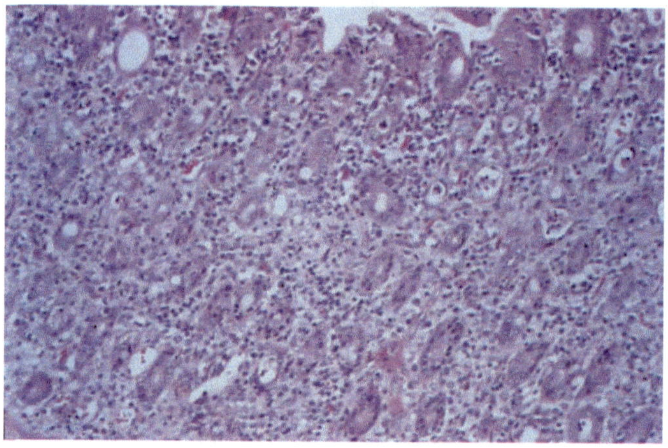

**Figure 6.115.** Horse. Colon. Potomac Horse Fever. Mononuclear Colitis. Microscopic features are moderate numbers of lymphocytes and macrophages in the lamina propria separating crypts sometimes containing inflammatory cells. (H&E) (Reprinted with permission from the Animal Technology Institute of Taiwan, Republic of China.)

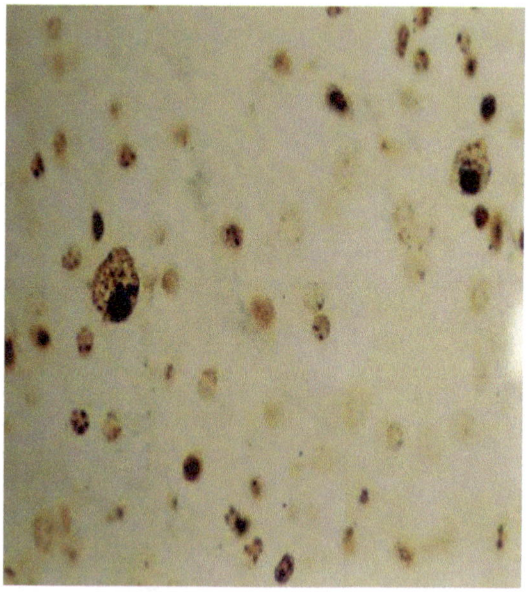

**Figure 6.116.** Horse. Colon. Potomac Horse Fever. A silver stain demonstrates clusters of morulae in the cytoplasm of macrophages (Steiner's silver)

## Potomac horse fever – Fact sheet

**Definition:** Infectious disease caused by *Neorickettsia risticii*

### Incidence, occurrence, and transmission

- Sporadic and seasonal (summer)
- United States, Canada, and Europe
- Flukes and arthropod-containing flukes

**Mortality:** 15–30%

### Gross findings

- Multifocal hemorrhagic erosions in colon and cecum mucosa
- Edema of subcutis along ventral abdomen

### Microscopic findings

- Moderate infiltration of lamina propria of colon and cecum by lymphocytes and macrophages

### Diagnosis

- Special silver stain (Steiner's) of colon
- Indirect fluorescent antibody of serum or ELISA
- PCR of feces or peripheral blood
- PCR on fresh or formalin-fixed, paraffin-embedded colon tissue

### Differential diagnosis

- *Salmonella*
- *Burkholdaria cepacio*
- Fungal and alimentary pythiosis
- NSAID toxicosis, antibiotics

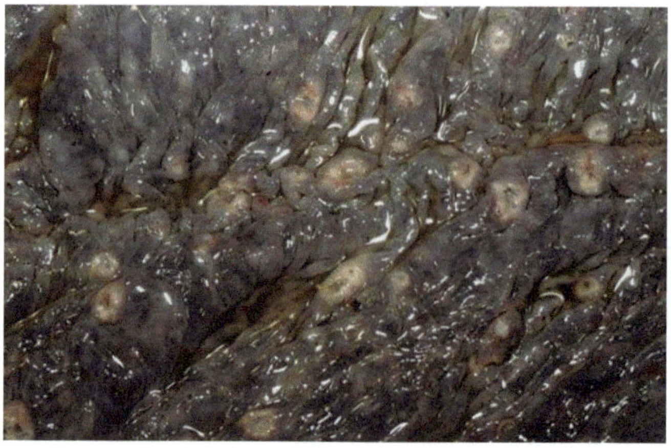

**Figure 6.117.** Horse. Colon. Ulcerative Colitis. The mucosa is studded with multiple small ulcers. *Burkholderia cepacia* (formerly *Pseudomonas cepacia*) was isolated. The lesions have to be differentiated from PHF salmonellosis and lymphoma. (Courtesy J. Roberts, National Zoo, Washington, DC.)

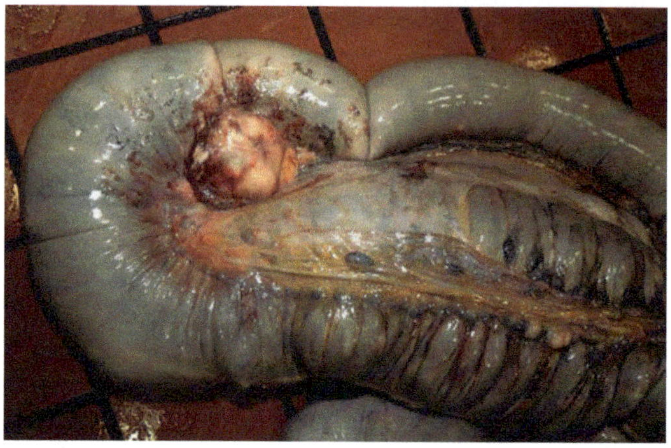

**Figure 6.118.** Horse. Colon. Mural Abscess. *Burkholderia cepacia*. Necrotizing and ulcerative transmural colitis with abscesses. There is evidence of segmental transmural inflammation and formation of an abscess in the mesocolon. (Courtesy Dr. J. Roberts, National Zoo, Washington, DC.)

*e. Granulomatous enteritis*

In addition to diarrhea, this type of enteritis leads to clinical signs of weight and muscle loss, malabsorption, malassimilation, and intermittent anorexia indicating chronicity of illness. Typical disease examples include equine intestinal mycobacteriosis, the enteric form of *Rhodococcus equi* infection, *Lawsonia intracellularis* proliferative enteritis, and less common idiopathic granulomatous enteritis and intestinal mycosis (histoplasmosis).

Equine Intestinal Mycobacteriosis. This rare equine disease affecting ileum, colon, and associated lymph nodes can be considered the morphologic analog to bovine paratuberculosis (Johne disease) and like Johne disease is caused by an acid-fast bacterium belonging to the *Mycobacterium avium-intracellulare* complex. The source of infection is likely from a reservoir of *M. avium* in the environment such as water or soil. Horses that are susceptible usually develop the intestinal form suggesting oral uptake of the bacilli.

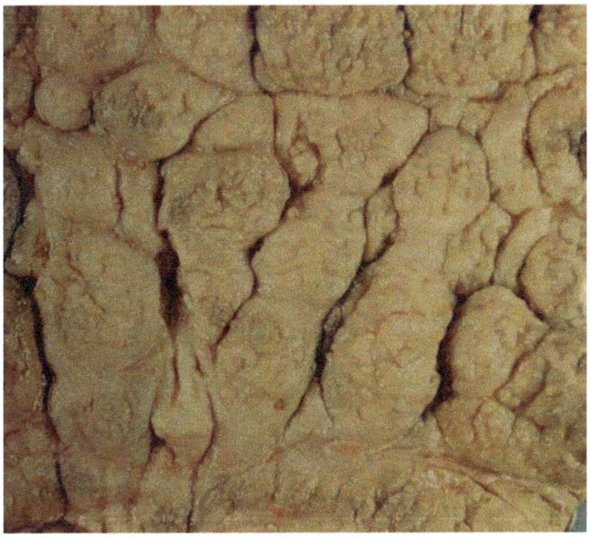

**Figure 6.119.** Horse. Colon. Equine Mycobacteriosis. Granulomatous Colitis. Like cobblestones, thick, leathery, plaques are covering the mucosa. (Reprinted with permission from the Animal Technology Institute of Taiwan, Republic of China.)

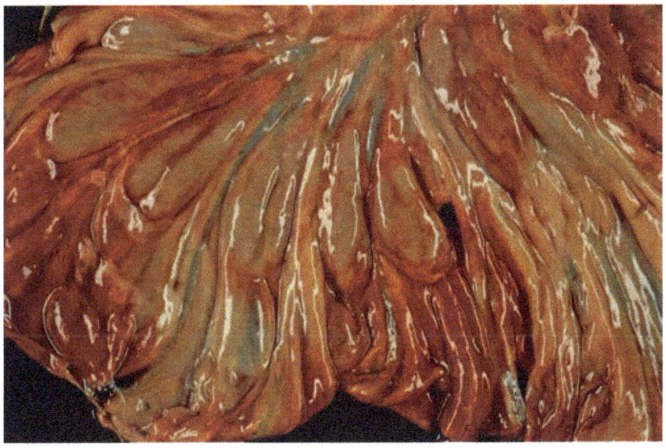

**Figure 6.120.** Horse. Mesenteric Lymph Nodes. Equine Mycobacteriosis. Lymphadenomegaly. Granulomatous lymphadenitis causing lymphadenomegaly. Draining lymph nodes are markedly enlarged. (Reprinted with permission from the Animal Technology Institute of Taiwan, Republic of China.)

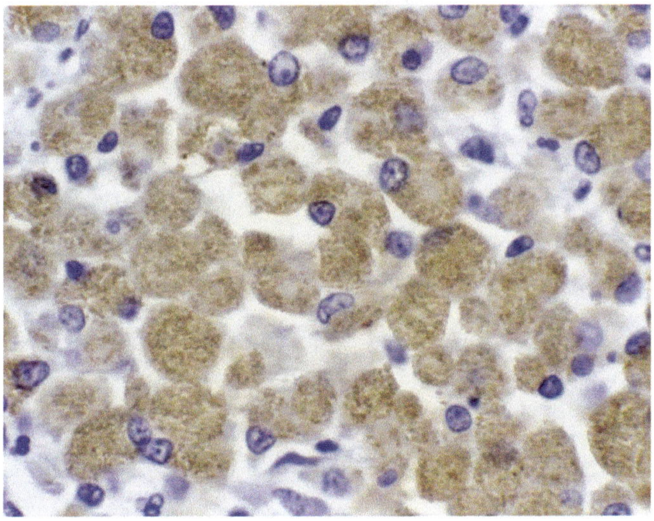

**Figure 6.121.** Horse. Colon. Equine Mycobacteriosis. The presence of a plethora of intracellular bacilli can be demonstrated with indirect immunohistochemistry. (IHC). Acid-fast staining will yield the same result.

Intestinal *Rhodococcus Equi* Infection. The alimentary form of *R. equi* develops in the ileum, colon, and cecum of mainly young horses. The portal of entry is likely oral. The inflammatory reaction to the bacillus is both granulomatous and ulcerative. There is concurrence of a significant adenopathy of adjacent lymph nodes draining macrophages containing intracellular organisms.

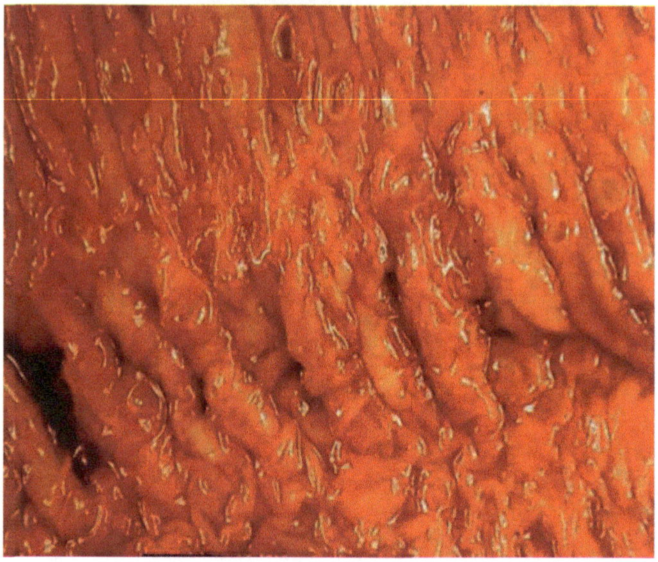

**Figure 6.122.** Horse. Colon. Pyogranulomatous Colitis. *Rhodococcus Equi*. The mucosa is diffusely thickened and is affected by multiple small ulcers.

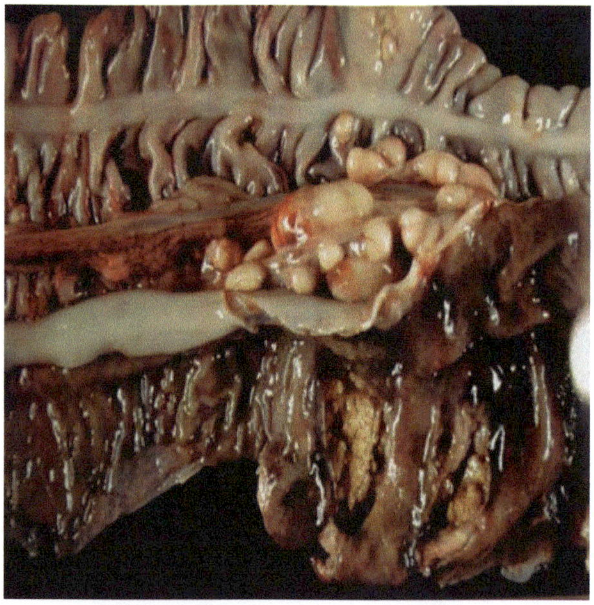

**Figure 6.123.** Horse. Colon. Intestine and Colonic Lymph Nodes. *Rhodococcus Equi* Pyogranulomatous Colitis. The opened part of the colon exposes a thickened mucosa covered by a fibrinonecrotic exudate. Small button-like ulcers can also be present. Draining lymphoid tissue is prominent. Chronic salmonellosis should be considered as the main differential diagnosis. (Reprinted with permission from the Animal Technology Institute of Taiwan, Republic of China.)

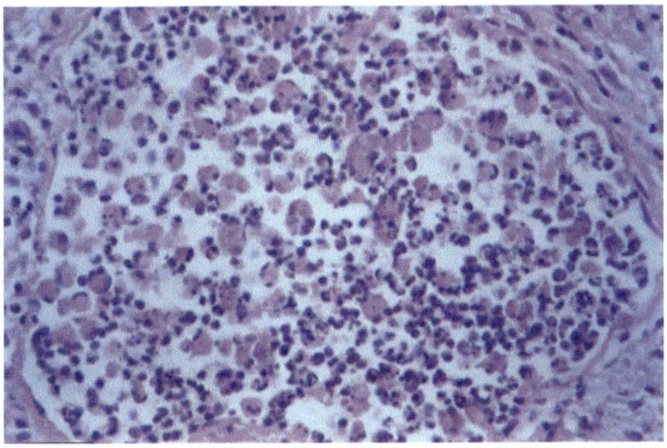

**Figure 6.124.** Horse. Colon. *Rhodococcus Equi* Enteritis. The typical change of infection by this bacterium is a pyogranulomatous inflammation. (H&E) (Reprinted with permission from the Animal Technology Institute of Taiwan, Republic of China.)

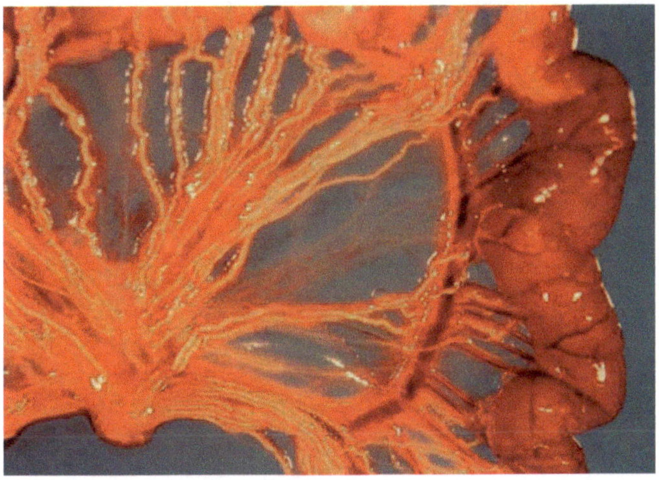

**Figure 6.125.** Horse. Mesenteric Lymphatics. Rhodococcal Lymphangitis. A string of thickened mesenteric lymph vessels is the result of a granulomatous inflammation with thrombosis. This reaction can also be seen in infection with *Streptococcus equi* subsp. *zooepidemicus* and has been lately reported with *Actinobacillus equuli* subsp. *hemolyticus*. Stasis of lymph in normal mesenteric lymphatics can be encountered postprandially.

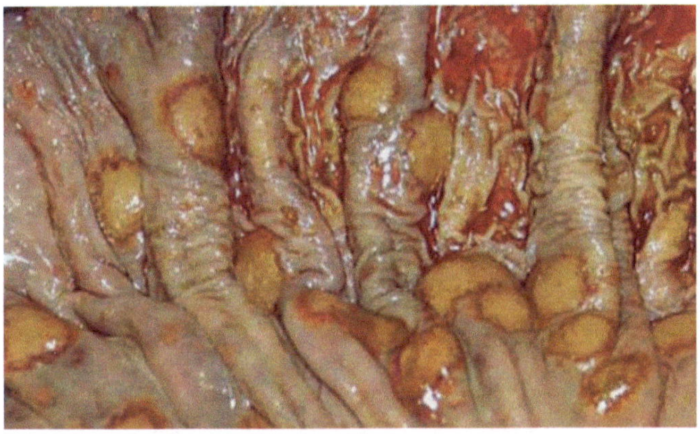

**Figure 6.126.** Horse. Colon. Mycotic Pyogranulomatous Angiocentric Colitis. Elevated yellow nodules in the mucosa resulted from a fungal infection. Fungal specification was not attempted other than visualization of septate hyphae in thrombosed arterioles. Fungi should be considered as differential agent in cases of pyogranulomatous enterocolitis. (Courtesy Dr. J. Roberts, Washington, DC.)

*f. Hyperplastic enteritis*

*Lawsonia Intracellularis* Enteropathy (Proliferative Enteritis). Infection by this thermophilic gram-negative obligatory intracellular organism can be demonstrated by silver stain within the enterocytes. In the horse, the ileum is usually affected by diffuse mucosal thickening.

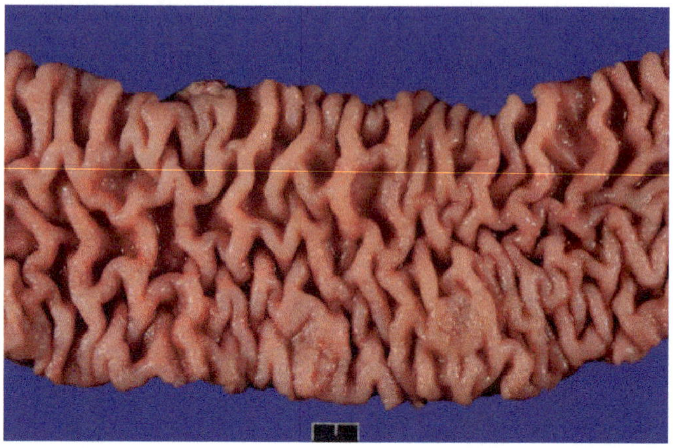

**Figure 6.127.** Horse. Ileum. *Lawsonia Intracellularis* Hyperplastic Enteropathy. The entire mucosa is thickened by mucosal hypertrophy forming rugae. Differential diagnoses are idiopathic equine granulomatous enteritis, likely a hypersensitivity reaction to feed elements, intestinal histoplasmosis, or alimentary tract lymphoma. (Courtesy Dr. J. Cooley, Mississippi State University.)

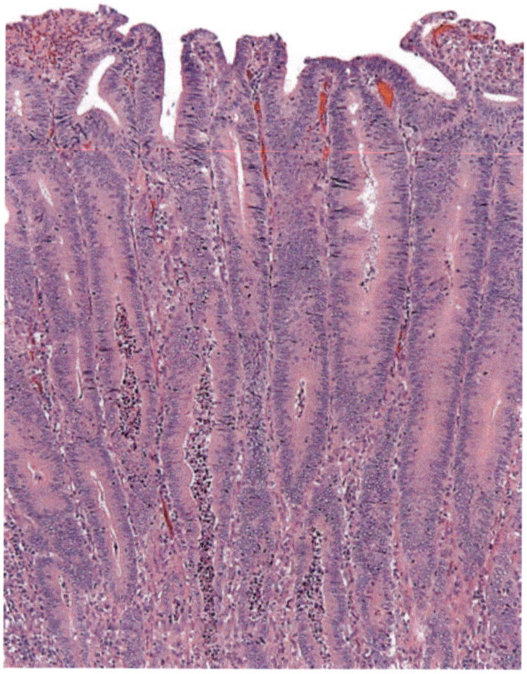

**Figure 6.128.** Horse. Ileum. *Lawsonia Intracellularis* Hyperplastic Enteropathy. Ileal crypts are markedly elongated by the enterocyte hypertrophy and hyperplasia. (H&E) (Courtesy J. Cooley, Mississippi State University.)

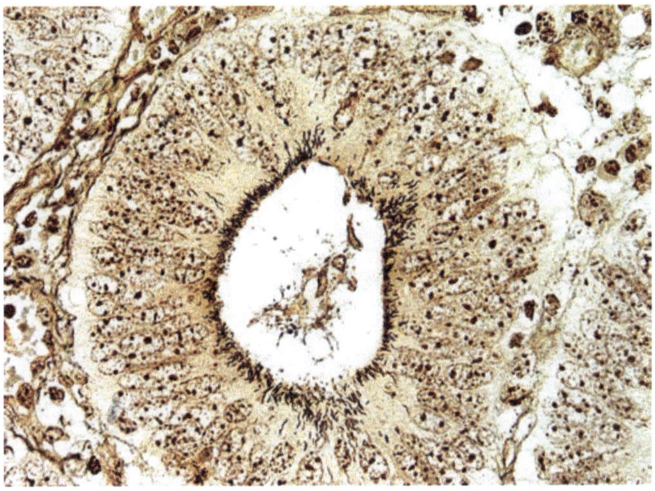

**Figure 6.129.** Horse. Ileum. *Lawsonia Intracellularis* Hyperplastic Enteropathy. A silver stain shows a dense single line of positive small rods of bacteria lined up within the cytoplasm of the cross section of the enterocyte-packed crypt. (Courtesy Dr. J. Cooley, Mississippi State University.)

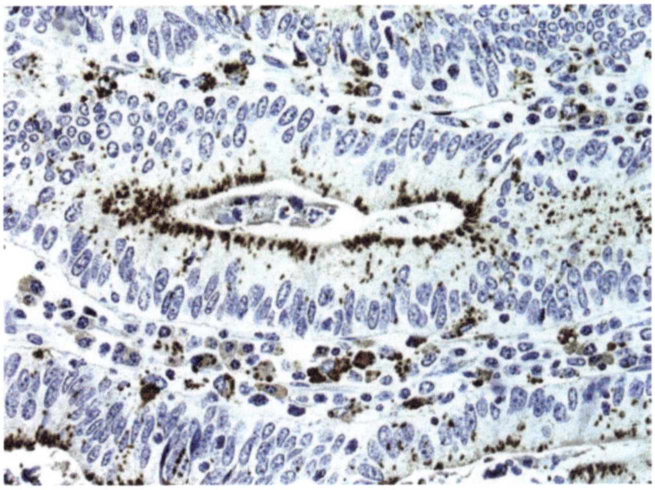

**Figure 6.130.** Horse. Ileum. *Lawsonia Intracellularis* Hyperplastic Enteropathy. Indirect immunohistochemistry demonstrates the localization of the intracellular bacteria mainly toward the surface of the mucosa. (IHC) (Courtesy Dr. J. Cooley, Mississippi State University.)

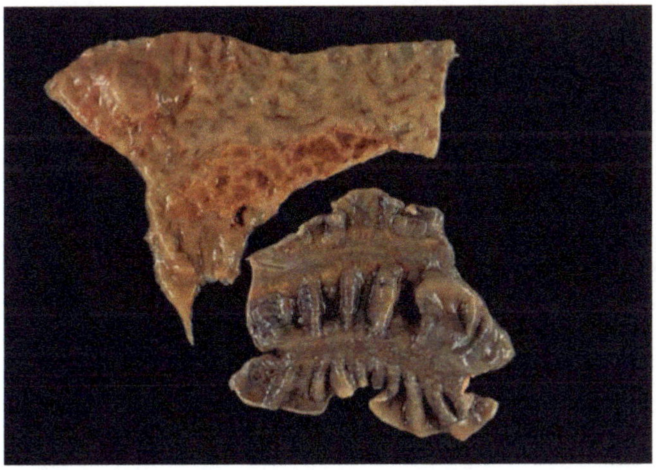

**Figure 6.131.** Horse. Colon. Pythiosis. Hyperplastic, Ulcerative Colitis. Proliferation of mucosa and presence of multiple small ulcers. Hyphae of the oomycete *Pythium insidiosum* were detected microscopically. This case is an example of the alimentary form of pythiosis, which unlike in the dog, is rare in horses.

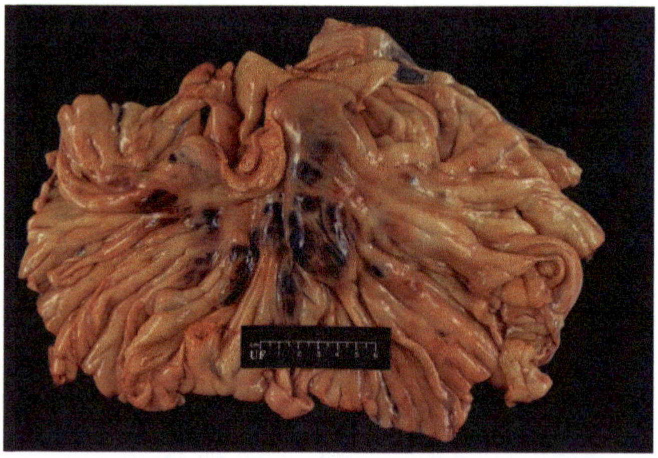

**Figure 6.132.** Horse. Mesenteric Lymph Nodes. Lymphadenopathy. Enlargement and hemorrhage indicate chronic reactive changes induced by the presence of enteric pathogens.

### g. *Inflammatory bowel diseases*

Individual examples of chronic inflammatory bowel diseases (IBDs) in the horse with no identifiable cause include (idiopathic) granulomatous enteritis (GE) frequently encountered in young Standardbreds, multisystemic eosinophilic epitheliotropic disease (MEED), lymphocytic-plasmacytic enterocolitis (LPE), and idiopathic eosinophilic enterocolitis (EC). Hypotheses for IBD in horses consider an abnormal immune response to infectious agents, small intestinal bacterial overgrowth, parasites, or food antigens. The hallmark inflammatory cells for these disorders are eosinophils. Weight loss, abdominal pain, malabsorption, and maldigestion are key clinical signs. Most horses do not survive despite treatment and management adjustment.

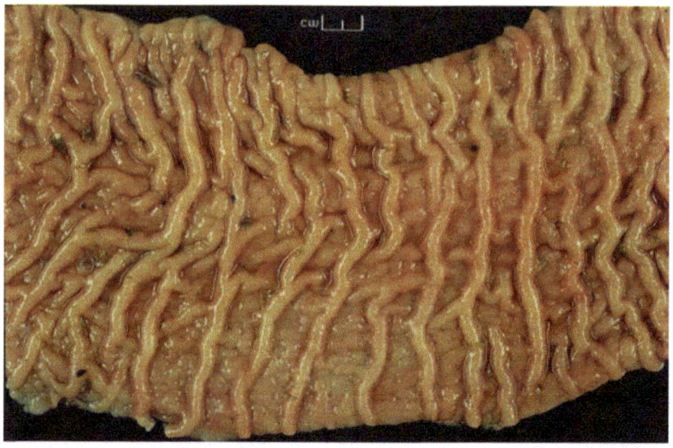

**Figure 6.133.** Horse. Jejunum. Chronic Enteropathy. The mucosa exhibits reduced folds and appears stretched out.

## Chronic enterocolitis – Fact sheet

### Clinical signs

- Weight loss
- Anorexia
- Diarrhea
- Malabsorption

### Gross findings

- Mucosal rugal thickening and ulceration
- Adenopathy of draining lymph nodes

### Microscopic findings

- Granulomatous and pyogranulomatous inflammation
- Proliferation of enterocytes

### Etiology

- *Mycobacterium avium-intracellulare* complex
- *Rhodococcus equi*
- *Lawsonia intracellularis*
- *Histoplasma capsulatum*
- *Aspergillus fumigatus*
- *Pythium insidiosum*

## 2. *Drug-induced enteropathy*

Toxic Right Dorsal Colitis. An astute observation made at necropsy led to the recognition of a unique ulcerative colitis affecting only the right dorsal colon. It was ultimately identified as a side effect of treatment with high doses of NSAIDs. Investigations into the mechanism of action revealed a significant reduction of blood flow into the right dorsal colon after administration of NSAIDs. Clinical signs of affected horses include colic, diarrhea, and weight loss.

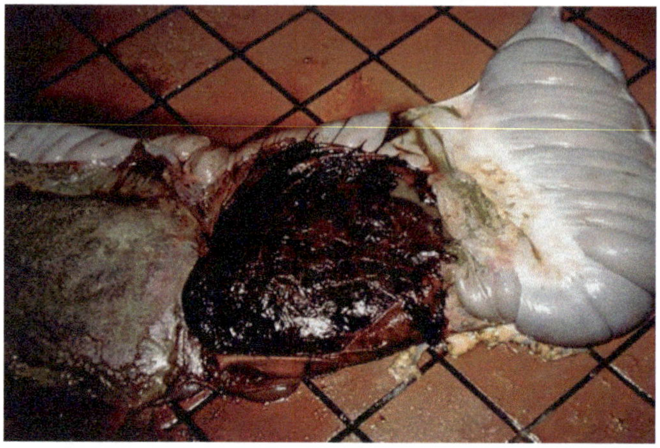

**Figure 6.134.** Horse. Right Dorsal Colon. Hemorrhage. Massive bleeding has occurred into the lumen. The horse had a history of repeated treatment with NSAIDs.

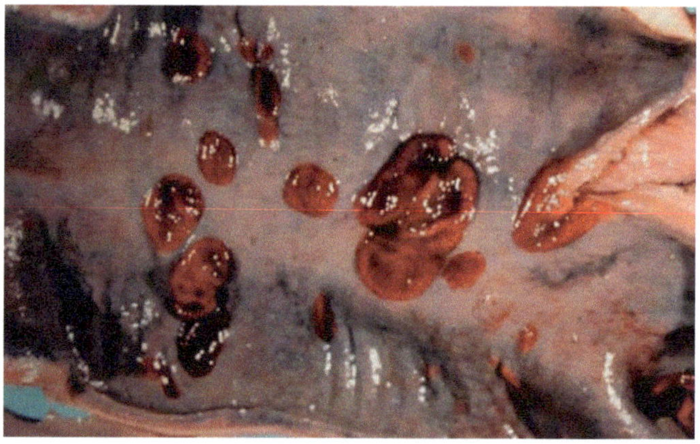

**Figure 6.135.** Horse. Right Dorsal Colon. Diffuse Ulceration and Multifocal Regenerative Hyperplasia. The mucosa is lost over extensive areas of deep ulceration into the submucosa. Only islands of hyperplastic mucosa are left. (Reprinted with permission from the Animal Technology Institute of Taiwan, Republic of China.)

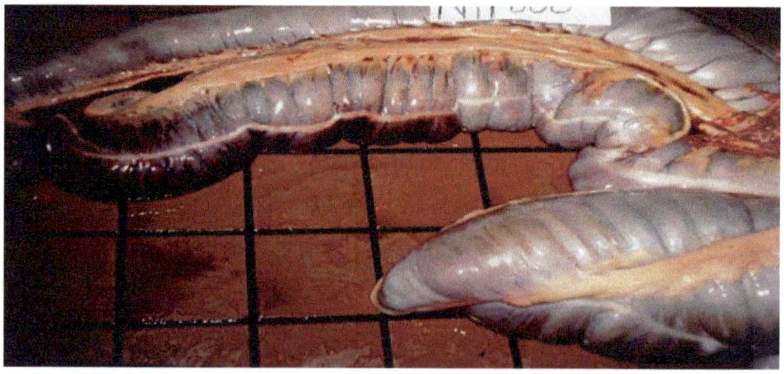

**Figure 6.136.** Horse. Colon. Mural Hemorrhagic Discoloration. Severe transmural drug-induced hemorrhagic necrosis and inflammation.

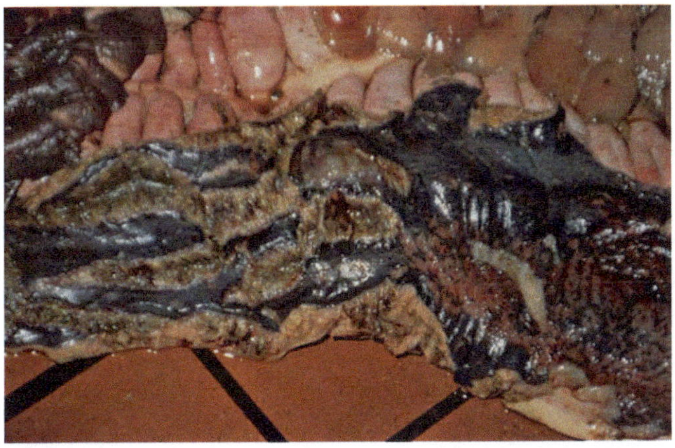

**Figure 6.137.** Horse. Colon. Severe Necrohemorrhagic and Ulcerative Colitis. Mucosal folds are covered by a fibrinonecrotic exudate and thickened from edema. Drug-induced (NSAIDs). Differential diagnosis: Salmonellosis.

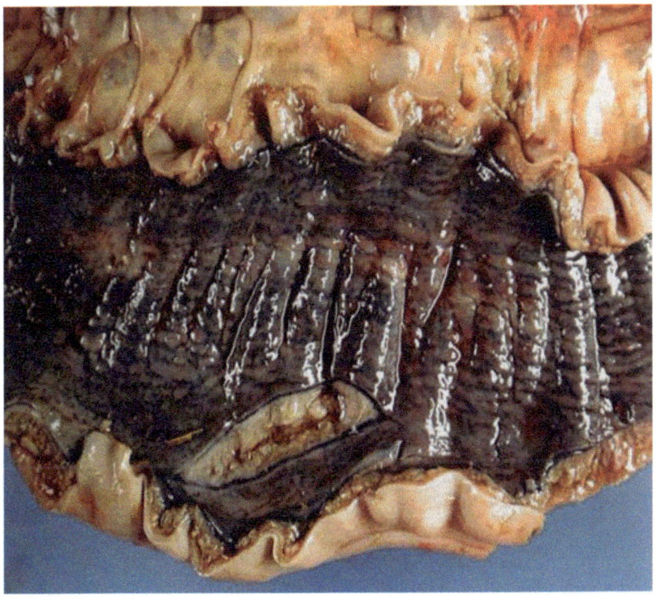

**Figure 6.138.** Horse. Colon. Severe Necrohemorrhagic Colitis. Most of the mucosa is denuded. No specific agents were isolated. The condition is thought to be the result of antibiotic treatment (antimicrobials) against enterocolitis with drugs such as gentamycin or streptomycin. No specific agents were isolated in this case, but *Clostridium* sp. has been identified in other cases.

## 3. *Endoparasites*

Equine endoparasites largely have disappeared since the introduction of effective antihelminthics. Nonetheless, they are still lurking, as they may be treatment-resistant or may affect horses not on regular parasite protocols. Nematodes, cestodes, trematodes, and protozoa can be expected when parasites occur in the horse.

### *a. Nematodes*

i. Ascariasis. Adult ascarids have a tendency to accumulate in the lumen of the small intestine, particularly in young horses. In these situations intestinal rupture and perforation with subsequent septic peritonitis can occur. Larval migration through various internal organs (kidneys, liver, or lung) may cause tissue destruction. *Parascaris equorum* is the species affecting horses.

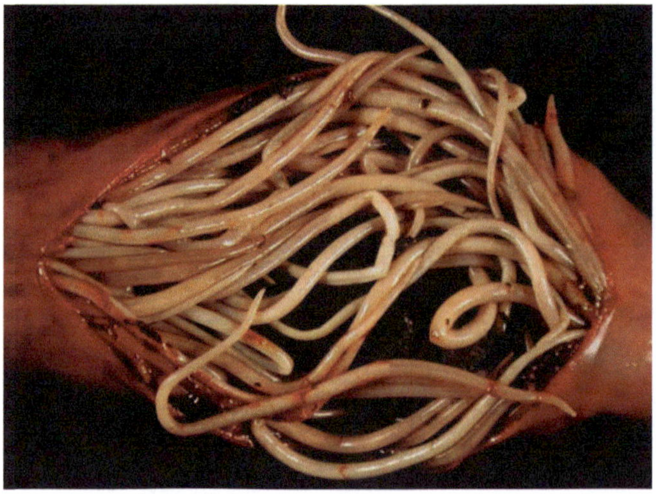

**Figure 6.139.** Horse. Jejunum. Catarrhal Enteritis. *Parascaris equorum.* Massive burden of intraluminal adult ascarids is evident throughout the lumen. The parasite may act as soft foreign bodies. Other complications may be intussusception and bile or pancreatic duct obstruction.

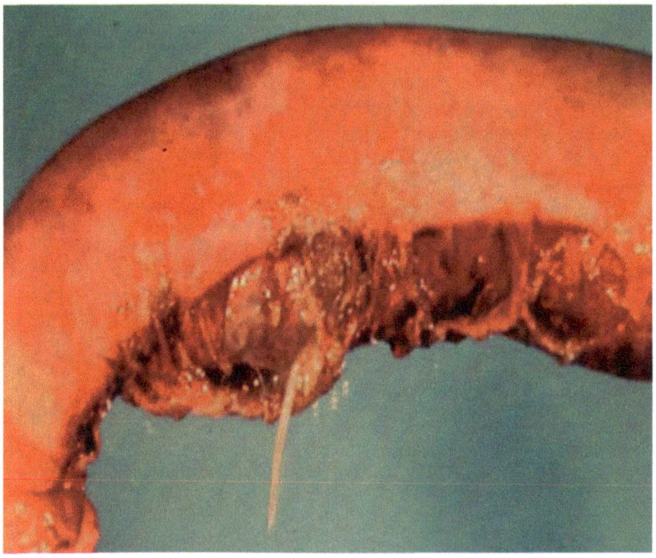

**Figure 6.140.** Horse. Jejunum. Perforation. *Parascaris equorum*. Rupture with spillover of adult worm and feces. (Reprinted with permission from the Animal Technology Institute of Taiwan, Republic of China.)

## ii. Oxyurosis

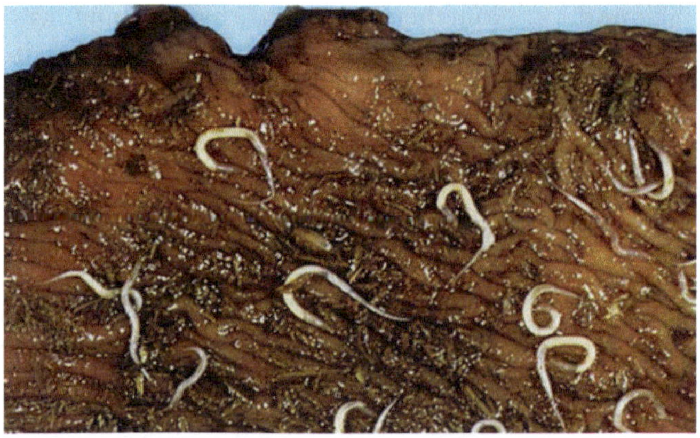

**Figure 6.141.** Horse. Colon. *Oxyuris equi*. Oxyuris also known as pinworm is located in the distal colon. Egg-producing female worms cause anal pruritus. Adults invoke no pathologic changes.

iii. Equine strongyles. Equine strongylosis can be the result of small or large strongyles. Small strongyles are known as Cyathostominae. Large strongyles are represented by *Strongylus vulgaris*, *Strongylus edentatus*, and *Strongylus equinus*. The life cycle is direct. Strongyles are hematophagous nematodes and cause hypoproteinemia.

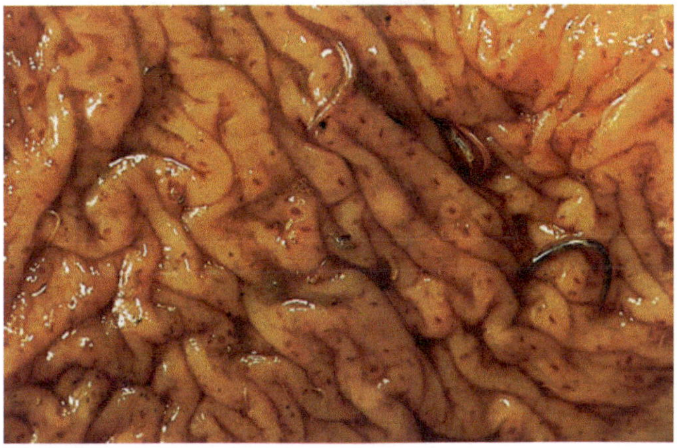

**Figure 6.142.** Horse. Cecum. Mucosal Edema. Strongyles. Adults of large (*Strongylus*) and small strongyles (*Cyastostominae*) and numerous encysted small coiled and reddish strongyle larvae. Adults of small strongyles are not pathogenic. Emergence of small strongyle larvae from the mucosa and submucosa causes ulceration and bacterial infection as complication. More than 50 species are known.

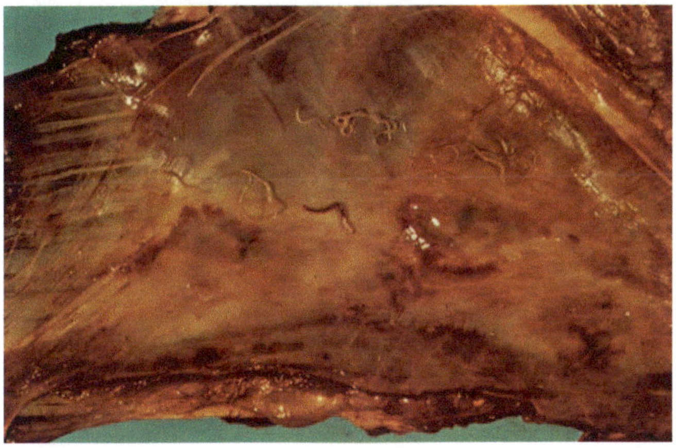

**Figure 6.143.** Horse. Peritoneum. Hemorrhage. *Strongylus edentatus*. Blood-fed adults are on and burrowed underneath the serosa. (Reprinted with permission from the Animal Technology Institute of Taiwan, Republic of China.)

iv. *Strongyloides westeri*. The small nematode resides in the small intestine of foals. It occasionally causes diarrhea. Larvae can be found burrowed within the mucosa microscopically.

*b. Cestodes*

The three species of equine tapeworms can be differentiated by size: *Anoplocephala magna* is the largest (7–8 cm), with *Anoplocephala perfoliata* significantly smaller (25–40 mm) and *Paranoplocephala mamillana* (6–50 mm). Equine tapeworms have been identified as a risk factor for colic predisposing horses to intussusception in the ileocecal area. Mites serve as intermediate hosts infecting horses while grazing.

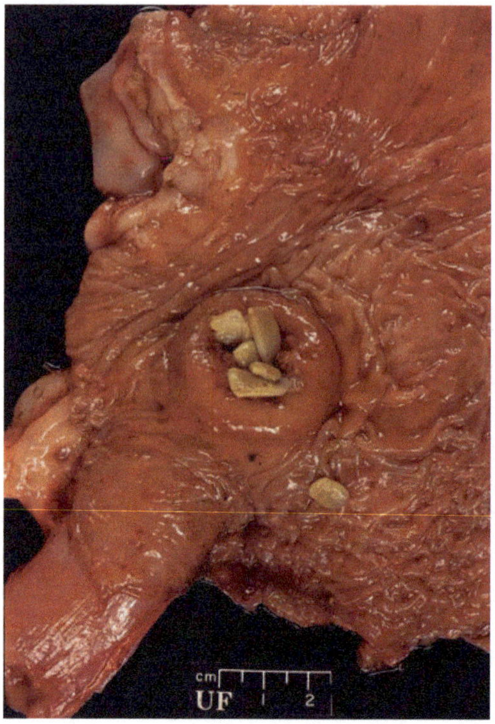


**Figure 6.144.** Horse. Ileocecal Valve. Hyperemia. *Anoplocephala Perfoliata*. A cluster of adult tapeworms inducing an erosive focal typhlitis. Histologically, numerous lymphocytes, plasma cells, and eosinophils can be observed.

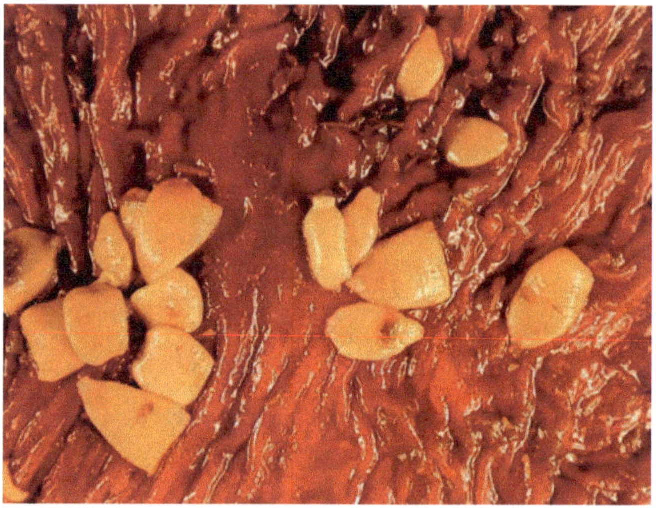

**Figure 6.145.** Horse. Colon. Catarrhal Colitis with Hyperemia. *Anoplocephala perfoliata*. Most of the adults reside within the cranial colon attached to the mucosa.

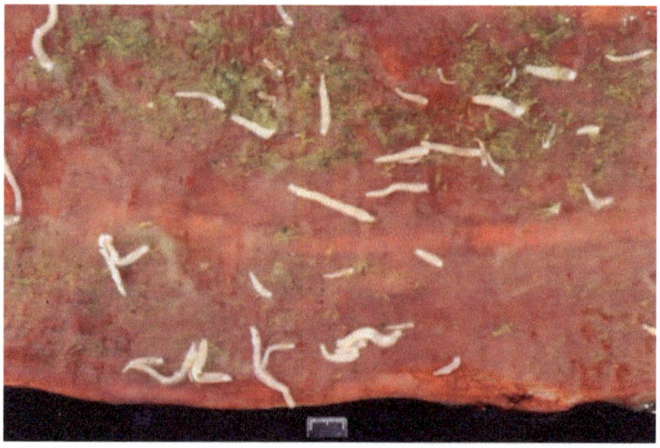

**Figure 6.146.** Horse. Small Intestine. Presence of *Paranoplocephala mamillana* adult worms. (Reprinted with permission from Noah's Archive, Dr. W.K. Read, Texas A&M University.)

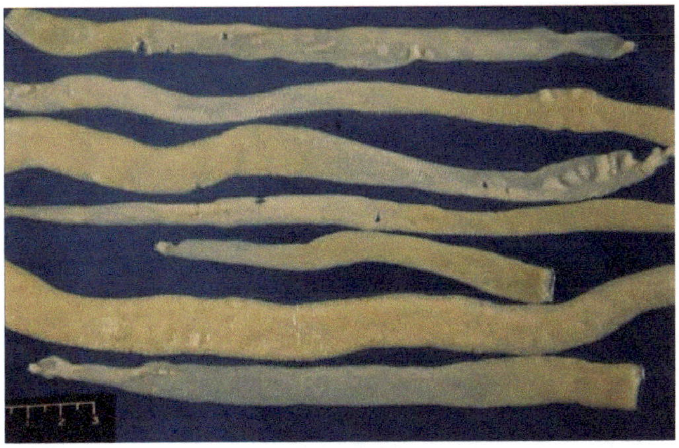

**Figure 6.147.** Demonstration of size of *Anoplocephala magna* adult tapeworms.

### *c. Trematodes*

In the Southeast of the United States, horses standing in swampy pastures with water reaching the abdomen exhibited firm mineralized white plaques on the intestinal serosa and within the liver as a mainly incidental finding at necropsy. These nodules were originally attributed to *Schistosoma* sp. and have been now identified as *Heterobilharzia americana* by DNA extraction, PCR amplification, and gene sequencing. Microscopically the nodules are composed of fibrosing granulomas with occasional schistosomula eggs and ghost larvae present in the center. Adults are very difficult to identify in mesenteric veins. The life cycle remains elusive after investigation of snails as the presumptive intermediate hosts found in these swampy pastures failed to contain cercariae.

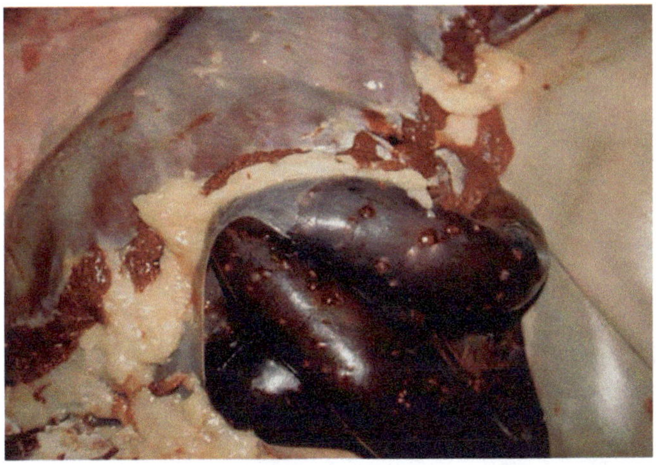

**Figure 6.148.** Horse. Small Intestine. *Heterobilharzia Americana* Mineralized Granulomas. The serosa contains several white plaques that feel firm to the touch.

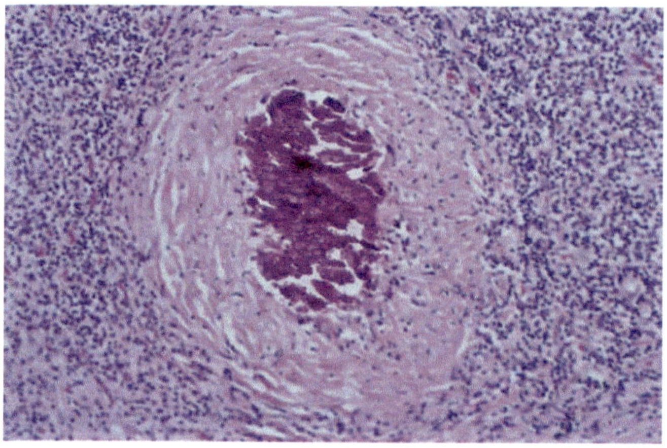

**Figure 6.149.** Horse. Small Intestine. *Heterobilharzia Americana* Fibrosing Granuloma. Microscopically, the plaques are composed of dense collagen with a small rim of inflammation and central mineralization. Intense search may reveal an occasional fragmented eggshell with a brown to black pigmented wall. (H&E)

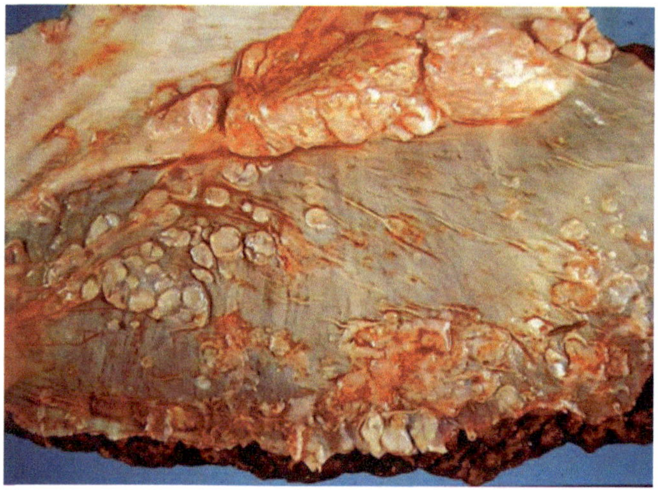

**Figure 6.150.** Horse. Abdominal Surface of Diaphragm. *Heterobilharzia Americana* Granulomas. Differential diagnosis: neoplasia.

*d. Enteric coccidiosis*

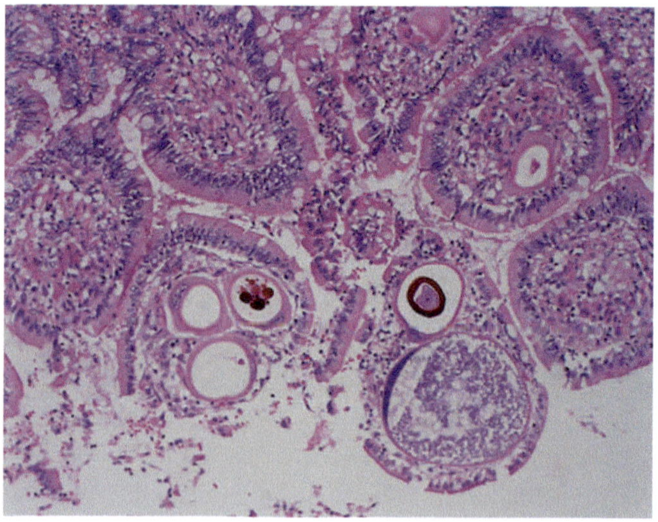

**Figure 6.151.** Horse. Small Intestine. *Eimeria Leuckarti.* Various stages of coccidial development are visible in the lamina propria of the tips of the intestinal villi in cross section. Emerging enteric protozoal diseases to consider are giardiasis and cryptosporidiosis. (H&E)

## Equine intestinal parasites – Fact sheet

| Species | Location of Adults |
|---|---|
| • *Parascaris equorum* | Small intestine |
| • *Strongyloides westeri* | Small intestine |
| • *Strongylus vulgaris* | Colon |
| • *Strongylus edentates* | Colon, cecum |
| • *Strongylus equinus* | Cecum |
| • *Cyathostominae* | Colon, cecum |
| • *Anoplocephala perfoliata* | Colon, cecum |
| • *Anaplocephala magna* | Small intestine |
| • *Paranoplocephala mamillana* | Small intestine |
| • *Heterobilharzia americana* | Mesenteric veins |
| • *Oxyuris equi* | Colon, cecum |
| • *Eimeria leukarti* | Small intestine |

### 4. *Intestinal neoplasia*

These are generally mesenchymal in origin and are mainly fibrosarcomas, leiomyosarcomas, and gastrointestinal stromal tumors or the alimentary form of lymphoma. Intestinal (adeno)carcinomas or polypoid adenomas are rare in horses. Because most of them look very similar at necropsy, microscopic examination is necessary for the specific diagnosis. Tumor phenotyping is helpful by applying tumor markers on tissue sections for microscopic identification.

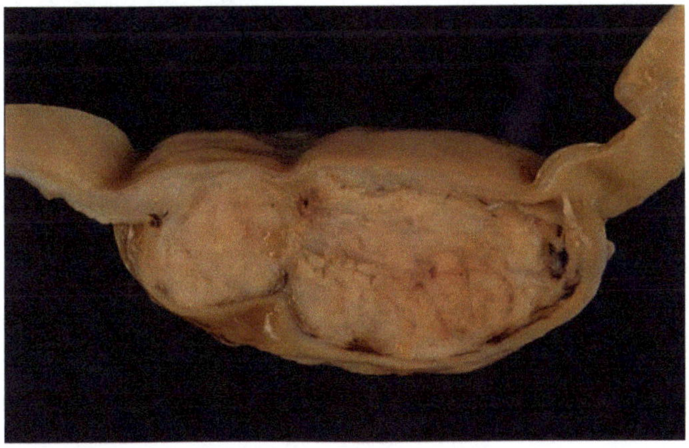

**Figure 6.152.** Horse. Jejunum. Leiomyoma. A lobulated, nodular white growth is expanding within the wall.

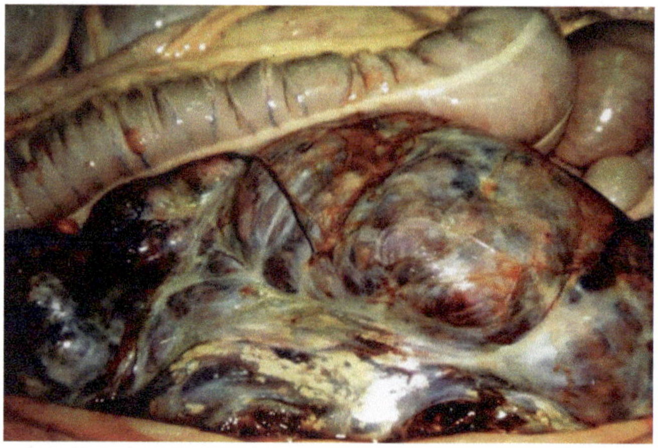

**Figure 6.153.** Horse. Colon. Leiomyosarcoma. A lobulated, fleshy growth protrudes from the wall of the colon. Other mesenchymal tumors have to be considered in the differential diagnosis. The mesenchymal tumors may become quite large, growing around and compressing neighboring organs.

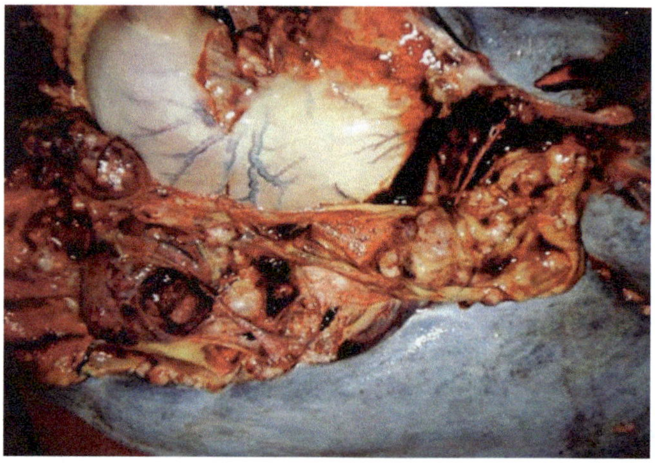

**Figure 6.154.** Horse. Mesentery. Fibrosarcoma. A multinodular growth has expanded into the mesentery.

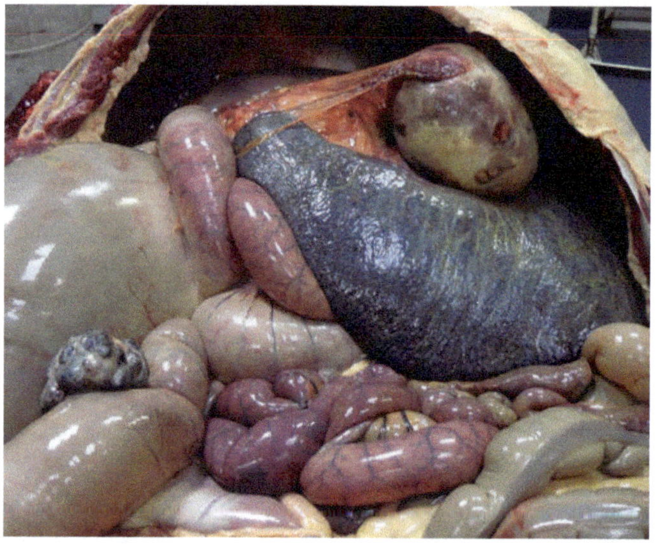

**Figure 6.155.** Horse. Abdomen. Gastrointestinal Stromal Tumor (GIST). Above the spleen and attached to the small intestinal serosa is a round tumor comprised of loosely arranged spindle cells expressing mesenchymal, muscular, and neural markers and c-Kit (CD117).

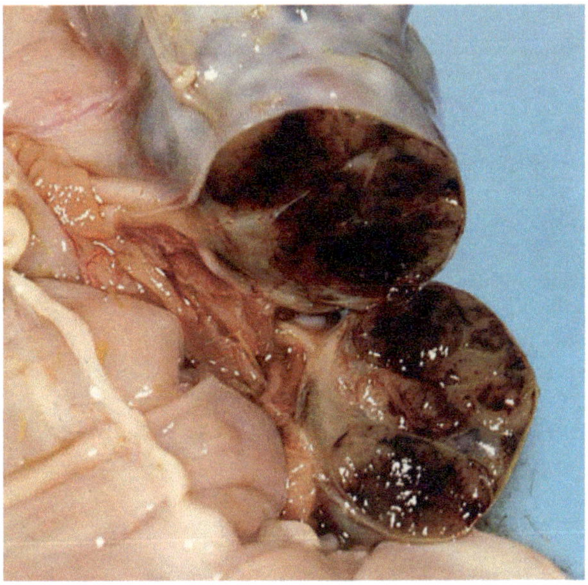

**Figure 6.156.** Horse. Colon. Gastrointestinal Stromal Tumor (GIST). On cross section the cigar-shaped tumor is lobulated, gelatinous, fleshy, and encapsulated.

Grossly, the mostly mural tumors are solitary or multifocal and may arise in the stomach and the small and large intestines. At times they are closely associated with the serosal surfaces of the intestinal tract. The nonmalignant tumors are fleshy and glistening with gelatinous cystic spaces intermixed and lobulated on cross section.

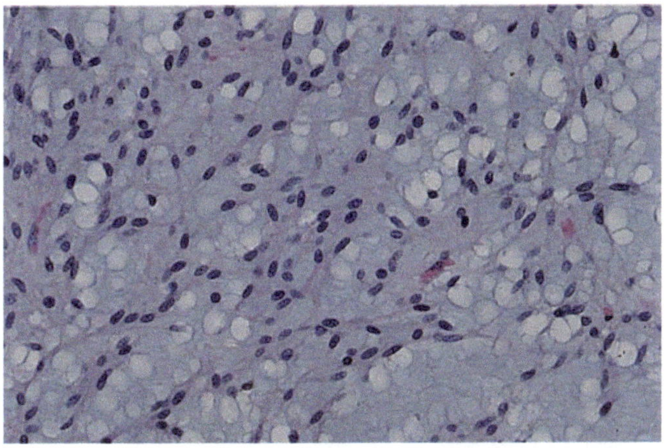

**Figure 6.157.** Horse. Small Intestine. Gastrointestinal Stromal Tumor (GIST). Microscopically the tumor is composed of a network of loosely arranged spindled and stellate cells separated by a mucinous stroma. (H&E)

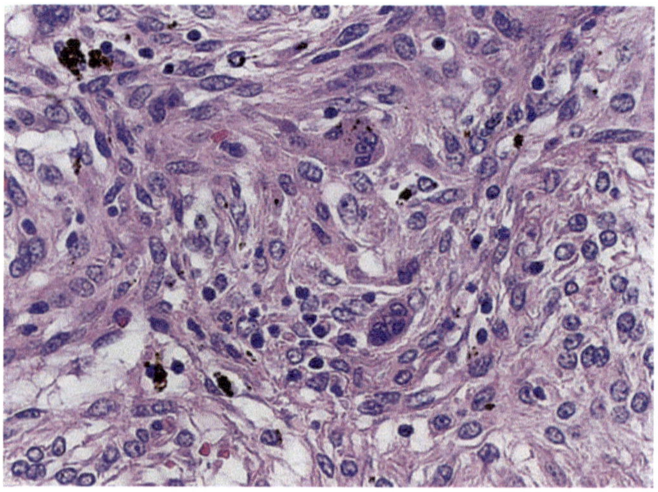

**Figure 6.158.** Horse. Small Intestine. GIST. Other areas have the appearance of a wavy formation of spindled cells with multinucleate cells intermingled. (H&E)

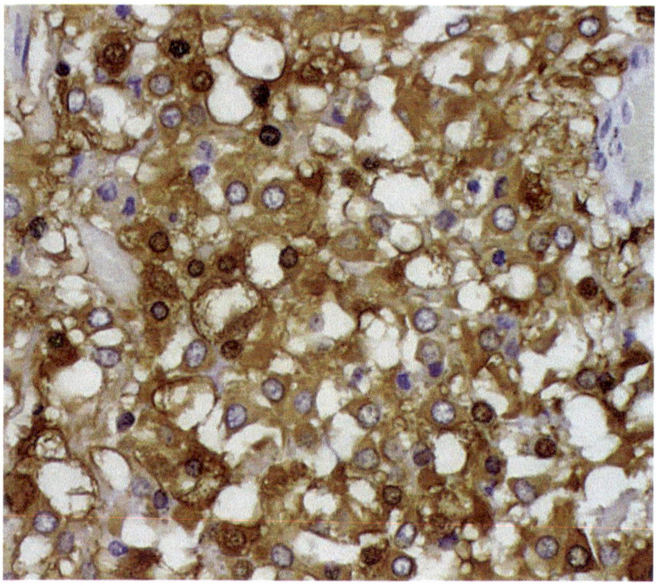

**Figure 6.159.** Horse. GIST. This neoplasm expresses vimentin (in the image), smooth muscle actin, desmin, S-100, neuron-specific enolase, and c-Kit (CD117). (IHC for vimentin)

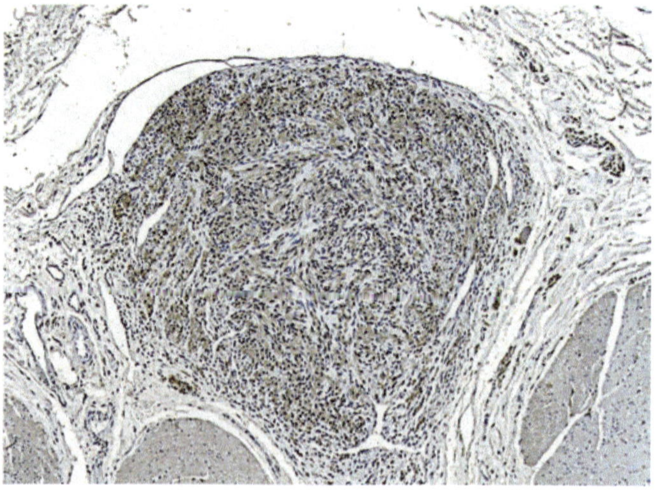

**Figure 6.160.** Horse. GIST. In this multifocal presentation of the tumor some neoplastic cells express smooth muscle actin, others S-100. Ultrastructurally, their morphology was myoid and Schwann-cell like. Here cells express S-100. (IHC)

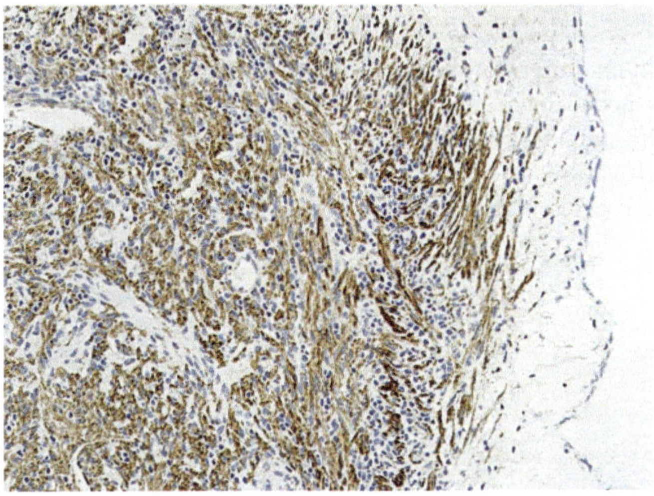

**Figure 6.161.** Horse. GIST. Other neoplastic cells express smooth muscle actin. Ultrastructurally, their morphology was myoid. (IHC)

By virtue of positive indirect immuohistochemistry for vimentin, and occasionally for actin and S-100, gastrointestinal tumors are composed of myogenic, neurogenic, and mesenchymal cells. It has been suggested that the cell of origin for GIST is the intramural pacemaker interstitial cell of Cajal.

Examples of alimentary lymphoma are presented in Chapter 15, "Diseases of the Hemolymphatic System."

### *5. Miscellaneous*

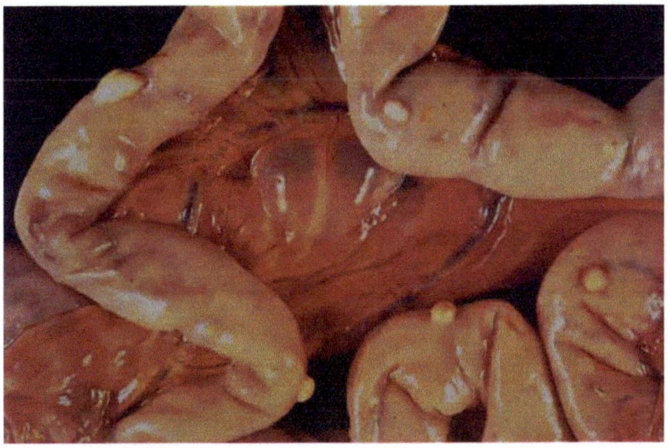

**Figure 6.162.** Horse. Jejunum. Serosal Nodules. The diagnosis was that of sterile granulomas or equine sarcoidosis, not to be confused with equine sarcoid. Similar granulomatous changes can affect multiple internal organs that are covered by serosal surfaces. In some cases mycobacterial DNA was identified by PCR in these granulomas.

## VI. Diseases of the peritoneum

The normal peritoneum is a smooth, thin, translucent, glistening membrane kept moist by small amounts of fluid.

If excessive, the abdominal fluid is diagnosed as abdominal effusion. Distinction should be made between antemortem and postmortem effusions. Depending on the nature of the excessive fluid, antemortem diagnosis includes hydroperitoneum, hemoperitoneum, and uroperitoneum.

## 1. *Inflammation*

Inflammation leading to peritonitis is nearly always septic. Inflammation may be focal or generalized. Focal inflammation leads to adhesions through fibrous tissue interfering with intestinal motility. Underlying causes are rupture, perforation, or leakage of a viscous direct extension through an inflamed gastrointestinal wall, or hematogenous or lymphatic spread.

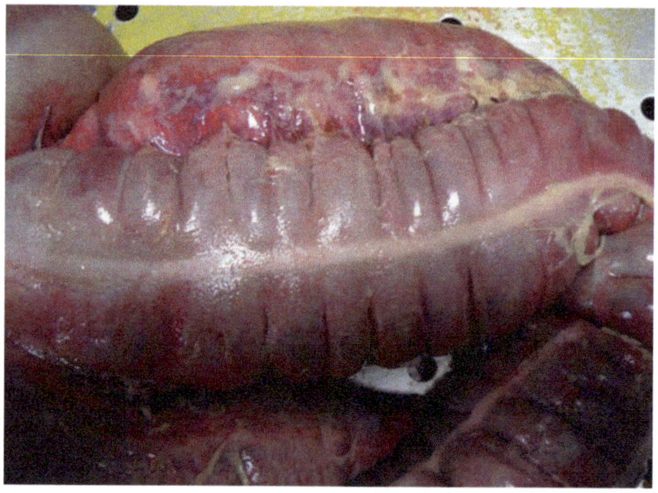

**Figure 6.163.** Horse. Abdomen. Colon. Peritonitis. Fibrinohemorrhagic inflammation resulting from colitis.

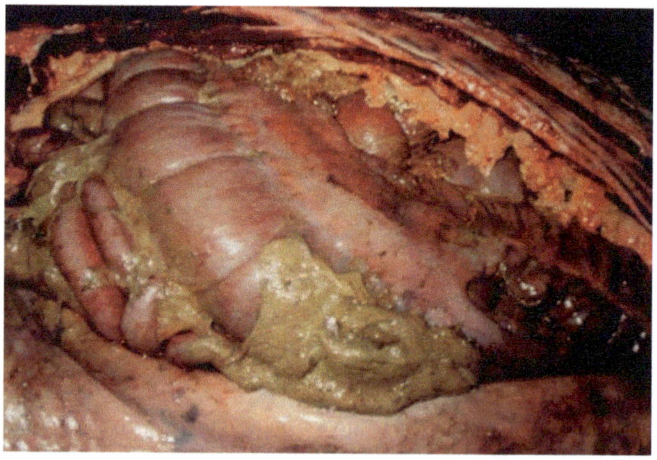

**Figure 6.164.** Horse. Abdomen. Peritonitis. Fibrinopurulent peritonitis resulting from rupture of the stomach or cecum is usually involved. (Reprinted with permission from the Animal Technology Institute of Taiwan, Republic of China.)

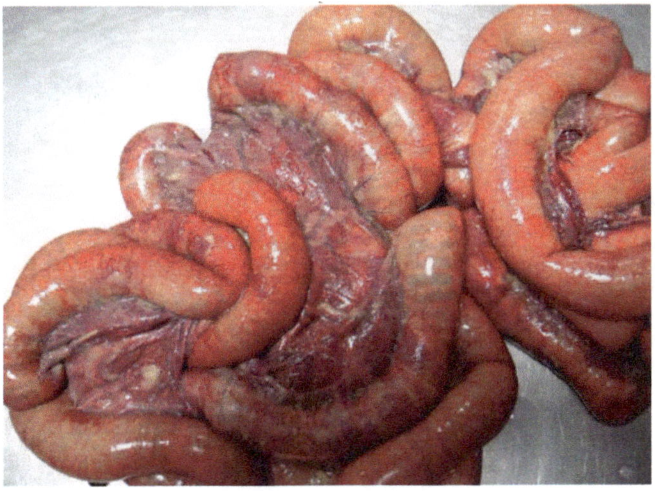

**Figure 6.165.** Horse. Small Intestine. Uroperitonitis. Resulted from ruptured infected urinary bladder. Serosal surfaces are hyperemic.

## 2. Neoplasia

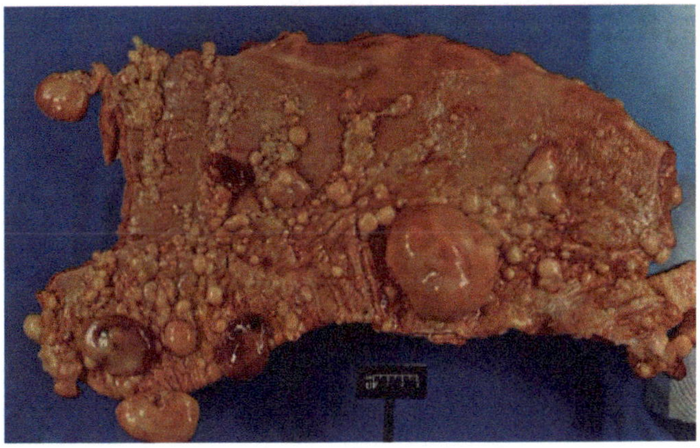

**Figure 6.166.** Horse. Diaphragm. Abdominal Mesothelioma. A massive, soft, yellow, grapelike growth was removed from the abdominal cavity.

Despite its benign term these are malignant tumors in the horse spreading within the abdominal cavity, causing ascites and metastasis to the lung. Individual cases of mesothelioma have been reported from the thorax and pericardium. Tumors arise from the cells of the serosal surfaces such as the peritoneum. Tumor markers are available for phenotyping. The neoplasm may express both cytokeratin and vimentin. Other tumor markers that can be used are calretinin, Wilms tumor (WT)-1 and carcinoembryonic antigen (CEA).

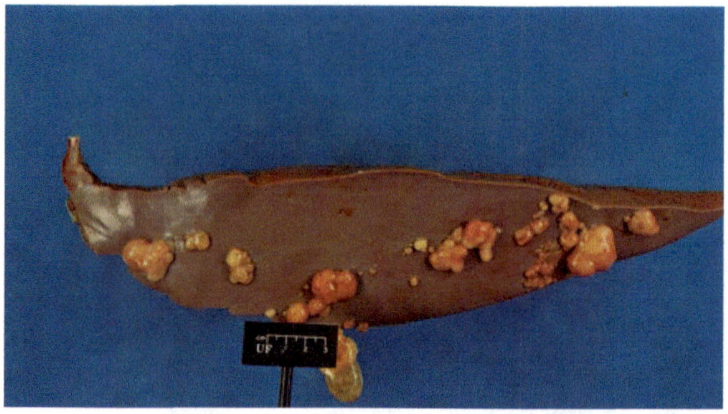

**Figure 6.167.** Horse. Liver. Malignant Mesothelioma. The growth spread to the Glisson's capsule of the liver by way of abdominal transplantation.

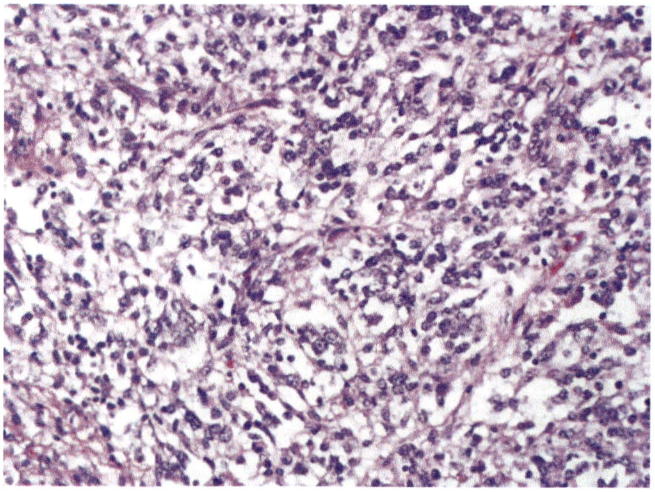

**Figure 6.168.** Horse. Abdomen. Malignant Mesothelioma. Histology may reveal a biphasic mass. In one of the phases it may be composed of pleomorphic, stellate round cells that are embedded in a clear, slightly myxoid stroma. (H&E)

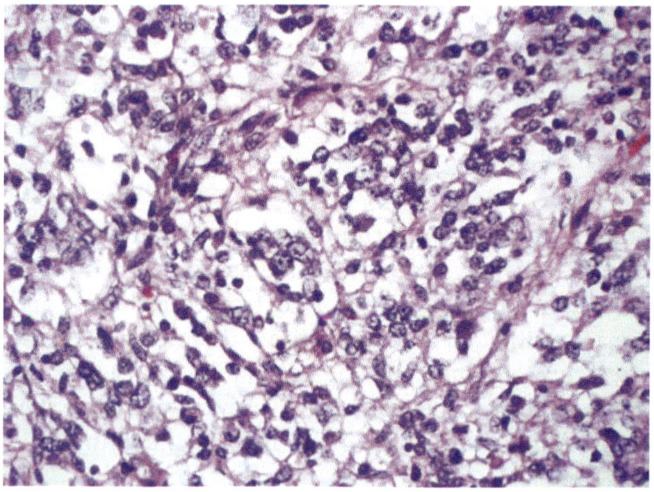

**Figure 6.169.** Horse. Abdomen. Malignant Mesothelioma. The other phase may exhibit epithelioid neoplastic cells connecting with each other as a network. (H&E)

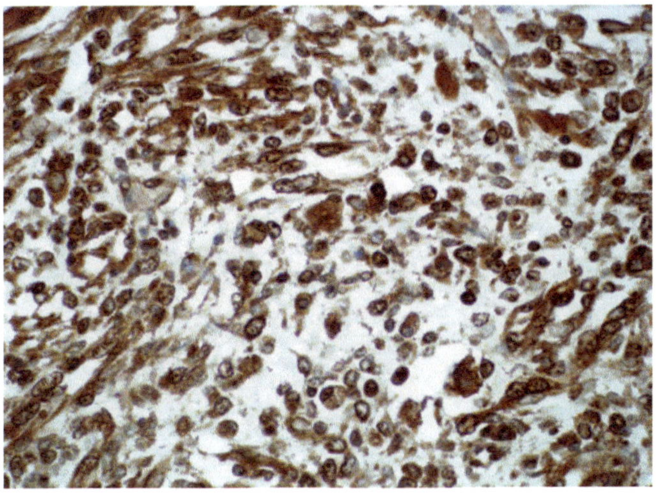

**Figure 6.170.** Horse. Abdomen. Malignant Mesothelioma. Epithelioid mesothelioma cells express intracytoplasmic carcinoembryonic antigen (CEA). (IHC)

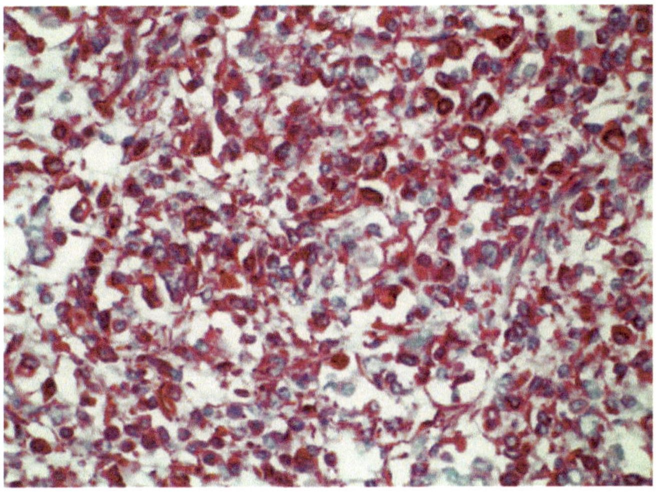

**Figure 6.171.** Horse. Abdomen. Malignant Mesothelioma. Vimentin. The neoplastic cells show strong cytoplasmic labeling for vimentin. (IHC)

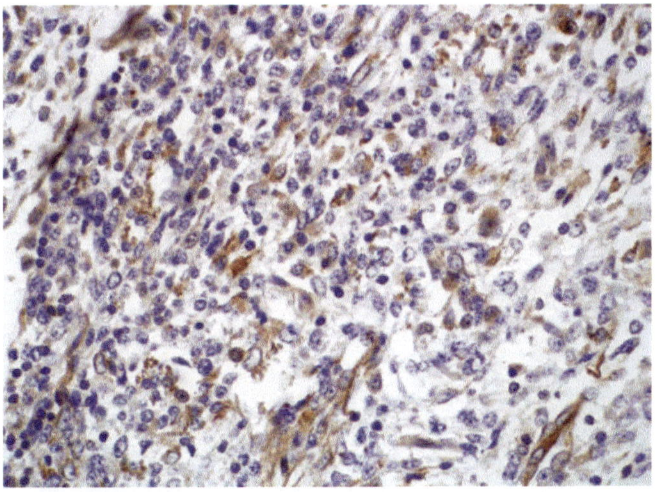

**Figure 6.172.** Horse. Abdomen. Malignant Mesothelioma. Wilms tumor-1 (WT1). Cytoplasmic labeling is moderate in spindled neoplastic cells. (IHC)

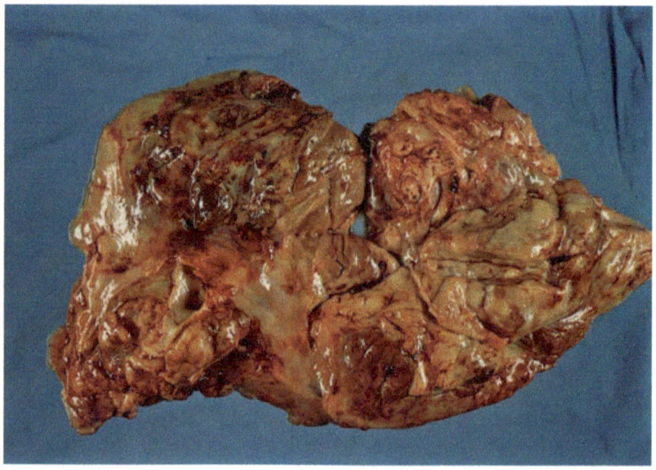

**Figure 6.173.** Horse. Abdomen. Malignant Mast Cell Tumor. This horse presented with fever of unknown origin and eosinophilia on hematology. At necropsy a fist-sized tumor was found in the cranioventral abdomen close to the liver. The tumor disseminated to the liver.

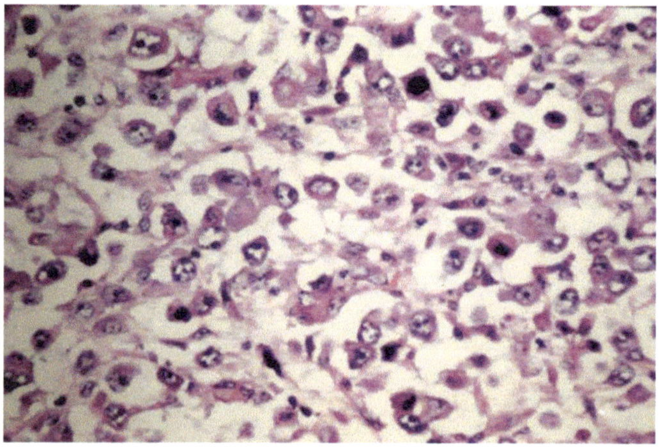

**Figure 6.174.** Horse. Abdominal Mast Cell Tumor. Cellular pleomorphism with prominent variable-sized nuclei and faint eosinophilic to vacuolic cytoplasm were the histologic features. A Giemsa stain shows evidence of faint metachromasia of individual cells.

### *3. Miscellaneous*

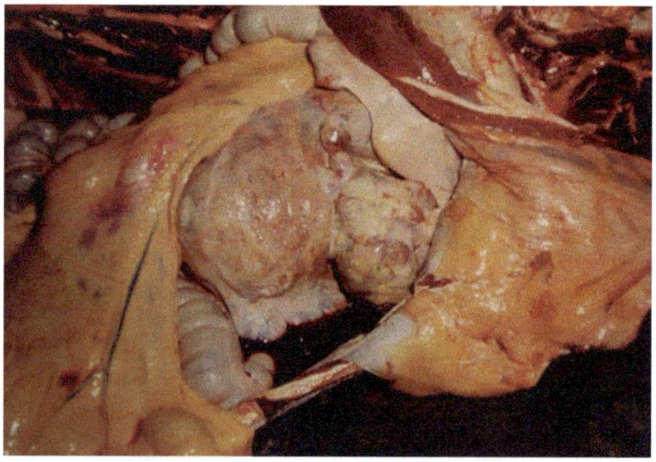

**Figure 6.175.** Horse. Abdomen. Amyloidosis. A large bulging mass within the ventral abdomen and adjacent to abundant abdominal adipose tissue considered an abdominal neoplasm was diagnosed microscopically to be massive amyloid deposition. The amyloid deposits are of AA type.

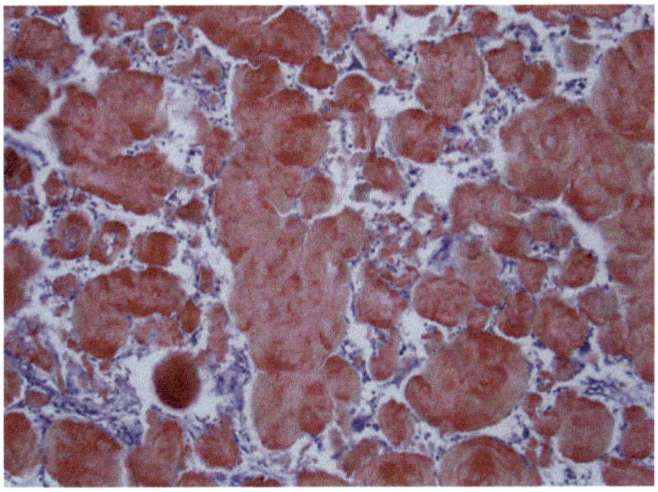

**Figure 6.176.** Horse. Abdomen. Amyloidosis. A Congo red special stain is positive for amyloid. (Congo red)

## Selected references


Andrews FM, Reinemeyer CR, McCracken MD, et al. 2002. Comparison of endoscopic, necropsy and histology scoring of equine gastric ulcers. *Equine Vet J* 34(5):475–478.

Arroyo LG, Staempfli HR, Weese JS. 2006. Potential role of *Clostridium difficile* as a cause of duodenitis-proximal jejunitis in horses. *J Med Microbiol* 55(Pt 5):605–608.

Begg LM, O'Sullivan CB. 2003. The prevalence and distribution of gastric ulceration in 345 racehorses. *Aust Vet J* 81(4):199–201.

Bell RJ, Mogg TD, Kingston JK. 2007. Equine gastric ulcer syndrome in adult horses: a review. *New Zealand Vet J* 55(1):1–12.

Benders NA, Veldhuis Kroese EJ, van der Kolk JH. 2004. Idiopathic muscular hypertrophy of the oesophagus in the horse: a retrospective study of 31 horses. *Equine Vet J* 36(1):46–50.

Broekman LE, Kuiper D. 2002. Megaesophagus in the horse. A short review of the literature and 18 own cases. *Vet Q* 24(4):199–202.

Chandra AMS, Buergelt CD, Ethell MT. 1999. Odontogenic myxoma of the mandible in a filly. *J Vet Diagn Invest* 11:224–277.

Corapi WV, Birch SM, Carlson KL, Chaffin MK, Snoden KF. 2011. *Heterobilharzia americana* infection as a cause of hepatic parasitic granulomas in a horse. *J Am Vet Med Assoc* 229(8):1117–1122.

Donaldson MT, Palmer JE. 1999. Prevalence of *Clostridium perfringens* enterotoxin and *Clostridium difficile* toxin A in feces of horses with diarrhea and colic. *J Am Vet Med Assoc* 215(3):358–361.

Ekiri AB, MacKay RJ, Gaskin JM, et al. 2009. Epidemiologic analysis of nosocomial Salmonella infections in hospitalized horses. *J Am Vet Med Assoc* 234(1): 109–119.

Feary DJ, Hassel DM. 2006. Enteritis and colitis in horses. *Vet Clin North Am Equine Pract* 22(2):437–479.

Feige K, Schwarzwald C, Fuerst A, Kaser-Hotz B. 2000. Esophageal obstruction in horses: a retrospective study of 34 cases. *Can Vet J* 41(3):2007–2010.

Frederick J, Giguere S, Sanchez LC. 2009. Infectious agents detected in the feces of diarrheic foals: a retrospective study of 233 cases (2003–2008). *J Vet Intern Med* 23(6):1254–1260.

Hackett RP. 1983. Nonstrangulated colonic displacement in horses. *J Am Vet Med Assoc* 182(8):235–240.

Helman RG, Edwards WC. 1997. Clinical feaures of blister beetle poisoning in equids: 70 cases (1983–1996). *J Am Vet Med Assoc* 211(8):1018–1021.

Howerth DG, Mead DG, Mueller PO, Duncan L, Murphy MD, Stallknecht DE. 1996. Experimental vesicular stomatitis virus infection in horses: effect of route of inoculation and virus serotype. *Vet Pathol* 43(6):943–955.

Hunter JO. 2009. Do horses suffer from irritable bowel syndrome? *Equine Vet J* 41(9):836–840.

Jeffcott LB, Colles CM. 1977. Phenylbutazone and the horse—a review. *Equine Vet J* 9(3):105–110.

Kalk KA. 2009. Inflammatory bowel disease in horses. *Vet Clin North Am Equine Pract* 25(2):303–315.

Karchner LF, Dill SG, Anderson WI, King JM. 1990. Right dorsal colitis. *J Vet Intern Med* 4(5):247–263.

Kiper ML, Traub-Dargatz J, Curtis JR. 1990. Gastric rupture in horses: 50 cases (1979–1987). *J Am Vet Med Assoc* 196(2):333–336.

Loehr CV, Polster U, Kuhnert P, Karger A, Rurangirwa FR, Teifke JP. 2012. Mesenteric lymphangitis and sepsis due to RTX toxin-producing *Actinobacillus* spp in 2 foals with hypothyroidism-dysmaturity syndrome. *Vet Pathol* 49(4): 592–601.

Magdesian KG, Dujowich M, Madigan JE, Hansen LM, Hirsh DC, Jang SS. 2006. Molecular characterization of *Clostridium difficile* isolates from horses in an intensive care unit and association of disease severity with strain type. *J Am Vet Med Assoc* 228(5):751–755.

Martineau H, Thompson H, Taylor D. 2009a. Pathology of gastritis and gastric ulceration in the horse. Part 1: range of lesions present in 21 mature individuals. *Equine Vet J* 41(7):638–644.

Martineau H, Thompson H, Taylor D. 2009b. Pathology of gastritis and gastric ulceration in the horse. Part 2: a scoring system. *Equine Vet J* 41(7):646–651.

McConnico RS, Morgan TW, Williams CC, Ubert JD, Moore RM. 2008. Pathophysiologic effects of phenylbutazone on the right dorsal colon in horses. *Am J Vet Res* 69(11):1496–1505.

McGurrin MK, Vengust M, Arroyo LG, Baird JD. 2007. An outbreak of Lawsonia intracellularis infection in a standardbred herd in Ontario. *Can Vet J* 48(9): 927–930.

Mulville P. 1991. Equine monocytic ehrlichiosis (Potomac horse fever): a review. *Equine Vet J* 23(6):400–404.

Murray M. 1996. Salmonellosis in horses. *J Am Vet Med Assoc* 209(3):558–560.

Murray M. 2001. Endoscopic findings of the gastric antrum and pylorus in horses: 162 cases (1996–2000). *J Vet Intern Med* 15(4):401–406.

Oliveira-Filho JP, Monteiro LN, Defiol DJ, Sequeira JL, Amorim M, Fabris VE, Del Piero F, Borges AS. 2012. Mycobacterium DNA detection in liver and skin of a horse with generalized sarcoidosis. *J Vet Diagn Invest* 24(3):596–600.

Oliver OE, Staempfli H. 2006. Acute diarrhea in the adult horse: case example and review. *Vet Clin North Am Equine Pract* 22(1):73–84.

Palmer JE. 1993. Potomac horse fever. *Vet Clin North Am Equine Pract* 9(2): 399–410.

Schmitt B. 2002. Vesicular stomatitis. *Vet Clin North Am Anim Pract* 18(3):453–459.

Schmitz DG. 1989. Cantharidin toxicosis in horses. *J Vet Intern Med* 3(4):208–215.

Schumacher J, Edwards JF, Cohen ND. 2000. Chronic idiopathic inflammatory bowel disease of the horse. *J Vet Intern Med* 14(3):258–265.

Schumacher J, Mullen J, Shelby R, Lenz S, Ruffin DC, Kemppainen BW. 1995. An investigation of the role of *Fusarium moniliforme* in duodenitis/proximal jejunitis of horses. *Vet Hum Toxicol* 37(1):39–45.

Songer JG, Trinh HT, Dial SM, Brazier JS, Glock RD. 2009. Equine colitis X associated with infection by *Clostridium difficile* NAP1/027. *J Vet Diagn Invest* 21(3): 377–380.

Taylor SD, Haldorson GJ, Vaughan B, Pusterla N. 2009. Gastric neoplasia in horses. *J Vet Intern Med* 23(5):1097–1102.

Thean S, Elliot B, Riley T. 2011. *Clostridium difficile* in horses in Australia – a preliminary study. *J Med Microbiol* 60(Pt 8):1188–1192.

Todhunter RJ, Erb HN, Roth L. 1986. Gastric rupture in horses: a review of 54 cases. *Equine Vet J* 18(4):288–293.

Traub-Dargatz JL, Jones RL. 1993. Clostridia-associated enterocolitis in adult horses and foals. *Vet Clin North Am Equine Pract* 9(2):411–421.

Ulrich R, Eydner M, Gruen A, Haydn J, Baumgaertner W. 2009. A biphasic malignant mesothelioma of the peritoneum and pleura in a horse. *Dtsch Tieraerztl Wochenschr* 116(5):186–191.

Van den Wollenberg L, Sloet van Oldruitenborgh-Oosterbaan MM. 2000. Gastric ulceration in horses: etiology, diagnosis, and therapy: a review. *Tijdschr Diergeneeskd* 125(21):642–647.

Van Rensburg IB, Jardine JE, Carstens JH, van der Walt ML. 1995. The prevalence of intestinal Salmonella infection in horses submitted for necropsy. *Onderstepoort J Vet Res* 62(1):65–67.

Whitlock RH. 1986. Colitis: differential diagnosis and treatment. *Equine Vet J* 18(4):278–283.

# 7 Diseases of the Liver and Pancreas

- I. Liver
  1. Hemodynamic changes
     a. Lobar atrophy
     b. Portosystemic shunt
     c. Chronic congestive heart failure
     d. Focal ischemia
  2. Metabolic, necrotic, and toxic diseases
     a. Lipidosis
     b. Amyloidosis
     c. Idiopathic acute hepatic disease
     d. Degeneration and necrosis
  3. Infectious hepatitis and hepatic abscesses
     a. Herpesvirus hepatitis
     b. Tyzzer's disease
     c. Leptospirosis
     d. *Rhodococcus equi* hepatitis
     e. Abscesses
     f. Equine infectious anemia virus hepatitis
     g. Cholangitis
  4. Endoparasitism
     a. Trematodes
     b. Cestodes
     c. Nematodes
  5. Primary and secondary hepatic neoplasia
  6. Liver biopsy
- Summary
- II. Pancreas
  1. Pancreatitis
  2. Pancreatic hypertrophy

*Color Atlas of Equine Pathology*, First Edition. Claus D. Buergelt and Fabio Del Piero.

## The equine liver

The liver is the largest single organ in the horse, weighing between 10 and 20 pounds (4.5–9.0 kg). Physiologically, the liver is involved in a variety of metabolic and detoxification functions. It possesses large functional reserve and regeneration capacities. When the liver fails, a variety of organ systems fail. Liver disease may be present long before liver failure develops. Equine liver diseases are relatively infrequent when compared with other animal species despite the many diseases primarily affecting the equine gastrointestinal tract. Predictable clinical signs of liver failure in the horse are icterus, hypoalbuminemia, coagulopathy, hypoglycemia, hyperlipoproteinemia, and hepatic encephalopathy. This chapter summarizes liver diseases unique to the equine animal species. Pathologic entities include metabolic disorders, toxic and immunologic insults, infectious agents, endoparasites, neoplastic disorders, and incidental findings.

# I. Liver

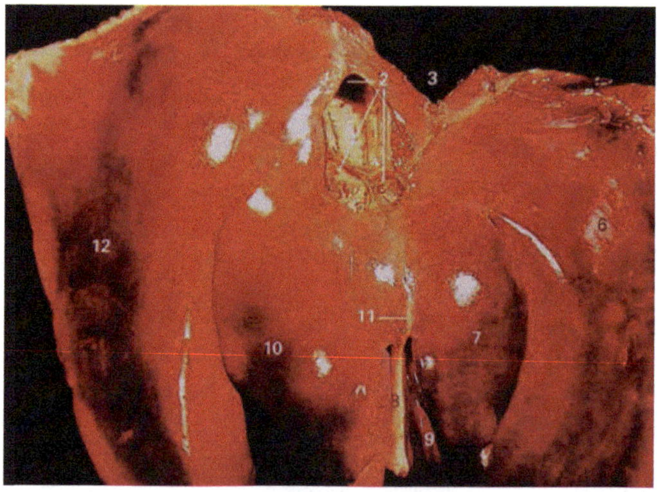

**Figure 7.1.** Horse. Liver. Diaphragmatic Surface. Normal. Color as expected. Numbers denote the anatomic identification of the hepatic lobes.

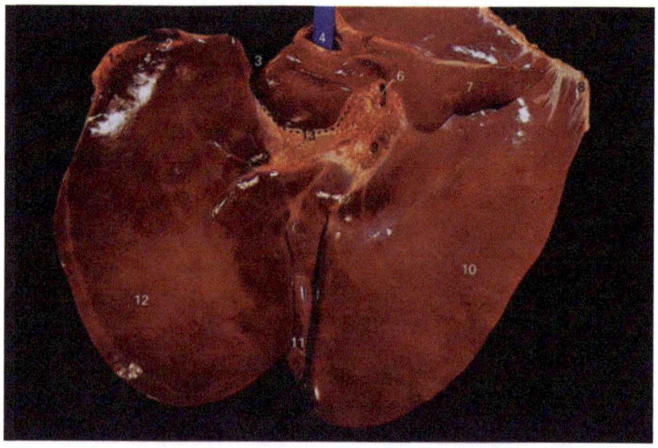

**Figure 7.2.** Horse. Liver. Visceral Surface and Hilus. Normal. Numbers identify anatomic configurations. The equine liver lacks a gallbladder.

## 1. *Hemodynamic changes*

### *a. Lobar atrophy*

In clinically normal horses, the right liver lobe constitutes half of the total liver weight. The condition of lobar atrophy is believed to be the result of ischemia in this part of the liver from long-standing atony of the adjacent right dorsal colon and base of the cecum.

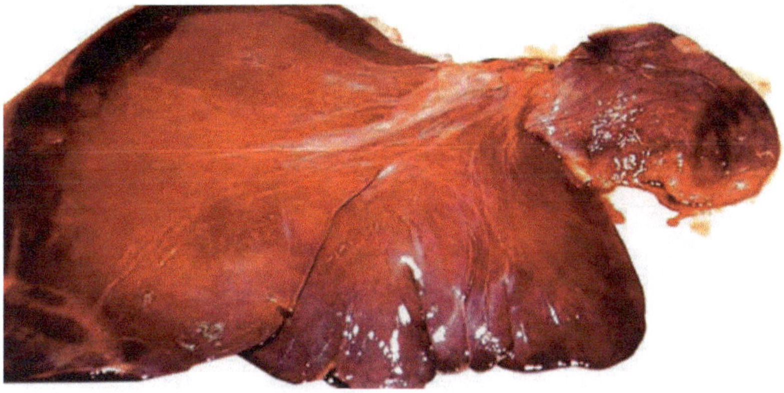

**Figure 7.3.** Horse. Liver. Hepatic Atrophy. The right liver lobe is markedly reduced in size. Differential diagnosis is generalized liver atrophy due to starvation.

### *b. Portosystemic shunt*

Foals and juvenile horses are mainly affected. Clinical signs are vague and may include depression, lethargy, and ataxia due to hepatic encephalopathy. Livers may be grossly reduced on size.

### *c. Chronic congestive heart failure*

Back flow and insufficient return of venous blood from the liver results in hepatomegaly and excessive flow of blood from the cross section.

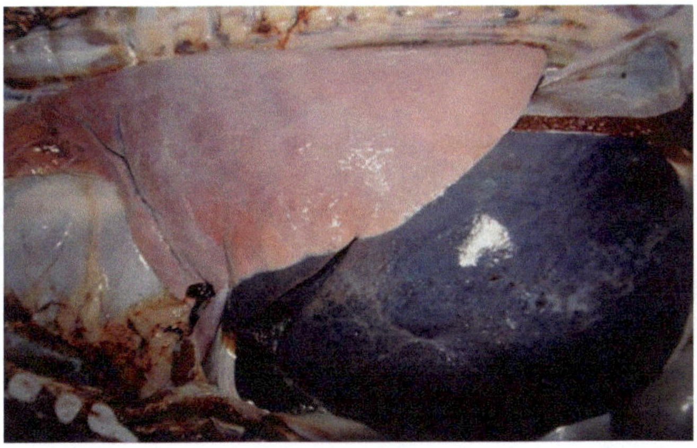

**Figure 7.4.** Horse. Liver In-situ. Passive Hepatic Congestion. Right-sided Heart Failure. The liver is dark blue and markedly enlarged indicating congestion. Pulmonary edema and hydropericardium are also visible. Ascites can be expected.

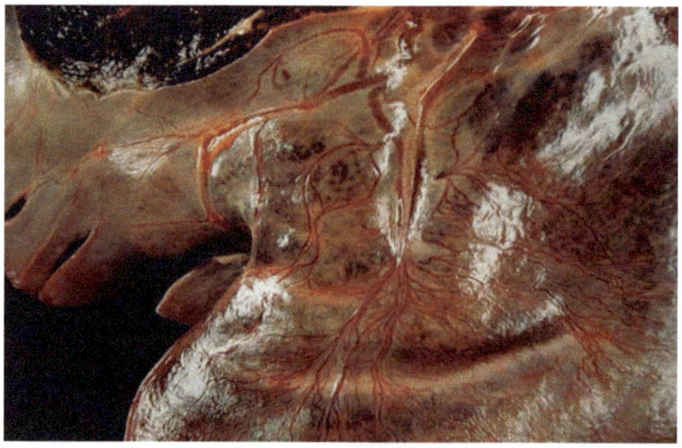

**Figure 7.5.** Horse. Liver. Venous Congestion ("Spider Veins"). Right-sided Heart Failure. Enlarged liver with spiderweb-like congestion of stretched Glisson capsule vessels.

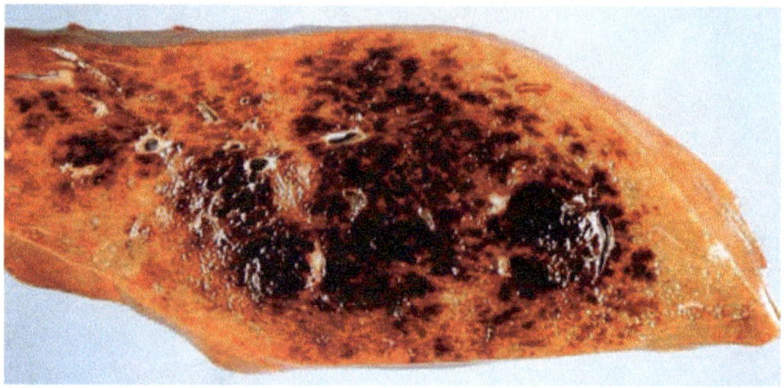

**Figure 7.6.** Horse. Liver Cross Section. Passive Venous Congestion. Right-Sided Heart Failure. Stagnating blood has caused a mottled pattern sometimes compared with a nutmeg.

*d. Focal ischemia*

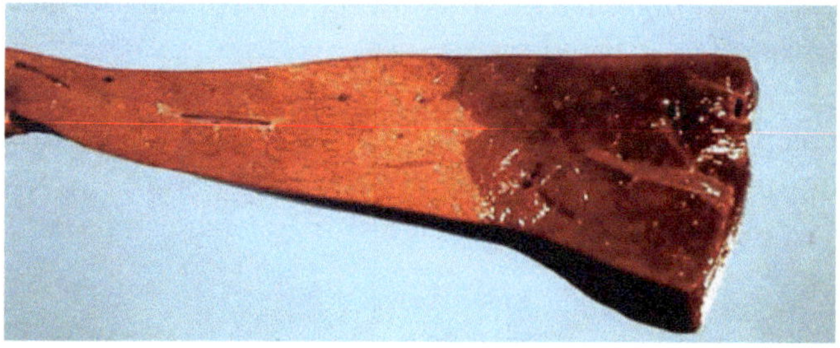

**Figure 7.7.** Horse. Liver. Focal Ischemic Lipidosis. This is an incidental finding on the diaphragmatic surface of the liver and the result of focal inflammatory adhesion between the liver surface and diaphragm surface. The condition is also coined as tension lipidosis. (Courtesy Dr. J. King, Cornell University.)

## 2. Metabolic, necrotic, and toxic diseases

*a. Lipidosis*

This metabolic disorder occurs mainly in ponies, donkeys, and Miniature horses. Anorexia and lethargy are clinical signs. Hepatic encephalopathy may ensue. The condition is associated with hyperlipidemia and hyperlipemia indicative of an underlying disturbance of the lipid metabolism. Hepatic lipidosis results when the rate of hepatic triglyceride synthesis exceeds the formation and release of very low density lipoprotein substance into the circulation. The two major hormones regulating lipid metabolism are glucocorticoids and insulin. Insulin resistance may play a role in the pathogenesis of hyperlipidemia.

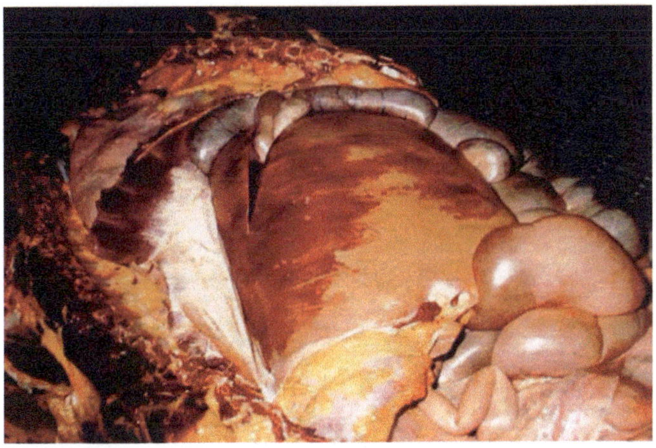

**Figure 7.8.** Horse. Liver In-situ. Hepatic Lipidosis. The liver exhibits large areas of yellow discoloration.

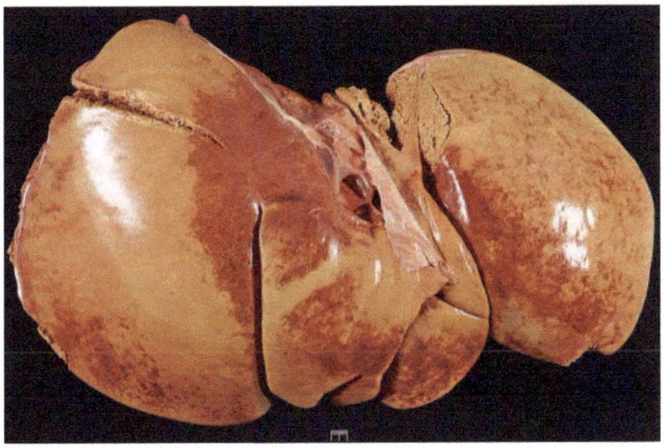

**Figure 7.9.** Horse. Liver. Hepatic Lipidosis. The entire liver is enlarged and yellow. Edges are rounded. On touch the parenchyma may easily rupture. Differential diagnosis: amyloidosis.

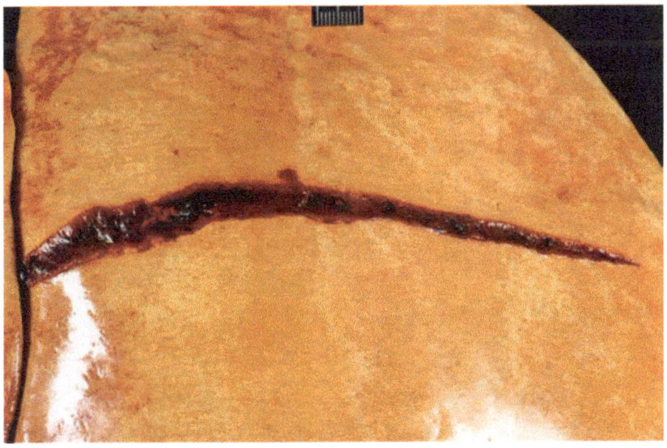

**Figure 7.10.** Horse. Liver. Surface Rupture in Hepatic Lipidosis. Hemoperitoneum may be a fatal complication.

*b. Amyloidosis*

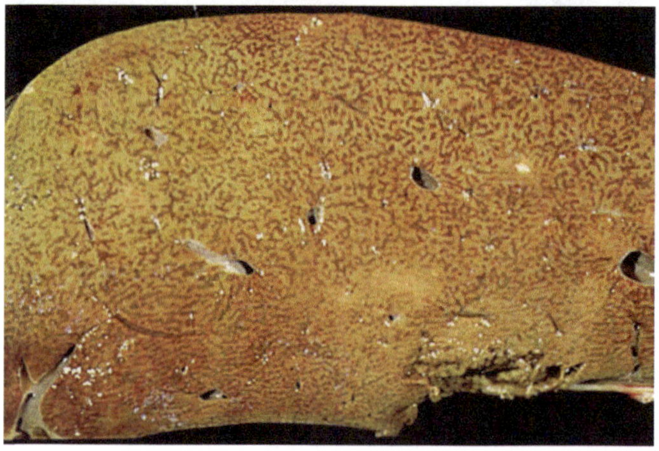

**Figure 7.11.** Horse. Liver. Amyloidosis. The interstitial accumulation of amyloid (yellow) progressively compresses and atrophies the hepatic parenchyma (brown). Hepatic amyloidosis typically is encountered in serum-producing horses and is of AA-type. (Courtesy Dr. P. Habecker, University of Pennsylvania.)

*c. Idiopathic acute hepatic disease*

A recent publication suggested a divergent virus belonging to the Flaviviridae family as possible etiologic cause. Synonyms for this condition are Theiler's disease or serum hepatitis. It is mainly a sporadic disease and typically occurs 40–60 days after injection of an equine-based product (e.g., tetanus antitoxin). Affected horses may show signs of hepatic failure. A type III hypersensitivity reaction originally had been suggested as the cause. Acute mortality may be as high as 50–60%. Affected horses present anorexia, hepatic encephalopathy, and icterus. Hepatic liver enzyme levels are increased. Serum total bile acid concentration will be elevated. Differential diagnoses include hepatotoxins and acute infectious diseases.

At necropsy, the liver is usually small and flattened. It may be bile-stained. Microscopic changes are characterized by severe panlobular necrosis and a mild to moderate mixed inflammatory infiltrate.

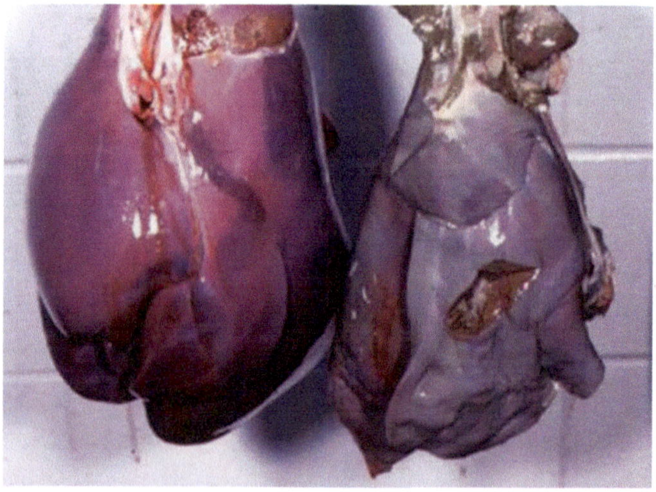

**Figure 7.12.** Horse. Liver. Acute Hepatic Necrosis. Theiler's disease. The affected liver is on the right and has a shrunken, flat profile with indentations on the capsular surface. A healthy liver is depicted on the left. (Courtesy Dr. J. King, Cornell University.)

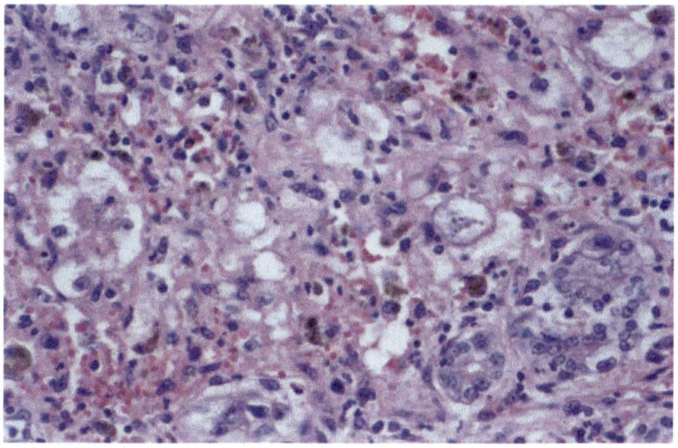

**Figure 7.13.** Horse. Liver. Acute Hepatic Necrosis. Theiler's disease. There is distortion of the hepatic lobular pattern due to a loss of intrinsic hepatocytes. A few remaining hepatocytes show vacuolar swelling. Intermixed are mainly mononuclear inflammatory cells. (H&E)

*d. Degeneration and necrosis*

The liver is highly susceptible to unspecific and specific toxins. Despite a high threshold toward toxins, long exposure to these induces degenerative and necrotic changes. Histologically, there are specific lobular patterns of response to bloodborne toxic injuries to the liver. Recognition of these patterns may be indicators of and may lead to narrowing the nature of the toxins involved. Depending on the duration, sequence, and dosage of the toxins, the liver will respond to toxic injury with fibrosis, cirrhosis, or regeneration.

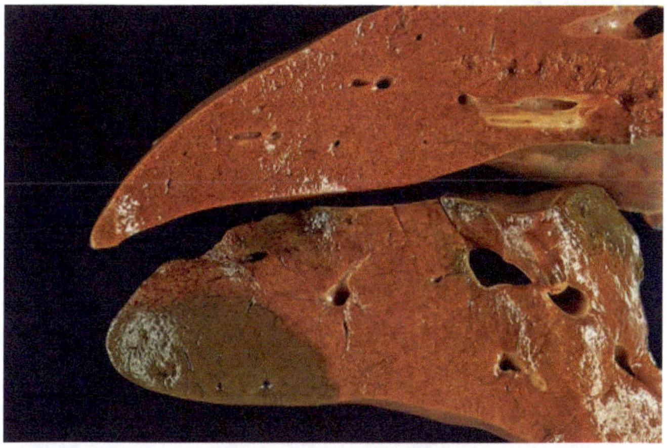

**Figure 7.14.** Horse. Liver. Focal Necrosis. The green brown areas of discoloration indicate the anatomic site of the necrosis.

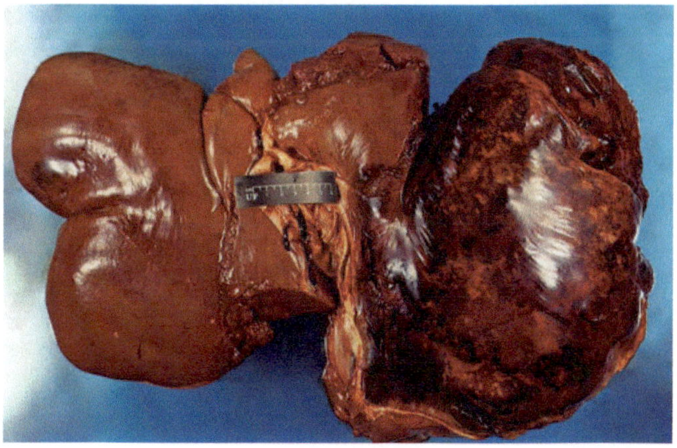

**Figure 7.15.** Horse. Liver. Lobar and Multifocal Necrosis. One lobe is markedly swollen and discolored. The other lobes reveal focal involvement of necrosis. Depending on blood flow and susceptibility of the detoxifying enzyme, the pattern of injury is not uniform in this case.

Toxins affecting the equine liver generally are derived from plants, fungi, chemicals, drugs, and heavy metals. Most commonly plants producing pyrrolizidine alkaloids (PAs) are responsible for liver failure in horses. These alkaloids are found in *Crotalaria, Amsinkia, Senecio* spp., and others.

i. Crotalaria toxicosis. Crotalaria, found predominantly in the South and Southeast of the United States has been the cause of many pastured horse losses. Known as wild pea or rattlebox, Crotalaria is planted as an agricultural cover crop. Two species, *Crotalaria sagittalis* and *Crotalaria spectabilis,* are particularly toxic to the equine liver. Horses, unlike small ruminants, are 30–40 times more susceptible to PA poisoning due to a poor capability to detoxify alkaloids in the liver.

Alkaloids are metabolized to toxic pyrrol esters in the liver by the hepatic PFO system (cytochrome P450). The pyrrol esters act as alkylating agents and ligate to hepatocellular nuclear proteins and nucleic acid (DNA) to become anti-mitotic. Cellular division occurs, but no DNA replication leading to nuclear DNA accumulation and increased nuclear size resulting in the formation of megalocytes. The megalocytes eventually die and are replaced by fibrous connective tissue. Reactive PA metabolites may also damage the lung alveolar and renal tubular epithelium, albeit to a lesser degree. Photosensitivity dermatitis develops as clinical complication.

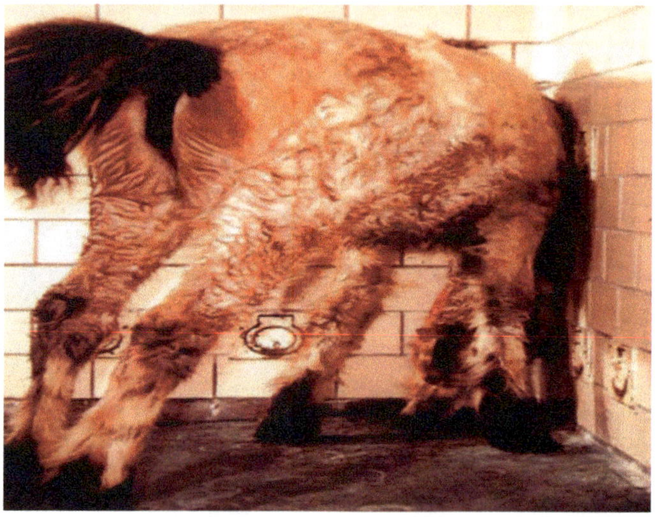

**Figure 7.16.** Horse. Equine Body. Head Pressing. Hepatic Encephalopathy from PA Toxicosis. The posture is a typical clinical sign seen in this condition.

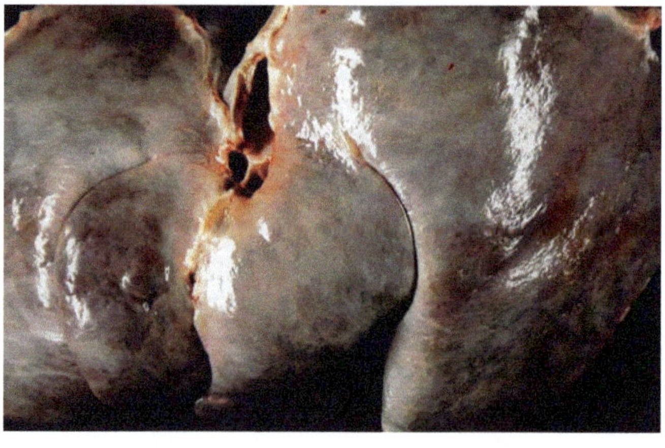

**Figure 7.17.** Horse. Liver. Fibrosis/ Cirrhosis. PA Toxicosis. The liver is pale, firm, and slightly enlarged with mild capsular surface irregularities.

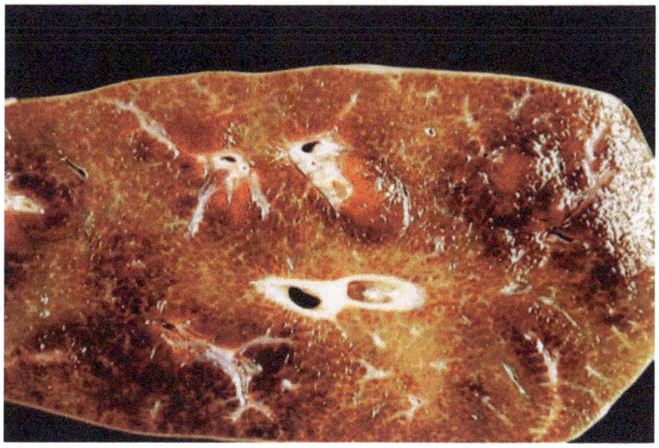

**Figure 7.18.** Horse. Liver. Fibrosis/ Cirrhosis. PA Toxicosis. On cross section the liver is mottled due to fibrosis/ cirrhosis resulting from long-standing PA consumption.

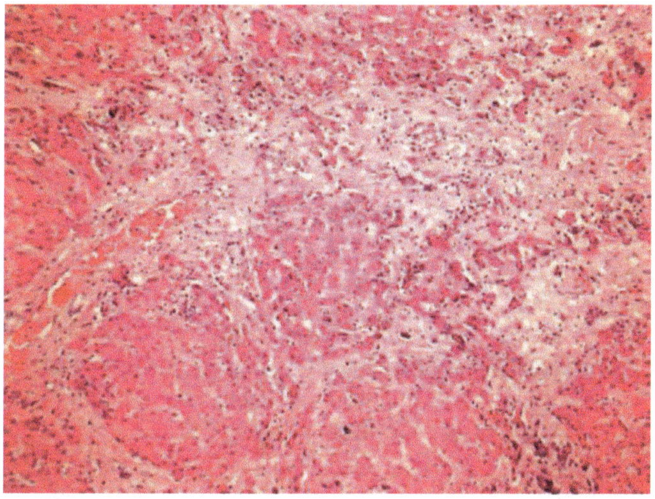

**Figure 7.19.** Horse. Liver. Peri- and Intralobular Fibrosis. PA Toxicosis. Peripheral hepatocytes have been replaced by dense collagen with some lobular bridging fibrosis. Inflammation is not a feature. (H&E)

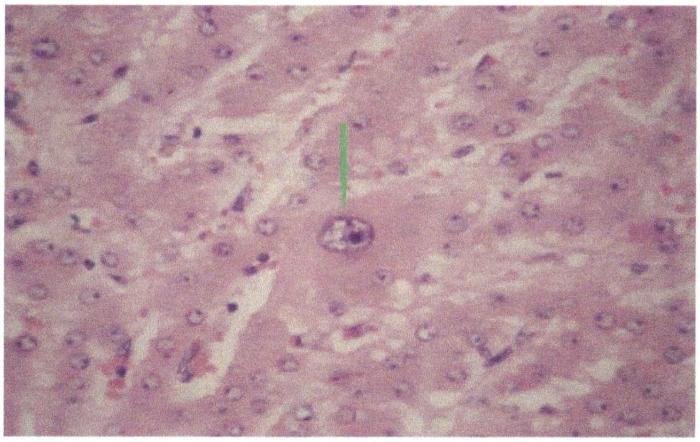

**Figure 7.20.** Horse. Liver. Megalocyte. PA Toxicosis. Hepatic megalocytosis (arrow) is characterized by nuclear enlargement and increased cytoplasmic volume. It is suggestive of PA but not pathognomonic for it. (H&E)

## Hepatic pyrrolizidine alkaloid (PA) toxicosis – Pathologic features

### Gross findings

- The liver usually maintains its weight and shape. It changes its color to pale gray and its texture to firm. On cut section the liver is mottled with colors ranging from brown to yellow-green.

### Microscopic findings

- Acute PA toxicosis is characterized by centrilobular necrosis and hemorrhage.
- Chronic PA toxicosis produces hepatocellular necrosis in the portal zones with fibrosis, biliary hyperplasia, and obstruction of hepatic veins. There is minimal inflammation, but bile ductular hyperplasia is an additional feature. Megalocytosis of hepatocytes is a hallmark for the presumptive diagnosis of PA toxicosis. Hepatocellular megalocytosis is by no means pathognomonic for PA toxicosis because it also occurs with nitrosamines and mycotoxins.

## Hepatic pyrrolizidine alkaloid (PA) toxicosis – Fact sheet

### Definition

- Hepatotoxicosis is caused by consumption of plants such as *Crotalaria* sp.
- Toxins cause severe hepatic fibrosis and liver failure

### Incidence

- In the United States toxic plants of concern are *Crotalaria* sp., *Amsinkia* sp., and *Heliotropium* sp.
- Horses are 30–40 times more susceptible to PAs than sheep and goats

### Differential diagnosis

- Mycotoxicosis
- Chronic (right-sided) heart failure

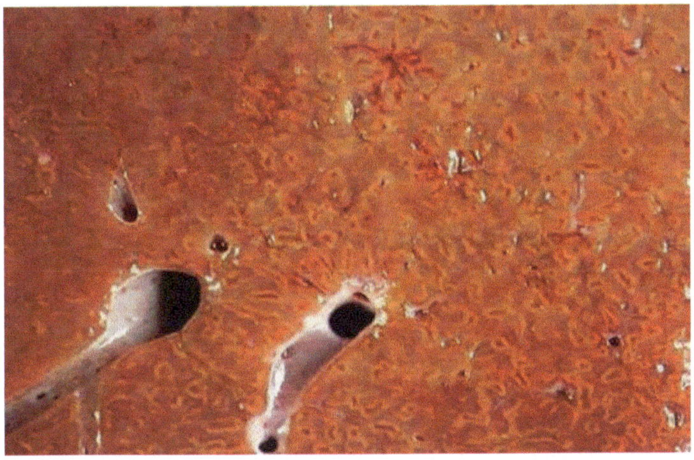

**Figure 7.21.** Horse. Liver. Necrosis and Cholestasis. Acute *Indigofera Spicata* Toxicosis. Toxic plant with potential to cause liver necrosis with mild inflammation clinically leading to hepatic encephalopathy known as Grove poisoning. (Courtesy Dr. J. Roberts, National Zoo, Washington, DC.)

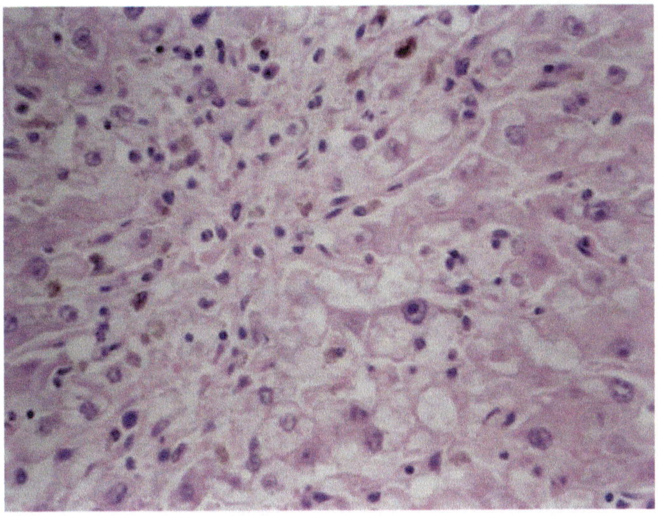

**Figure 7.22.** Horse. Liver. Cytoplasmic Vacuolation. *Indigofera Spicata* Toxicosis. There is evidence of cytoplasmic vacuolic degeneration of hepatocytes with loss of nuclei. Hepatocytes are swollen and dissociated reducing the sinusoidal space. Nuclei vary in size with some evidence of megalocytosis. Mononuclear cell inflammation is mild and random. There is cholestasis. (H&E) (Courtesy Dr. J. Roberts, National Zoo, Washington, DC.)

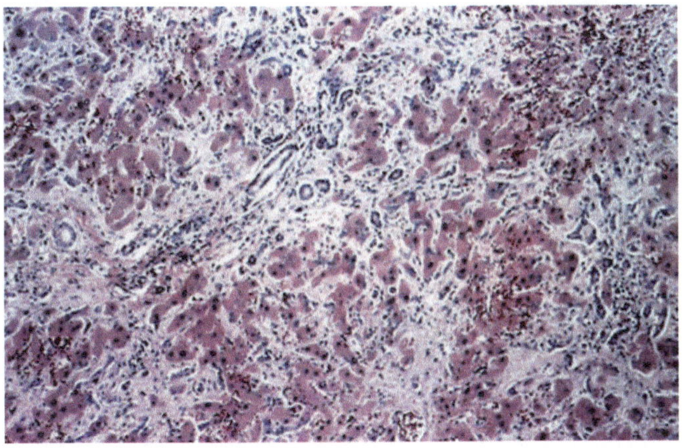

**Figure 7.23.** Horse. Liver. Fibrosing Hepatitis. Chronic Ragwort (Senecio) Poisoning. Hepatocellular Dropout. Individual and groups of hepatocytes are surrounded by inflammatory cells and early collagen formations. (H&E)

### Toxic plants with potential for liver failure in horses

- Kleingrass toxicosis
- Alsike clover toxicosis
- Ragwort (*Senecio jacobea*) toxicosis
- Mycotoxic lupinosis
- Cocklebur (Xanthium) toxicosis
- Creeping Indigo (*Indigofera spicata*) toxicosis
- *Lantana camara* toxicosis

ii. Aflatoxicosis. Aflatoxins are metabolic products of fungi such as *Aspergillus flavus* that may contaminate feed. Affected livers are enlarged and swollen grossly. Microscopic features may include fatty degeneration, necrosis of hepatocytes, biliary hyperplasia, and cellular pleomorphism of hepatocytes including megalocytosis.

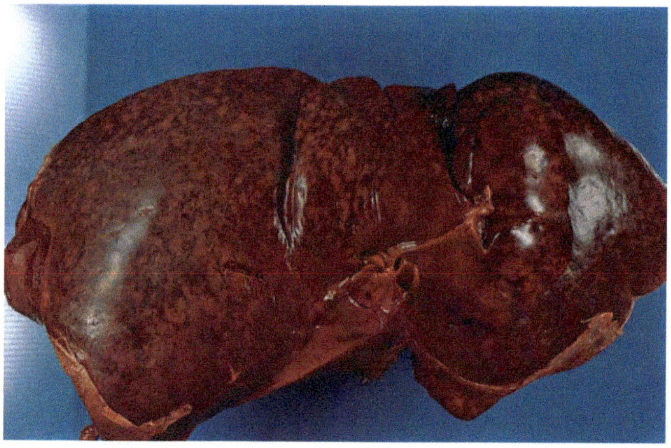

**Figure 7.24.** Horse. Liver. Hepatomegaly. Aflatoxicosis. The liver is tan, enlarged, and swollen indicated by rounded edges.

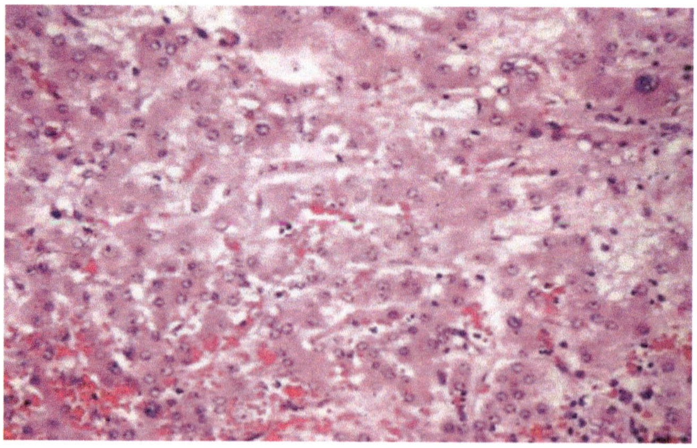

**Figure 7.25.** Horse. Liver. Hepatocellular Disorientation. Aflatoxicosis. Hepatic plates are disorganized. Sinusoids are distended. An occasional megalocyte is present. (H&E)

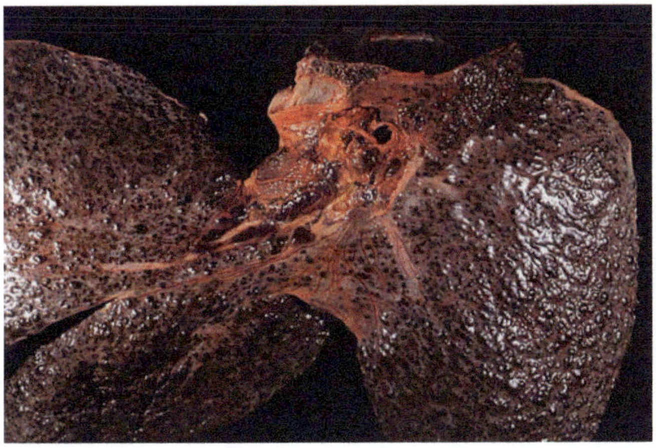

**Figure 7.26.** Horse. Liver. Cirrhosis. Diffuse postnecrotic micronodular to macronodular regeneration with intranodular fibrosis. (Courtesy Dr. P. Habecker, University of Pennsylvania.)

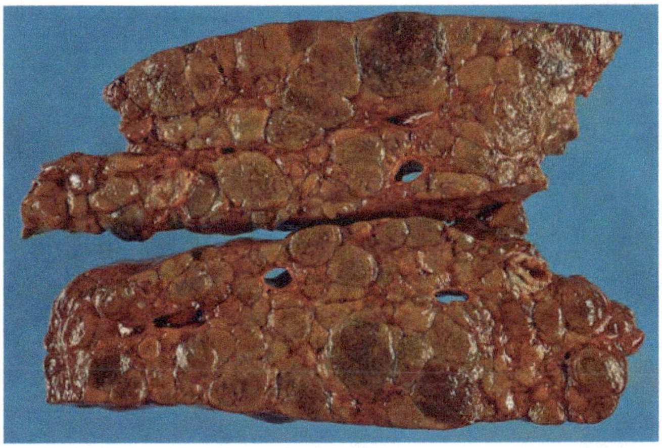

**Figure 7.27.** Horse. Liver. Postnecrotic Macronodular Regeneration. Regeneration of parenchymal hepatocellular loss is a potential of the liver to respond to injury. If the injurious process persists, scarring as the result of fibrosis and nodular regeneration ensues. End-stage liver with cirrhosis may develop.

### 3. *Infectious hepatitis and hepatic abscesses*

*a. Herpesvirus hepatitis*
Discussed in Chapter 2, "Diseases of Foals and Juveniles."

*b. Tyzzer's disease*
Caused by *Clostridium piliformis* and discussed in Chapter 2, "Diseases of Foals and Juveniles."

*c. Leptospirosis*
Discussed under "Equine Bacterial Abortions" in Chapter 12.

*d.* Rhodococcus equi *hepatitis*
Has been occasionally described in conjunction with disseminated *R. equi* infection.

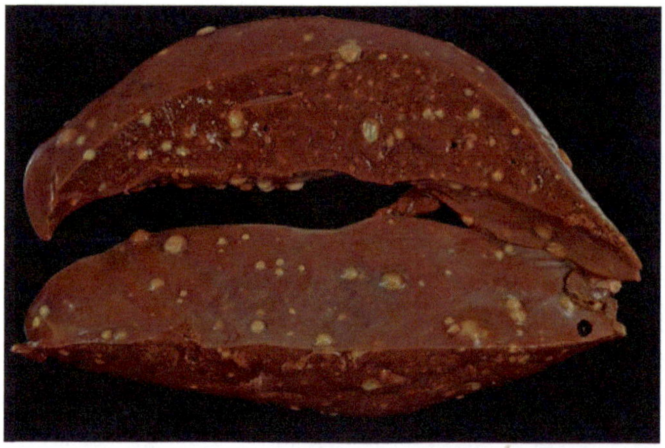

**Figure 7.28.** Horse. Liver. Caseous Hepatitis. *Rhodococcus Equi*. Discrete yellow foci are randomly distributed through the hepatic parenchyma. Differential diagnosis is disseminated infection with *Mycobacterium avium* subsp. *avium*.

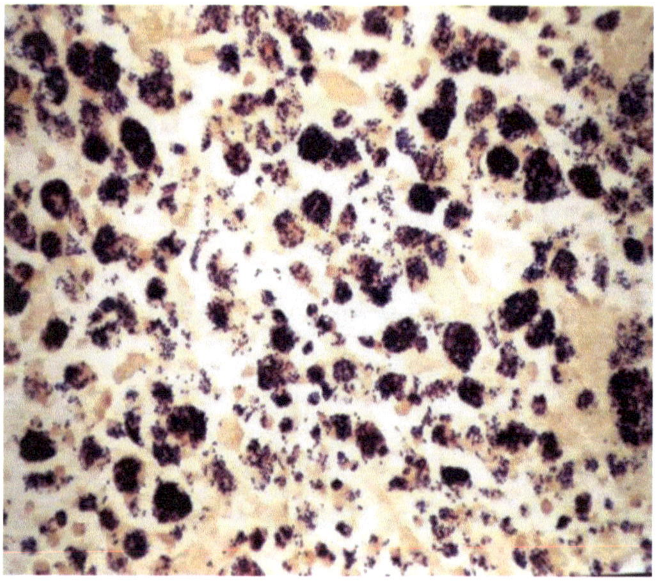

**Figure 7.29.** Horse. Liver. Caseous Hepatitis. *Rhodococcus Equi*. Microscopically, myriads of gram-positive intrahistiocytic intracytoplasmic cocci are scattered within hepatic lobules. (Brown and Brenn)

*e. Abscesses*

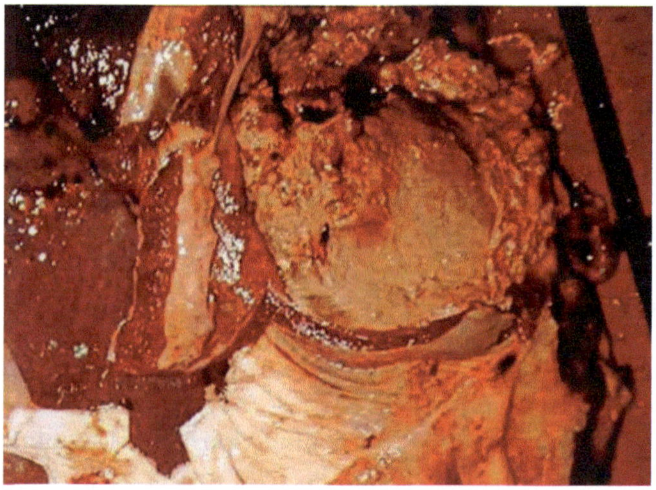

**Figure 7.30.** Horse. Liver. Hepatic Abscess. Bacterial abscesses are rare in horses, unlike in cattle. This local abscess between the diaphragm and the liver lobe is partially sealed off by a capsule, but the inflammation has extended into the liver parenchyma. *Escherichia coli*, *Salmonella*, and *Streptococcus equi* subsp. *zooepidemicus* are commonly isolated.

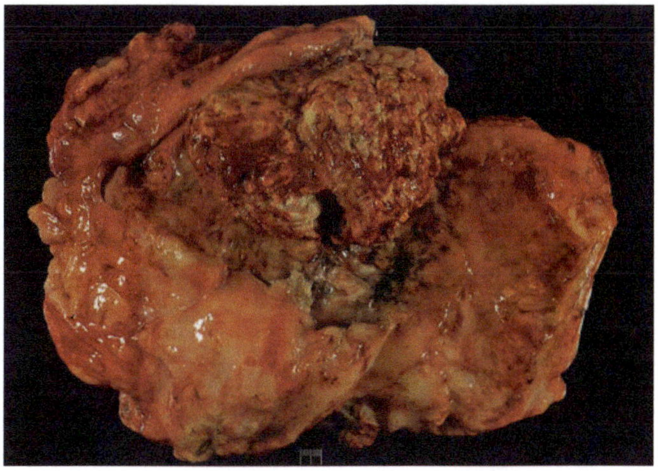

**Figure 7.31.** Horse. Liver. Hepatic Abscess. The liver surface is covered by fibrous material that has sealed an abscess in the center. *Corynebacterium pseudotuberculosis*, the organism of "pigeon fever," was isolated in this case. The musculature of the horse is the usual target organ system for this organism.

*f. Equine infectious anemia virus hepatitis*

The liver may be grossly enlarged and hilar lymph nodes are increased in size. Hemosiderosis gives the liver parenchyma a tan appearance. The disease is best diagnosed microscopically by the presence of small clusters of lymphocytes randomly distributed within sinusoids. (See "Equine Infectious Anemia" in Chapter 15, "Diseases of the Hemolymphatic System.")

*g. Cholangitis*

Considered the result of an ascending infection of enteric pathogens.

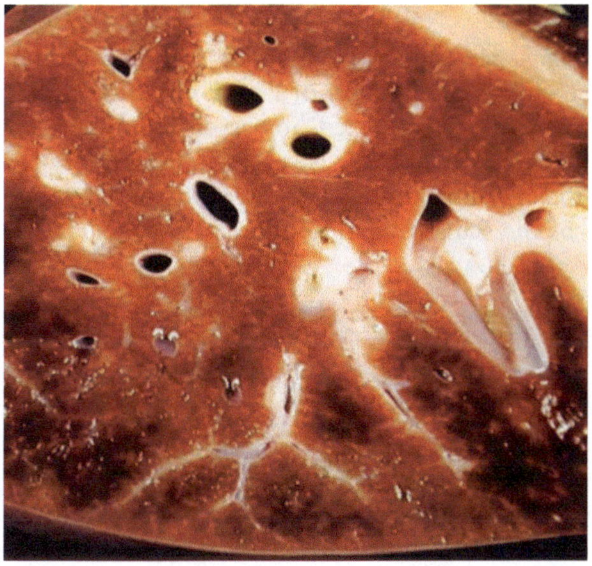

**Figure 7.32.** Horse. Liver. Pericholangitis. The biliary tree system on cross section is pronounced (white foci) suggesting chronic inflammation.

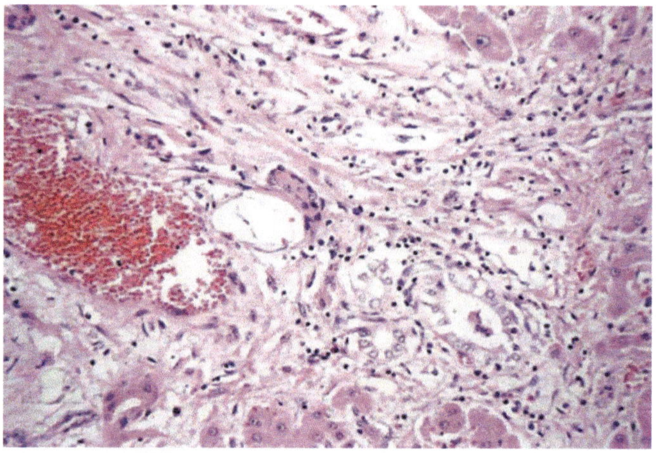

**Figure 7.33.** Horse. Liver. Pericholangitis. Microscopically, the portal tract is distended by infiltrating mononuclear cells. Bile ductules are loosely surrounded by similar inflammatory cells. (H&E)

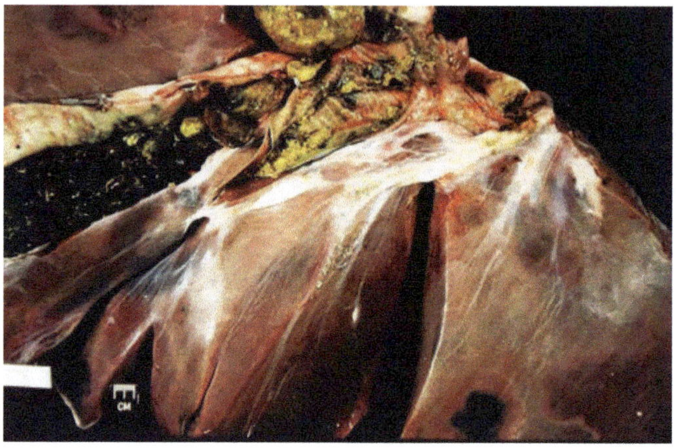

**Figure 7.34.** Horse. Liver. Cholangitis and Choleliths. Dark green inspissated bile-stained concretions distend the common bile duct. Obstruction of bile flow leads to intrahepatic cholestasis.

### 4. *Endoparasitism*

#### *a. Trematodes*

Schistosomiasis has been mentioned under "Gastrointestinal Parasitism." Schistosomes belong to the phylum of Platyhelminthes and are trematodes. The liver when involved in affected horses develops fibrosing granulomas. Liver failure can occur when there is severe inflammatory reaction to parasitic overload. Recent publications have incriminated *Heterobilharzia americana* as source of the schistosomal nodules.

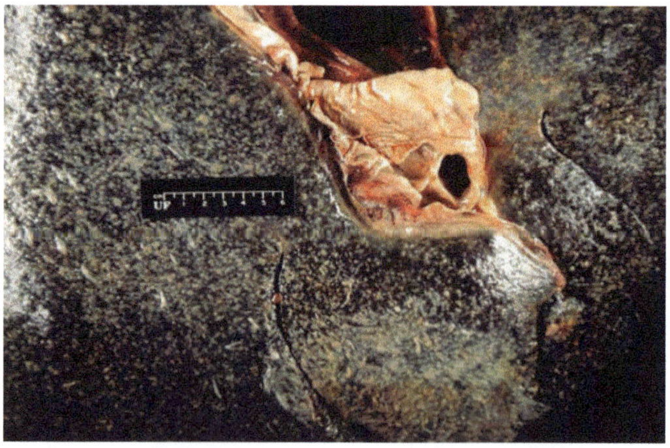

**Figure 7.35.** Horse. Liver. Granulomatous Fibrosing Hepatitis. *Heterobilharzia Americana*. (Schistosomiasis).The entire liver is seeded with white, firm, bulging nodules. This horse died because of liver failure.

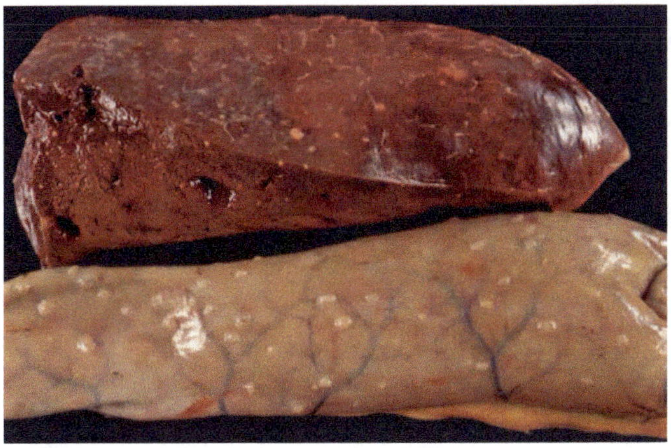

**Figure 7.36.** Horse. Liver and Intestinal Serosa. Granulomatous Fibrosing Hepatitis and Serositis. *Heterobilharzia Americana*. White nodules are seen in the liver capsule. They also are present on the intestinal serosa.

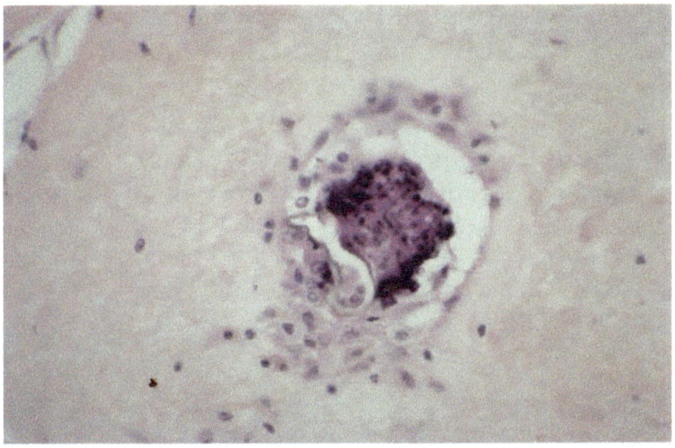

**Figure 7.37.** Horse. Liver. Fibrosing Granuloma. There is evidence of a mineralized central core with fibrosis in the periphery. The center on occasion may contain residual trematode eggshells or miracidia (H&E)

*b. Cestodes*

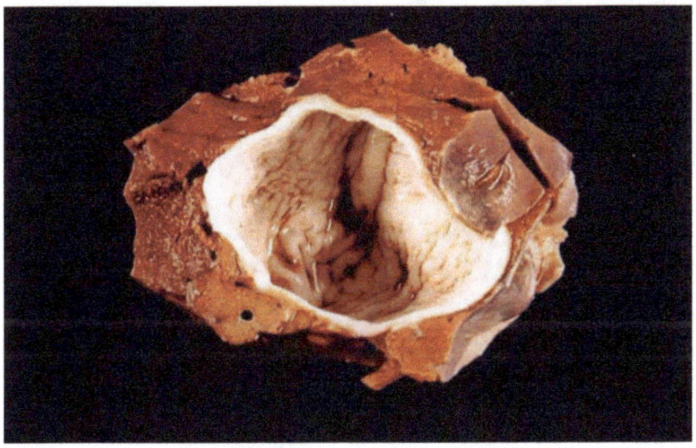

**Figure 7.38.** Horse. Liver. Cut Surface. Hydatidosis. A cyst demarcated by a white thick-walled capsule was the site of *Echinococcus granulosus*, larval stage, equine strain. It was filled with numerous protoscoloces. This was an incidental finding at necropsy. Canids are the definitive host for this cestode. The horse is considered an intermediate host.

*c. Nematodes*

Ascarid and strongyle larvae have a tendency to migrate through the liver. The migration path is identified by small fibrous scars. As they break through the Glisson's capsule at the diaphragmatic surface of the liver and the adjacent abdominal diaphragm surface, the healing of the migration tracts results in fibrous tags thought to be indicative of such larval migration.

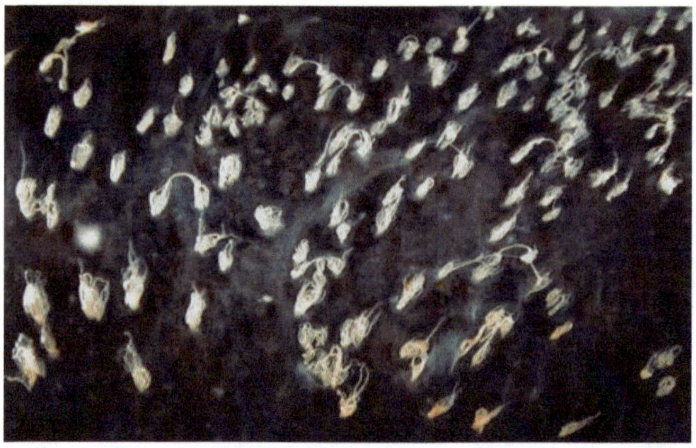

**Figure 7.39.** Horse. Liver. Diaphragmatic Surface. Fibrous Tags. Thought to be the result of migration of nematode larvae. With these having disappeared through preventive antihelminthic treatment, the fibrous liver tags are still seen as incidental findings at necropsy perhaps resulting most likely from friction rubs.

### *5. Primary and secondary hepatic neoplasia*

Primary neoplasms of the equine liver are rare and generally consist of hepatoblastomas seen in late-term aborted fetuses and young horses up to 3 years and cholangiocarcinomas seen in older horses. Hepatocellular carcinomas are extremely rare. Only three cases of these have been reported in the literature since 1969. Miscellaneous other tumors involving the equine liver have been reported to be carcinoids, mast cell tumors, and lymphomas.

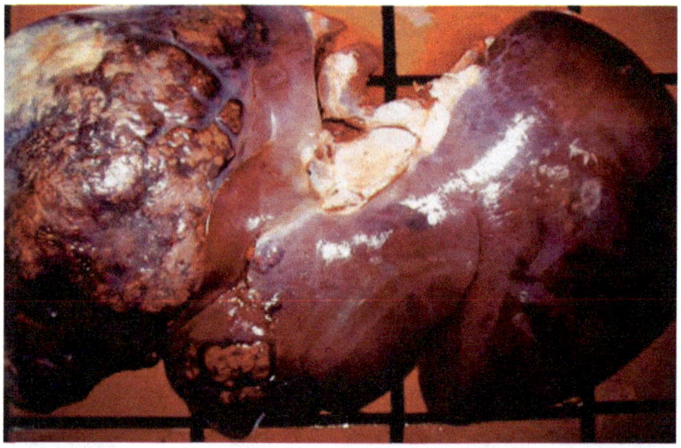

**Figure 7.40.** Horse. Juvenile. Liver. Hepatoblastoma. The liver is enlarged and has fleshy elevations on the surface of the right lobe.

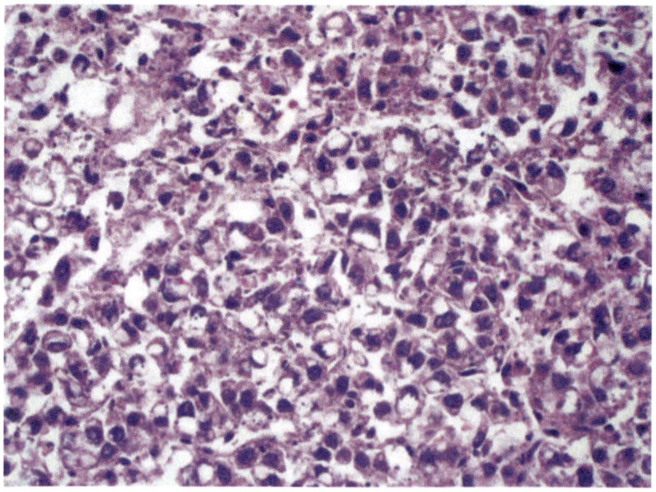

**Figure 7.41.** Foal. Liver. Hepatoblastoma. The neoplastic cells are composed of sheets of pleomorphic, vacuolic epithelial cells resembling embryonal hepatocytes, lacking features or differentiated hepatic lobules. (H&E)

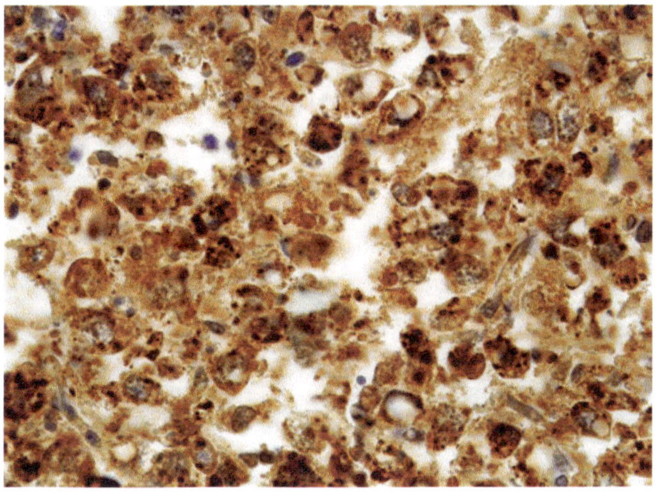

**Figure 7.42.** Foal. Liver. Hepatoblastoma. The tumor cells show strong cytoplasmic labeling for Hep Par 1. (IHC)

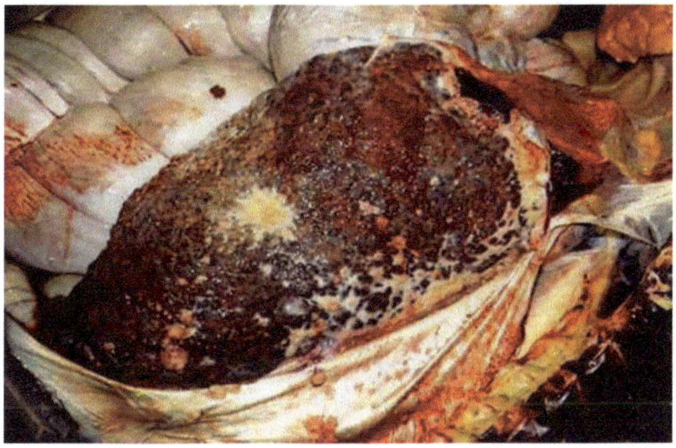

**Figure 7.43.** Mule. Liver. Hepatocellular Carcinoma. Numerous, various-sized growths have seeded the hepatic surface. Aflatoxicosis may be a possible cause. (Courtesy Dr. J .Roberts, National Zoo, Washington, DC.)

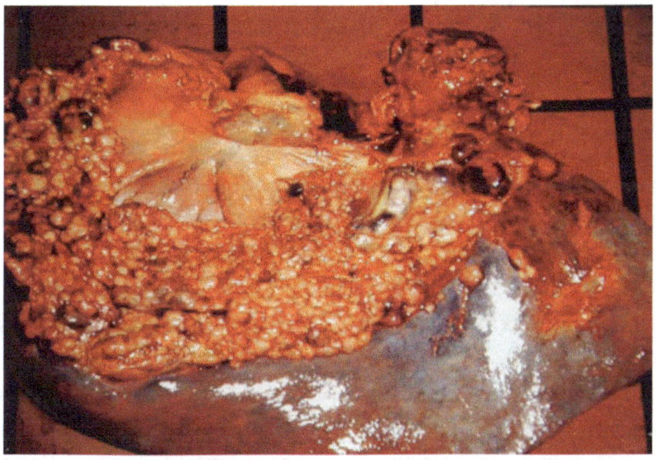

**Figure 7.44.** Horse. Liver. Cholangiocarcinoma. Multiple firm yellow nodules are randomly distributed throughout the parenchyma and are seeding the abdominal surface of the diaphragm.

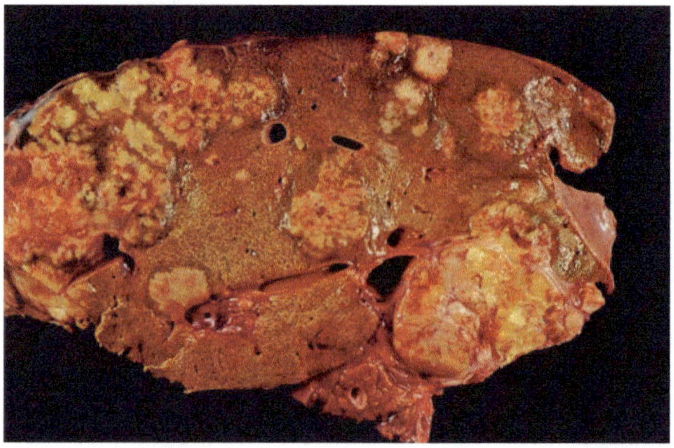

**Figure 7.45.** Horse. Liver. Carcinoid. Multiple, varying sized tan growths are invading the liver parenchyma. Some of these are confluent. This tumor has been diagnosed as carcinoid based on its microscopic epithelioid features and by immunohistochemistry for neurosecretory granules, performed with labels for chromogranin A, CEA, calcitonin, synaptophysin, and S-100.

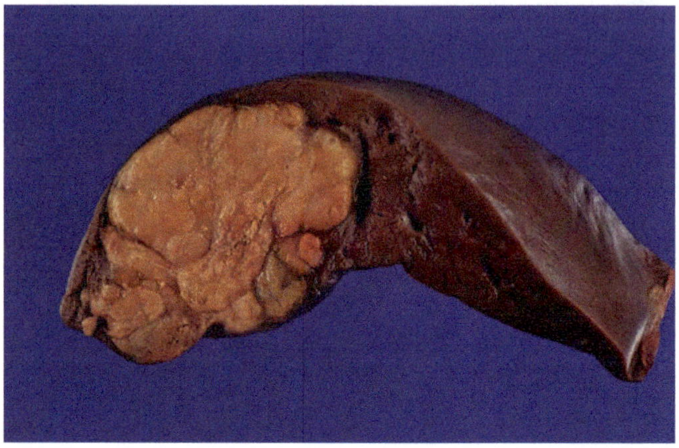

**Figure 7.46.** Horse. Liver. Lymphoma. Multicentric or alimentary forms of lymphoma can involve the equine liver. At the gross level, the nodular tumors are indistinguishable from other types of primary or metastatic neoplasms.

### *6. Liver biopsy*

A biopsy can be taken for antemortem diagnosis of suspected liver disease. The tissue obtained via needle biopsy is adequate for histopathology evaluation. The site of performing a liver biopsy is between ribs 12 and 13 of the right flank of a sedated standing horse.

## Summary

The liver has an impressive potential to regenerate but responds to insults in only a limited number of ways. Random foci of necrosis are the result of infectious agents. Examples are infection with alpha herpesvirus and *C. piliformis*, the agent of Tyzzer's disease. Diffuse necrosis with dropout of hepatocytes occurs in conjunction with idiopathic hepatic disease (Theiler's disease/serum hepatitis). Megalocytosis develops in PA toxicosis and mycotoxicosis. Fibrosis and cirrhosis are hallmark lesion of toxic injuries and for the most part are irreversible as regeneration as initial response is limited in duration. Hepatic endoparasitism is a rare event in horses. Primary hepatic neoplasms are rare; metastases of tumors from different primary sites are more frequent. The liver biopsy is a diagnostic tool for antemortem liver disease diagnosis.

## II. Pancreas

The equine pancreas located between the base of the cecum and the right dorsal colon has exocrine and endocrine functions. Pancreatic disease in the horse is not frequently diagnosed as a pathologic entity. Possible pathologic findings are calculi, parasitic granulomas, and eosinophilic pancreatitis (idiopathic eosinophilic disease).

### *1. Pancreatitis*

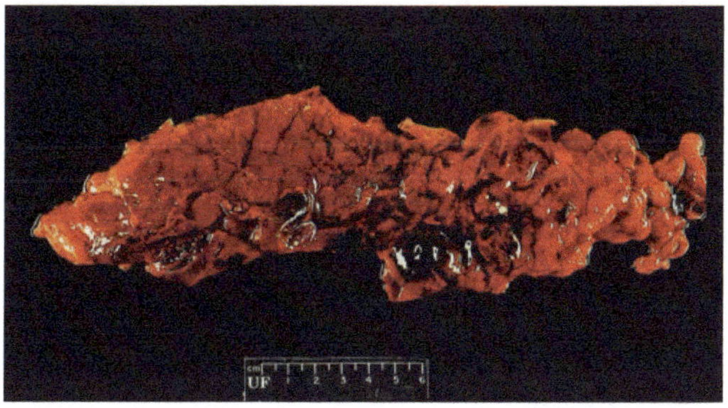

**Figure 7.47.** Horse. Pancreas. Acute, Hemorrhagic Pancreatitis. The lobules are severely reddened. The cause of the hemorrhage remained unknown. Immune-mediated disease, toxins, drugs, or deficiency of an essential nutrient remain etiologic possibilities.

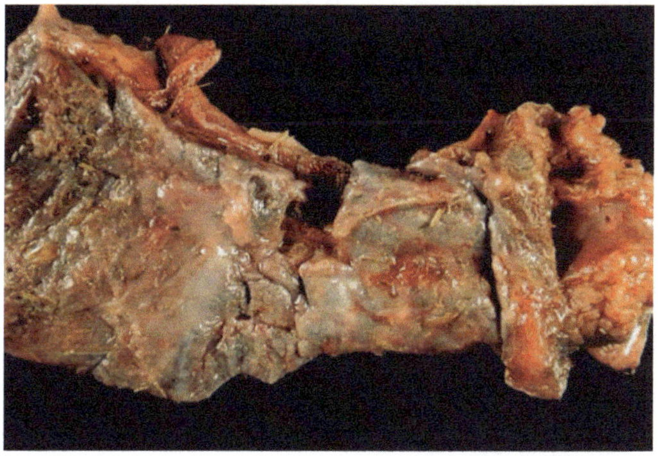

**Figure 7.48.** Horse. Pancreas. Chronic, Fibrosing Pancreatitis. Inflammation. The lobular architecture is distorted by fibrin deposition, pus pockets, and fibrosis. Parasitic migration has been implicated, mainly *Strongylus equinus* larvae. The inflammation leads to destruction of both the exocrine and endocrine pancreas.

As a differential diagnosis for chronic pancreatitis, the multisystemic, eosinophilic, epitheliotropic disease of horses has to be considered in which lymphoplasmacytic and eosinophilic infiltrates together with eosinophilic granuloma formations can be found.

### 2. Pancreatic hypertrophy

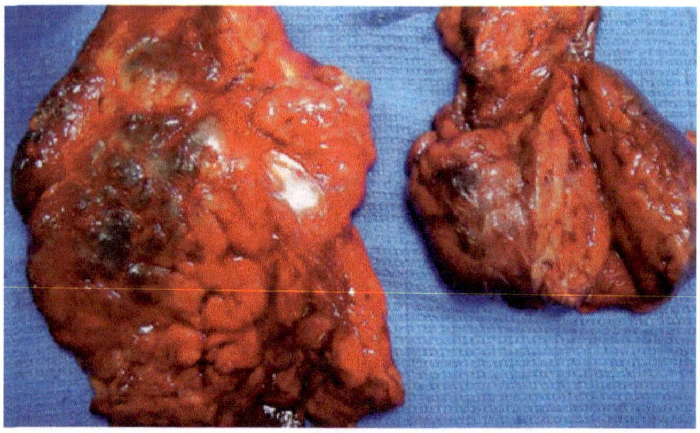

**Figure 7.49.** Horse. Pancreas. Hypertrophy. Both pieces combined to one enlarged pancreas.

## Selected references


Acland HM, Mann PC, Robertsen JL, Divers TJ, Lichtensteiger CA, Whitlock RH. 1984. Toxic hepatopathy in neonatal foals. *Vet Pathol* 21(1):3–9.

Beeler-Marfisi J, Arroyo L, Caswell JL, Delay J, Bienzle D. 2010. Equine primary liver tumors: a case series and review of the literature. *J Vet Diagn Invest* 22(2):174–183.

Chandriani S, Skewes-Cox P, Zhong W, Ganem DE, Divers ThJ, Van Blaricum AJ, Tennat BC, Kistler AL. Identification of previously undescribed divergent virus from the Flaviviridae family in an outbreak of equine serum hepatitis. Available at www.pnas.org/cgi/doi/10.1073/pnas.1219217110.

Corapi WV, Birch SM, Carlson KL, Keith-Chaffin M, Snowden KF. 2011. *Heterobilharzia americana* infection as a cause of hepatic parasitic granuloma in a horse. *J Am Vet Med Assoc* 239(8):1117–1122.

Guglick MA, MacAllister CG, Ely RW, Edwards WC. 1995. Hepatic disease associated with administration of tetanus antitoxin in eight horses.1995. *J Am Vet Med Assoc* 206(11):1737–1740.

Hepatotoxic plants. In: *The Merck Veterinary Manual*. 2011. Whitehouse Station, NJ: Merck Sharp & Dohme.

Jakowski RM. 1994. Right hepatic lobe atrophy in horses: 17 cases (1983–1993). *J Am Vet Med Assoc* 204(7):1057–1061.

Kato M, Higuchi T, Orita Y, Ishikawa Y, Kadota K. 1997. Combined hepatocellular carcinoma and cholangiocarcinoma. *J Comp Pathol* 116(4):409–413.

Messer NT, Johnson PJ. 1994. Idiopathic acute hepatic disease in horses: 12 cases (1982–1992). *J Am Vet Med Assoc* 204(12):1934–1937.

Mogg TD, Palmer JE.1995. Hyperlipidemia, hyperlipemia and hepatic lipidosis in American miniature horses: 23 cases (1990–1994). *J Am Vet Med Assoc* 207(5):604–607.

Rezabeck GB, Giles RC, Lyons ET. 1993. Echinococcus granulosus hydatid cysts in the livers of two horses. *J Vet Diagn Invest* 5(1):122–125.

West HJ. 1996. Clinical and pathological studies in horses with hepatic diseases. *Equine Vet J* 28(2):146–156.

# 8 Diseases of the Urinary System

I. Kidney
   1. Abnormalities
   2. Circulatory disturbances
      a. Hemorrhage
      b. Infarcts
   3. Metabolic disturbances
   4. Inflammatory and infectious diseases
   5. Necrosis/degeneration
   6. Renolithiasis
   7. Neoplasia

II. Lower urinary tract
   1. Inflammation
   2. Neoplasia

*Color Atlas of Equine Pathology*, First Edition. Claus D. Buergelt and Fabio Del Piero.

The kidney fulfills three major functions: (1) elimination of waste products, (2) homeostasis of water and acid/base balance, and (3) as an endocrine organ the production of erythropoietin, renin/angiotensin, and conversion of vitamin D to its most active form, 1,25-dihydroxycholecalciferol to aid in intestinal calcium resorption. Additional functions are activation/deactivation of polypeptide hormones such as insulin and glucagon, and the local production of prostaglandins.

The kidney is a filtration-resorption organ and relatively simple in its mode of operation in regulating the salt and water balance and excretion of nitrogen metabolites. The nephron is the basic functional unit of the kidney. The nephron consists of a single glomerulotubular unit. There are 1–2 million nephrons per human kidney giving it a large functional reserve; a loss of 75% of nephrons still maintains renal function.

The kidneys are richly supplied by blood vessels. In healthy human individuals, about a quarter of the cardiac output is delivered to the kidneys. Approximately 180 liters per 24 hours are filtered through the human glomerular capillaries.

In terms of primary renal pathologic processes, there are developmental abnormalities, glomerular diseases, tubular diseases, pelvic diseases, vascular diseases, and neoplasms.

## I. Kidney

### 1. Abnormalities

These include renal aplasia, hypoplasia, dysplasia, fused kidneys (horseshoe kidneys), persistent lobulation, and renal cysts.

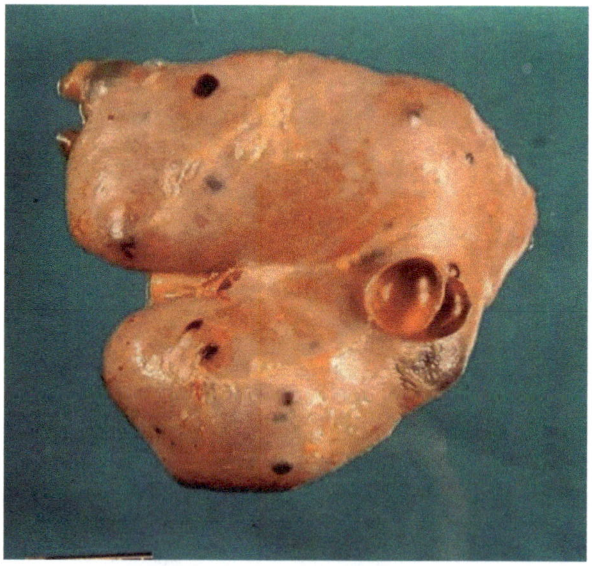

**Figure 8.1.** Horse. Kidney. Polycystic Kidney. Thin-walled clear fluid distensions are visible in the cortex. Multiple cysts are usually primary developmental abnormalities. Individual cysts may develop secondarily to inflammation and fibrosis.

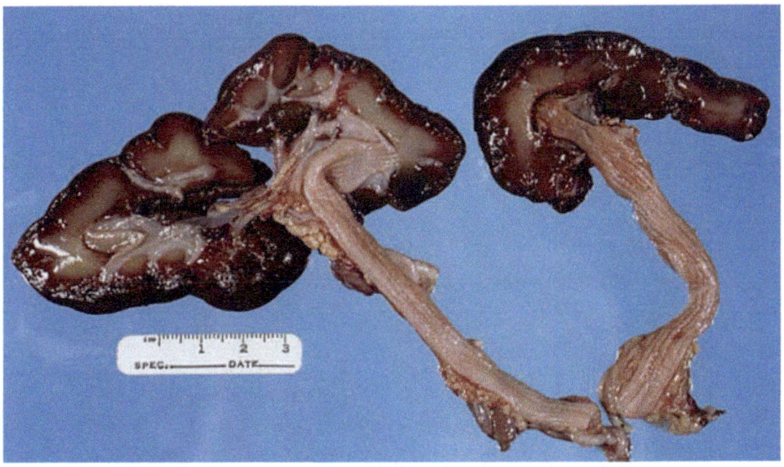

**Figure 8.2.** Horse. Kidneys. Bilateral Hypoplasia/Dysplasia. Various segments of the final kidney architecture arise from different embryologic components. Dysplasia has been defined as abnormal renal structural organization and differentiation. Dysplasia can be unilateral or bilateral. Bilateral in foals after EPM treatment of pregnant mare with trimetoprim sulfa supplemented with folic acid.

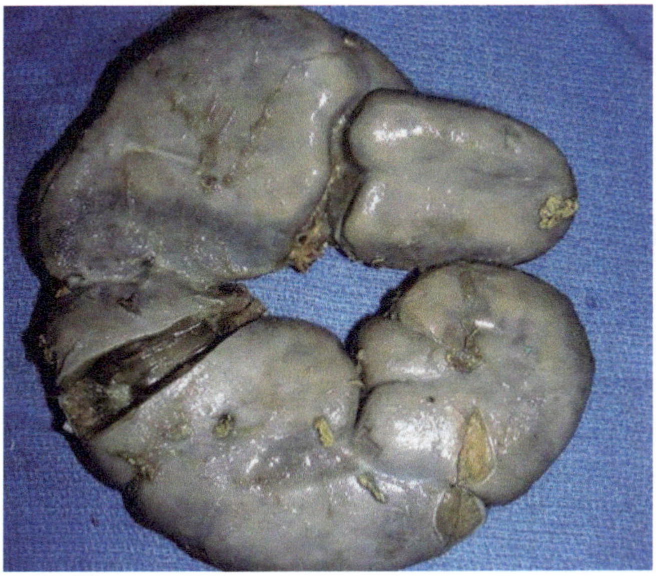

**Figure 8.3.** Horse. Kidney. Horseshoe Kidney. It is the result of fusion of the cranial or caudal poles of the two kidneys during organ development. Histology and function are normal.

## 2. *Circulatory disturbances*

### *a. Hemorrhage*

Hemorrhage results from trauma, bleeding disorders, or vascular insults. Petechiations are reflections of sepsis.

### *b. Infarcts*

Renal infarcts occur from vascular occlusions by thromboemboli showered from different sources, usually the heart. Infarcts are hemorrhagic when acute and white when chronic. They are typically wedge shaped. The size depends on the caliber of the occluded vessel.

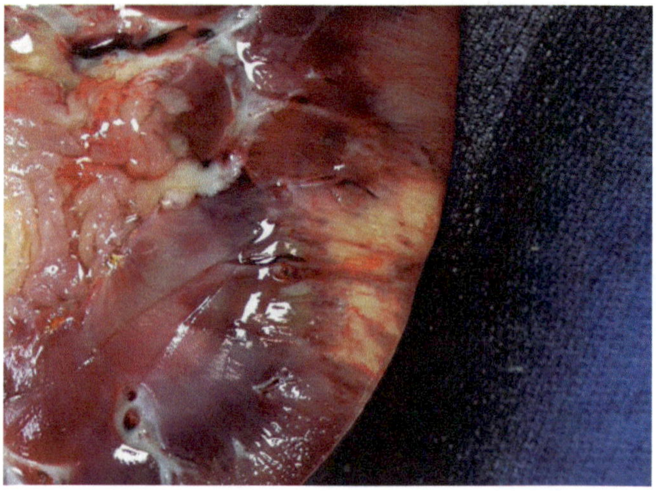

**Figure 8.4.** Horse. Kidney. Chronic Infarct. A yellowish triangular focus in the cortex is discretely delineated from the normal cortical parenchyma.

### *3. Metabolic disturbances*

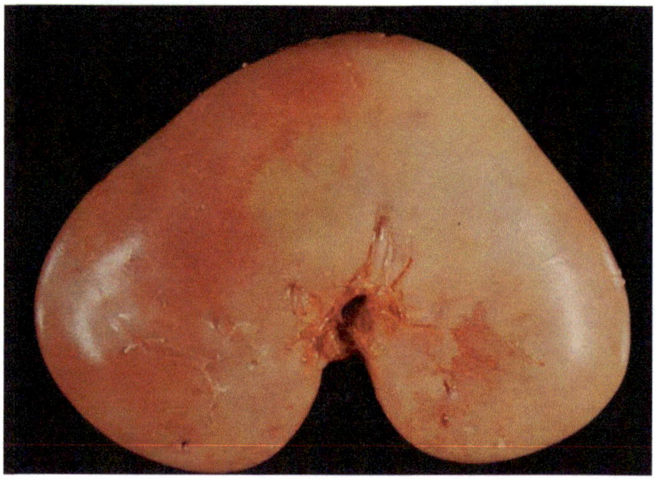

**Figure 8.5.** Horse. Kidney. Lipidosis. The kidney is yellow and soft on touch. It belonged to a pregnant mare with severe obesity. Differential diagnoses for pallor are nephrosis, anemia, fibrosis, and autolysis.

### *4. Inflammatory and infectious diseases*

Inflammatory disease may be acute and chronic. Inflammation in the kidney may involve glomeruli, the tubulointerstitial apparatus, and the pelvis. Overlapping forms are common. Glomerulitis may lead to glomerulonephritis and pyelitis to pyelonephritis. Clinical presentation of primary glomerular disease is proteinuria; primary tubular disease clinically results in uremia, polyuria, electrolyte loss, acid/base imbalance, and ultimately renal failure.

If infectious agents are involved, these can either reach the kidneys hematogenously or ascending from the lower urinary tract (urogenously). Infectious agents in horses usually are bacteria. Rarely are viruses, parasites, and fungi involved.

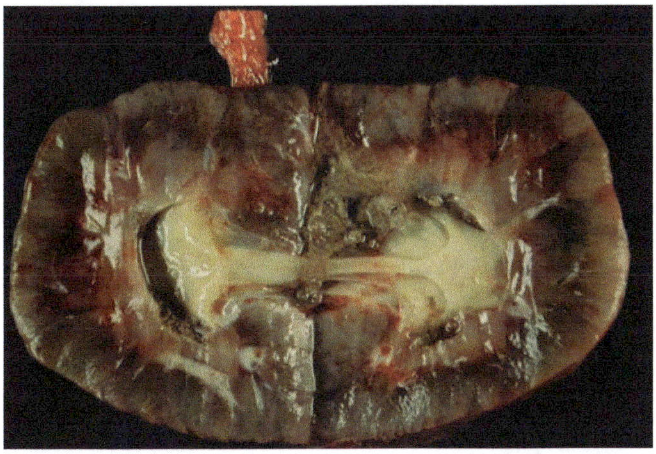

**Figure 8.6.** Horse. Kidney. Chronic Glomerulonephritis, Fibrosis, and Renal Calculi. The kidney is pale green and firm. Stripping the capsule will lead to tearing of the cortical surface. The cortex is poorly outlined. Small renal calculi are lodged in the pelvis. With no compensation possible, renal failure is the clinical outcome of these end-stage morphologic changes if both kidneys are involved.

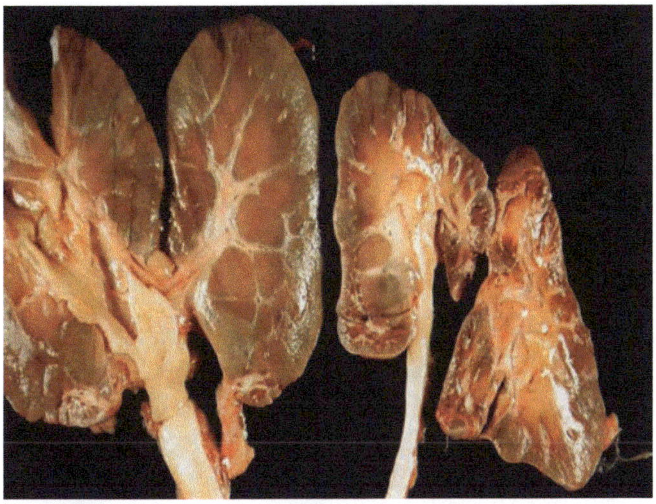

**Figure 8.7.** Horse. Kidneys. Glomerulosclerosis. Bilateral Atrophy. Asymmetry and greenish discoloration of the cortex and an irregular cortex are the changes in this set of kidneys.

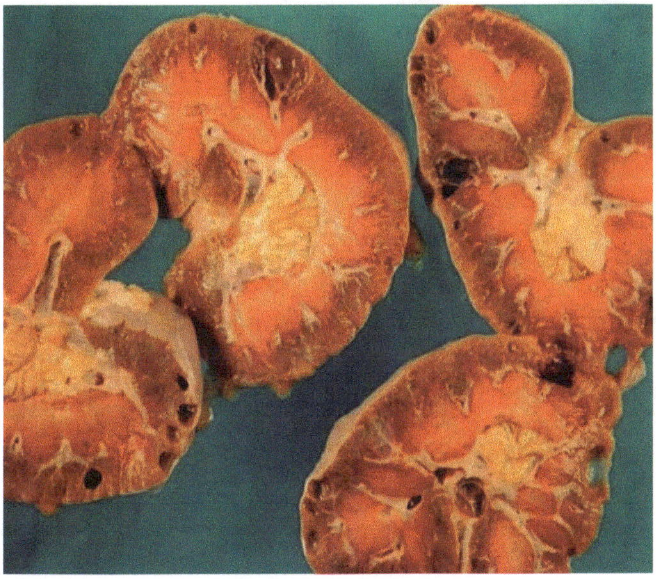

**Figure 8.8.** Horse. Kidneys. Membranoproliferative Glomerulonephritis. Cortical Cysts and Fibrosis. The cortex of both kidneys is irregular and contains multiple cysts. The surface of the kidney is wavy.

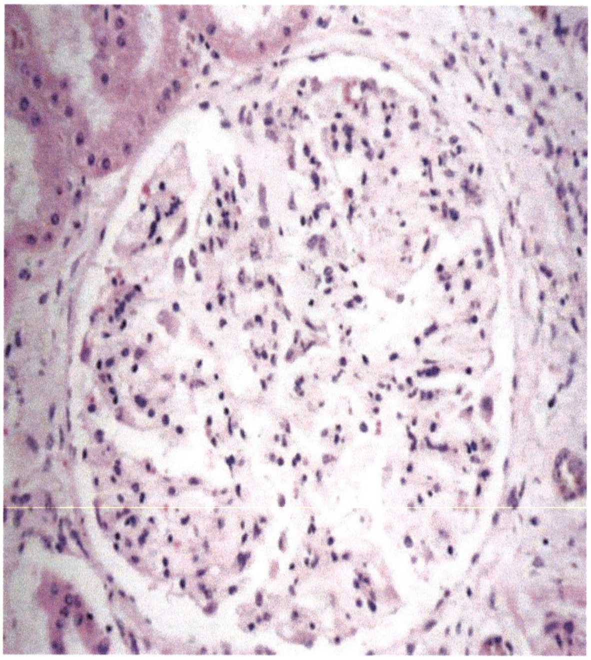

**Figure 8.9.** Horse. Kidney. Membranoproliferative Glomerulitis. Generalized thickening of basement membranes and prominent mesangium. (H&E)

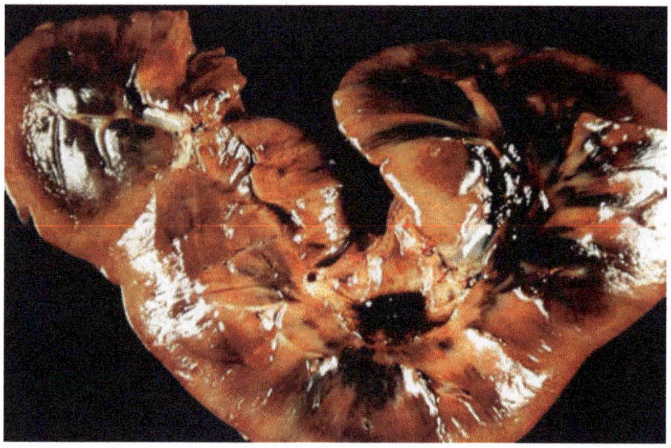

**Figure 8.10.** Horse. Kidney. Pyelonephritis. The lower medulla is characterized by hemorrhage sometimes expanding to the cortex. The medullary crest is ill-defined.

Although rare in horses, pyelonephritis is indicative of ascending inflammation from obstruction of the urinary passages or from the lower urinary tract bacterial infection. The inflammation, when chronic, results in deformation of the pelvis from scarring fibrosis, but it also ascends fingerlike into the lower medulla with similar tissue damage. A pyelitis should not be confused with the presence of intrapelvic mucin accumulation from goblet cells, which are normal, and excessive constituent cells of the urothelium lining the pelvis.

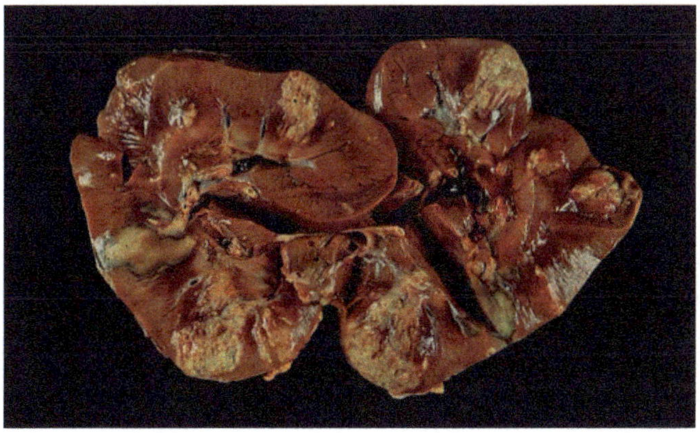

**Figure 8.11.** Horse. Kidneys. Pyogranulomatous Nephritis. Multiple caseating nodules have infiltrated the cortex and medulla. Bacteria such as *Corynebacterium* sp. and others should be considered as cause.

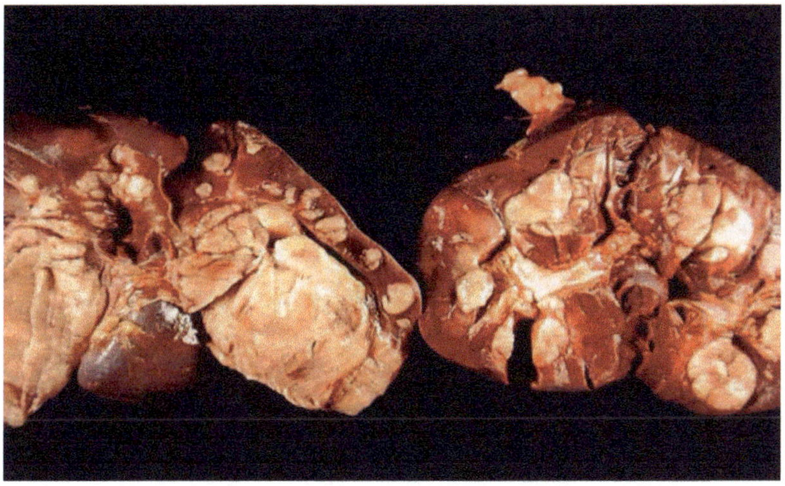

**Figure 8.12.** Horse. Kidneys. Parasitic Granulomatous Nephritis. Large areas of the kidney have been replaced by a tan solid, sharply demarcated tissue resembling neoplasia. This was a case of *Halicephalobus gingivalis* infestation.

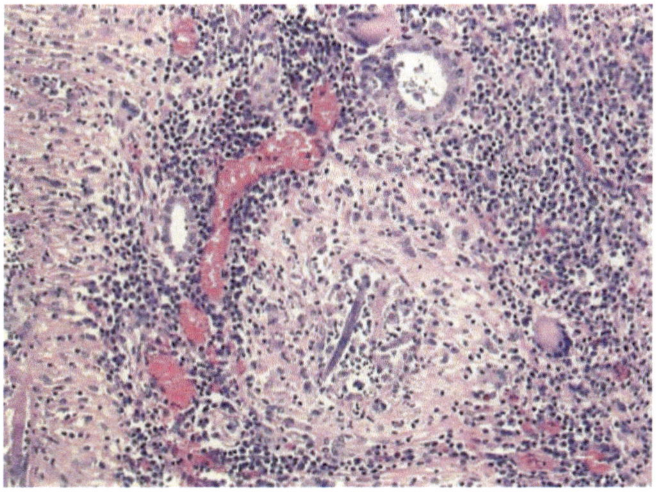

**Figure 8.13.** Horse. Kidney. Parasitic Granulomatous Nephritis. Microscopic examination shows granulomatous inflammation characterized by epithelioid macrophages, giant cells, lymphocytes, and plasma cells with embedded rhabditiform larvae identified as *Halicephalobus gingivalis*. (H&E)

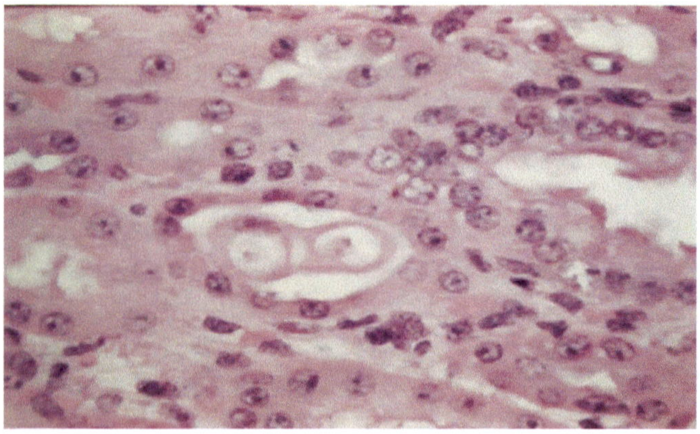

**Figure 8.14.** Horse. Kidney. Renal Coccidiosis. Schizonts of *Klossiella equi* are present in the epithelial cells of the proximal convoluted tubules. The finding of coccidia in the equine kidney is incidental. There are no gross lesions, and there is no inflammatory reaction to its presence. (H&E)

A recent discovery of polyomavirus infection in two horses recognized epithelial cell lysis with cytomegaly and karyomegaly in dilated distal tubules and collecting ducts. Viropathic changes included anisocytosis with cellular jumbling and enlarged nuclei with chromatin margination and basophilic intranuclear inclusions. Intermixed were inflammatory cells such as neutrophils, lymphocytes, plasma cells, and occasional multinucleate giant cells. Transmission electron microscopy of degenerating tubular cells demonstrated electron-dense, 40–50 nm diameter, icosahedral, nonenveloped viral particles. Viral antigen was demonstrated via immunostaining in nuclei and cytoplasm of collecting duct and distal tubular epithelium and also in 40–50% of glomeruli. The complete genome sequence of this polyomavirus has been isolated.

### *5. Necrosis/degeneration*

These changes in the kidney are generally referred to as nephrosis. Etiologic considerations are decreased renal perfusion (ischemia), exogenous toxins such as chemicals, drugs, plants, and metals, and endogenous toxins such as hemoglobin, myoglobin, and bilirubin. The proximal convoluted tubules are the most susceptible to toxins. Regeneration of affected tubular epithelium is only possible if the basement membranes are left intact. If tubulorrhexis occurs, then fibrosis and scarring will ensue.

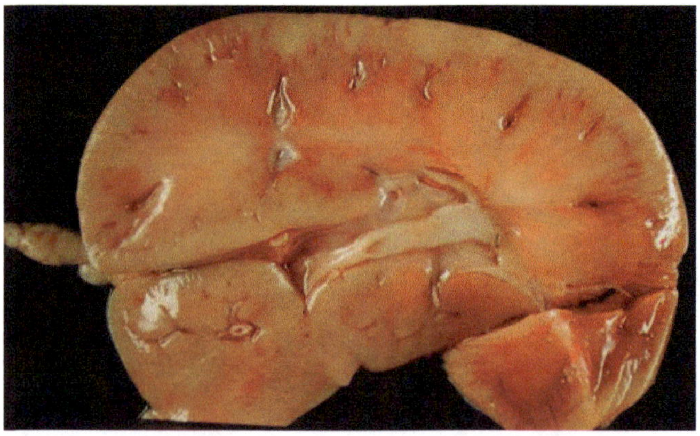

**Figure 8.15.** Horse. Kidney. Gentamicin Nephrosis. The kidneys are pale and moist. Therapeutic levels of gentamicin application are nephrotoxic to horses. Drug withdrawal reverses toxicity. Differential diagnoses: ischemia, lipidosis, EVA nephritis.

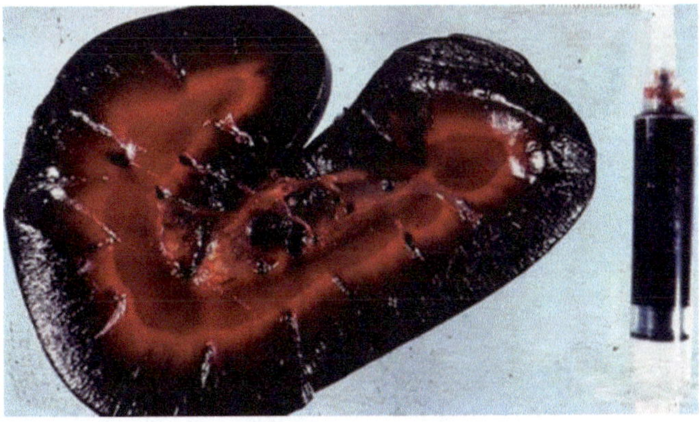

**Figure 8.16.** Horse. Kidney. Red Maple Leaf (*Acer rubrum*) Toxicosis. Pigmentary Nephrosis. The cortex is diffusely stained by hemoglobin. Hemoglobinuria is featured in the syringe. (Courtesy Dr. W. Crowell, Noah's Archive, University of Georgia.)

Ingestion of wilted leaves results in laboratory findings of severe hemolytic anemia, methemoglobinemia, and Heinz body formation (refer to Chapter 15, "Diseases of the Hemolymphatic System"). Consumption of red maple leaves has been incriminated for occasional abortions. Laminitis and colic can also develop clinically. Differential diagnosis should consider myoglobinuria.

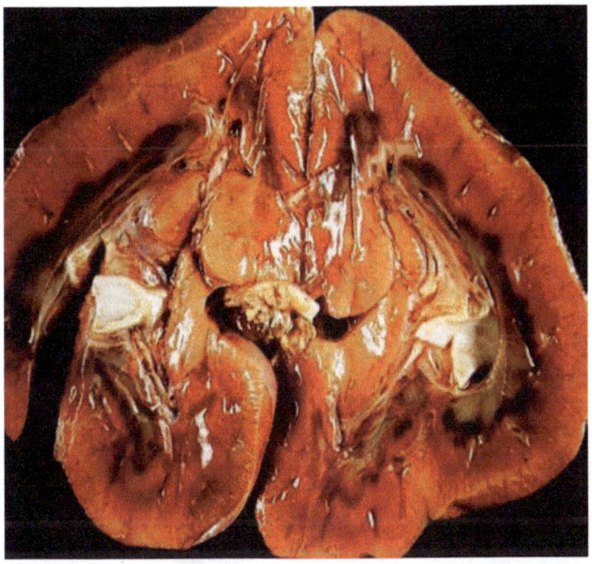

**Figure 8.17.** Horse. Kidney. Medullary Crest Necrosis. The application of nonsteroidal anti-inflammatory drugs will interfere with prostaglandin synthesis at the renal papillae and crest. Prostaglandins have a vasodilatory function at that renal location. Without prostaglandin protection, vasoconstriction and ischemia occur. The induced changes are characterized by greenish discoloration and are mostly incidental findings at necropsy. Occasionally, renal failure can ensue if changes are extremely severe.

### *6. Renolithiasis*

Calculi (stones) may form anywhere in the urinary tract. Renal calculi are mainly of calcium carbonate composition. Calculi may be incidental findings or lead to hydronephrosis, hydroureter, or total occlusion of the urinary passages resulting in anuria.

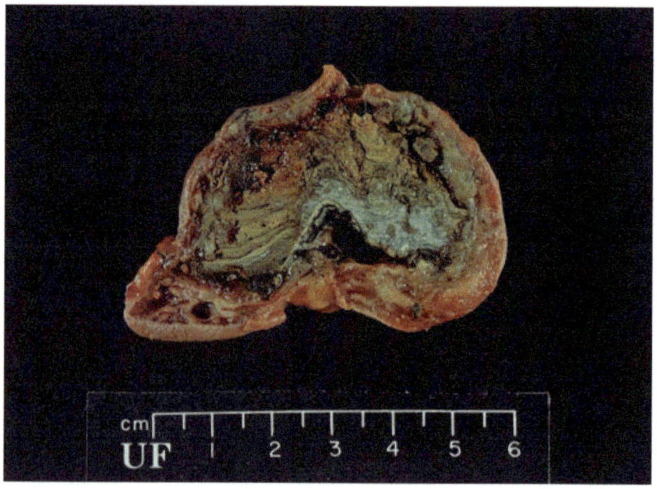


**Figure 8.18.** Horse. Kidney. Nephrolith. Laminated concretions occupy the entire pelvis with compression atrophy of the medulla and partially the cortex.

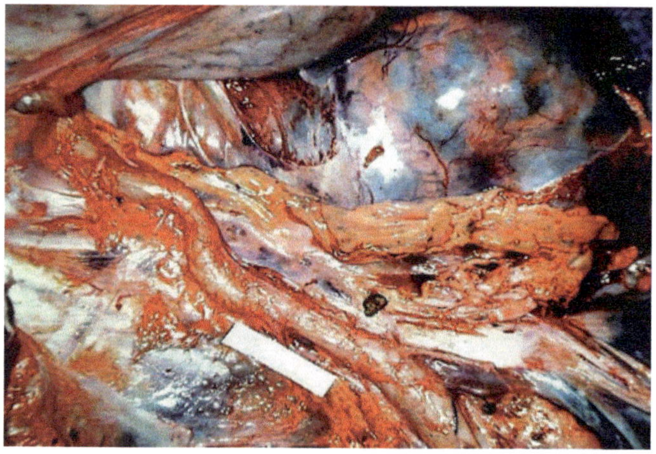

**Figure 8.19.** Horse. Kidney. Hydronephrosis and Hydroureter. If there is entrapment of calculi in the urinary passages, obstruction of urinary outflow leads to hydronephrosis and hydroureter.

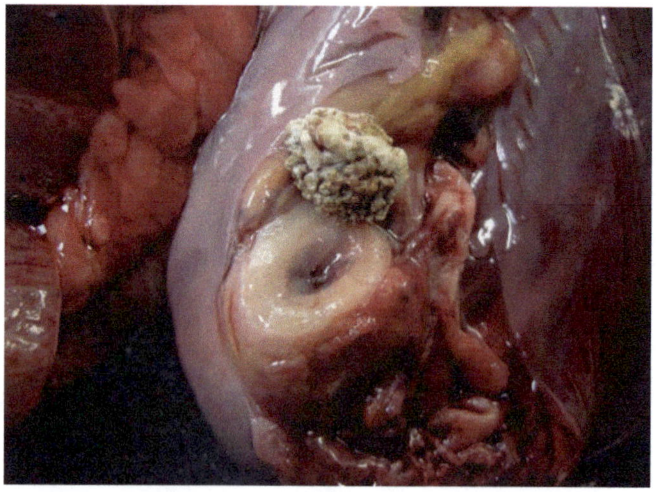

**Figure 8.20.** Horse. Ureter. Calculus. Chronic Ureteritis. Marked enlargement and thickening due to edema and fibrosis.

### 7. Neoplasia

These are rare and diagnosed as adenoma or carcinoma if primary and epithelial. They appear in older horses. Most of these tumors are unilateral and present in one pole of the kidney. Secondary tumors occur more frequently as metastases.

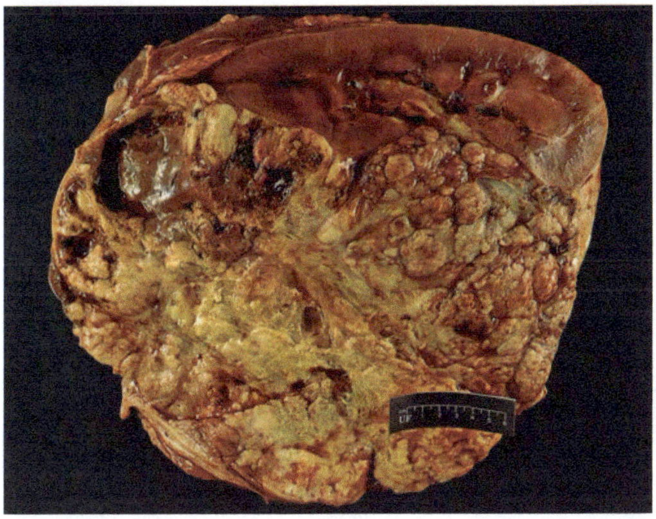

**Figure 8.21.** Horse. Kidney. Neoplasia. A renal carcinoma arising from one pole has replaced most of the renal parenchyma.

## II. Lower urinary tract

Organs of the lower urinary tract are the ureters, urinary bladder, and urethra. They have in common urothelium as mucosal lining. Most diseases in this system affect the urinary bladder.

### 1. Inflammation

Cystitis may be acute or chronic. Either form is rare. An example of acute cystitis is blister beetle poisoning with mucosal hemorrhage and erosions.

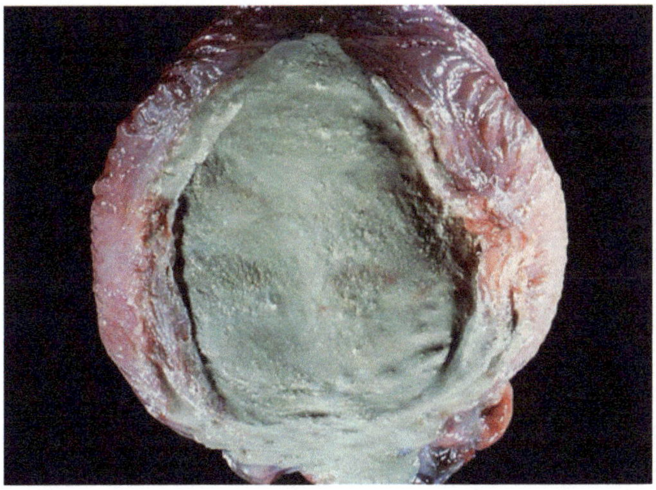

**Figure 8.22.** Horse. Urinary Bladder. Chronic Cystitis. Sorghum Poisoning. The entire wall is thickened, particularly the mucosa. The lumen is filled with a green sludge-like material. Ataxia and weakness are the first clinical signs observed in horses grazing on *Sorghum* sp. plants. Urinary incontinence and bladder paralysis follows nervous clinical signs. (Courtesy Dr. D. Meuten, North Carolina State University.)

**Figure 8.23.** Horse. Urinary Bladder. Apical Necrosis. This lesion is the result of damage to the nerves of the pelvic plexus or lumbosacral spinal cord leading to neurogenic ischemia and bladder paralysis. The devitalized tissue may rupture leading to uroperitoneum. Possible underlying causes are equine herpesvirus-1, polyneuritis, and spinal trauma.

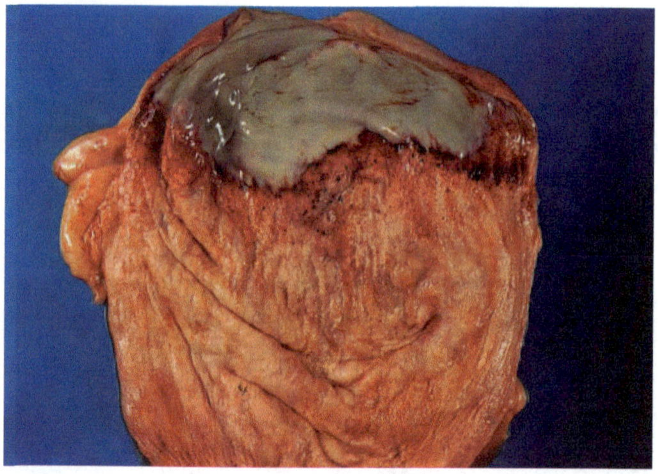

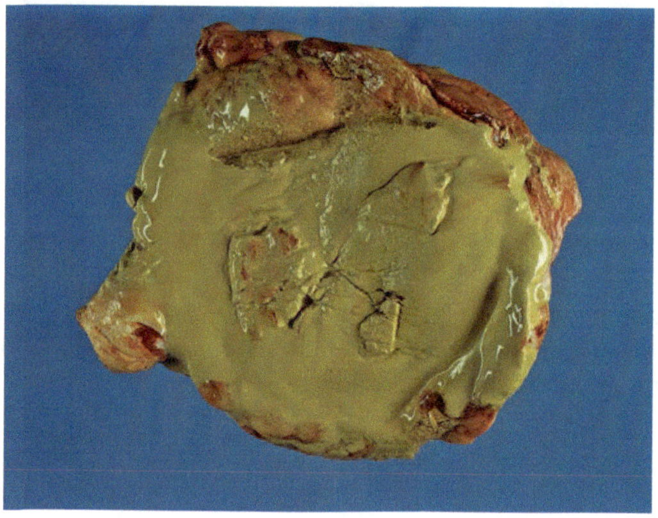

**Figure 8.24.** Horse. Urinary Bladder. Concretions. Yellow sandlike material with inspissation accumulated in the apical lumen results from reduction of urination; it is a common finding in older horses. The sludge is composed of calcium carbonate crystals and epithelial debris. This finding needs to be differentiated from purulent cystitis, which is rare in horses.

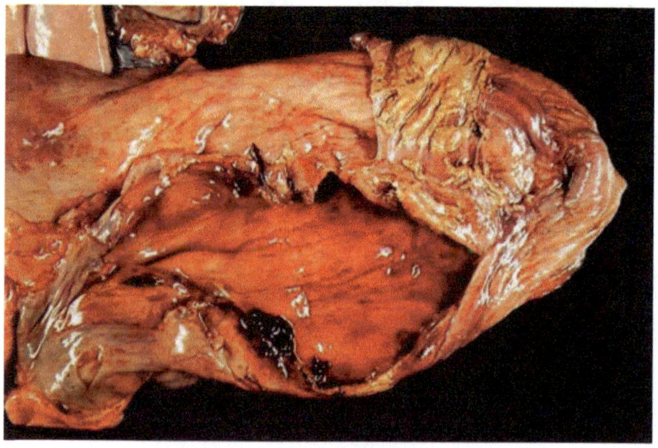

**Figure 8.25.** Horse. Urinary Bladder. Rupture. Obstruction of urinary flow due to calculi in the urinary passages was the cause.

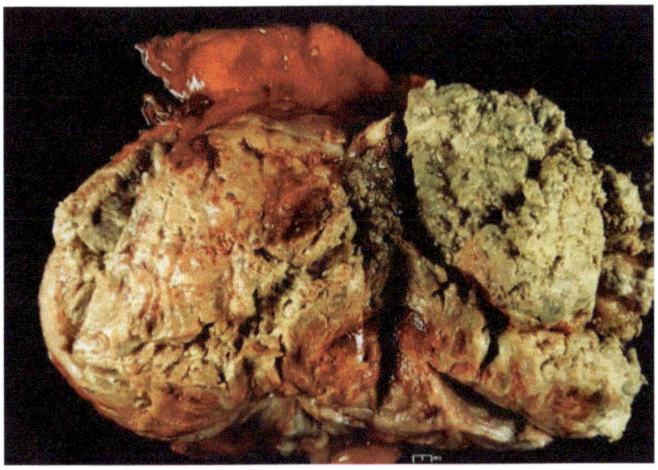

**Figure 8.26.** Horse. Urinary Bladder. Transitional Cell Carcinoma. A multilobular friable growth has caused a thickening of the entire bladder mucosa.

## Suggested references

Corriher AA, Barton MH, Sellon DC, Blikslager AT, Johnes SL. 2006. Red maple (*Acer rubrum*) leaf toxicosis in horses: a retrospective study of 32 cases. *J Vet Intern Med* 20(5):1197–1201.

Stair EL, Edwards WC, Burrows GE, Torbeck K. 1993. Suspected red maple (*Acer rubrum*) toxicosis with abortion in two Percheron mares. *Vet Hum Toxicol* 35(3):229–230.

# 9 Diseases of the Muscular System

I. Genetic muscle disorders
   1. Glycogen branching enzyme deficiency
   2. Polysaccharide storage myopathy
   3. Hyperkalemic periodic paralysis
   4. Malignant hyperthermia
   5. Recurrent exertional rhabdomyolysis
II. Myotonic myopathy
III. Dietary and conditioning-associated muscle diseases
   1. Exertional rhabdomyolysis
   2. Tying-up in equine athletes
   3. Azoturia in working horses
IV. Myonecrosis/myodegeneration
V. Myositis
VI. Neurogenic myopathy
VII. Immune-mediated myopathy
   1. Infarctive purpura hemorrhagica
   2. Streptococcal acute severe rhabdomyolysis
   3. Immune-mediated myositis
VIII. Hormonal imbalance myopathy
IX. Trauma
X. Neoplasia

*Color Atlas of Equine Pathology*, First Edition. Claus D. Buergelt and Fabio Del Piero.

Diseases affecting any muscle group can influence performance and intended function. Genetic muscle disorders, metabolic, nutritional, toxic, infectious, neurogenic, immune-mediated, traumatic, and even neoplastic etiologies have to be considered when diagnosing equine muscle disease.

There are two types of skeletal muscle fibers. Type 1, the red aerobic fiber, rich in myoglobin and oxidative enzymes, is slow contracting and resists fatigue. Type 2, the pale anaerobic fiber, rich in glycogen, is fast in contracting and rapidly fatigues. It follows a glycolytic pathway for energy supply. Type 2 muscle fibers can be subdivided into types 2A and 2B. Most muscles contain both type 1 and type 2 fibers.

A review article of equine muscle disorders proposed dividing muscle diseases into nonexertional and exertional entities. The presence or absence of rhabdomyolysis creates a subdivision and secondary classification. A third category includes myopathies resulting from altered membrane structures.

## I. Genetic muscle disorders

Genetic disorders of equine skeletal muscle include single gene abnormality or gene pool abnormality and follow either an autosomal or dominant mode of inheritance. Examples for such muscle disorders in the horse are two types of glycogenoses: (1) glycogen branching enzyme deficiency (GBED), recessive; and (2) types 1 and 2 polysaccharide storage myopathy (PSSM), dominant. Other examples of genetic disorders are hyperkalemic periodic paralysis (HYPP), dominant; malignant hyperthermia (MH), dominant; and recurrent exertional rhabdomyolysis (RER), dominant.

### *1. Glycogen branching enzyme deficiency*

Considered to be inherited as an autosomal recessive trait, GBED affects foals or aborted fetuses of Quarter horses or Paint horses and is the result of *GBE1* gene mutation. In addition to skeletal and cardiac muscles, liver and brain are affected by cytoplasmic storage of basophilic globular or crystalline material. The material reacts positively with periodic acid-Schiff (PAS). Genetic testing for *GBE1* mutation can be done on mane or tail hair of foals. Affected foals are born weak, may have flexural deformities, and usually die before the age of 8 weeks.

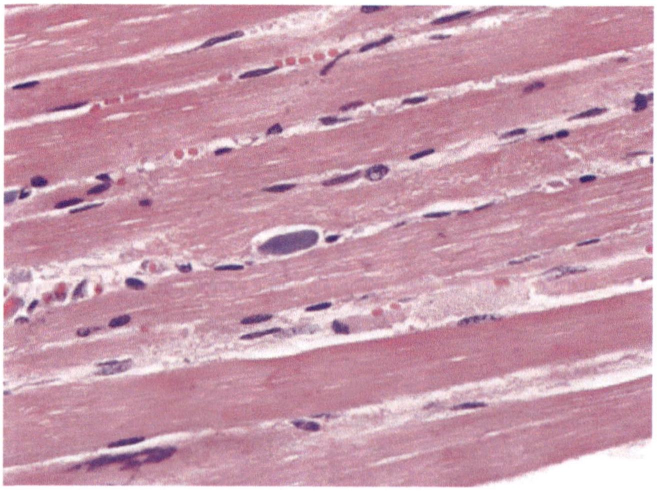

**Figure 9.1.** Horse. Skeletal Muscle. Glycogen-Branching Enzyme Deficiency (GBED). Spherical or oval basophilic inclusions are present in the sarcoplasm of myofibers. (H&E) (Courtesy Dr. N. Allison, RPL, Inc., North Carolina.)

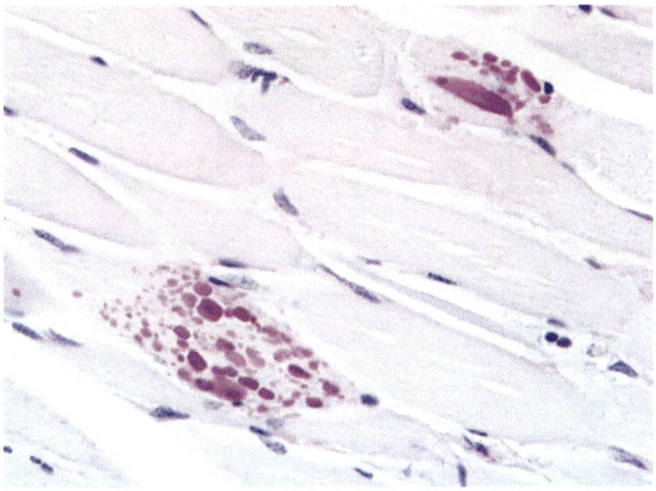

**Figure 9.2.** Horse. Skeletal Muscle. GBED. These inclusions stain positive with periodic acid-Schiff before and after digestion with diastase. (PAS) (Courtesy Dr. N. Allison, RPL, Inc., North Carolina.)

## *2. Polysaccharide storage myopathy*

Abnormal carbohydrate metabolism may lead to excess polysaccharide storage in the sarcoplasm and rhabdomyolysis in affected horses. The condition occurs in Quarter horses, Morgans, warmbloods, and draft horses. Type-1 PSSM is the result of a mutation in the glycogen synthase 1 gene and dominantly inherited. The genetic abnormality is not known for type 2 polysaccharide storage myopathy (PSSM), which, in addition to the breeds just listed, may also occur in Arabians and Thoroughbreds. Clinical signs are gait stiffness, muscle atrophy and generalized weakness, exercise intolerance, and reluctance to move. Serum muscle enzyme levels are usually increased with PSSM. Differential diagnoses include exertional rhabdomyolysis and postanesthetic myopathy. The condition may be inherited as an autosomal recessive trait.

In a skeletal-muscle biopsy of PSSM, the diagnosis is made by microscopically demonstrating accumulated PAS-positive, amylase-resistant glycogen in the sarcoplasm of mainly type 2A and type 2B myofibers. Sometimes there is evidence of fiber size variation.

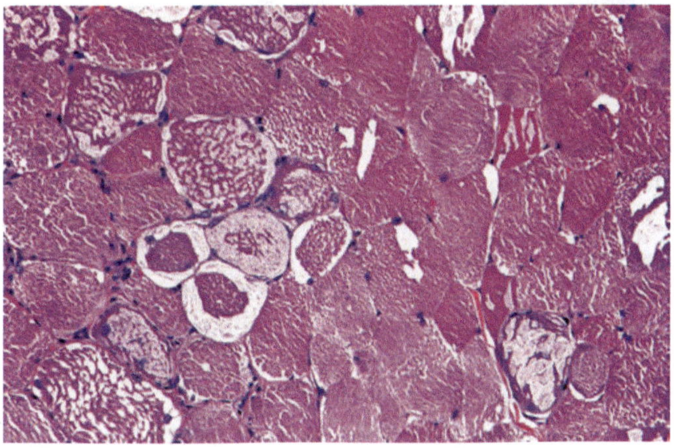

**Figure 9.3.** Horse. Skeletal Muscle. PSSM. Intracytoplasmic material has accumulated in the myocyte sarcoplasm as vacuoles and of eosinophilic, hyaline clusters. There is evidence of fiber size variation. (H&E) (Courtesy Dr. B. Valentine, Oregon State University.)

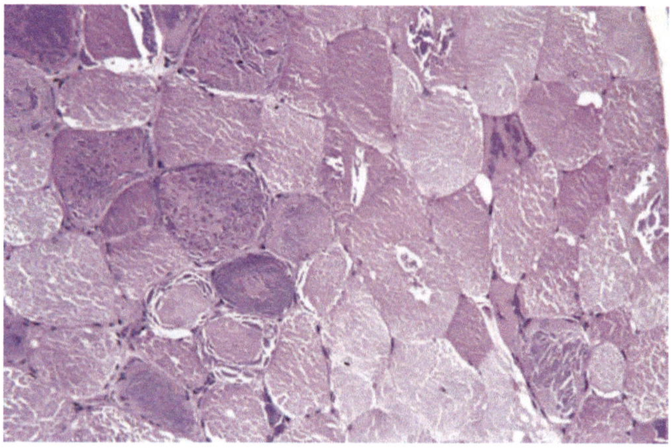

**Figure 9.4.** Horse. Skeletal Muscle. PSSM. Staining with PAS for glycogen shows that the eosinophilic myocyte clusters stain positive. (PAS) (Courtesy Dr. B. Valentine, Oregon State University.)

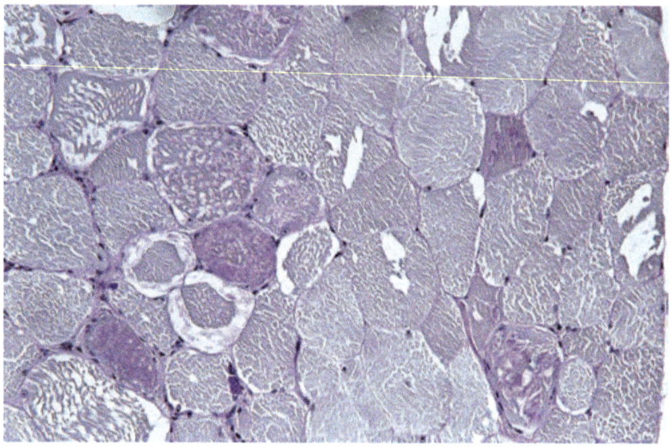

**Figure 9.5.** Horse. Skeletal Muscle. PSSM. After exposure to amylase, affected fibers resisted amylase treatment and react positive for glycogen. (PAS) (Courtesy Dr. B. Valentine, Oregon State University.)

### *3. Hyperkalemic periodic paralysis*

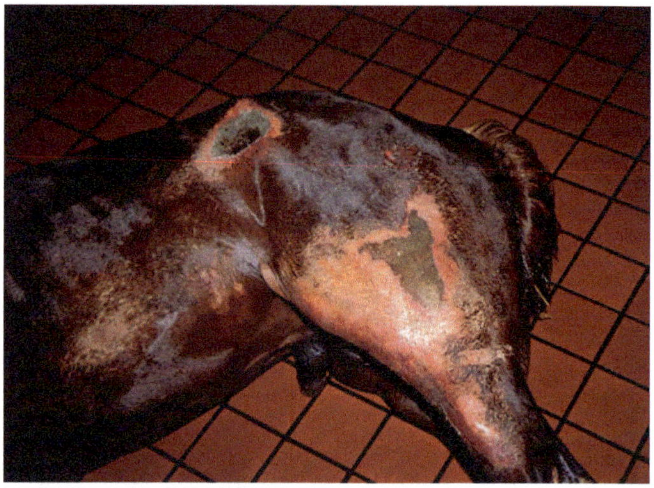

**Figure 9.6.** Horse. Body. Hyperkalemic Periodic Paralysis (HYPP). Multiple decubital skin ulcers are present due to multiple episodes of involuntary recumbency.

The biochemical disorder is the result of mutation in the sodium channel gene and affects Quarter horses, American Paint horses, and Appaloosas with episodes of generalized muscular fasciculation, laryngospasm, dysphagia, weakness, and emaciation. Clinical signs last from 15 to 60 minutes. Serum potassium concentrations are elevated during clinical manifestations (5 to 9 nmol/L; normal: 3–5.6 nmol/L). Doubling of or prominent muscles and minimal histopathologic changes such as vacuoles in type 2 fibers can be morphologically encountered in HYPP. Carriers of the mutant gene can be identified by DNA testing of blood or hair samples.

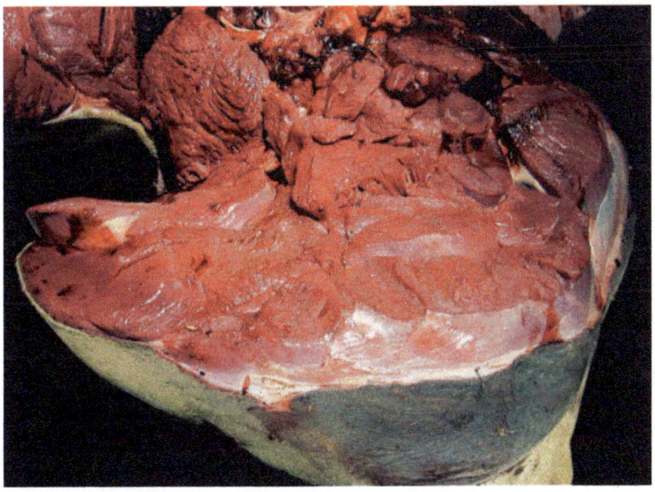

**Figure 9.7.** Horse. Skeletal Muscles. HYPP. Doubling of muscles and muscular prominence are present in the hind limb.

### *4. Malignant hyperthermia*

The inherited disorder occurs in Quarter horses and Paints during anesthesia with volatile anesthetics and can be determined by genetic testing. Malignant hyperthermia (MH) is the result of a single point mutation in the ryanodine receptor 1 gene (*RyR1*). It leads to rhabdomyolysis, metabolic acidosis, and sudden death in individual cases. Hyperthermia may reach 43°C. Specific staining abnormalities are not observed in myofibers of affected horses.

### *5. Recurrent exertional rhabdomyolysis*

RER has been described in 5–7% of Thoroughbreds, Standardbreds, and Arabians. Painful muscle cramping, stiff gait, and reluctance to move are clinical signs. Episodes are intermittent and associated with the elevation of muscle enzyme serum levels. Diagnosis is made by observing microscopically segmental necrosis and central location of the myofiber nucleus in skeletal muscle biopsies and by ruling out PSSM. Other differential diagnoses are MH and tetanus.

## Genetic muscle disorders – Fact sheet

**Definition:** Dysfunction of muscle fibers due to substance storage in sarcoplasm or due to single biochemical abnormality caused by gene mutation.

### Types

Glycogen branching enzyme deficiency (GRED)

Hyperkalemic periodic paralysis (HYPP)

Polysaccharide storage myopathy (PSSM)type 1 and 2

Malignant hyperthermia (MH)

Recurrent exertional rhabdomyolysis (RER)

## Genetic muscle disorders – Fact sheet continued

### Mode of inheritance

GRED: autosomal recessive

HYPP: autosomal dominant

PSSM:

Type 1: autosomal recessive

Type 2: unknown

MH: autosomal dominant

RER: autosomal dominant

### Breeds involved

Quarter Horse: GRED, HYPP, type 1, 2 PSSM, MH

Paint Horse: GRED, HYPP, MH

Appaloosa: HYPP

Morgans: Type 1, 2 PSSM

Standardbred: RER

Arabian: Type 2 PSSM, RER

Thoroughbred: Type 2 PSSM, RER

Draft horses: Type 1 PSSM

Warm blood: Type 1, 2 PSSM

### Gross pathology

GRED: None

HYPP: Doubling of muscle; muscle prominence

Type 1 PSSM: Muscle atrophy

Type 2 PSSM: Muscle atrophy

MH: Pallor

RER: Pallor, myoglobinemia, myoglobinuria

### Microscopic findings

GRED: basophilic globules, periodic acid-Schiff positive

HYPP: Vacuoles in type 2 myocytes

Type 1, 2 PSSM: Periodic acid-Schiff positive; amylase-resistant glycogen

MH: Hypercontracted muscle fibers. Coagulation necrosis of muscle fibers

RER: Centrally located nucleus in myocyte

## II. Myotonic myopathy

Complex 1 mitochondrial respiratory chain deficiency (mitochondrial myopathy) has been described in one Arabian horse. The horse developed exercise intolerance and lameness as well as lactic acidosis. Enlarged and distorted mitochondria in myofibers were noted by electron microscopy.

## III. Dietary and conditioning-associated muscle diseases

### *1. Exertional rhabdomyolysis*

The muscle injury typically occurs in horses fed a carbohydrate-rich diet that is continued when the horse is resting over a period of time. When the horse exercises again, a "burnout" effect takes place in the glycolytic fibers with pronounced myoglobinemia, myoglobinuria, and renal tubular pigmentary necrosis as result. Ensuing metabolic acidosis may be fatal.

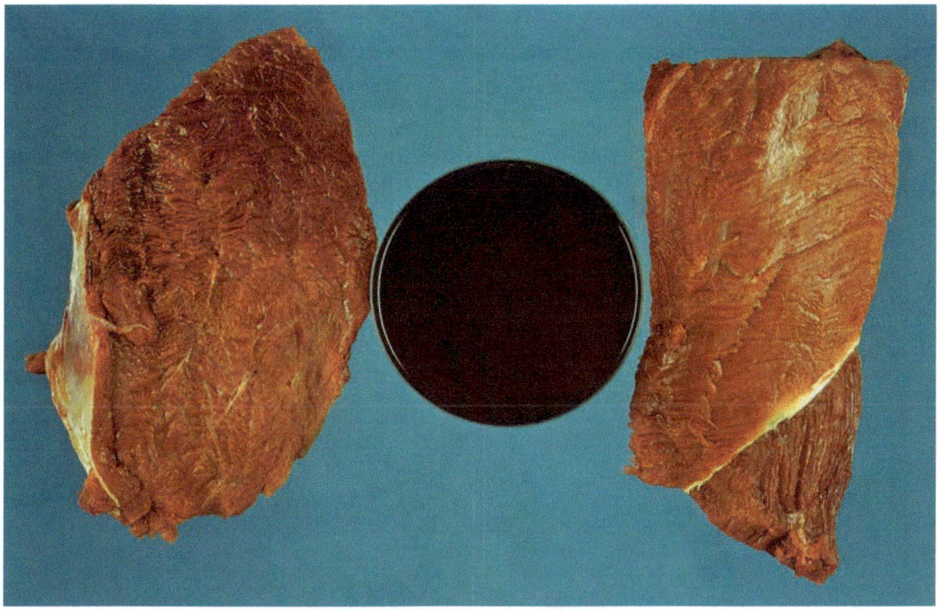

**Figure 9.8.** Horse. Skeletal Muscle. Exertional Rhabdomyolysis. Muscle pallor and red-tinged urine in the Petri dish resulted from lysis of myoglobin in muscle sarcoplasm and release into the urine (myoglobinuria). Gluteal muscles are usually involved.

### *2. Tying-up in equine athletes*

The condition is the result of acute rhabdomyolysis seen in riding and racing horses. It has clinical features in common with azoturia, but affected horses recover following a period of rest. Metabolic acidosis does not occur. Muscle lesions are subtle at the microscopic level.

### *3. Azoturia in working horses*

Paralytic myoglobinuria occurs very shortly after commencing work following some days of rest. Affected horses are stiff in hind limbs, and they sweat and tremble. Muscles of the girdle are rigid. Grossly, affected muscles may be pale, moist, swollen, and hemorrhagic. Histologically, there may be subtle hyaline changes in the myofibers; inflammation or mineralization is not observed.

## IV. Myonecrosis/myodegeneration

Nongenetic acquired primary degenerative changes of muscle fibers are mainly infectious, nutritional, or toxic in origin. In nutritional deficiency due to vitamin E/selenium shortage (white muscle disease), type 1 fibers with greater workload are affected in young animals.

Examples of toxic causes of myodegeneration are ionophores such as monensin, drugs such as ivermectin, or plants such as *Cassia occidentalis*, snakeroot (*Eupatorium rugosum*) in the Midwest of the United States, and others. Type 1 and type 2 myofibers may be affected. Affected muscles are pale grossly in monensin and *Cassia* toxicoses. Snakeroot toxicosis, the result of tremetone, leads to nonexertional rhabdomyolysis and severe myonecrosis of postural skeletal muscles.

A similar muscle condition is observed in Europe and is known as acute seasonal pasture myopathy (atypical myopathy) with signs of rhabdomyolysis. Histologic changes are similar to nutritional myodegeneration, but evidence of mild amylase-resistant polysaccharide accumulation similar to PSSM in myofibers and mild lipid storage are apparently additional features in pasture myopathy. A high mortality rate (up to 90%) is associated with the disorder. Preliminary results from Switzerland suggest that toxins produced by *Clostridium sordelli* and *Clostridium bifermentans* might be involved.

Postanesthetic myodegeneration is an example of ischemic myopathy due to prolonged recumbency while under anesthesia.

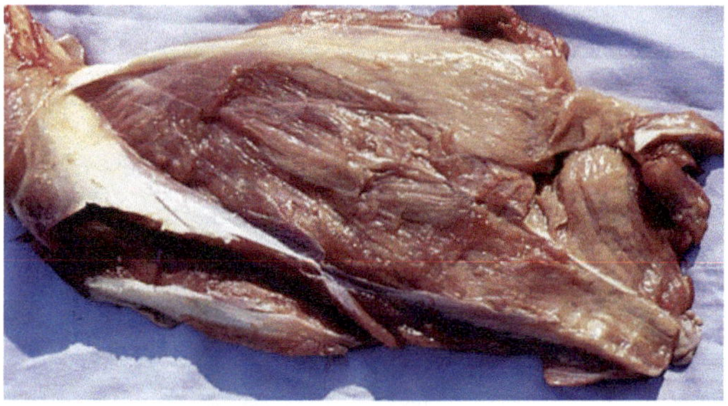

**Figure 9.9.** Foal. Skeletal Muscle. Pallor. Myodegeneration due to nutritional deficiency (white muscle disease). Selenium is a membrane antioxidant, whereas vitamin E protects membranes.

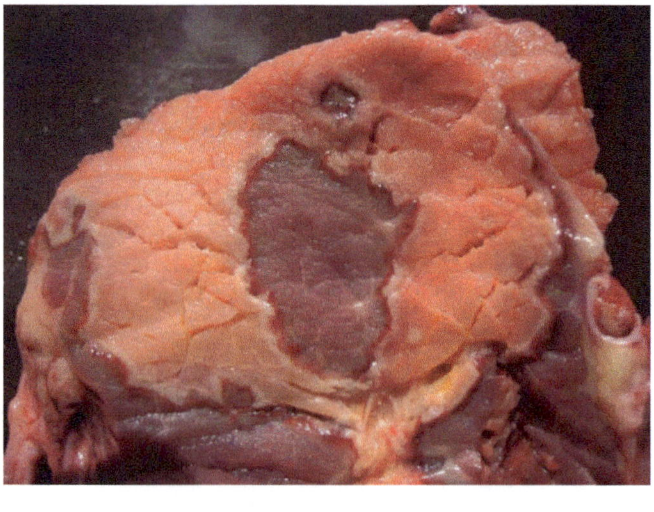

**Figure 9.10.** Horse. Perilaryngeal Muscle. Necrosis. This type of lesion can be infectious or traumatic in origin.

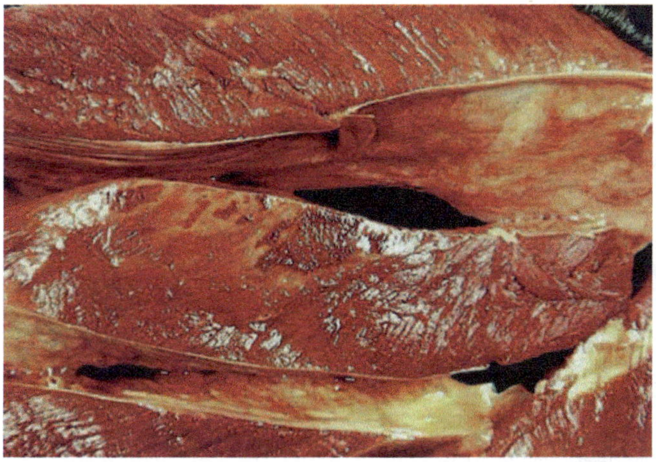

**Figure 9.11.** Horse. Skeletal Muscles. Myodegeneration and Infarcts. Pallor and sharply delineated red areas are indicative of vascular compromise.

## V. Myositis

Inflammation from bacteria and necrosis from bacterial toxins (clostridial) are the principal pathologic changes. Bacteria responsible for myositis are *Clostridium septicum* as the most common of clostridial myositis, *Corynebacterium pseudotuberculosis* (pigeon fever), and occasional other gram-positive or gram-negative bacteria (*Staphylococcus aureus, Salmonella*). Intramyocyte protozoa (*Sarcocystis* sp.) may also play a role in the pathogenesis of myositis. *Clostridium botulinum* responsible for botulism is discussed in Appendix A, "Diseases without Pathology."

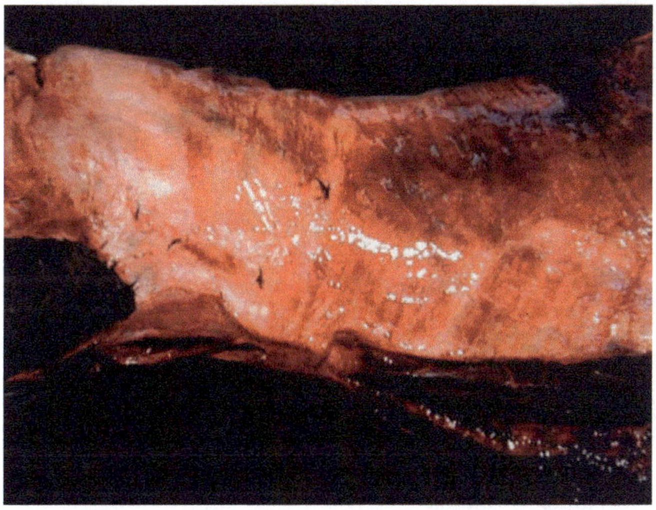

**Figure 9.12.** Horse. Neck. Skeletal Muscle. *Clostridium septicum* Malignant Edema. Often fatal in horses, it is frequently the result of a contaminated injection site or contaminated wound. Affected muscles are hemorrhagic, moist, and may contain some gas. Other species of *Clostridium* such as *C. perfringens* may be involved.

## VI. Neurogenic myopathy

Equine laryngeal hemiplegia from damage to the left recurrent laryngeal nerve is an example of denervation myofiber atrophy. Another example discussed in Chapter 3, "Diseases of the Nervous System and Peripheral Nerves," is muscle atrophy of the postural hindleg muscles.

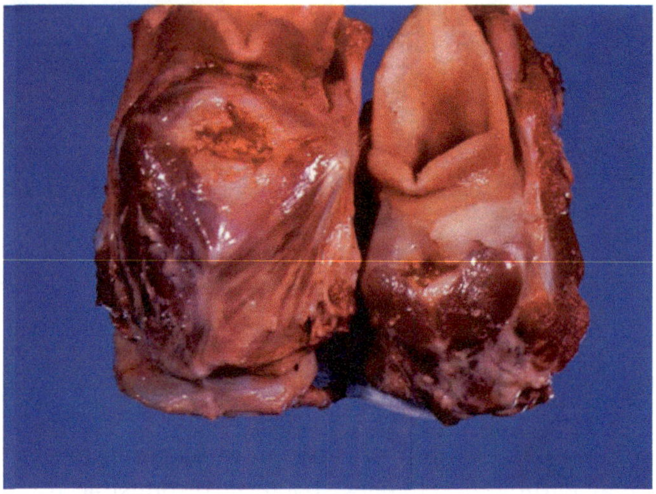

**Figure 9.13.** Horse. Larynx. Laryngeal Hemiplegia. Unilateral Muscle Atrophy. The larynx on the left has the left dorsal cricoarythenoideus (DCA) muscle pale and atrophic when compared with the opposite DCA muscle and the larynx of an unaffected horse on the right.

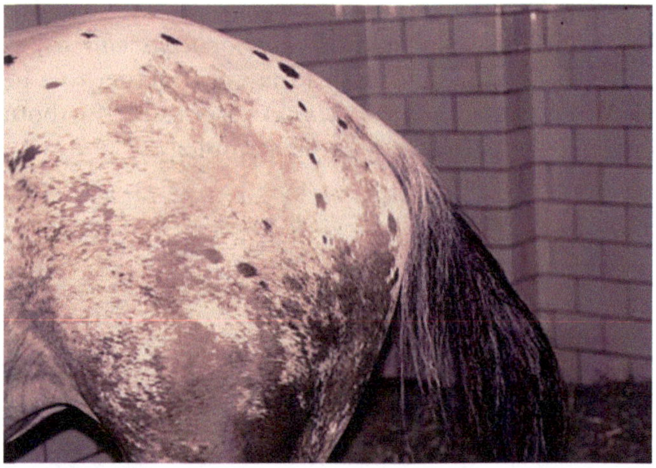

**Figure 9.14.** Horse. Tail Muscle. Denervation Atrophy. There is evidence of a dent in muscle contour. The tail is unusually low. The muscle atrophy resulted from Equine Motor Neuron Disease affecting coccigeal, femural, quadriceps, and triceps brachii muscles.

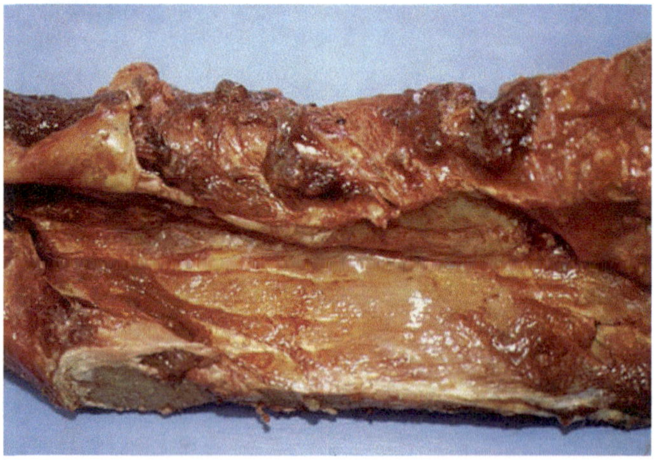

**Figure 9.15.** Horse. Lumbosacral Muscle. Denervation Atrophy. This lesion was secondary to trauma. Muscles are characterized by pallor and edema suggesting myodegeneration and atrophy.

## VII. Immune-mediated myopathy

Three different immune-mediated myopathies need to be distinguished in horses.

### 1. *Infarctive purpura hemorrhagica*

Horses exposed to *Streptococcus equi* subsp. *equi* may develop a postinfectious immune complex–induced vasculitis that is accompanied by hemorrhage, edema, and necrosis of mainly the muscles of the limbs. Subcutaneous edema of all four limbs and pitting edema of the ventral abdomen may be present as clinical signs. Hemorrhages and petechiations can be seen within the visible mucous membranes and in internal organs. Circulating immune complexes are deposited in the wall of small blood vessels rendering them "leaky." The deposits are composed of mainly immunoglobulin (Ig)M or IgA and streptococcal M protein.

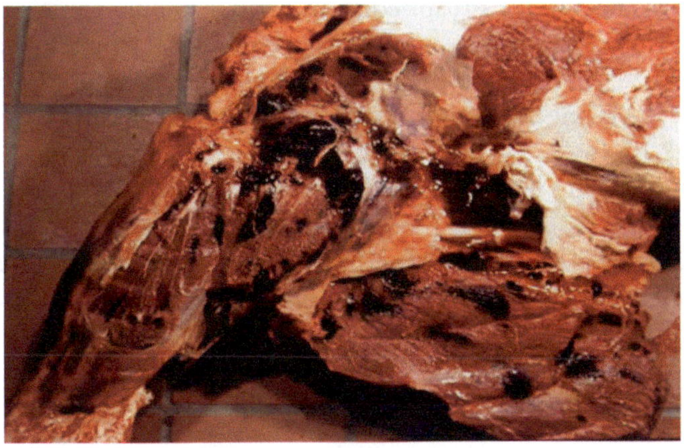

**Figure 9.16.** Horse. Limb. Skeletal Muscles. Multifocal Acute Intramuscular and Fascial Hemorrhages. Purpura Hemorrhagica. Differential diagnoses should include clostridial myositis and trauma.

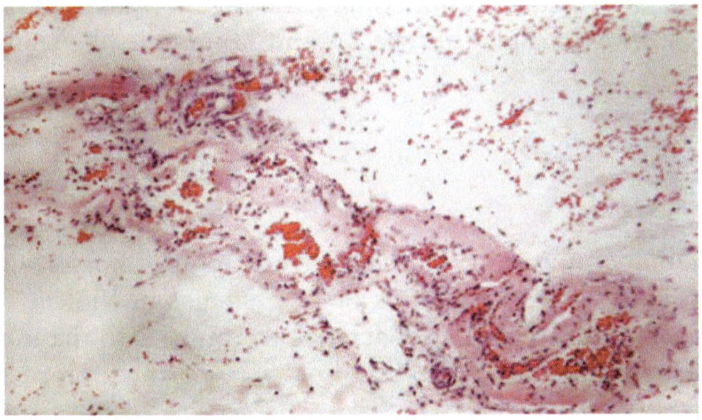

**Figure 9.17.** Horse. Blood Vessel. Subcutis. Purpura Hemorrhagica. Leukoclastic vasculitis with fibrinoid necrosis and red blood cell extravasation are microscopic criteria for the diagnosis of purpura hemorrhagica. (H&E)

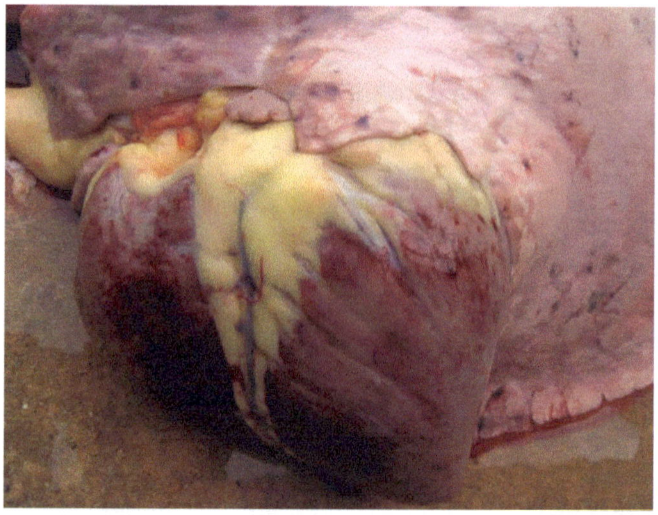

**Figure 9.18.** Horse. Heart. Petechiae. Purpura Hemorrhagica. Petechiae are disseminated on epicardium and lung. Differential diagnosis: sepsis.

### *2. Streptococcal acute severe rhabdomyolysis*

A variant form of *S. equi* subsp. *equi* myopathy includes microscopic myonecrosis and rhabdomyolysis resembling streptococcal toxic shock syndrome. *Streptococci* and *Streptococcal equi* myosin binding protein can be identified in these cases. Myonecrosis with inflammation can be quite extensive.

### *3. Immune-mediated myositis*

This form of muscle wasting is seen in Quarter horses. It affects epaxial and gluteal muscles that rapidly become atrophic. Affected muscles are infiltrated with histiocytes and T-lymphocytes. Myofibers do not react with immunoglobulin G staining.

## VIII. Hormonal imbalance myopathy

A myopathy with muscle wasting has been described in older horses with pituitary pars intermedia dysfunction. Muscle biopsies from the gluteus medius muscle show atrophy of type 2A and 2B muscle fibers and loss of 2B myofibers.

## IX. Trauma

External traumatic injuries to muscles are common in horses. On occasion, they are due to violent contractures or overextension. Violent contractures of muscles may result in hernias. Catastrophic injuries to the muscles of the forelimbs are typically encountered in horses performing on racetracks.

## X. Neoplasia



These have been described as rhabdomyoma, when benign, or rhabdomyosarcoma, when malignant, and as hemangiosarcoma when arising from the endothelial lining of the muscular vasculature. Intramuscular desmoid tumors originating from myofibroblasts (equine musculoaponeurotic fibromatosis) have been reported as sporadic tumors in epaxial muscles. Invasion by lipocytes into muscle fascia may constitute an infiltrating lipoma. Likewise, dermal melanomas or mastocytomas may extend into superficial muscles.

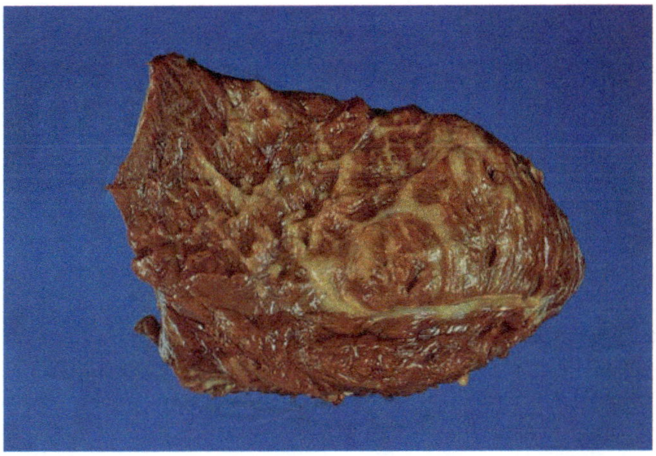

**Figure 9.19.** Horse. Skeletal Muscle. Infiltrating Lipoma. Bands of adipose tissue are intermixed with muscle fascia and muscle tissue.

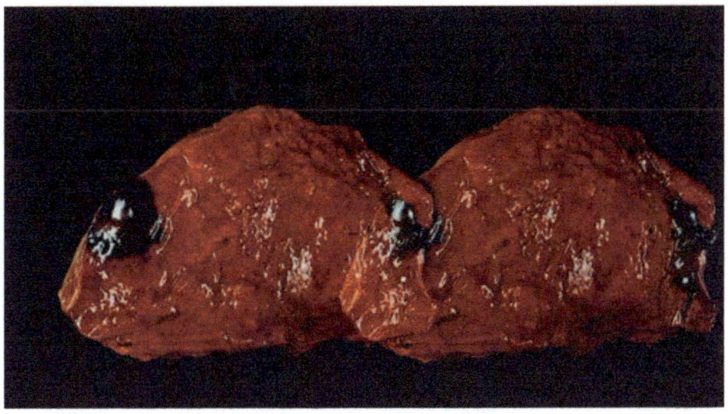

**Figure 9.20.** Horse. Skeletal Muscle. Hemangiosarcoma. Despite the benign gross appearance of the red foci, the tumor had malignant histologic features.

The few reported cases of equine rhabdomyosarcoma had a preference for legs, tongue, and tissues of the head. They revealed a locally invasive behavior, with metastasis being rare. Indirect immunohistochemistry was positive for desmin, myosin, and sarcomeric actin.

## Selected references


Aleman M. 2008. A review of muscular disorders. *Neuromuscular Disord* 18(4): 277–287.

Aleman M, Watson JL, Williams DC, LeCouteur RA, Nieto JE, Shelton GD. 2006. Myopathy in horses with pituitary pars intermedia dysfunction (Cushing's disease). *Neuromuscular Disord* 16(11):737–744.

Calore EE, Pellissier JF, Figarella-Branger D, deBarsy T, Pouget J, Serratice G. 1992. Polysaccharide amylopectin-type storage myopathy [in French]. *Rev Neurol (Paris)* 148(11):696–703.

Castleman WL, Toplon DE, Clark T, et al. 2011. Rhabdomyosarcoma in 8 horses. *Vet Pathol* 48(6):1144–1150.

Dranchak PK, Valberg StJ, Onan GW, et al. 2005. Inheritance of recurrent exertional rhabdomyolysis in Thoroughbreds. *J Am Vet Med Assoc* 227(5):762–767.

Finno CJ, Valberg SJ, Wuenschmann A, Murphy MJ. 2006. Seasonal pasture myopathy in horses in the Midwestern United States: 14 cases (1998–2005). *J Am Vet Med Assoc* 229(7):1134–1141.

Kaese HJ, Valberg SJ, Hayden DW, et al. 2005. Infarctive purpura hemorrhagica in five horses. *J Am Vet Med Assoc* 226(11):1893–1898.

Lewis SS, Valberg SJ, Nielsen IL. 2007. Suspected immune-mediated myositis in horses. *J Vet Intern Med* 21(3):495–503.

McCue ME, Armien AG, Lucio M, Mickelson JR, Valberg SJ. 2009. Comparative skeletal muscle histopathologic and ultrastructural features in two forms of polysaccharide storage myopathy in horses. *Vet Pathol* 46(6):1281–1291.

Meyer TS, Fedde MR, Cox JH, Erickson HH. 1999. Hyperkalaemic periodic paralysis in horses: a review. *Equine Vet J* 31(5):362–367.

Naylor JM. 1994. Equine hyperkalemic periodic paralysis: a review and implications. *Can Vet J* 35(5):279–285.

Nogradi N, Spier SJ, Toth B, Vaughan B. 2012. Musculoskeletal *Corynebacterium pseudotuberculosis* infection in horses: 35 cases (1999–2009). *J Am Vet Med Assoc* 241(6):771–777.

Quist EM, Dougherty JJ, Chaffin MK, Porter BF. 2011. Equine rhabdomyolysis. *Vet Pathol* 48(6):52–58.

Render JA, Common RS, Kennedy FA, Jones MZ, Fyfe JC. 1999. Amylopectinosis in fetal and neonatal Quarter Horses. *Vet Pathol* 36(2):157–160.

Valberg ST. 2011. The genetic basis for muscle disorders in horses. *The Practitioner* 5:23–25.

Valentine BA. 2008. Pathologic findings in equine muscle (excluding polysaccharide storage): a necropsy study. *J Vet Diag Invest* 20(5):572–579.

Valentine BA, Cooper BJ. 2005. Incidence of polysaccharide storage myopaty: necropsy study of 225 horses. *Vet Pathol* 42(6):823–827.

Valentine BA, Del Piero F, Edwards RB. 1999. Intramuscular desmoid tumor (musculoaponeurotic fibromatosis) in two horses. *Vet Pathol* 36(5):468–470.

# 10 Disease of the Skeletal System

Contributed by Julie B. Engiles



*Color Atlas of Equine Pathology*, First Edition. Claus D. Buergelt and Fabio Del Piero.

# I. Congenital/developmental lesions

## *1. Aplasia/hypoplasia/dysplasia*

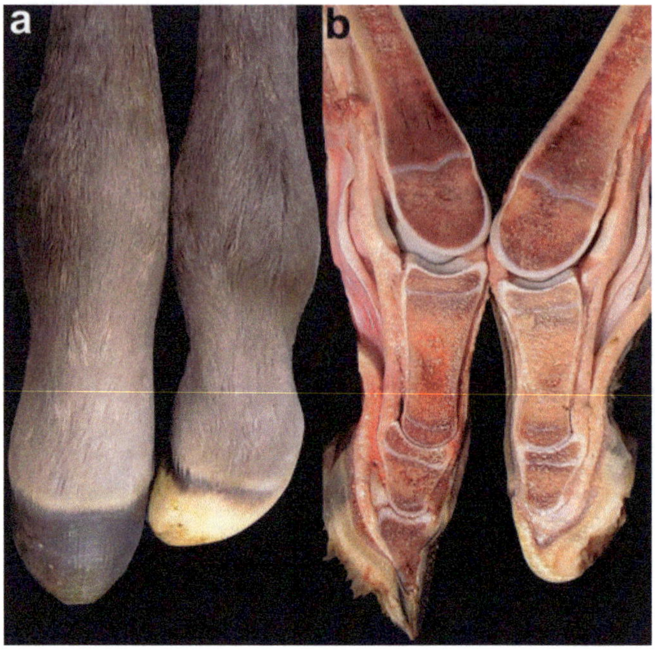


**Figure 10.1.** Foal. Neonate. (a) Distal forelimbs. Unilateral hemimelia with limb shortening and varus deformity. (b) Longitudinal sections reveal aplasia of the distal phalanx and navicular bone of the left forelimb.

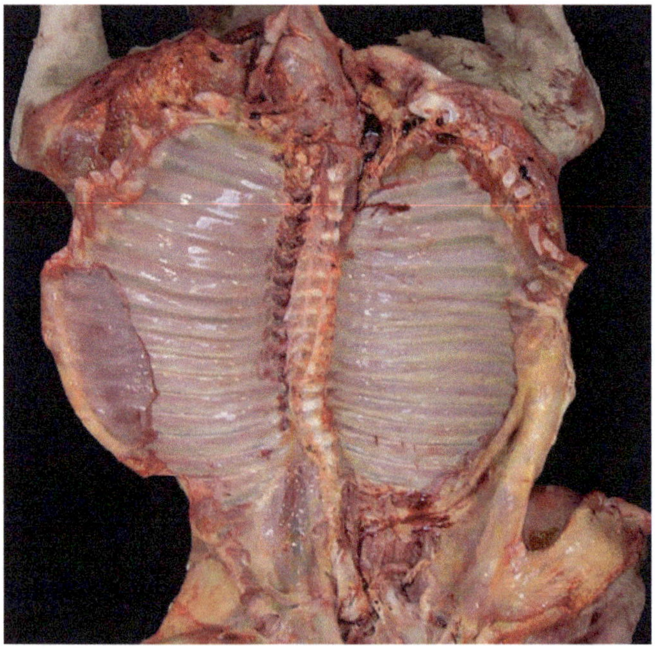

**Figure 10.2.** Foal. Neonate. Axial skeleton (ventral view of spine). Congenital scoliosis (right lateral curvature of the spine) involving the caudal thoracic segment. (Courtesy Dr. P. Habecker, New Bolton Center, University of Pennsylvania.)

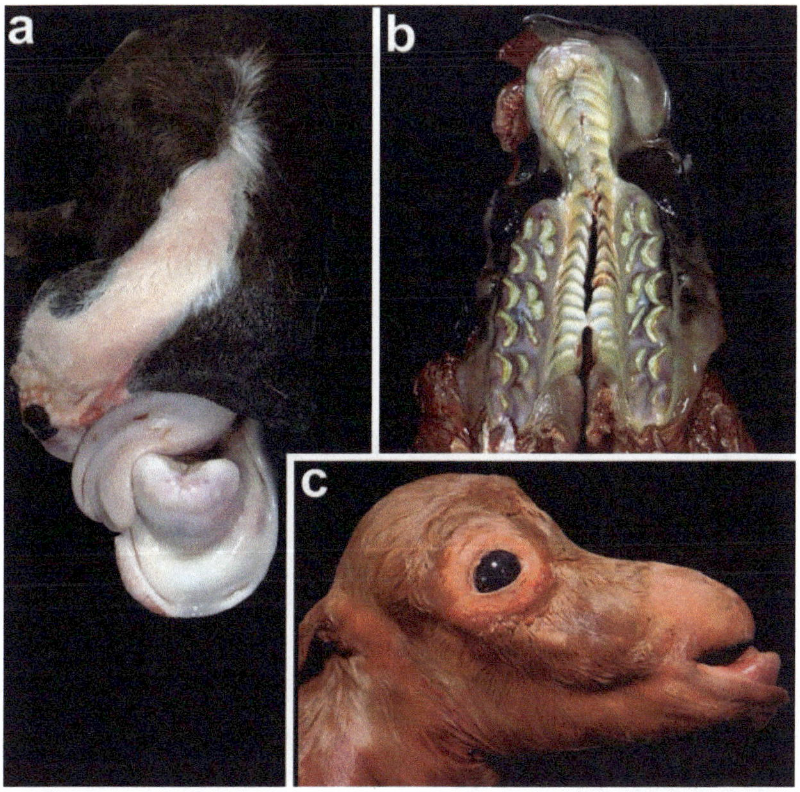

**Figure 10.3.** Foal. Neonates. Craniofacial dysplasias (i.e., malformations). (a) Lateral deviation of the rostral maxilla, (b) "Wry nose"; (b) palatoschisis, "cleft palate"; (c) maxillary brachygnathia. (Courtesy Dr. P. Habecker, New Bolton Center, University of Pennsylvania.)

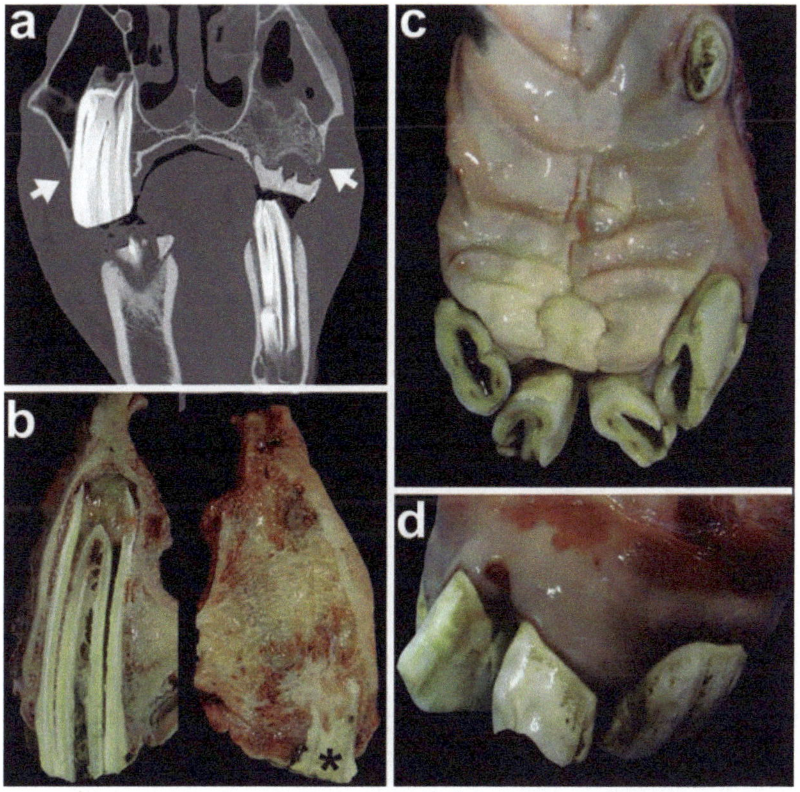

**Figure 10.4.** Horse. Regional hypodontia and odontodysplasia of the maxillary arcade.(a) Computed tomography (CT) scan reveals abnormal development of the right second maxillary molar (right arrow) as compared with the left second maxillary molar (left arrow). (b) Sagittal sections of both second maxillary molars (M2) show lack of enamel and dentin production of the right M2 with retention of the deciduous tooth, or "cap" (asterisk) when compared with the normal left M2. (c, d) Malformation and abnormal orientation of the maxillary incisors with aplasia of the left canine tooth.

## 2. *Osteochondrosis/osteochondritis dissecans*

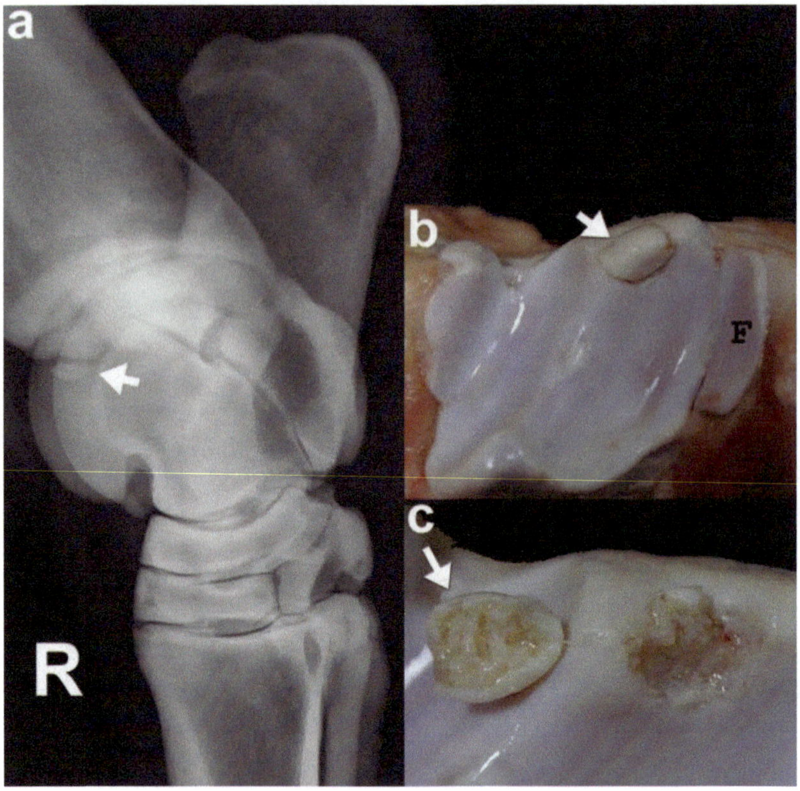


**Figure 10.5.** Horse. Juvenile. Osteochondritis dissecans (OCD), hock. (a) Digital radiograph reveals an osteochondral fragment (arrow) associated with the distal intermediate ridge of the tibia ("DIRT" lesion). (b, c) The osteochondral fragment is loosely associated with the subchondral bone (arrow) and manually dissects away from the subchondral bone, which has a soft, crumbly texture. (b) The distal fibula (F) is labeled for orientation. (Gross photos in [b] and [c] courtesy of Dr. P. Habecker, New Bolton Center, University of Pennsylvania)

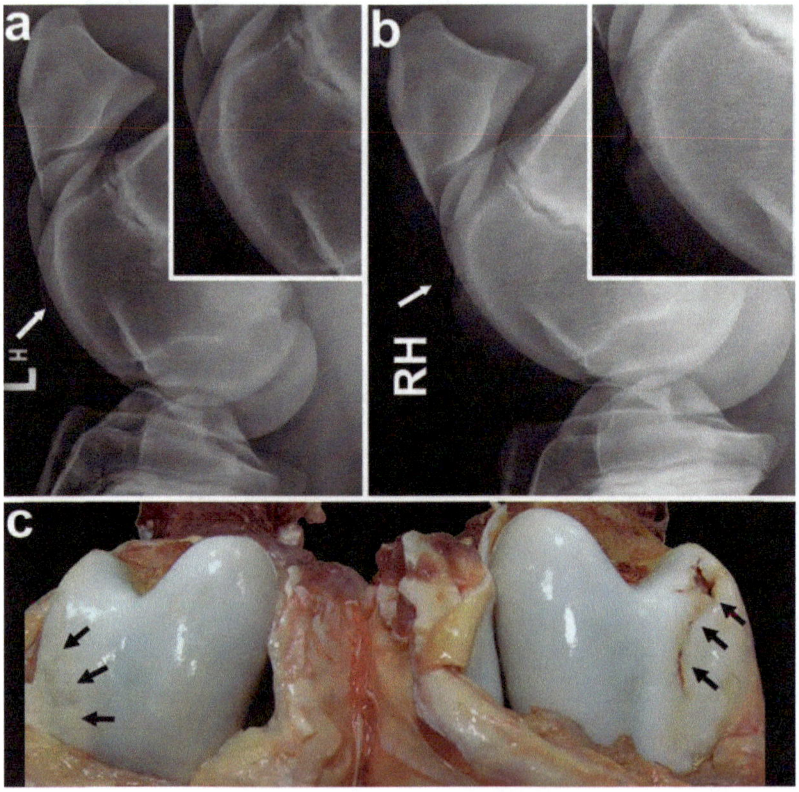


**Figure 10.6.** Horse. Juvenile. OCD, stifle. Oblique projection digital radiographs with enlarged insets of the (a) left and (b) right femoropatellar joints reveal an OCD lesion of the lateral trochlear ridge (LTR) of the right stifle (arrow) as compared with the normal LTR of the left stifle (arrow). (c) Gross photos show a large dissecting osteochondral defect in the left LTR (right arrows); however, a smaller nondissecting cartilage defect is within the LTR of the right stifle (left arrows). The animal was euthanized due to poor prognosis for future athletic performance. (Gross photo [c] courtesy of Dr. P. Habecker, New Bolton Center, University of Pennsylvania.)

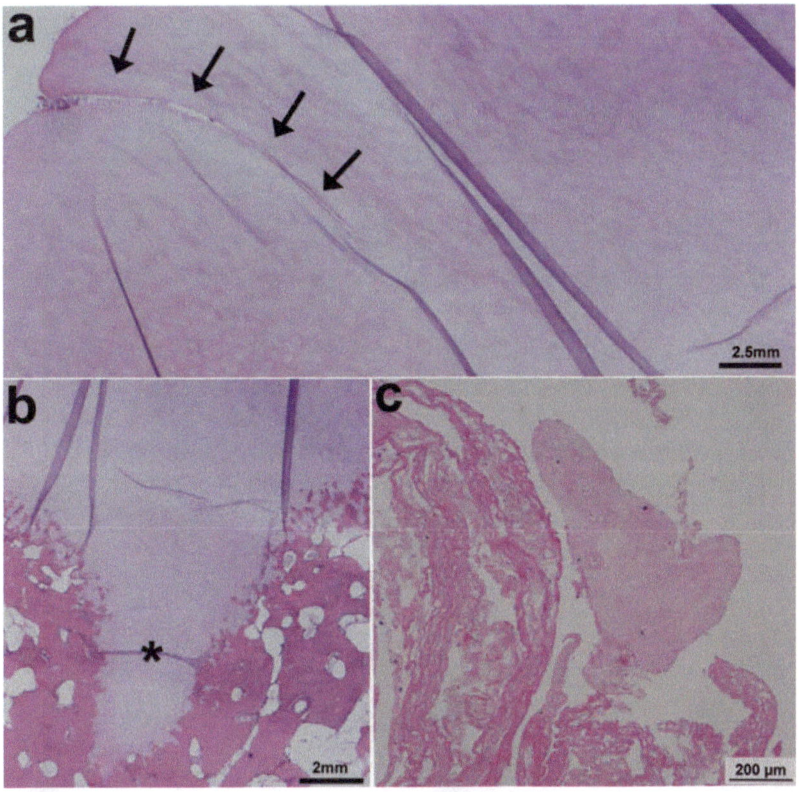


**Figure 10.7.** Horse. Juvenile. OCD, lateral trochlear ridge of distal femur. (a) Photomicrograph of the lesion shows a dissecting fissure through the articular cartilage (arrows; H&E) and (b) a retained core of hyaline cartilage (asterisk; H&E) surrounded by sclerotic subchondral bone. (c) A dissected fragment of cartilage, enmeshed in fibrin, is adjacent to the synovial membrane of a joint recess (H&E).

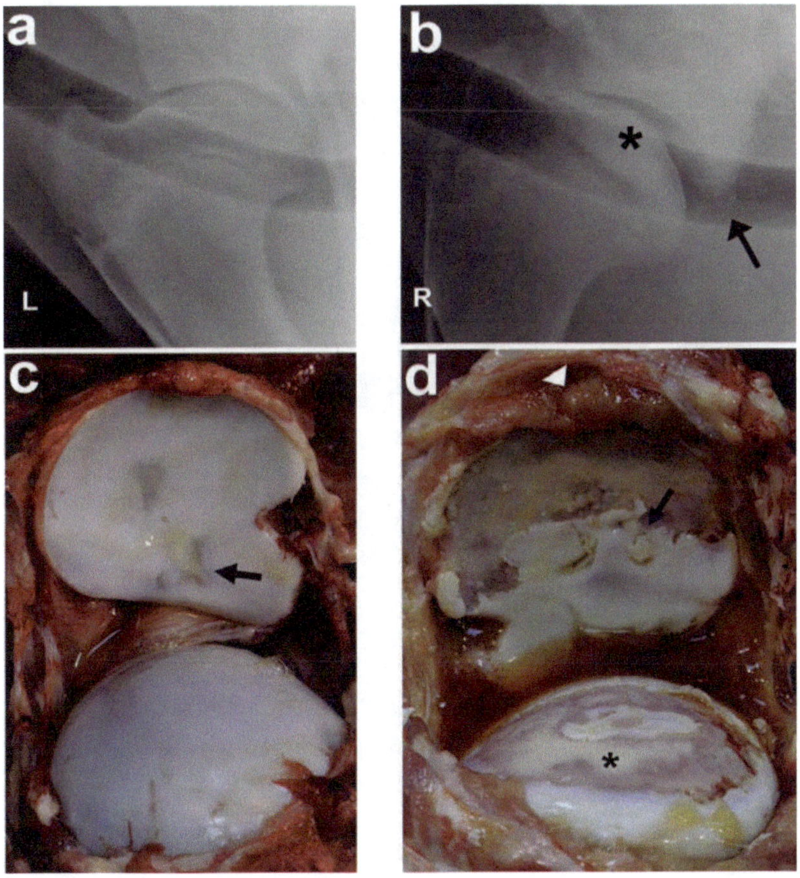


**Figure 10.8.** Horse. OCD, humeral head of glenohumeral (shoulder) joint. Digital radiographs of the (a) left and (b) right shoulder joints from an 8-month-old warmblood filly with chronic right forelimb lameness and shoulder joint effusion. (b) As compared with the left, the right shoulder shows an abnormal contour of the right humeral head with joint space incongruence, subchondral lysis (asterisk), subchondral sclerosis, and numerous free osteochondral fragments along the caudal distal aspect of the glenoid (arrow). (c) Gross evaluation reveals a small articular cartilage depression (mild OCD) within the left glenoid (arrow), but (d) the right glenoid has numerous depressions and dissecting cartilage flaps (arrow), with severe secondary degenerative osteoarthritis characterized by subchondral sclerosis and eburnation of the humeral head (asterisk), hyperplasia and hyperemia of the synovial membrane (arrowhead), and fibrous thickening of the joint capsule.

## 3. *Cervical vertebral instability (equine wobbler syndrome)*

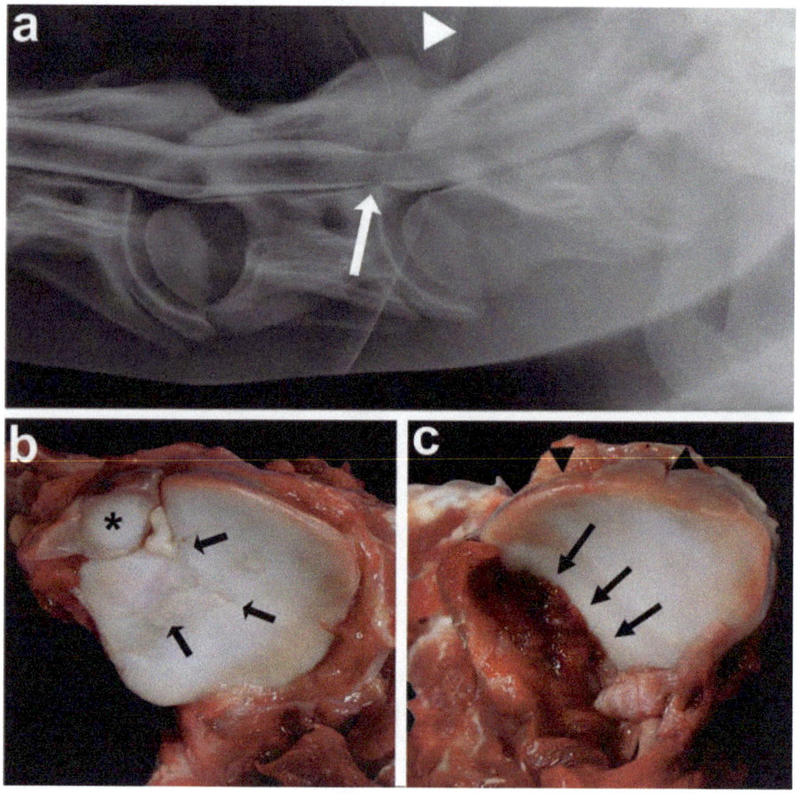


**Figure 10.9.** Horse. Dynamic cervical vertebral stenosis due to OCD and malarticulation of the cervical vertebral facets. (a) Digital radiograph with epidural contrast (myelogram) of the cervical spine shows vertebral canal stenosis with thinning of the dorsal and ventral dye columns (arrow) and enlarged facets (arrowhead). (b) Gross dissection of C4-C5 facet joint reveals articular cartilage fissures (arrows) and an isolated osteochondral island (asterisk) within the C4 caudal facet. Subchondral bone lipping along the articular margins of the cranial C5 facet (arrowheads) with synovial hyperplasia and hyperemia (arrows) indicates secondary degenerative osteoarthritis.

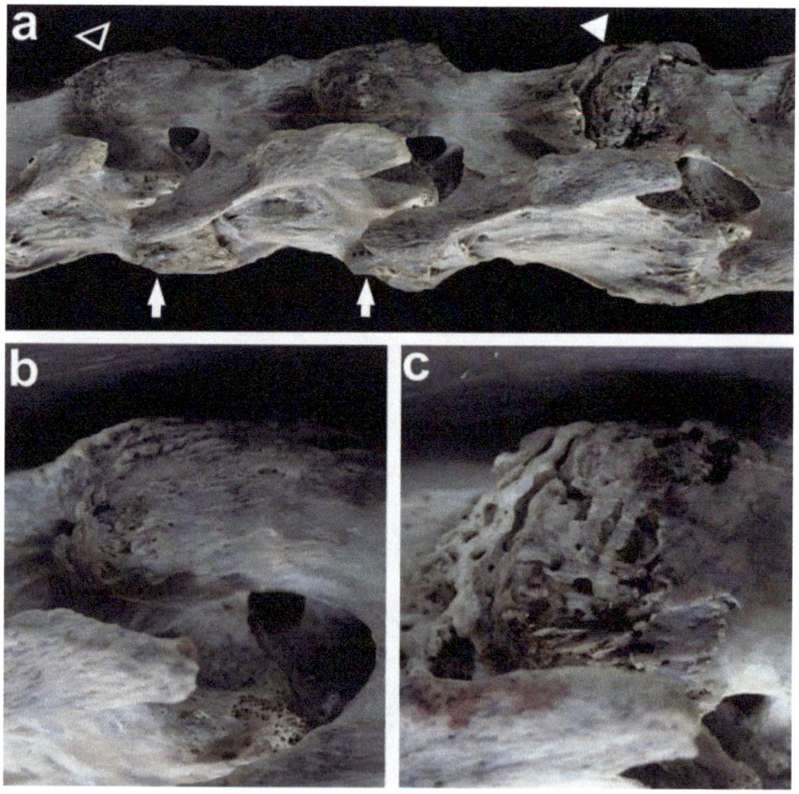


**Figure 10.10.** (a) Boiled specimen of a cervical spine from an 18-year-old Thoroughbred gelding that had dynamic cervical vertebral stenosis and prior arthrodesis with metallic basket surgical implants (arrows) placed as a juvenile. The surgically fused joints show smooth bony contours of the facet joints (a, open arrowhead; (b), whereas the adjacent, nonsurgically fused facet joint shows severe periarticular osteophytosis (a, arrowhead; (c) consistent with chronic vertebral instability and secondary severe degenerative osteoarthritis.

## II. Traumatic lesions (fractures)

### *1. Axial skeletal fractures*

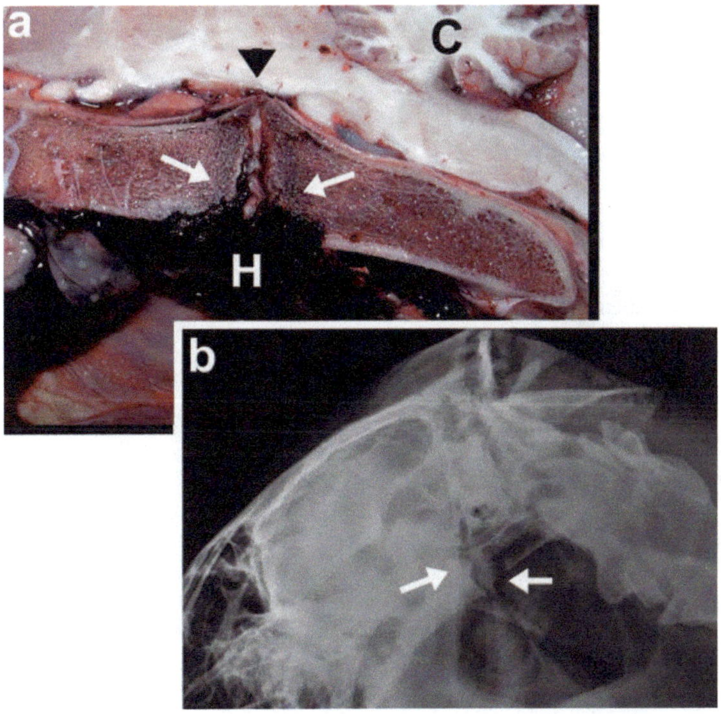


**Figure 10.11.** Horse. (a) Parasagittal section shows a fracture (arrows) with a hematoma (H) centered on the synarthrosis between the basisphenoid and basioccipital bone with dorsal subluxation and compression of the brainstem caudal to the hypothalamus (arrowhead). The cerebellum (C) is labeled for orientation. (b) Digital radiograph shows a linear lucency that extends ventrally from the nuchal crest and courses through the suture lines between the occipital and parietal bones, and basisphenoid and basioccipital bones (arrows), representing traumatic separation at the suture line. Early callus at the base of the basisphenoid bone is consistent with the duration of time since the injury was sustained.

The gross photo (Fig. 10.11a) is from a young foal that sustained a headlong fall into a paddock fence. In addition to seizures, the foal had central diabetes insipidus. The radiograph (Fig. 10.11b) is from a different foal that sustained a backward fall 2 months prior. The fractures visible on the radiograph represent similar injuries as highlighted in the gross photo (Fig. 10.11a) This fracture configuration is common in growing foals sustaining this form of trauma due to open or incompletely fused growth plates in the basisphenoid or basioccipital bones.

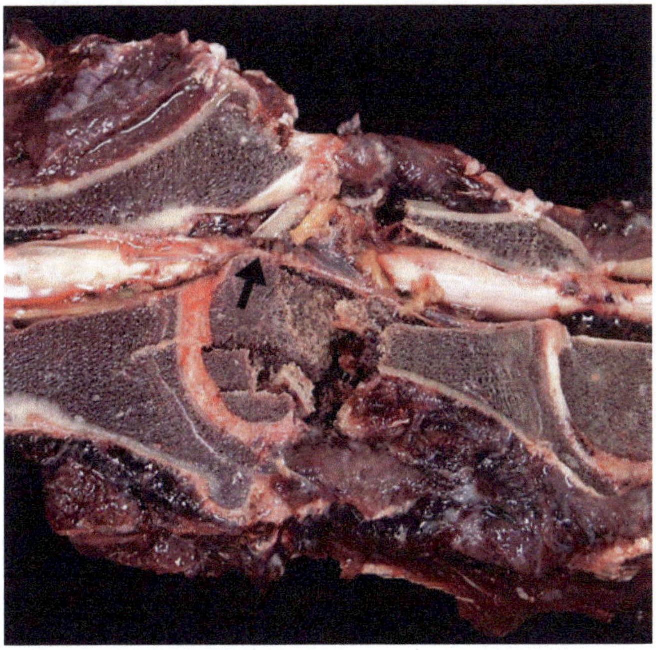

**Figure 10.12.** Parasagittal section of a fractured cervical spine from a 4-year-old Thoroughbred colt that occurred immediately following a breakdown injury of the forelimb. Displaced, comminuted fractures of the third cervical vertebral body and dorsal lamina resulted in subluxation of the C2-C3 vertebral endplates with compression and complete transection of the spinal cord (arrow). Surprisingly, the dura mater remained intact.

## *2. Growth plate fractures*

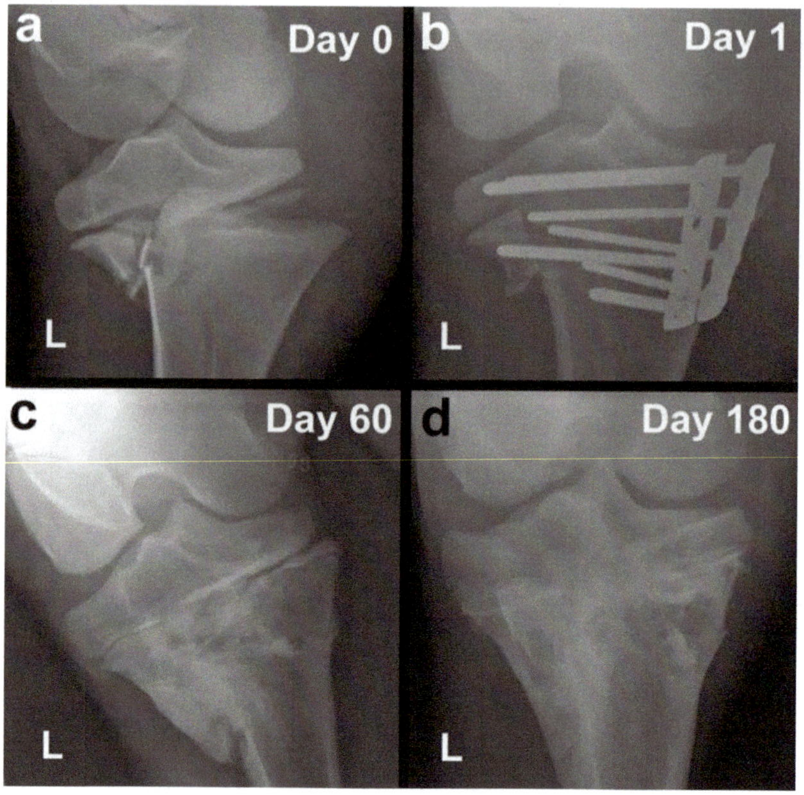


**Figure 10.13.** Horse. Physeal fracture of the left tibia from a foal with surgical fixation, implant infection and removal, and progressive fracture remodeling. (a) A Salter-Harris fracture type II (Day 0) is surgically repaired (b) using metallic plates and screws (Day 1). Due to complications, the surgical implants were removed. (c) Progressive modeling and ossification of the fracture is demonstrated (Day 60), and shows (d) gradual reduction and smoothing of the callus with eventual incorporation of the metaphyseal spike (Day 180).

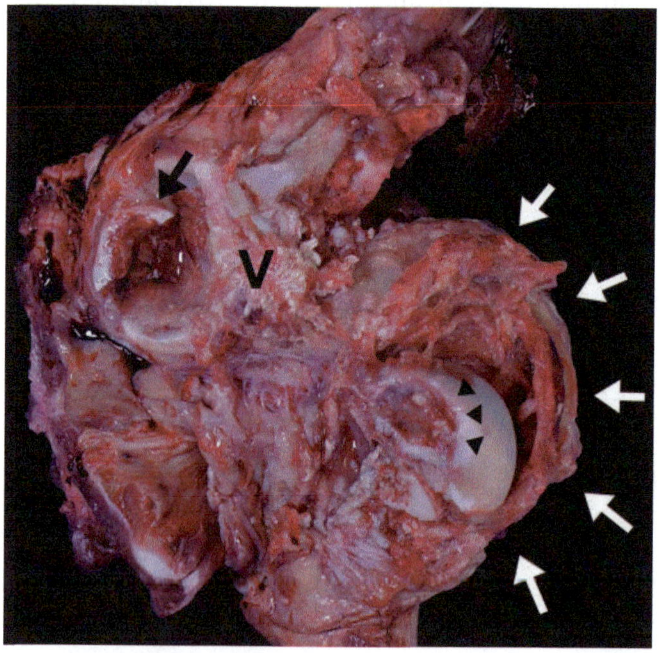


**Figure 10.14.** Foal. Chronic epiphyseal fracture of the femoral head with luxation and pseudoarthrosis. A portion of the epiphysis of the femoral head is fractured (arrowheads). The displaced fracture fragment is adhered within a fibrotic articular surface of the acetabular cup (black arrow) and surrounded by villous projections of a hyperplastic synovial membrane (V). The femoral head is luxated and sits within a soft tissue pocket, or "pseudoarthrosis," located dorsocranial to the acetabulum (white arrows).

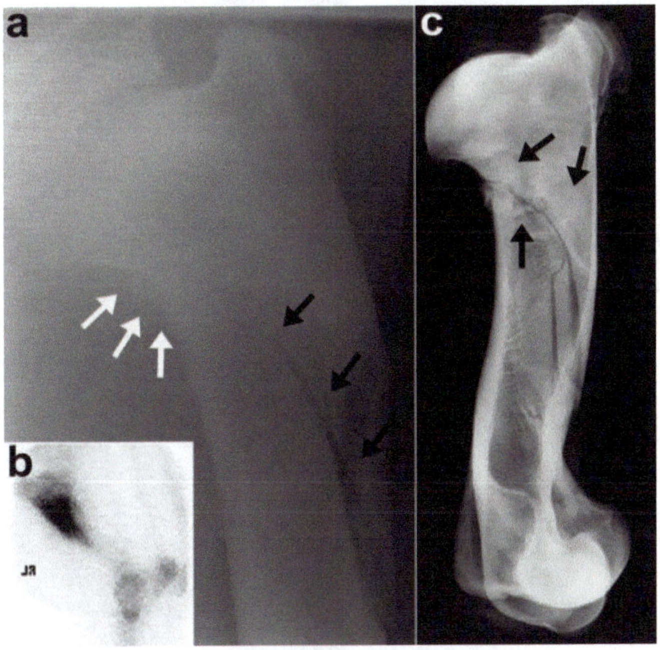


**Figure 10.15.** Racehorse. Juvenile. (a) Radiograph, antemortem. A displaced oblique fracture extends through the proximal to mid humeral diaphysis (black arrows). A slight periosteal proliferation is evident along the proximal caudal medial surface of the metaphysis (white arrows). (b) Nuclear scintigraphic scan: antemortem. Markedly increased radiopharmaceutical uptake within the proximal diaphyseal-metaphyseal junction, consistent with active bone remodeling, and indicative of a proximal humeral stress fracture. (c) Radiograph: postmortem. A diaphyseal fracture line extends into the caudal aspect of the metaphysis. Patchy medullary radiopacities (black arrows) surround this portion of the fracture, indicative of endosteal callus.

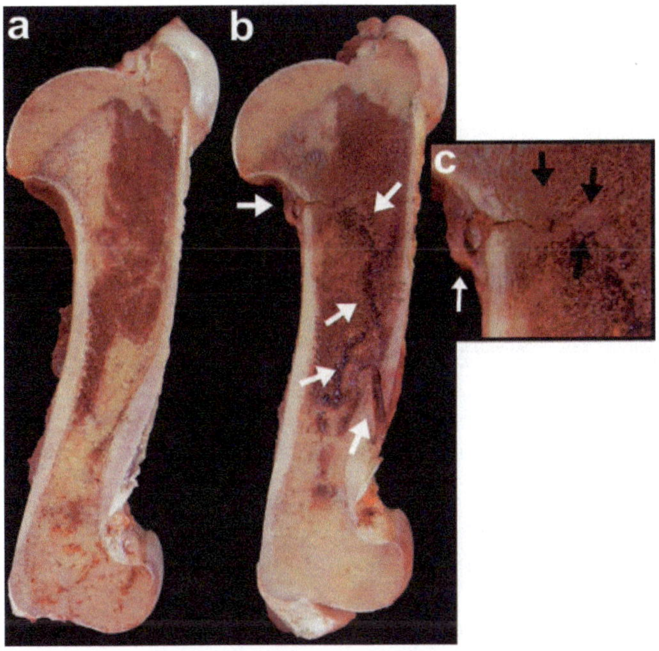


**Figure 10.16.** Racehorse. Juvenile. Gross photos of the humeral fracture imaged in Figure 10.15. (a) The normal left humerus is compared with (b) the right humerus that shows a displaced dorsal distal diaphyseal fracture bridged by hemorrhage that extends proximally through the medullary cavity and out through the caudal proximal diaphyseal-metaphyseal junction (white arrows). (c) Inset of the metaphyseal region shows intramedullary foci of new bone (e.g., endosteal callus) that surround the fracture line (black arrows), as well as slight periosteal callus along the caudal metaphysis (white arrow).

Stress fractures can result in catastrophic failure that necessitates humane euthanasia. Stress fractures are relatively common in young Thoroughbred racehorses and can be difficult to diagnose without the use of nuclear scintigraphy. Although the onset of lameness can be acute and severe, it can resolve quickly with stall rest, is difficult to localize, and response to diagnostic nerve blocks of the distal limb is negative. Endosteal callus or minimal periosteal callus (indicative of prior bone injury with a repair response) is often present, but often difficult to detect on radiographs.

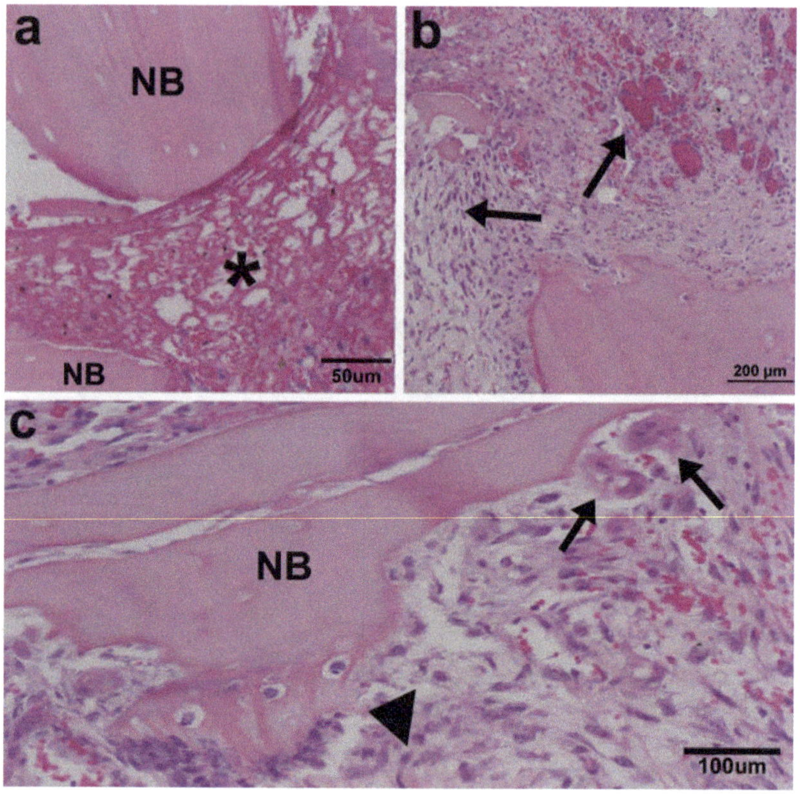


**Figure 10.17.** Racehorse. Juvenile. H&E photomicrographs of acute fracture and early phases of fracture healing. (a) Fracture fragments of necrotic bone (NB) are embedded within a hematoma (asterisk). (b) With time, the hematoma will organize into granulation tissue with proliferation of mesenchymal stem cells (arrows). (c) Osteoclasts (arrows) begin to resorb necrotic bone spicules (NB), as osteoblasts begin to produce woven "repair" bone (arrowhead). This process is also known as "creeping substitution."

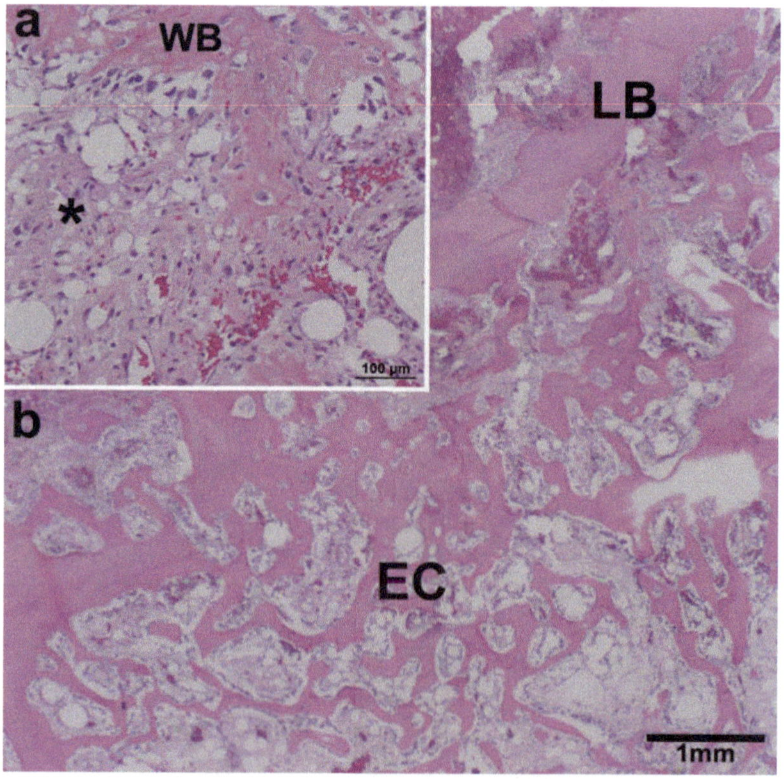


**Figure 10.18.** Racehorse. Juvenile. Photomicrographs (H&E) of later phases of fracture healing. (a) Woven bone (WB) produced by osteoblasts from differentiated osteoprogenitor cells (asterisk) forms (b) an endosteal callus (EC) adjacent to (c) partially resorbed fragments of compact lamellar bone (LB).

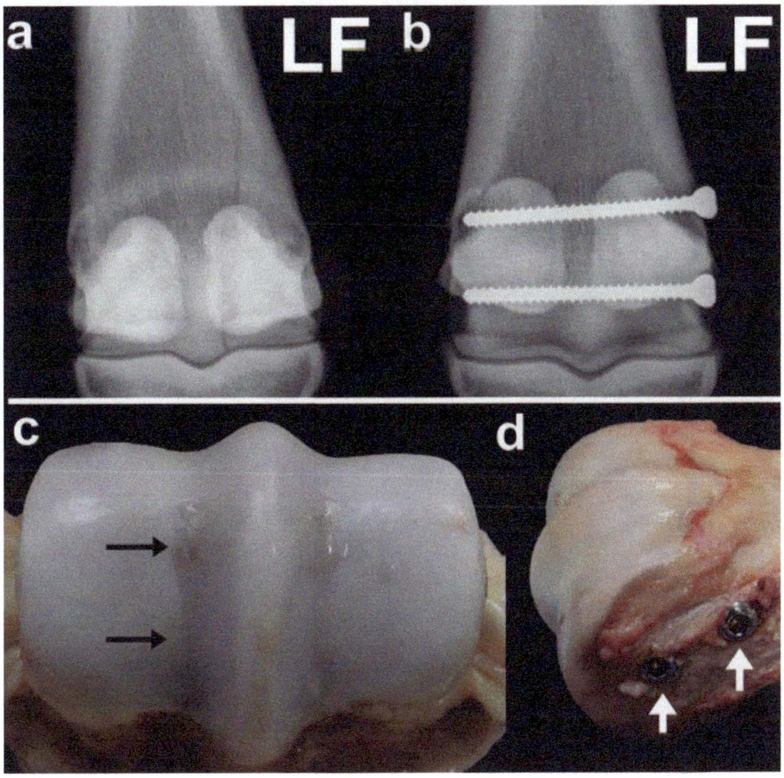


**Figure 10.19.** Horse. Lateral condylar fracture of the left third metacarpus with internal fixation surgical repair. (a) Preoperative and (b) postoperative digital radiographs of a Thoroughbred racehorse that sustained an incomplete simple, nondisplaced lateral condylar fracture. (b–d) Excellent anatomic reduction of the fracture was achieved by internal fixation using cortical bone screws placed in lag fashion, and articular cartilage damage is minimal. An excellent prognosis to return to racing was given; however, the horse was euthanized due to development of postoperative pneumonia.

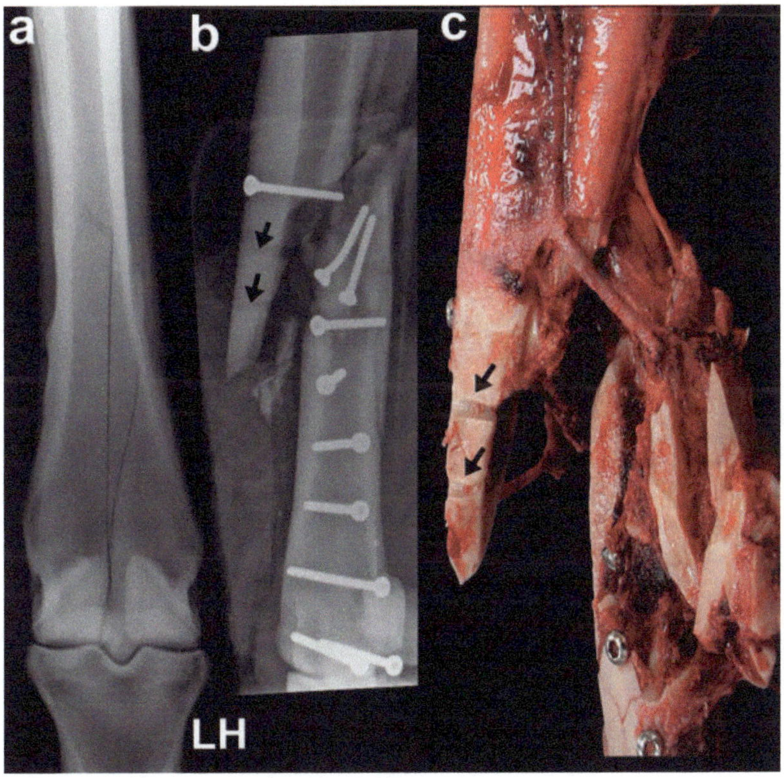


**Figure 10.20.** Horse. Medial condylar fracture (Y configuration) of (a) the left hind limb with (b, c) surgical internal fixation and subsequent catastrophic failure. The postoperative fracture extends through two proximal screws placed in the mid-diaphyseal region (arrows).

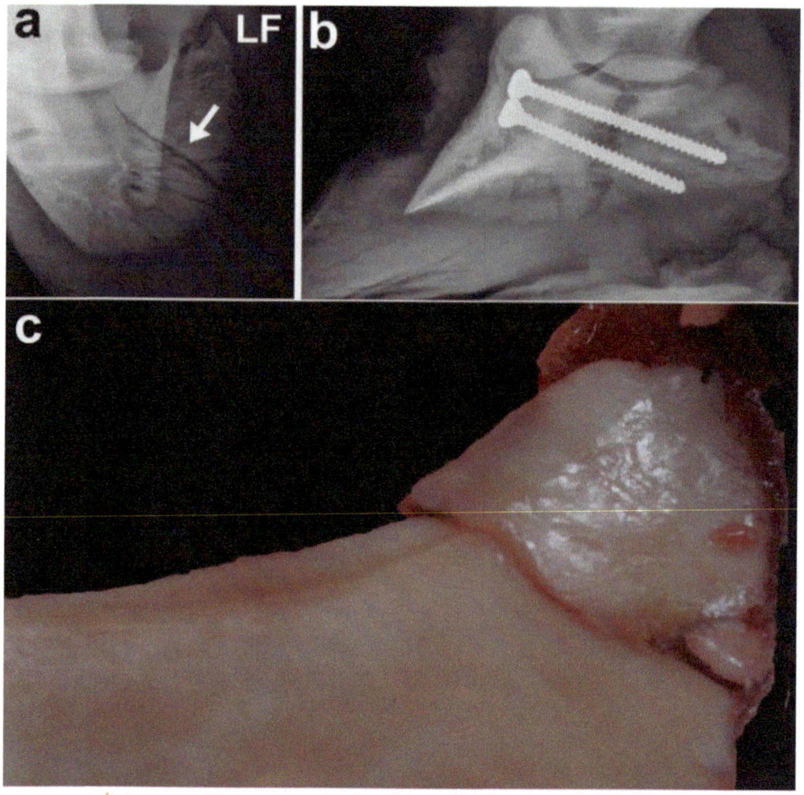


**Figure 10.21.** Horse. Chronic articular wing fracture of the distal phalanx with surgical implant infection and fibrous nonunion. (a) Preoperative digital radiographs of a mildly displaced articular wing fracture (arrow). (b) Digital radiographs obtained 3 months postoperatively reveal widening of the fracture line and mild lysis surrounding the surgical implants. (c) Dissection of the distal phalanx shows poor anatomic reduction with proximal and caudal displacement of the largest fracture fragment forming a prominent "step" in the articular cartilage surface.

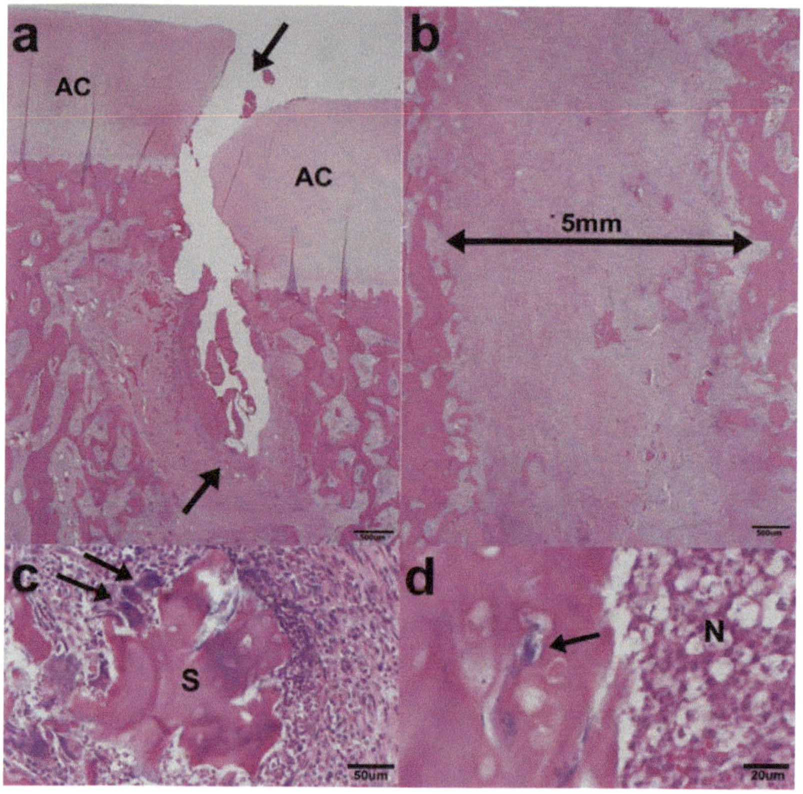


**Figure 10.22.** Horse. Photomicrographs (H&E) show (a) persistence of the fracture (arrows) with incongruence of the articular cartilage surface (AC). (b) A section through the deeper portion of bone shows fracture fragments bridged by 5 mm of fibrous connective tissue (arrow). (c) Small necrotic bone fragments, sequestra (S) are surrounded by suppurative inflammation and multinucleate osteoclasts (arrows). (d) Persistent infection is evidenced by bacteria observed within necrotic bone fragments (arrow) surrounded by neutrophils (N).

## III. Infectious/inflammatory lesions

### *1. Septic arthritis*

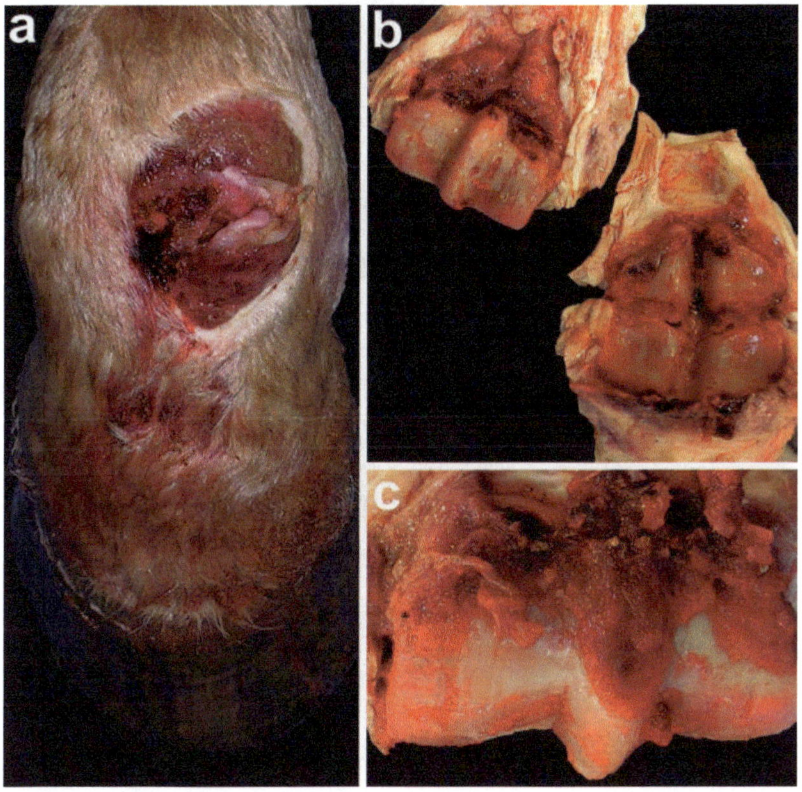


**Figure 10.23.** Horse. Traumatically induced chronic septic arthritis of the metacarpophalangeal joint. (a) A cutaneous ulcer and bud of granulation tissue surrounds a chronic fistula that communicates with the metacarpophalangeal joint. (b) The synovium is severely hyperplastic and hyperemic, and the articular cartilage is thinned and yellow. (c) Pannus extends from the periarticular margins over portions of the articular cartilage, which has an irregular "scored" surface.

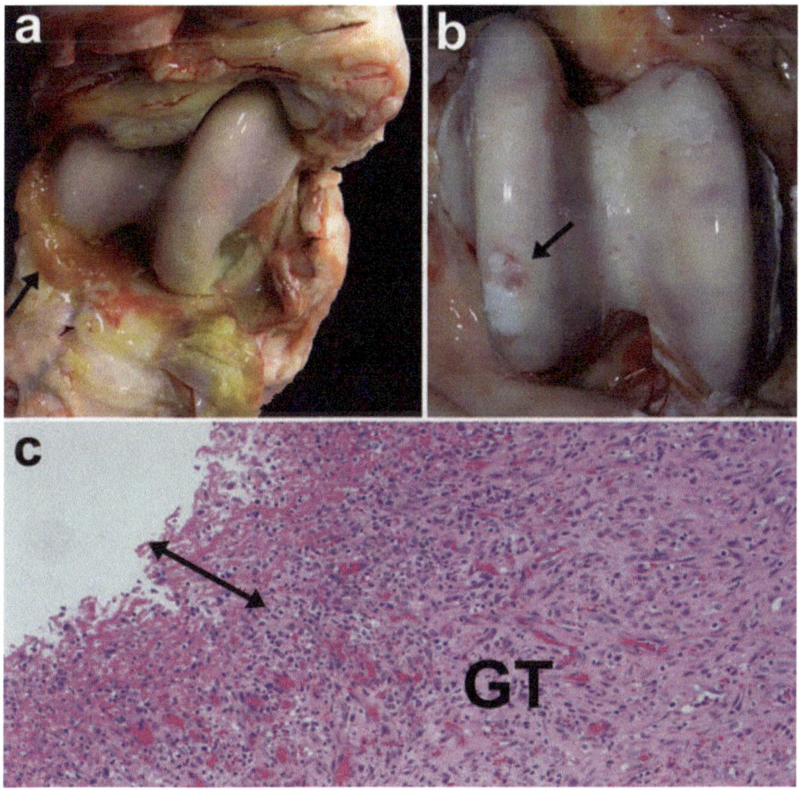


**Figure 10.24.** Septic arthritis of the tarsocrural (hock) joint in a young foal with recent history of enterocolitis. (a) Prolonged suppurative inflammation resulted in diffuse cartilage atrophy and synovial hyperplasia (arrow) with fibrinous exudate. (b) Close inspection reveals few remaining islands of articular cartilage (arrow). (c) Photomicrograph of the synovial membrane effaced by an exudate of fibrin and inflammatory cells (double-headed arrow) and subtended by granulation tissue proliferation (GT).

## 2. Septic osteomyelitis: neonates and juvenile horses

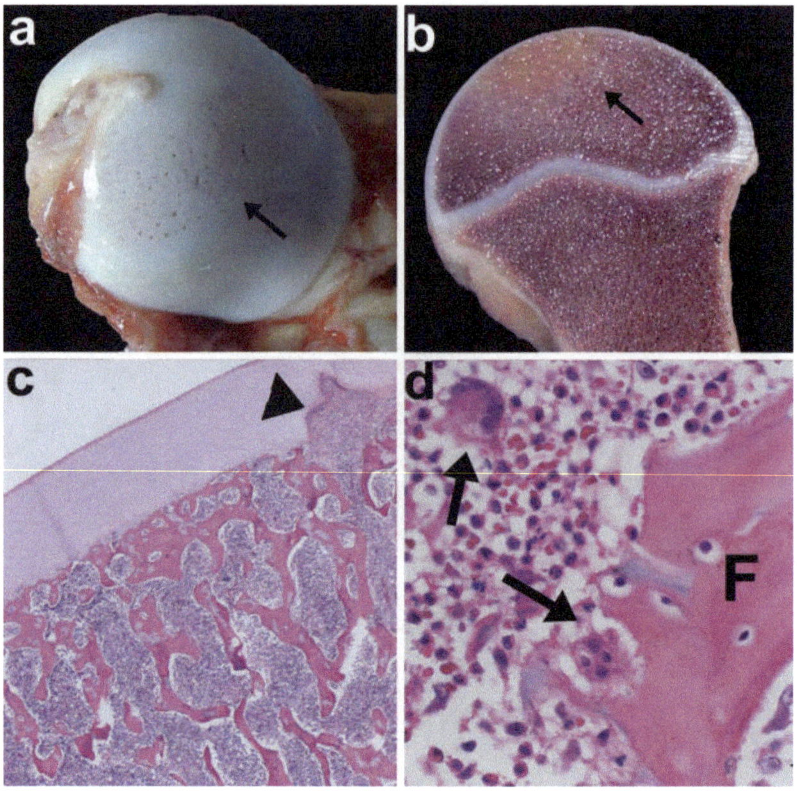


**Figure 10.25.** Septic epiphysitis of the femoral head in a young foal. (a) Articular cartilage atrophy exposes the vascular channels that feed the deeper layers of cartilage (arrow). (b) Sagittal section reveals a discrete yellow-tan focus of inflammation within the subchondral bone of the femoral capital epiphysis (arrow). Low (c) and high (d) magnification H&E photomicrographs of the inflammatory focus in (b) show suppurative inflammation filling the medullary spaces and (c) extending into an expanded vascular canal within the overlying cartilage. (d) Fractured primary trabeculae (F) are surrounded by neutrophils and multinucleate osteoclasts (arrows).

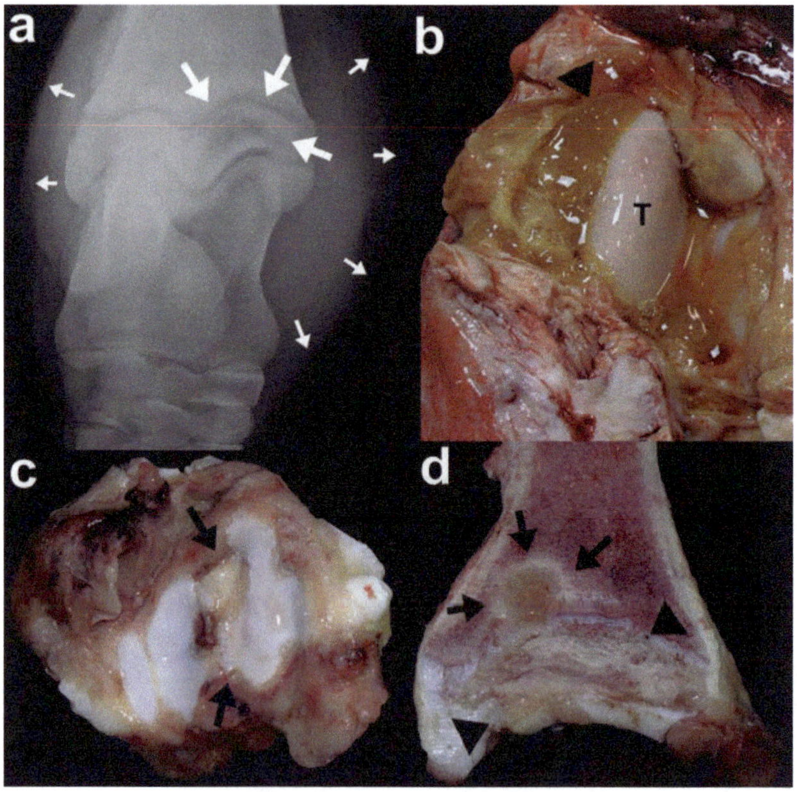


**Figure 10.26.** Septic arthritis and osteomyelitis of the distal tibia with physeal abscess and sequestrum in a young foal. (a) A digital radiograph reveals soft tissue swelling involving the tarsocrural joint (small outer arrows) and a well-defined radiolucency adjacent to the distal tibial physis (large arrows). (b) The joint is packed with gelatinous, fibrino-suppurative exudate (arrowhead), and there is articular cartilage atrophy of the talus (T). (c) The distal tibia contains a well-demarcated dull yellow focus of necrotic bone, that is, sequestrum (arrows). (d) A sagittal section reveal a well-demarcated abscess proximal to the metaphyseal physis surrounded by a sclerotic rim (arrows). The abscess crosses the physis, extending to the sequestrum (arrowheads).

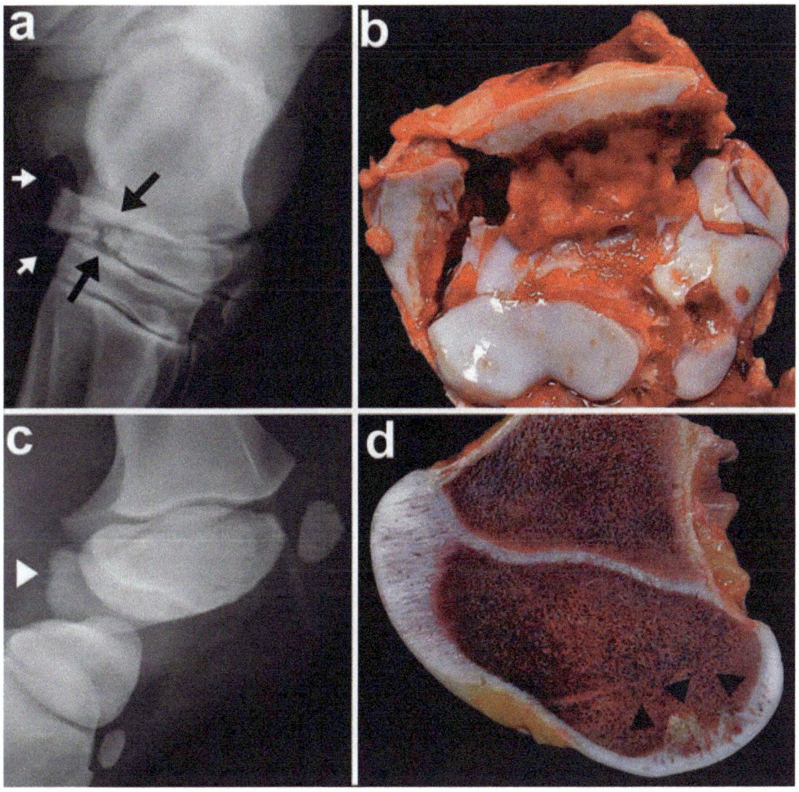


**Figure 10.27.** (a) Septic osteomyelitis of the central tarsal bone with pathologic fracture (black arrows) and displaced comminuted fracture fragments (white arrows) in a foal. (b) This fracture was initially thought to be of traumatic origin; however, necropsy revealed suppurative inflammation within the joint that extended from the inner portions of the bone. (c) Septic epiphysitis of the lateral femoral condyle of a foal can resemble an OCD lesion on a radiograph (arrowhead); however, the predilection site was inappropriate for OCD, and (d) necropsy revealed a wedge-shaped yellow suppurative focus at the site of the osteochondral defect (arrowheads), indicative of infectious etiology.

### *3. Septic osteomyelitis: adult horses*

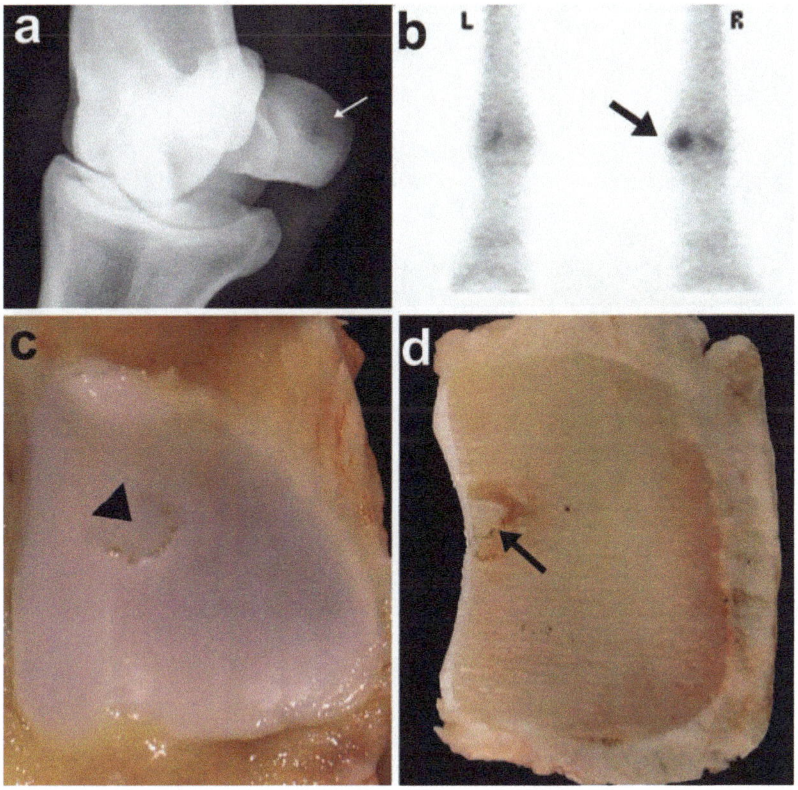


**Figure 10.28.** Septic osteomyelitis of the right hind medial sesamoid bone from a Thoroughbred racehorse euthanized for chronic intermittent grade 1-3 lameness. (a) A wedge-shaped radiolucency within the medial sesamoid bone seen on the dorsomedial-plantarolateral oblique projection (arrow) corresponds to (b) severe increased radiopharmaceutical uptake within the same sesamoid bone (arrow).
(c) Metatarsophalangeal (fetlock) joint dissection reveals a semi-lunar depression within the central articular surface of the medial sesamoid bone (arrowhead) with mild clear-yellow effusion and synovial hyperplasia.
(d) Sagittal sections reveal a wedge-shaped sequestrum (arrow) surrounded by an involucrum.

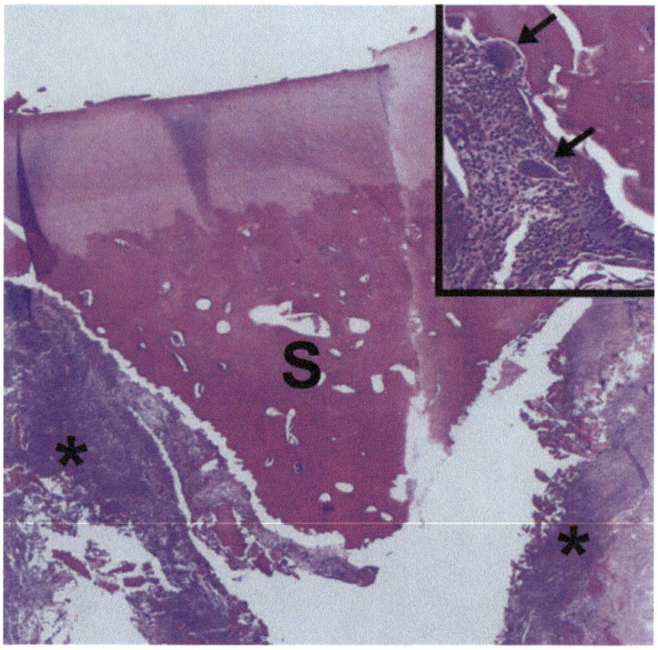


**Figure 10.29.** Horse. Photomicrographs (H&E) of a sagittal section from the medial sesamoid bone in Figure 10.28 reveals the bony sequestrum (S) rimmed by suppurative inflammation (asterisks) and smaller fragments of necrotic bone. Higher magnification inset reveals necrotic neutrophils and multinucleate osteoclasts (arrows) surround the necrotic bone fragment devoid of nuclei within osteocyte lacunae.

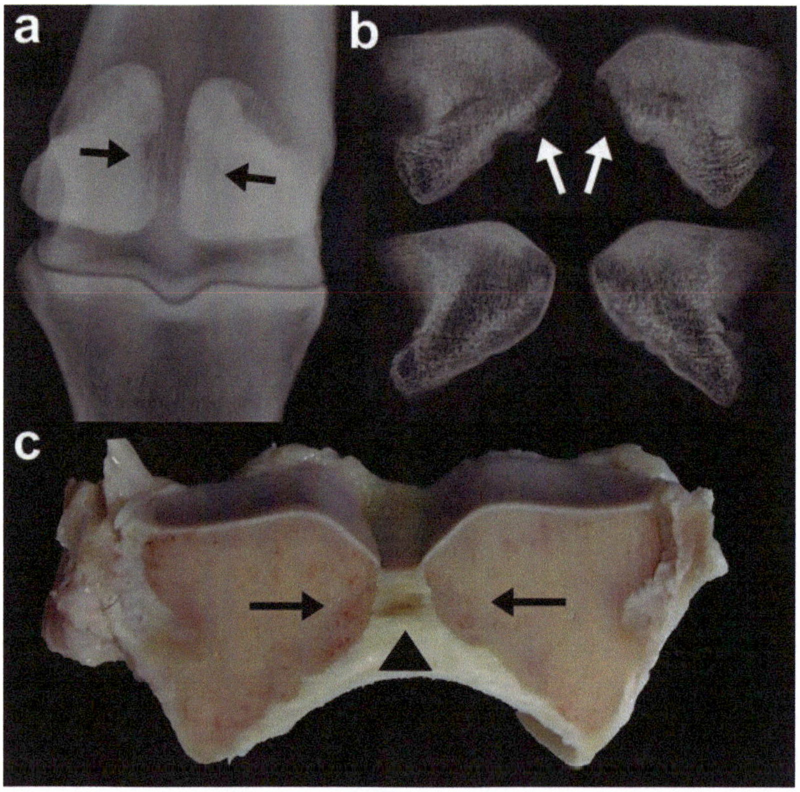


**Figure 10.30.** Biaxial mycotic intersesamoidean enthesitis and sesamoid osteomyelitis in a horse with severe chronic right forelimb lameness due to septic fetlock arthritis nonresponsive to systemic and intra-articular antimicrobials. (a) Fetlock joint: antemortem. Biaxial radiolucencies involve the medial and lateral proximal sesamoid bones (arrows). (b) Postmortem radiographs of disarticulated, transverse sections of the affected right (b, upper) and normal left (b, lower) sesamoid bones highlight the biaxial radiolucencies (arrows) identified in (a). (c) Gross photo of this section shows a discrete green-yellow focus within the intersesamoidean ligament (arrowhead) surrounded by hyperemic bone (arrows).

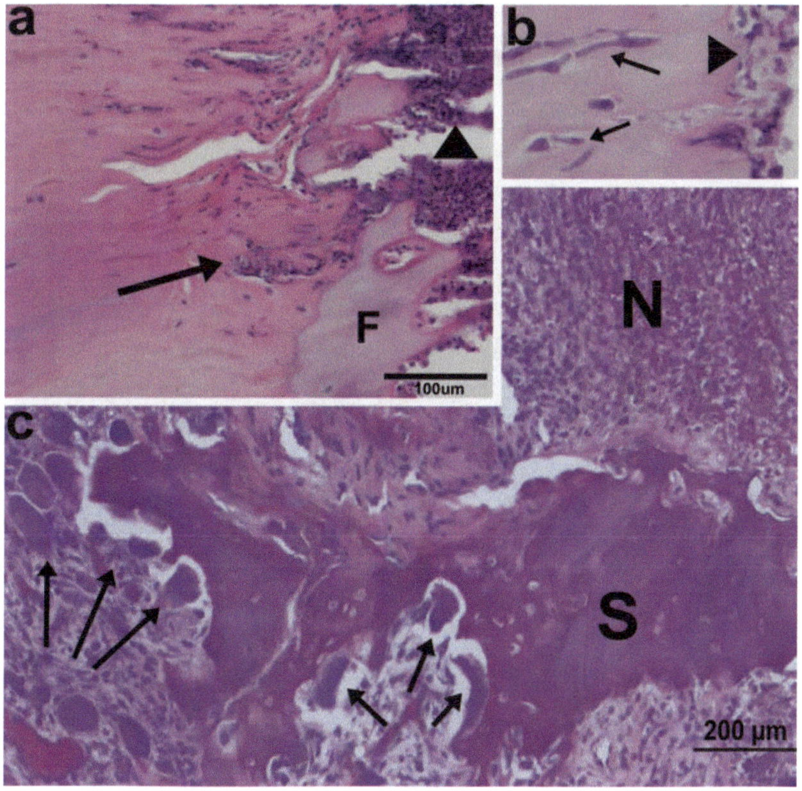


**Figure 10.31.** Horse. Photomicrographs (H&E) of mycotic intersesamoidean desmitis and biaxial sesamoid osteomyelitis (Figure 10.30). *Mucor* sp. fungi were isolated from cultures of synovial fluid; bacteria cultures were negative. (a) Suppurative inflammation (arrow; arrowhead) dissects between collagen fibers of the intersesamoidean ligament and separates avulsion fragments (F) from the axial aspects of the sesamoid bones. (b) Higher magnification of the intersesamoidean ligament reveals septated and branching fungal hyphae (arrow) adjacent to suppurative inflammation (arrowhead). (c) Avulsed bony sequestra (S) are surrounded by neutrophils (N) and partially rimmed by multinucleate osteoclasts within Howship lacunae (arrows).

### 4. *Surgical implant-associated osteomyelitis*

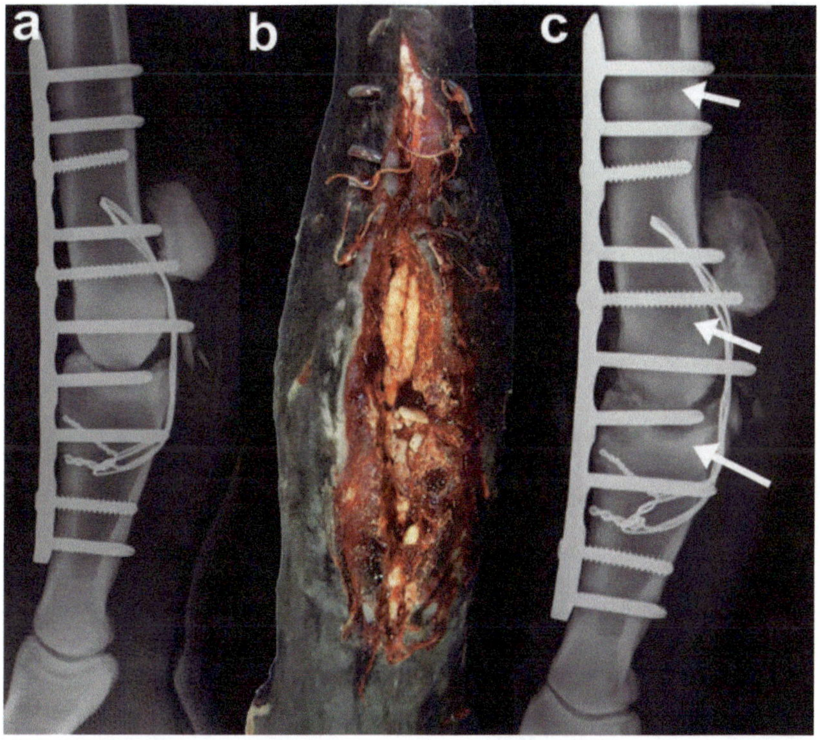


**Figure 10.32.** Fetlock arthrodesis with postsurgical implant infection in a Thoroughbred racehorse with a breakdown injury. (a) Immediate postoperative radiographs show successful surgery. However, within a few days the horse developed significant lameness and cellulitis with dehiscence of the surgical incision. (b) Suspected surgical implant infection was treated with regional and systemic intravenous antimicrobials and placement of antimicrobial impregnated polymethyl methacrolate beads into the wound. (c) Sequential postoperative radiographs revealed progressive osteolysis of the bone surrounding the proximal screw as well as the joint (arrows). The plate was removed but the horse was euthanized a few days later due to intractable pain and poor prognosis.

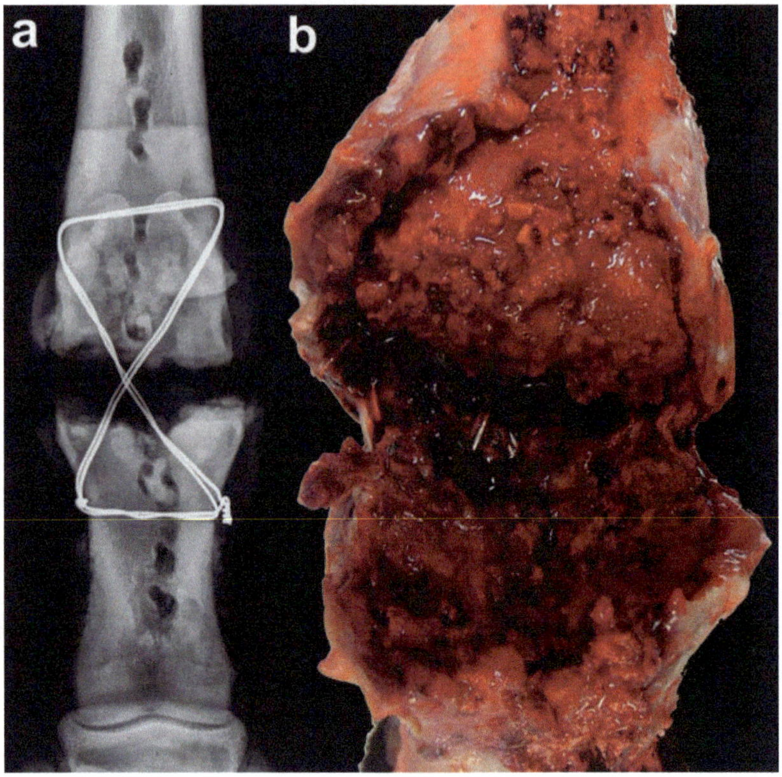


**Figure 10.33.** Horse. Chronic osteomyelitis with progressive osteolysis from a postsurgical implant infection. (a) A postmortem radiograph of the distal limb (Figure 10.32) demonstrates severe osteolysis of the bone surrounding the fetlock joint and a cuff of periosteal new bone along the proximal phalanx. (b) Gross inspection of the fetlock joint reveals lytic bone covered by a thick bed of granulation tissue. Postsurgical implant infection is a serious complication of orthopedic surgery and is predisposed by trauma to the soft tissues sustained at the time of the injury that often compromises the vascular supply and introduces contaminated foreign material.

### *5. Nonseptic (autoinflammatory) arthritis*

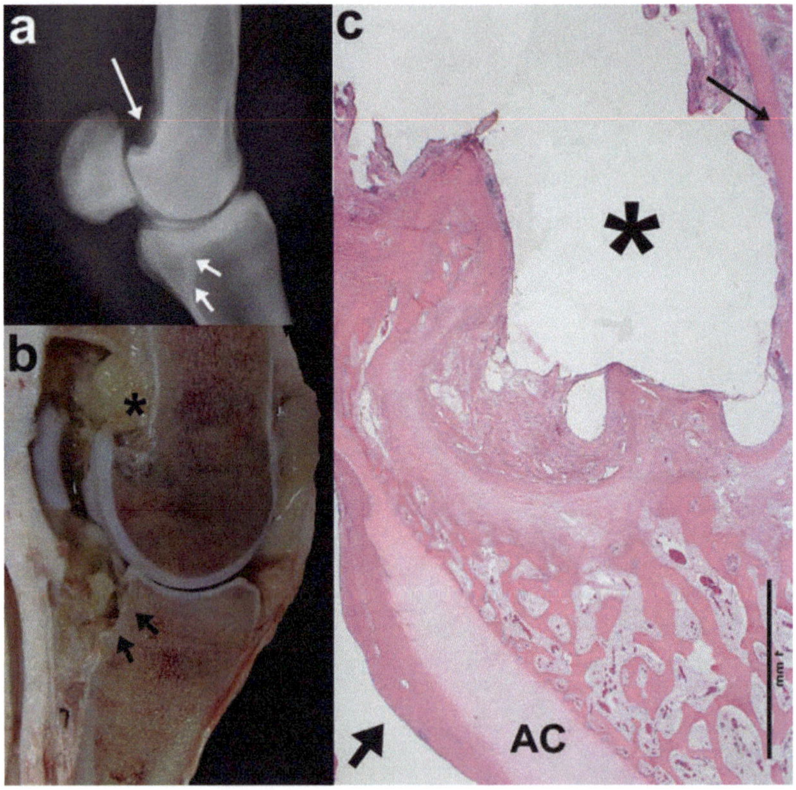


**Figure 10.34.** Idiopathic, nonsuppurative, erosive, and deforming arthritis in a yearling Thoroughbred colt. There was a history of a wound over the fetlock 6 months prior to developing sudden severe effusion in the right front fetlock joint. The horse was sound at the walk and trot. (a) Radiographs reveal massive joint swelling with osteolysis of the palmar aspects of distal MCIII and proximal P1 (arrows). (b) There is severe hyperplasia of the synovium (asterisk) and deforming osteolysis (arrows). (c) Histopathology (H&E) shows margins of articular cartilage (AC) coated by pannus (thick arrow). Cyst-like invaginations of the synovium extend into palmar periarticular margins of bone (asterisk) with subsequent cortical thinning (thin arrows).

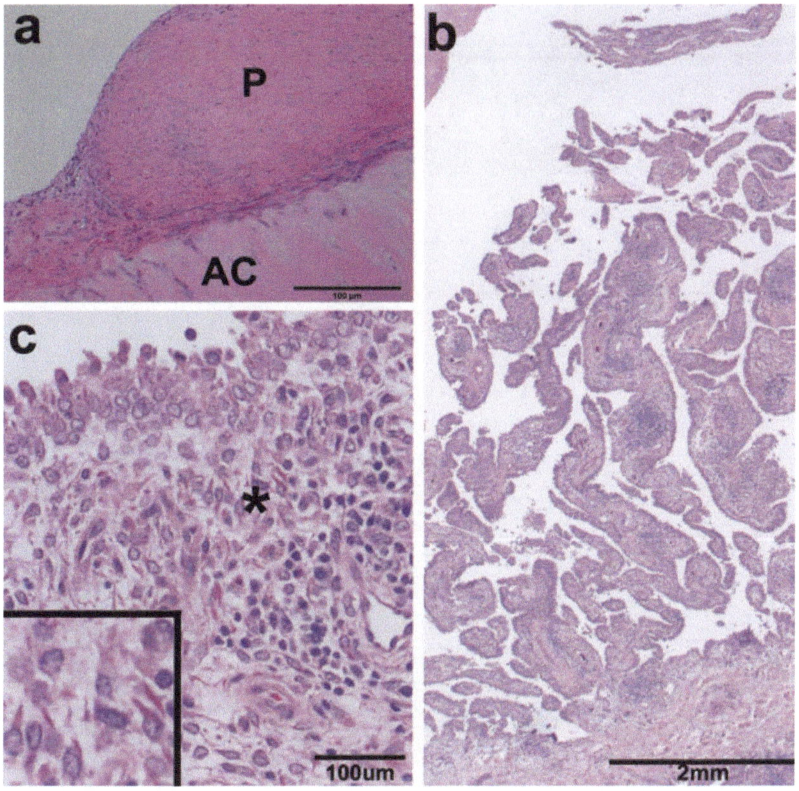


**Figure 10.35.** Horse. Higher magnification H&E photomicrographs of Figure 10.34.c. (a) The pannus (P), composed of a thick layer of dense fibrovascular connective tissue, extends into the superficial layers of articular cartilage (AC) that shows features of degeneration, including matrix hypereosinophilia and chondrocyte depletion. (b) The synovium is inflamed and demonstrates villous hypertrophy. (c) The synovial membrane is lined by multiple layers of plump synoviocytes and the subsynovial stroma is infiltrated by lymphocytes, plasma cells, and macrophages, many of which contain needle-like eosinophilic crystals (asterisk and inset). The origin or composition of the crystals was not identified. The lesion is presumped to represent a nonseptic (autoinflammatory) process.

## IV. Idiopathic, ischemic/vascular-associated lesions and laminitis

### *1. Osteonecrosis*

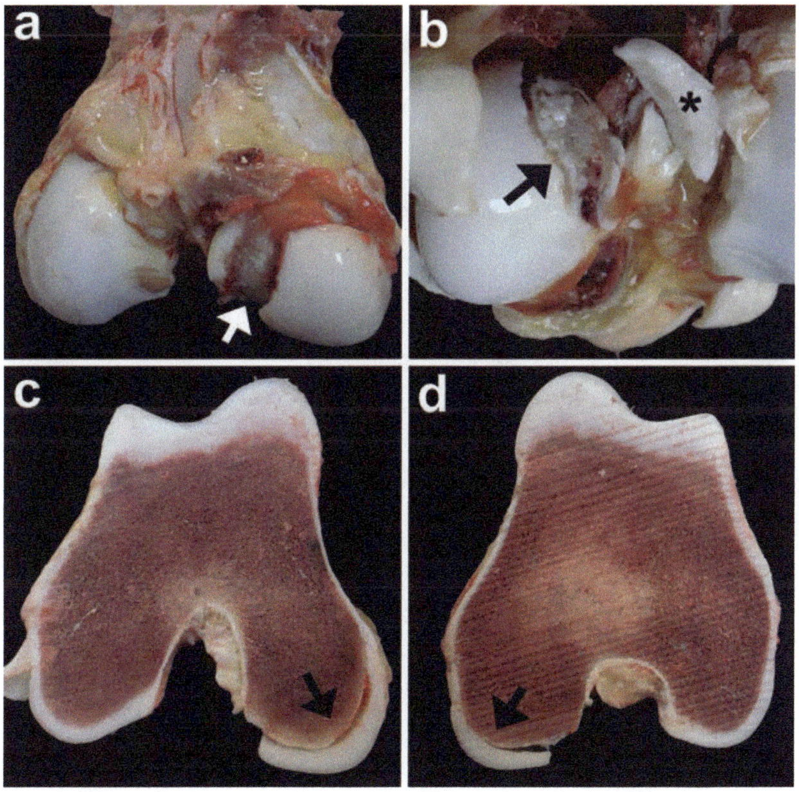


**Figure 10.36.** Bilateral osteonecrosis (avascular necrosis) of the medial femoral condyles from a foal with stifle effusion and hind end lameness. (a, b) Gross photos of the caudal aspects of the distal femurs reveal large fissures within the articular cartilage (a, white arrow; b, black arrow) with a free osteochondral fragment (b, asterisk). (c, d) Transverse sections through the distal femurs show dissecting cartilaginous flaps affecting both medial femoral condyles (arrows) with pallor of the subchondral bone (left more severely affected than the right).

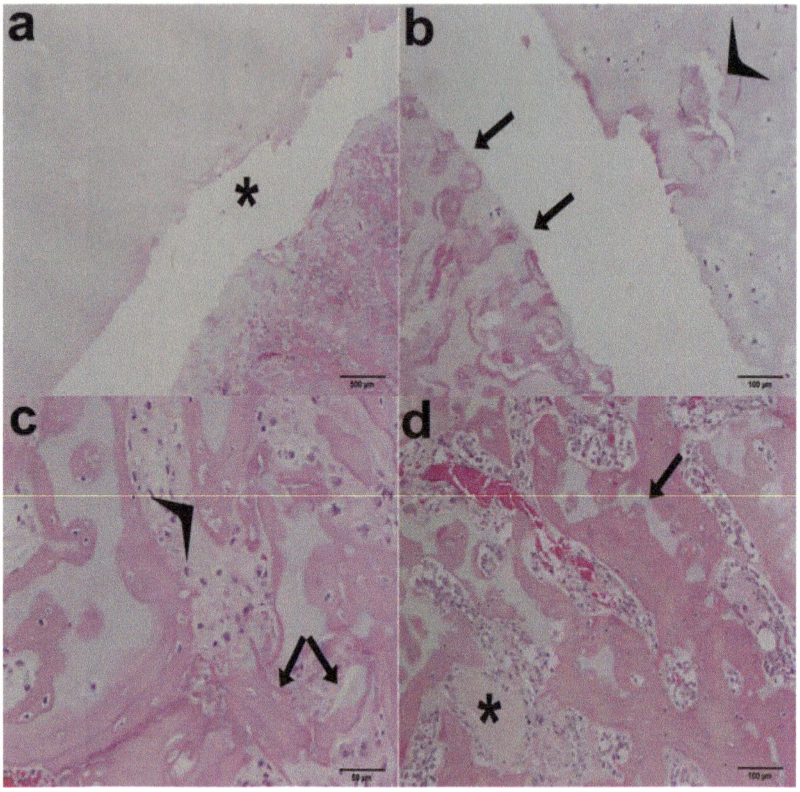


**Figure 10.37.** Horse. Bilateral (avascular) osteonecrosis of the medial femoral condyles. Photomicrographs (H&E) from the lesion in Figure 10.36c. (a) A large cleft (asterisk) dissects across the epiphyseal growth plate. (b) Higher magnification shows necrotic medullary spaces between fractured primary trabeculae (arrows) and a necrotic vascular canal within the overlying cartilage (arrowhead). (c) Recent necrosis and infractions within the superficial regions of subchondral bone evidenced by lacunae devoid of osteocyte nuclei (arrowhead), medullary spaces devoid of capillaries, and skewed orientation of fragments of primary trabeculae (arrows). (d) Deeper ("recovered") regions of subchondral bone contain few viable medullary blood vessels and new layers of woven bone deposited on necrotic primary trabeculae (arrow). Note, a single necrotic blood vessel persists in this region (asterisk).

## *2. Enostosis-like lesions*

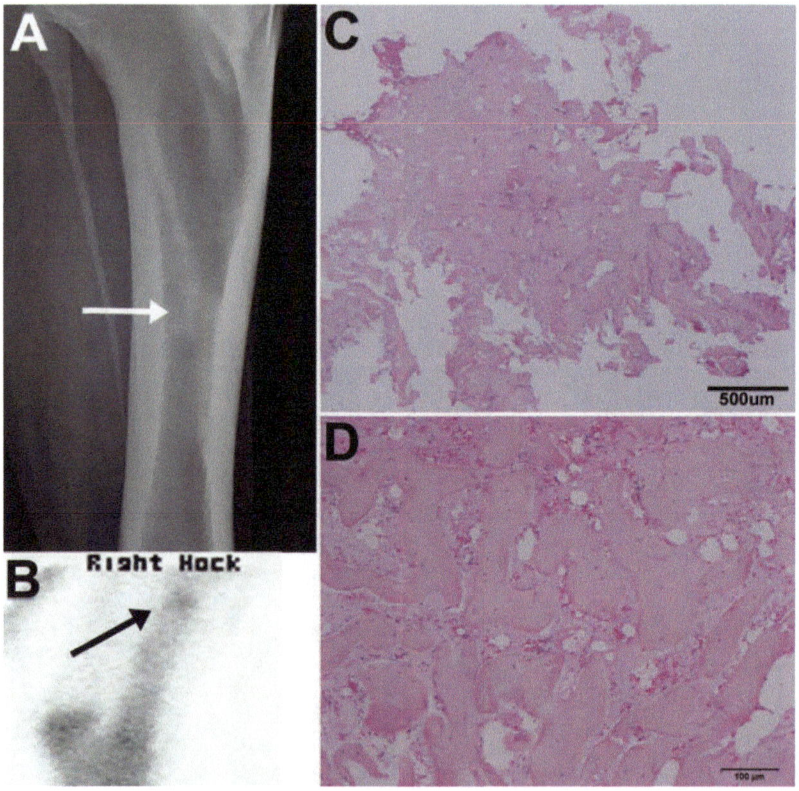


**Figure 10.38.** Enostosis-like lesion in the tibia of a horse with chronic intermittent, mild to severe, hind limb lameness. (a) Digital radiograph of the tibia shows a well-defined radiopacity within the medullary cavity of the mid-diaphysis (arrow). (b) Nuclear scintigraphic scan shows focal increased radioisotope uptake within a region that corresponds to the radiopacity, consistent with active bone remodeling (arrow). (c, d) Photomicrographs of H&E-stained sections from a Tru-Cut biopsy specimen show sclerotic islands of woven bone trabeculae containing small amounts of intervening fibrovascular tissue. Although the cause for this lesion was not determined, potential etiologies include an infarct of the medullary compartment.

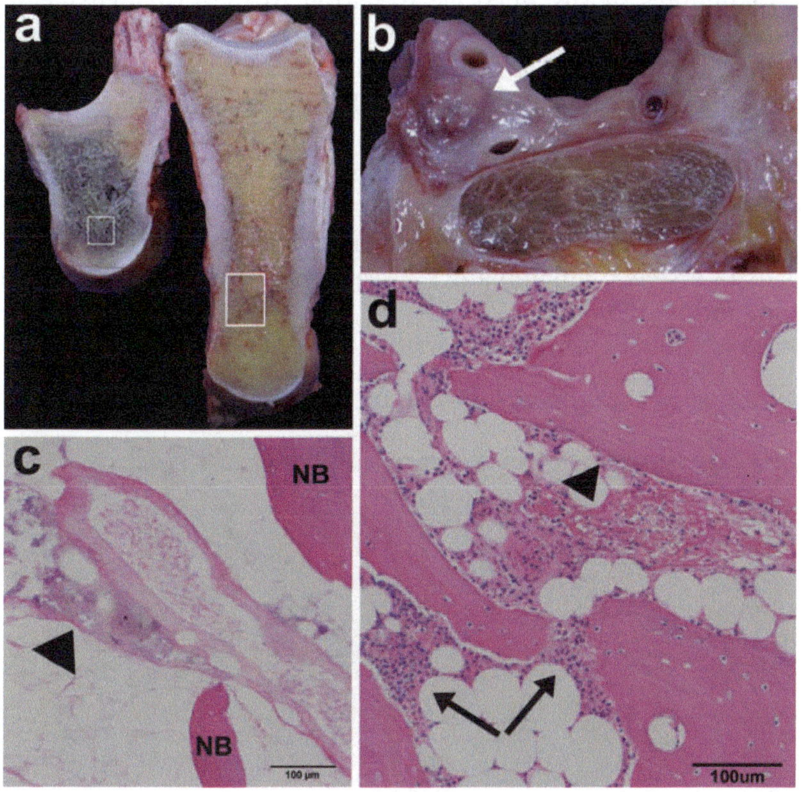


Figure 10.39. Gangrenous distal limb necrosis in an adult mare with chronic laminitis and subsolar abscess that resulted in ascending digital thrombophlebitis (a) Gangrenous necrosis of P2 (left) evidenced by green-gray discoloration of the medullary cavity, as compared with P1 (right). (b) The lumen and wall of the lateral digital vein is effaced by a thrombus (arrow). (c, d) H&E photomicrographs of the framed regions of P2 (a,left; c) and P1 (a, right;d) show spicules of necrotic bone (NB) and advanced autolysis of medullary spaces with proliferations of large bacilli (arrowhead), consistent with dry gangrene. (d) Within P1, are foci of acute necrosis with fibrin deposition (arrowhead) and suppurative inflammation (arrows), corresponding to grossly hyperemic foci, and consistent with embolic osteomyelitis.

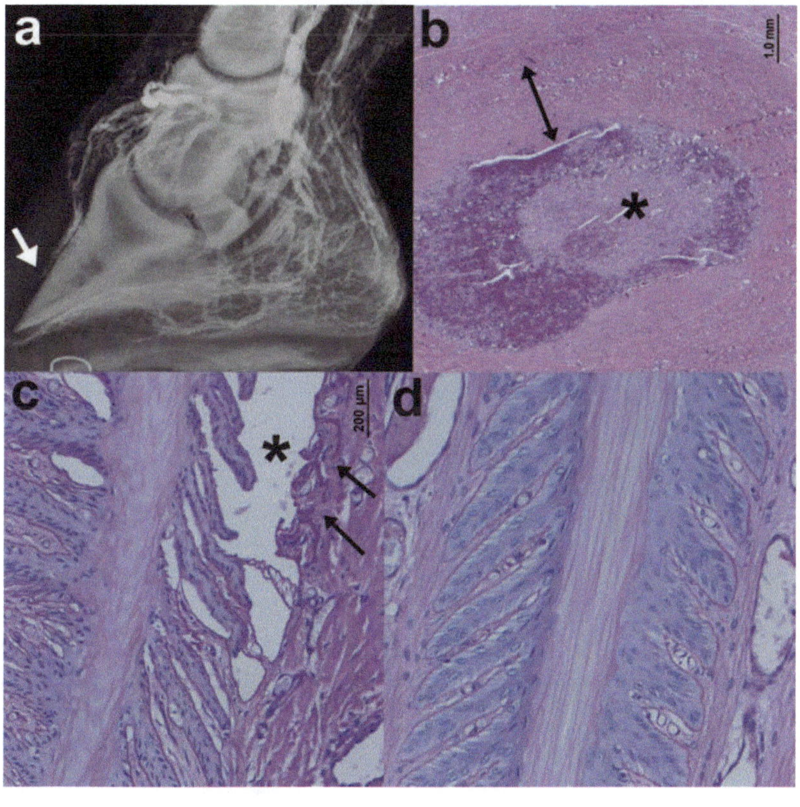


Figure 10.40. Peracute, developmental equine laminitis. (a) Contrast venogram shows loss of contrast dye along the sublamellar corium (arrow). (b) H&E photomicrograph of the medial digital artery shows an organized thrombus (asterisk) and a thickened, sclerotic wall (double-headed arrow) composed of proliferating smooth muscle cells and myofibroblasts. (c, d) PAS-stained photomicrographs reveal acute necrosis of secondary epidermal lamellae (SELs) with early basement membrane separation (c, asterisk). Contorted remnants of basement membrane persist within the dermal lamellae (c, arrows). (d) Comparison is made with normal lamellae from the contralateral limb.

Two weeks prior, the horse became entangled in an electric wire fence resulting in 15 minutes of sustained electrocution to the proximal metatarsus. Clinical signs of laminitis (e.g., bounding digital pulses, shifting limb lameness) were not observed prior to euthanasia, consistent with the developmental, "clinically silent" stages of laminitis. The electrocution injury resulted in a progressive, sclerosing vascuolopathy causing distal limb ischemia with unilateral laminitis (the contralateral lamellae were histologically normal). Although the inciting cause (electrocution) in this case of laminitis is unusual, the lamellar histologic changes are similar to acute laminitis from other etiologies (e.g., systemic inflammatory disease, supporting limb overload, carbohydrate-induced laminitis).

### 4. *Laminitis and laminitis-associated distal phalangeal osteolysis*

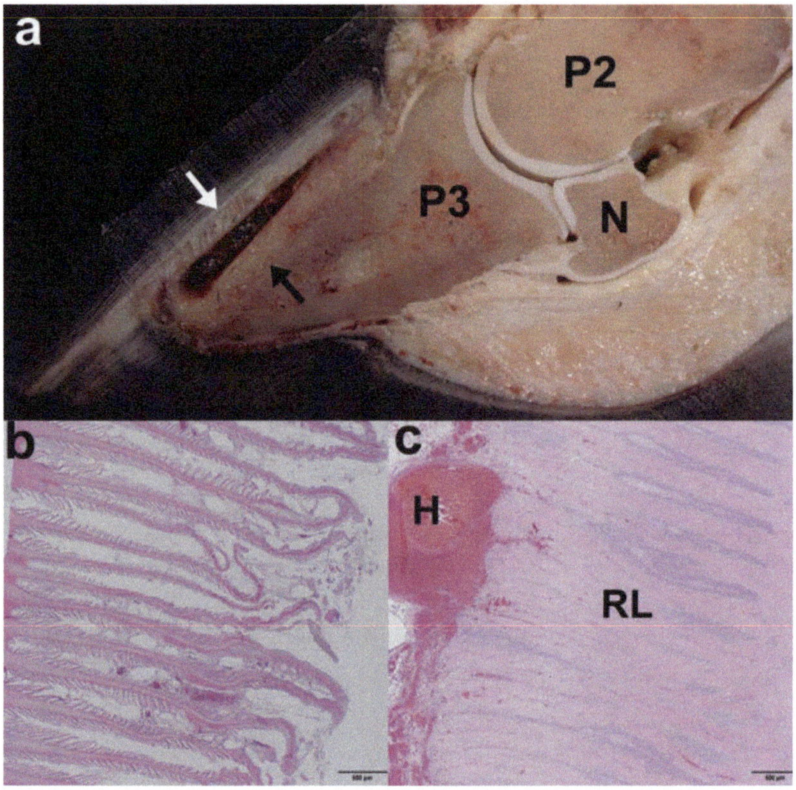


**Figure 10.41.** (a) Severe acute laminitis with separation (arrows), ventral rotation, and sinking of the distal phalanx in a horse with systemic inflammatory disease (colitis with pulmonary thromboemboli). Middle phalanx (P2), distal phalanx (P3), and navicular bone (N) are labeled for orientation. (b,c) H&E photomicrographs corresponding to tissue demarcated by the white and black arrows (a), respectively. (b) Primary and secondary epidermal lamellae are completely separated from the underlying corium. (c) A large hematoma (H) corresponds to hemorrhage accumulated within the region of hoof wall separation (a, arrows); regenerating (dysplastic) lamellae (RL) can be seen in the corium.

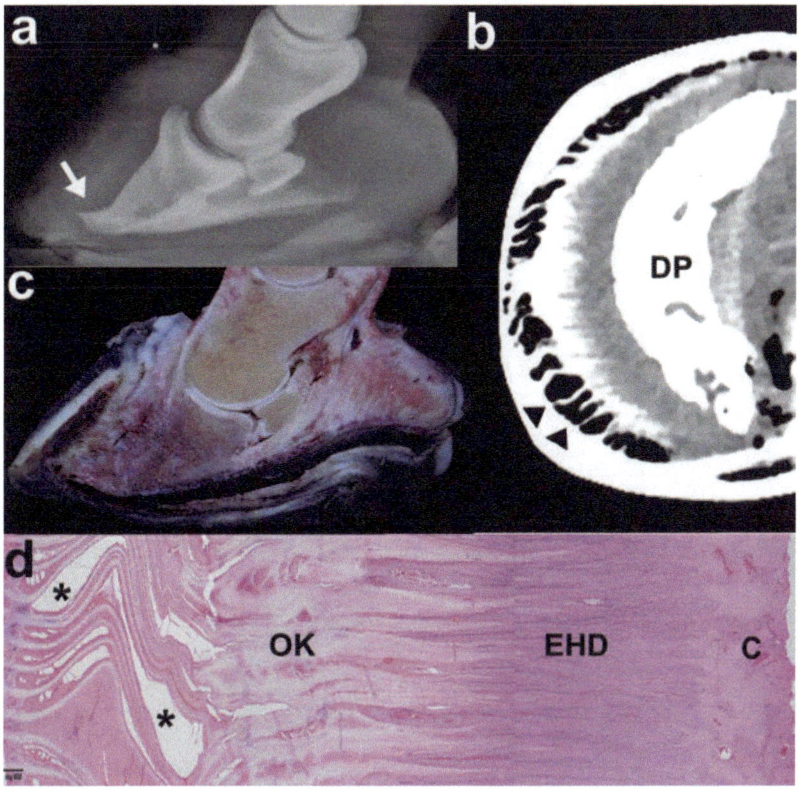


**Figure 10.42.** Chronic-recurrent laminitis with lamellar wedge formation in a mare with a functional pituitary adenoma. (a) Digital radiograph of one forefoot shows severe ventral rotation and sinking of the distal phalanx with P3 remodeling and fracture of the solar margin (arrow). (b) Computed tomographic (CT) transverse images of the distal foot show lamellar separation with serum accumulation (arrowheads) and aberrant lamellar proliferation dorsal to the distal phalanx (DP). (c) Sagittal section gross photo of the foot shows the abnormal hoof-lamellar configuration with lamellar wedge formation and purple-red discoloration of the distal phalanx. (d) Composite photomicrograph (H&E) shows abaxial (outer) separation with clefting (asterisks) and serum accumulation, orthokeratotic hyperkeratosis (OK) and epidermal lamellar hyperplasia/dysplasia (EHD) with underlying corium (C), all of which comprise the lamellar wedge.

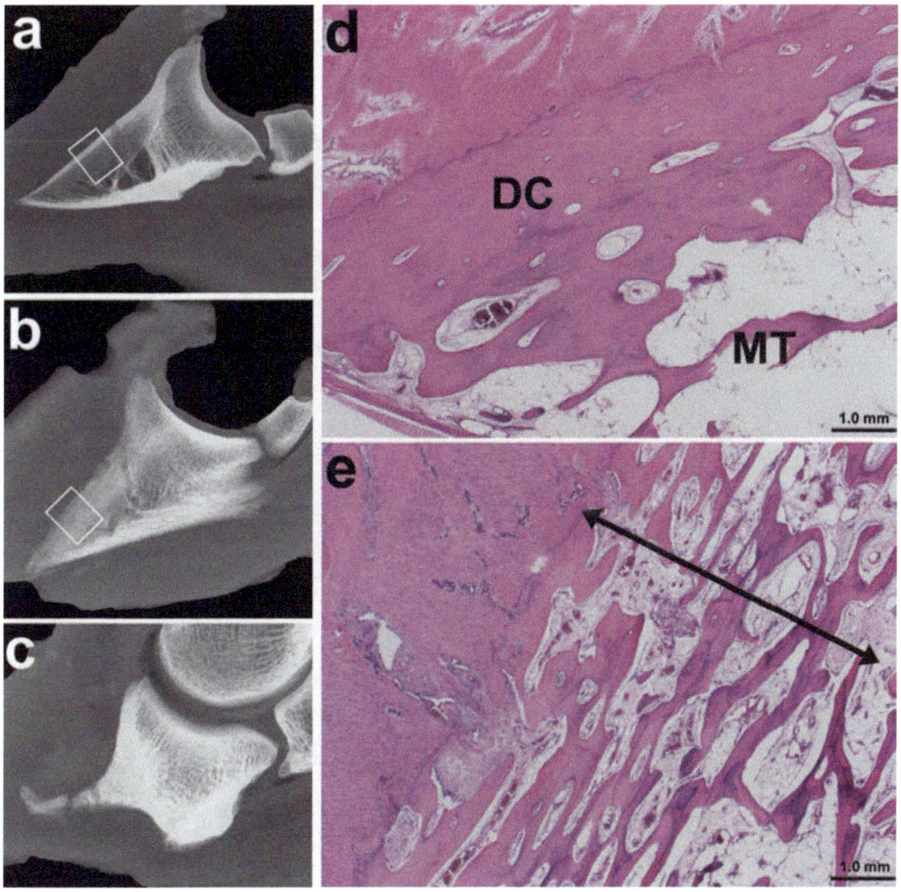


**Figure 10.43.** Distal phalangeal pathology associated with equine laminitis. Digital radiographs of 1-cm-thick sagittal sections from (a) a nonlaminitic foot, (b) a laminitic foot (1-month duration) due to contralateral limb lameness (i.e., supporting limb laminitis), and (c) a laminitic foot (10-year duration) initially due to grain-overload–induced colitis. The panel shows progressive remodeling of the compact and trabecular bone (b, c) with deforming osteolysis and solar margin fractures (c). H&E photomicrographs of (d,e) of the region of bone framed in panels a and b. The nonlaminitic foot has a well-defined dorsal cortex of lamellar compact bone (d, DC) with medullary trabeculae (MT) interspersed by medullary spaces composed of adipocytes and blood vessels; inflammation is not a feature. (e) In contrast, the laminitic foot shows dorsal cortical bone loss and increased porosity that merge into medullary trabeculae (double-headed arrows). The medullary spaces are edematous and hyperemic with increased vascular profiles.

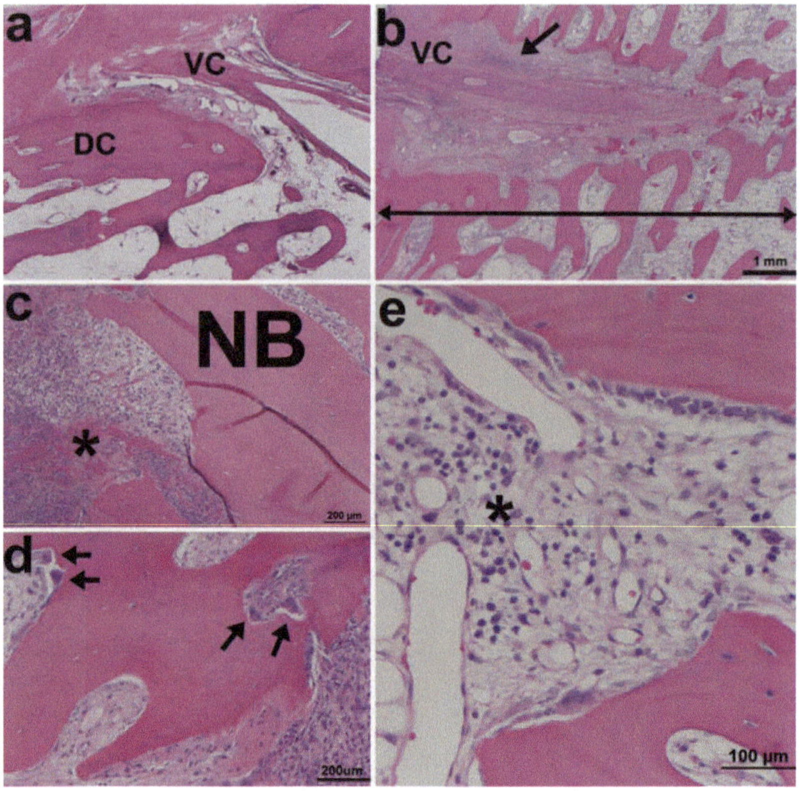


**Figure 10.44.** Laminitis-associated distal phalangeal osteopathology. Photomicrographs of H&E-stained sections from a nonlaminitic horse (a), and laminitic horses (b–e) showing the normal dorsal cortex (a, DC) and perforating vascular canal (a, VC) compared with the laminitic horse that shows dorsal cortical bone loss and trabeculation (b, double arrowhead) with perivascular fibrosis and inflammation (b, arrow) of the vascular canal and medullary spaces. Higher magnification shows necrotic bone trabeculae (c, NB) with fibrin (c, asterisk) and inflammation of the medullary spaces, and osteoclastic osteolysis (d, arrows). (e) Increased vascular profiles with predominantly mononuclear inflammatory cells (asterisk) infiltrate and replace normal medullary fibroadipose tissue.

## V. Degenerative lesions

### *1. Degenerative osteoarthritis/degenerative joint disease*

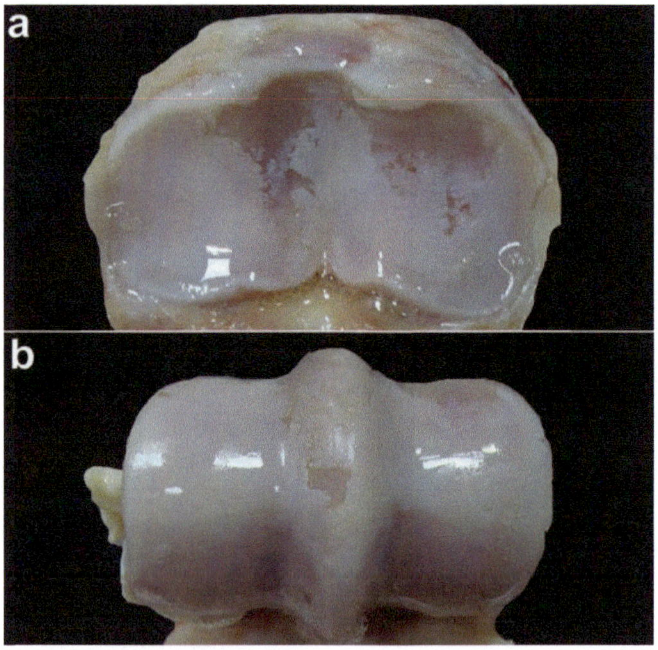


**Figure 10.45.** Moderate degenerative osteoarthritis of the metacarpophalangeal (fetlock) joint from a Thoroughbred racehorse. There is cartilage thinning (atrophy) and ulceration involving (a) the articular surfaces of proximal P1, (b) the midsagittal ridge and dorsal aspect of the condyles of the distal third metacarpus. Mild osteophyte proliferation is observed along the dorsal articular margin of proximal P1 in (a).

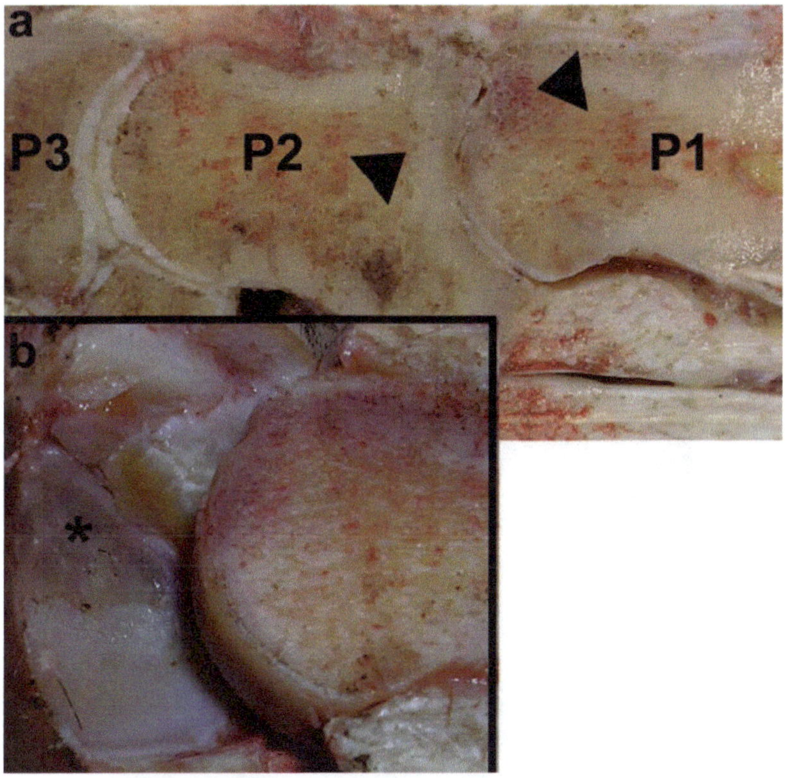


**Figure 10.46.** Severe degenerative osteoarthritis of the proximal interphalangeal (pastern) joint from a pleasure horse. (a) Degenerative changes include ulceration and loss of articular cartilage with bone-on-bone contact between the proximal (P1) and middle (P2) phalanges. Subchondral bone remodeling is evident by hyperemia of distal P1 (right arrowhead) and sclerosis of proximal P2 (left arrowhead). (b) Disarticulation reveals the focal cartilage ulcer concentrated along the dorsal aspect of the joint (asterisk).

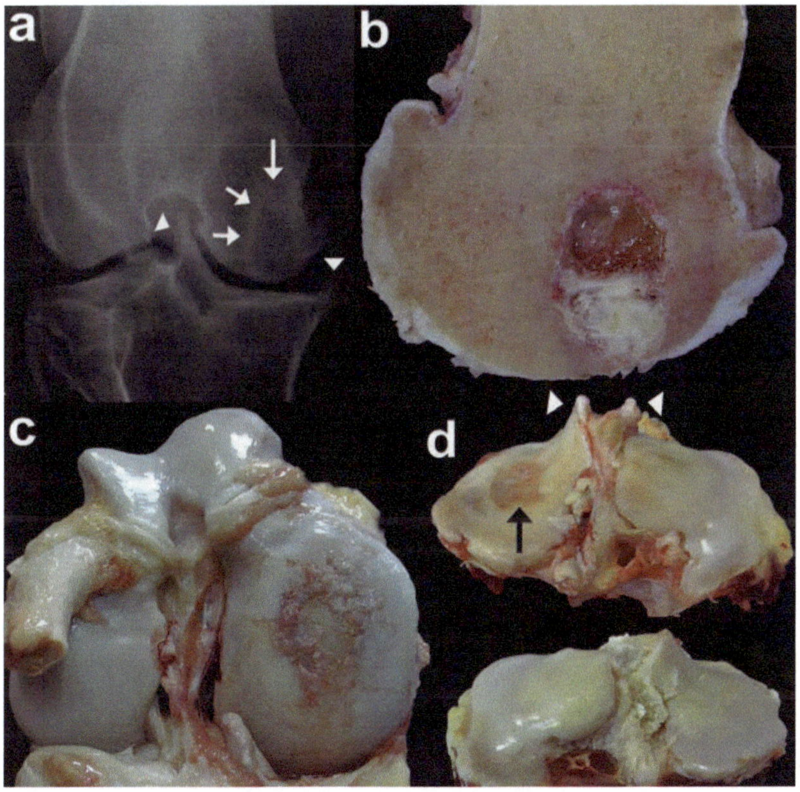


**Figure 10.47.** Horse. (a) Digital radiograph shows a large well-demarcated oval radiolucency circumscribed by a radiopaque (sclerotic) rim of bone within the medial femoral condyle (arrows). Reduced joint space and large osteophytes (arrowheads) of the intercondylar eminence and medial proximal tibia are present. (b) Sagittal sections from the medial femoral condyle show a large osseous cyst-like lesion filled with gelatinous mesenchyme extending from the articular surface into the deep subchondral bone. (c) A large ulcer is within articular surface of the medial femoral condyle, (d) and surface of the medial tibial condyle (arrow). (d) Large osteophytes extend from the intercondylar eminence and medial margin of the proximal tibia (arrowheads). Comparisons can be made with the contralateral (normal) tibia below.

Subchondral bone cyst of the medial femoral condyle with severe chronic degenerative osteoarthritis in a sport horse (Fig. 10.47). These lesions can be congenital or may result from a full-thickness defect through the articular cartilage into the subchondral bone. Indications of the later consistent with severe, chronic, degenerative osteoarthritis, include reduced joint space and osteophytosis. The cause of the arthritis may be associated with a medial meniscal tear creating joint instability (Fig. 10.48).

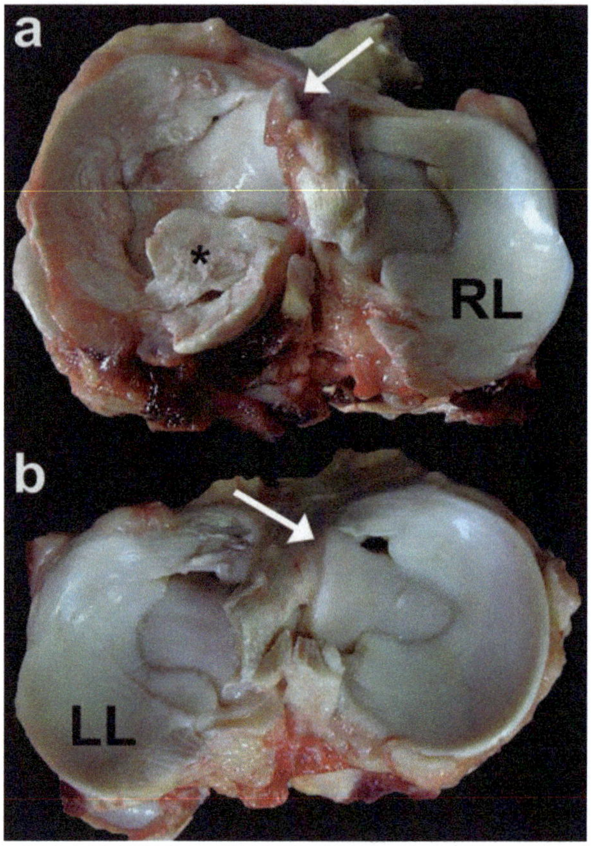


**Figure 10.48.** (a) Medial meniscal tear in the right femorotibial joint from the same sport horse shown in Figure 10.47. Frayed ligament fibers surround a large flap-like tear within the medial meniscus (asterisk). (b) The degenerative changes (arrow) in the right medial meniscus are compared with the right lateral meniscus (RL) and both medial (arrow) and lateral (LL) menisci of the contralateral (left) femorotibial joint.

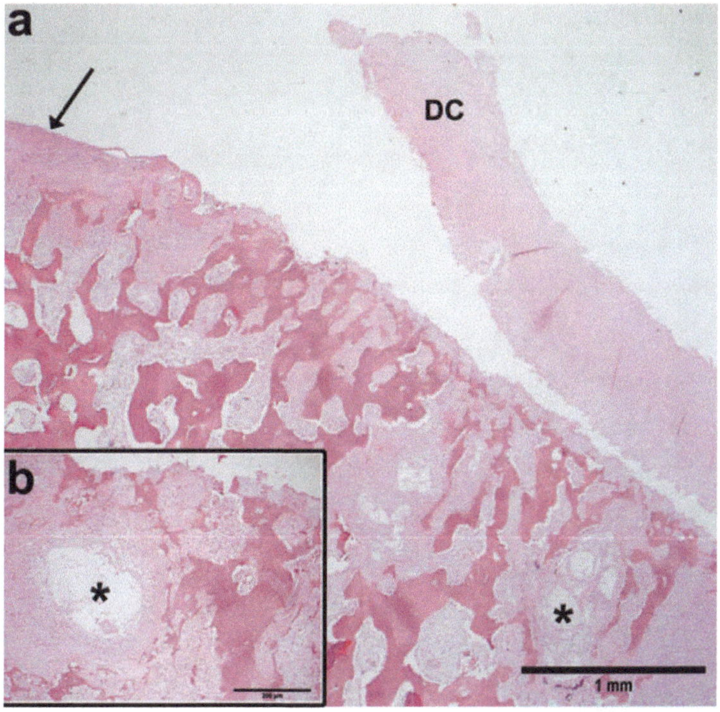


**Figure 10.49.** Degenerative osteoarthritis secondary to OCD of the glenohumeral joint. Low (a) and high (b) magnification H&E photomicrographs of the humeral head from the horse in Figure 10.8d. A flap of cartilage (a, DC) dissects from the underlying articular-epiphyseal complex. There is ulceration of the adjacent articular cartilage with exposure of the subchondral bone interface, which is coated by a fibrinous to fibrous membrane (a, arrow). Proliferating spindle cells embedded in a myxoid to loose collagenous extracellular matrix fill subchondral medullary spaces, and there is formation of cyst-like structures (e.g., subchondral bone cysts) (a, b, asterisk).

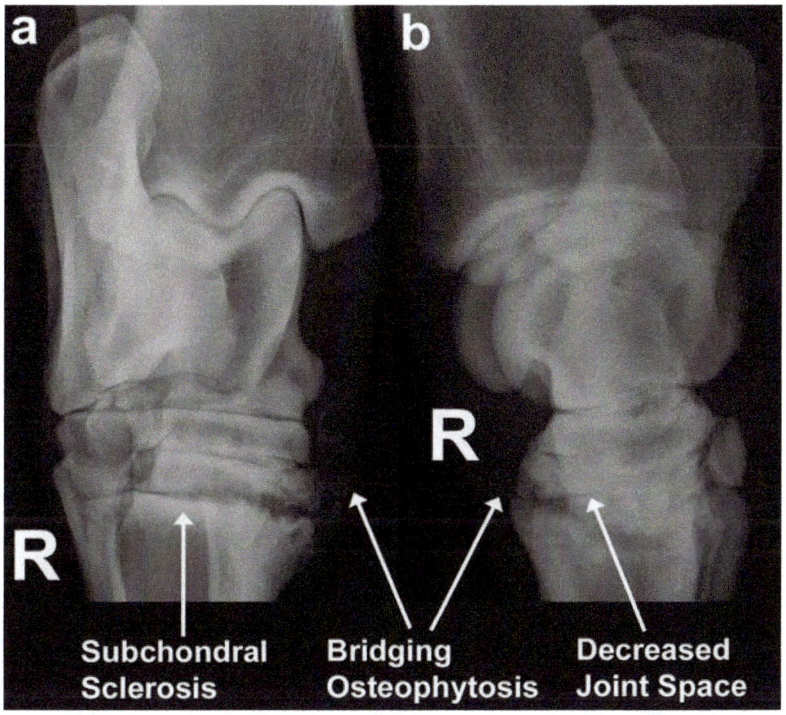


**Figure 10.50.** Bridging ankylosis of the metatarsophalangeal joint in the hock of a horse with chronic septic arthritis from an iatrogenically induced infection. (a) Oblique lateral and (b) medial digital radiographic projections show end-stage degenerative changes with bridging osteophytes and "self-fusion" of the joint (arrows). Other chronic degenerative features include subchondral sclerosis and decreased joint space due to articular cartilage loss.

## 2. Navicular disease

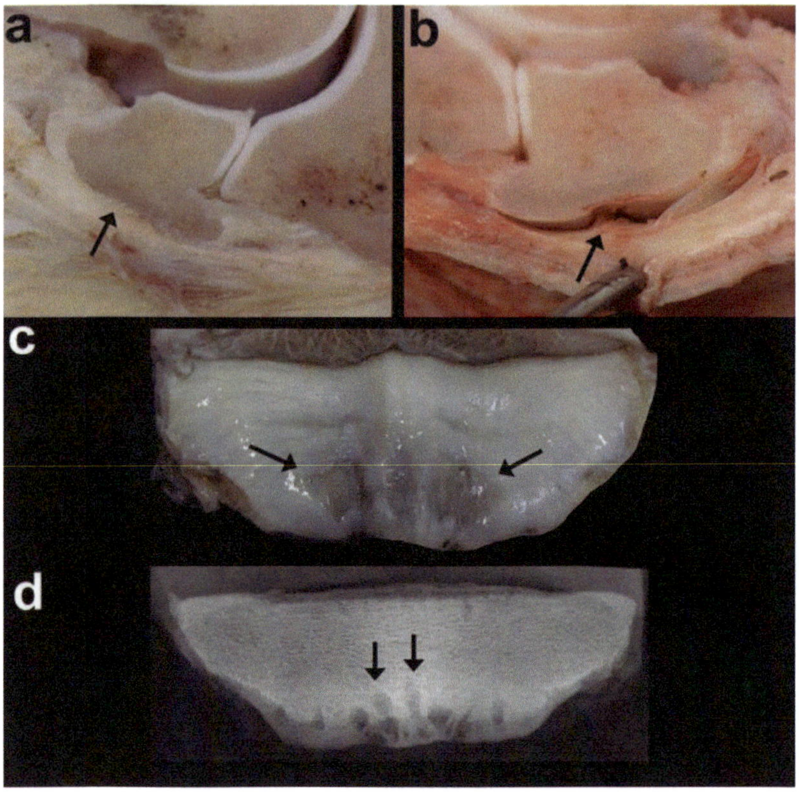


**Figure 10.51.** Navicular disease in a pleasure horse. (a) Gross photographs show loss of the flexor surface (arrow), with (b) adhesions to the deep digital flexor tendon (arrow). (c) Isolation of the navicular bone shows discrete ulcers within the fibrocartilage (arrows). (d) "Lollipop" lesions (arrows) consistent with enlargement of the synovial fossae are characteristic radiographic indications of navicular disease. An osteophyte at the left margin of the bone is also present.

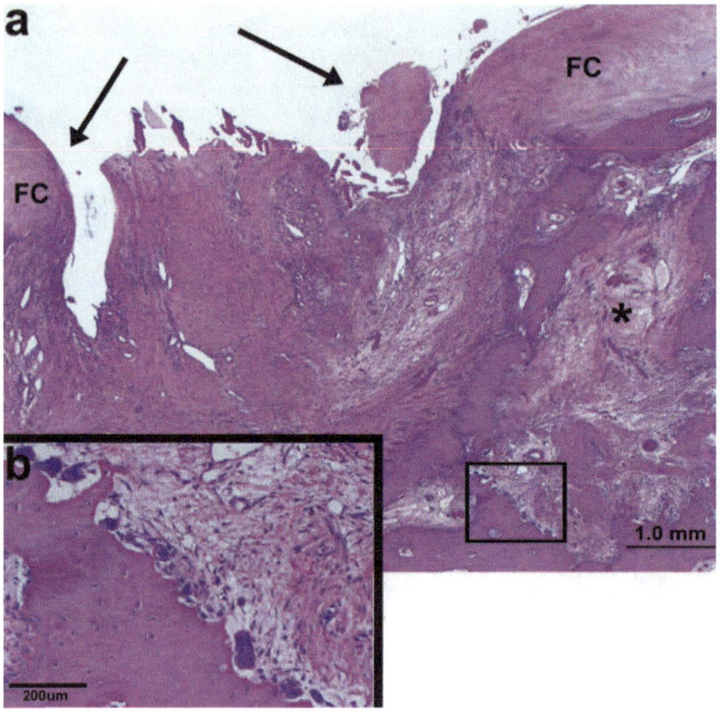


**Figure 10.52.** Horse. Navicular disease. (a) Low and (b) high magnification H&E photomicrographs corresponding to sagittal sections of the ulcerated regions of flexor surface fibrocartilage in Figure 10.51.c show focal fibrillation and ulceration (arrows) of the fibrocartilage (FC). There is lysis of subchondral bone (asterisk) and active osteoclastic osteolysis (frame). (b) Higher magnification of framed region reveals numerous multinucleate osteoclasts within Howship lacunae that line the surfaces of subchondral bone, indicative of active osteoclastic osteolysis.

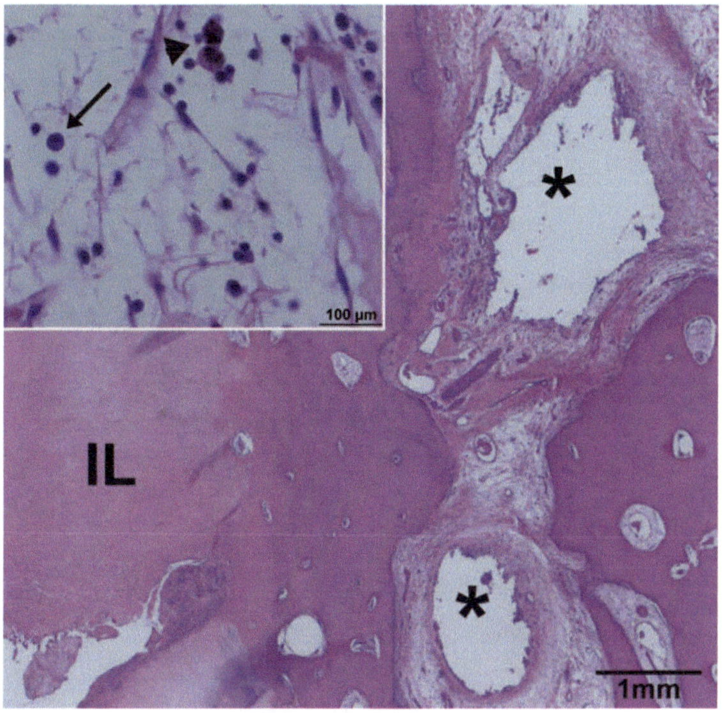


**Figure 10.53.** Horse. Navicular disease. Low and high (inset) magnification H&E photomicrographs of the distal margin of the navicular bone corresponding to enlarged synovial fossae depicted in Figure 10.51d. The bone proximal to the impar ligament (IL) shows large osseous cyst-like lesions lined by synovium (asterisks). The surrounding connective tissues (inset) contain inflammatory cells including plasma cells (arrow) and hemosiderophages (arrowhead) within a myxoid proliferation of spindle cells.

### 3. *Temporohyoid osteoarthropathy*

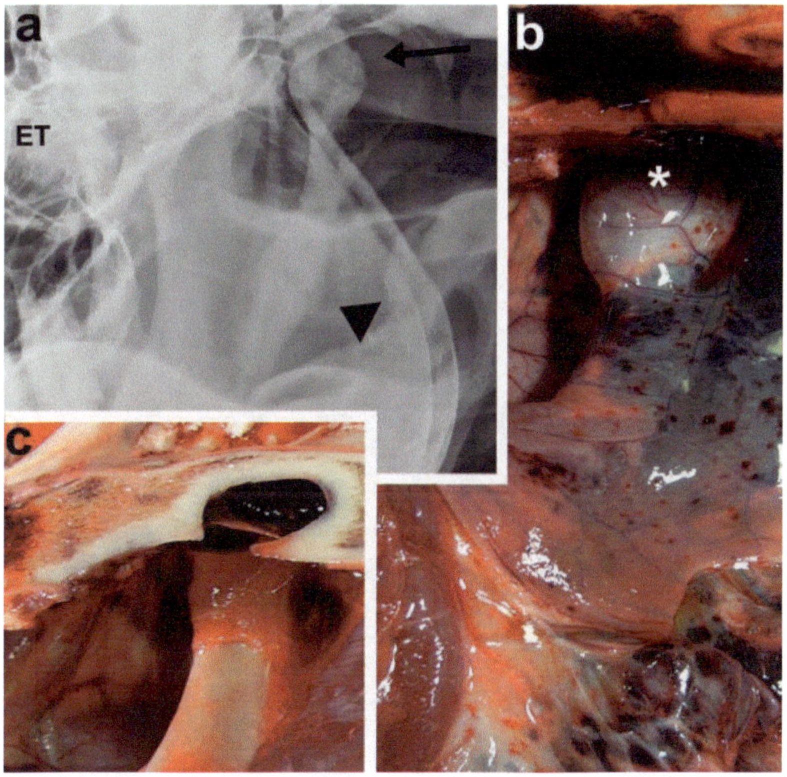


**Figure 10.54.** Temporohyoid osteoarthropathy in a horse that developed acute right-sided facial nerve paralysis and head tilt. (a) Oblique projection digital radiograph of the skull reveals chronic fractures of the proximal (arrow) and midbody (arrowhead) portions of the right stylohyoid bone with associated fracture calluses. Ethmoid turbinates (ET) are labeled for orientation. The articulation between the stylohyoid bone and osseous tympanic bulla was markedly enlarged with sclerosis of the tympanic bulla. (b) Gross photos taken at necropsy confirm the radiographic findings in the right stylohyoid bone (asterisk) as compared with (c) the unaffected left stylohyoid bone.

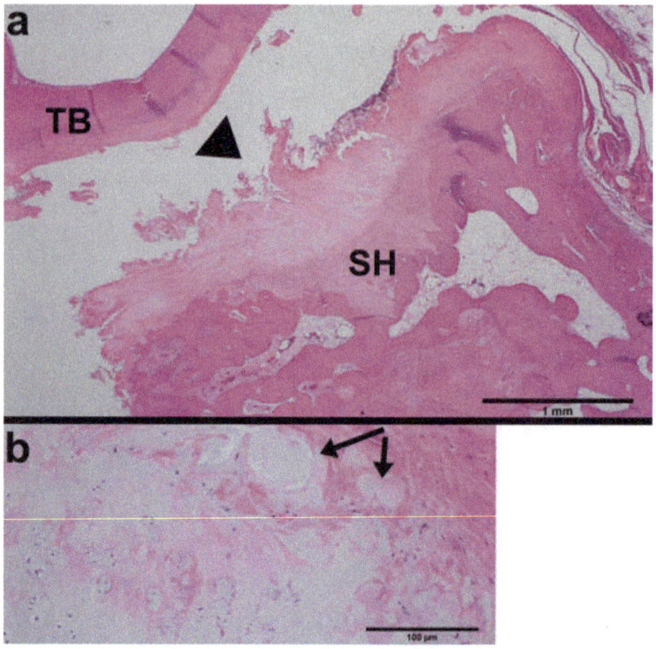


**Figure 10.55.** Temporohyoid osteoarthropathy: degenerative histologic changes. (a) Low and (b) high magnification H&E photomicrographs of the right temporohyoid joint from the horse in Figure 10.54 reveal matrix degeneration with fibrillation and fissures (arrowhead) of the articular cartilage of the stylohyoid bone (SH). Tympanic bulla (TB) of the petrous temporal bone is labeled for orientation. (b) Higher magnification of the cartilage shows loss of matrix staining and dropout of chondrocytes (arrows).

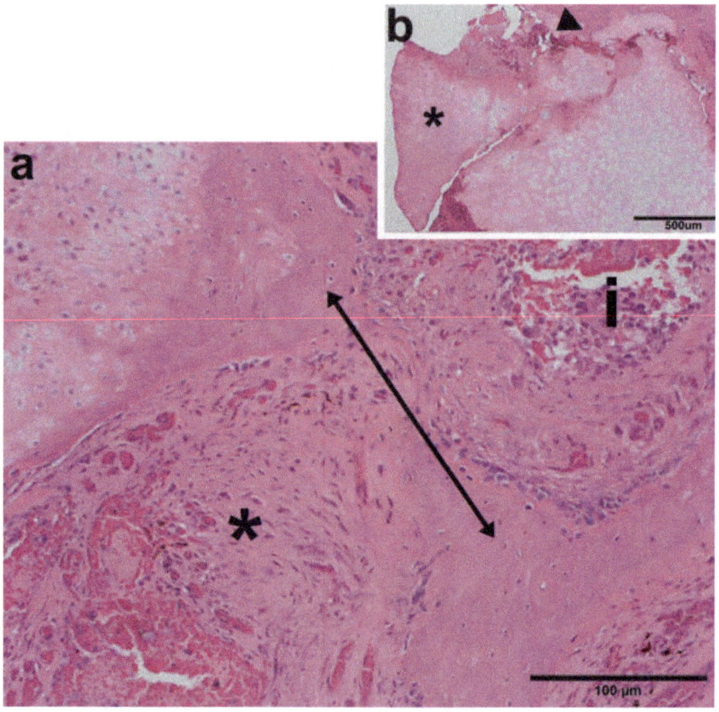


**Figure 10.56.** Horse. Temporohyoid osteoarthropathy with partial ankylosis and fracture of the articulation between the stylohyoid and temporal bones. (a) Low and (b) high magnification H&E photomicrographs of the right temporohyoid joint show the articulation is spanned by a proliferation of woven bone (double-headed arrow), and organizing fibrovascular connective tissue (asterisk). A pocket of fibrin with non-suppurative inflammatory cells (i) is adjacent to the fused portion. (b) High magnification inset shows fractured cartilage (asterisk) and acute hemorrhage (arrowhead).

### *4. Distal third metacarpal/metatarsal subchondral (maladaptive) bone disease*

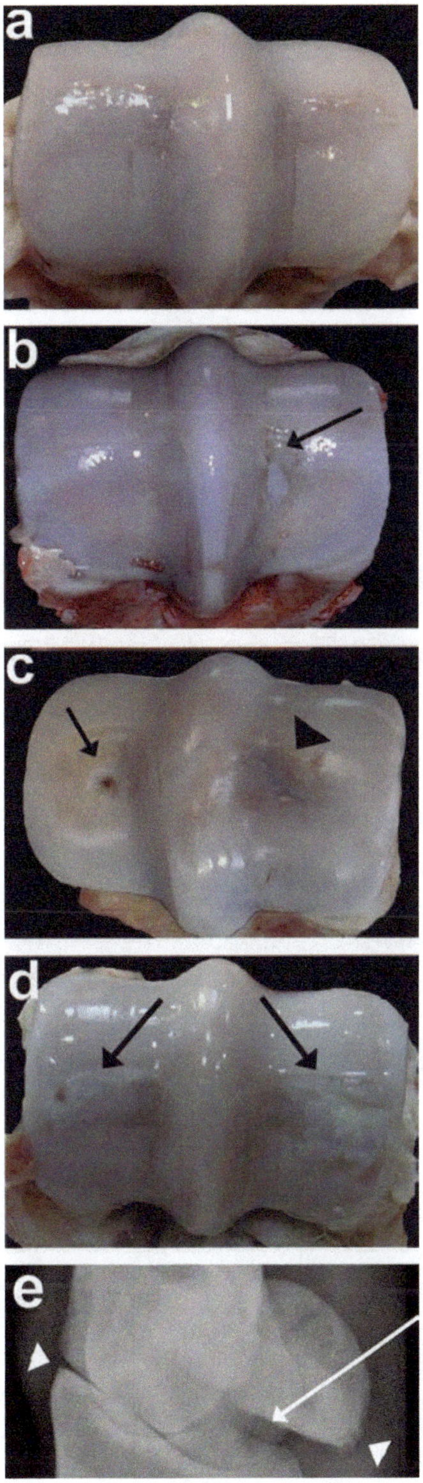


**Figure 10.57.** Subchondral (maladaptive) bone disease in racehorses. (a–c) Four gross photographs of the distal third metacarpus (MCIII) show progressive degenerative changes characterized by shallow cartilage depressions and parallel linear grooves within the medial and lateral condyles, adjacent to the midsagittal ridge (a). A linear cartilage fissure has developed axial to cartilage erosion within the lateral condyle (b, arrow). More severe pathology is demonstrated by a large wedge-shaped purple depression within the articular cartilage of the lateral condyle (c, arrowhead), consistent with subchondral bone bruising and mild collapse, and a punctate cartilage depression within the medial condyle (c, arrow), consistent with more severe subchondral bone collapse. Lesions in a retired racehorse used in light work reveal healing of subchondral bone lesions by fibrocartilaginous "scars" (d, double arrows). Radiographic lesions indicative of subchondral bone disease include subchondral sclerosis and lysis of the condyles (e, arrow). Other degenerative changes, such as osteophytosis seen along the distal margin of the sesamoid bone and dorsal proximal margin of the proximal phalanx (e, arrowheads), are also common. These lesions are thought to arise from high impact repetitive osseous stress to subchondral bone sustained during training and racing.

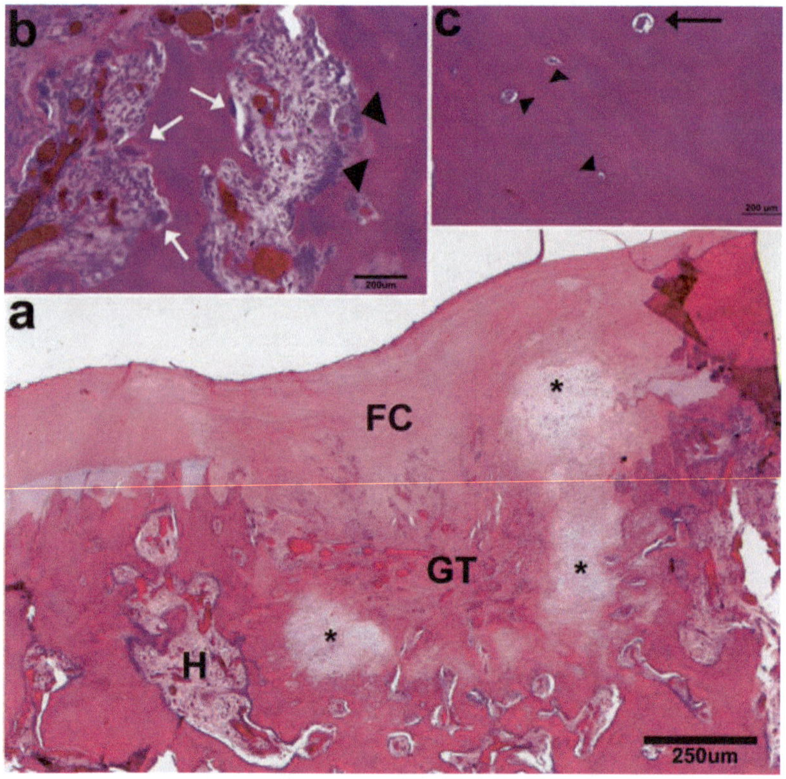


**Figure 10.58.** (a) Low and (b,c) high magnification H&E photomicrographs of the MCIII distal lateral condyle from a horse with subchondral bone disease. A focal depression in the articular cartilage surface (Fig. 10.57c, arrowhead) corresponds to a defect within the articular-epiphyseal complex. (a) The normal tissue architecture is replaced by a superficial region of fibrocartilage (FC), subtended by organizing granulation tissue (GT), and islands of hyaline cartilage (asterisks) that extend deep into the subchondral bone, which contains hyperemic medullary spaces (H). (b) Hyperemic medullary spaces correspond to active bone remodeling with bone lined by numerous osteoclasts within Howship lacunae (arrows) and plump polygonal osteoblasts (arrowheads). (c) The defect is surrounded by regions of sclerotic compact bone that contain sparse and extremely small osteonal canals (arrowheads).

### *5. Dorsal metacarpal disease with microcracks ("bucked shins")*

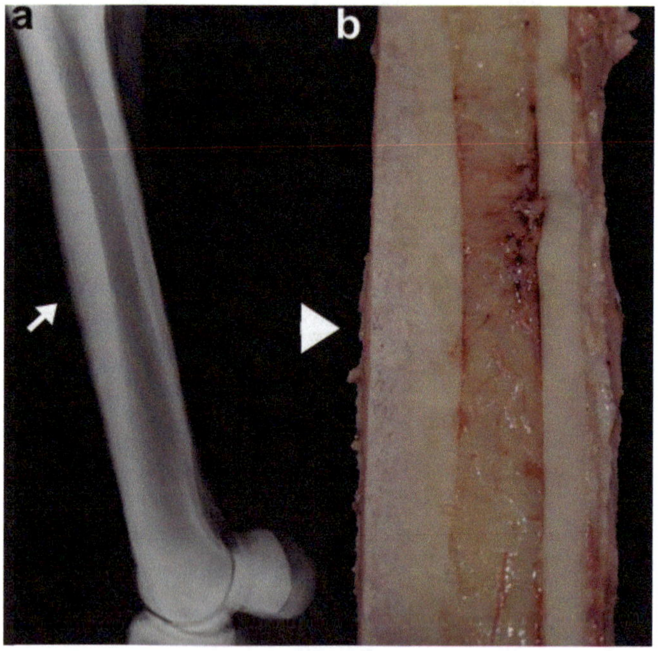


**Figure 10.59.** Dorsal cortical remodeling and microcracks, also known as "bucked shins," in the third metacarpal (cannon) bone of a juvenile racehorse. (a) Lateral digital radiographic projection of the mid-metacarpus reveals thickening of the dorsal cortex with the formation of oblique linear radiolucencies, for example, microcracks (arrow). (b) Gross photograph of this region confirms thickening of the dorsal cortex with prominent, hyperemic osteonal canals evident grossly (arrowhead).

## VI. Proliferative and neoplastic disease

### *1. Benign and nonneoplastic proliferative lesions*

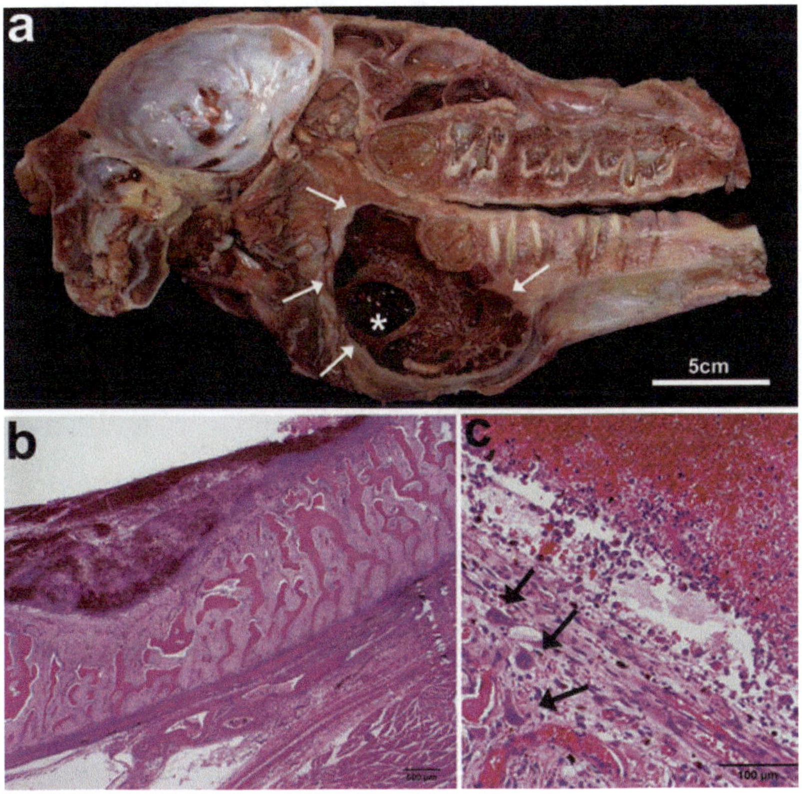


**Figure 10.60.** Aneurysmal bone cyst in a neonatal foal presented with a large intraosseous swelling of the left mandibular ramus. (a) Expanding and effacing the bone is a large well-demarcated, multiloculated cavity (arrows) divided into smaller cystic compartments (asterisk) by thin fibrous septae. (b) Low and (c) high magnification photomicrographs of sections taken from the margin of the lesion reveal (b) an outer layer of radiating woven bone trabeculae interspersed by loose collagenous stroma, a middle layer of fibrovascular connective tissue, and an inner cavity filled with blood. (c) Within the blood filled cavity and surrounding connective tissue are numerous hemosiderophages and multinucleated osteoclasts (arrows).

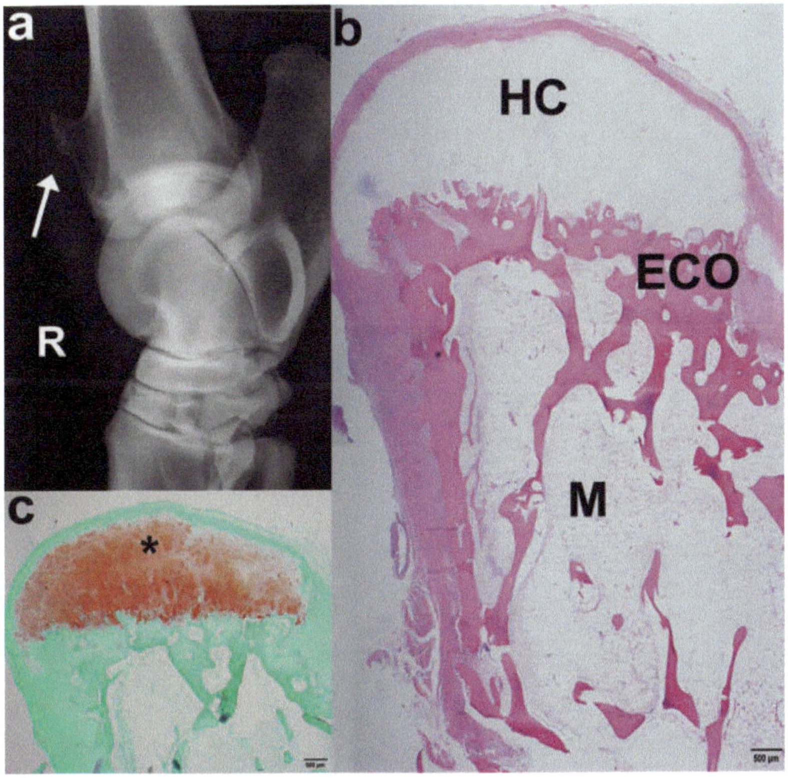


**Figure 10.61.** Osteochondroma of the tibia in a juvenile horse. (a) Digital radiograph of the right distal tibia and hock shows a focal well-demarcated exostosis that extends from and is contiguous with the dorsal cortex (arrow). (b) H&E low magnification composite photomicrograph of the surgically excised lesion shows a distal cap of hyaline cartilage (HC) that merges with an ossified growth plate (prior zone of endochondral ossification; ECO) that extends into bone trabeculae interspersed by medullary spaces (M). (c) A Safranin-O stained section shows intense red staining of the hyaline cartilage cap, consistent with the proteoglycan-rich matrix (asterisk) of hyaline cartilage.

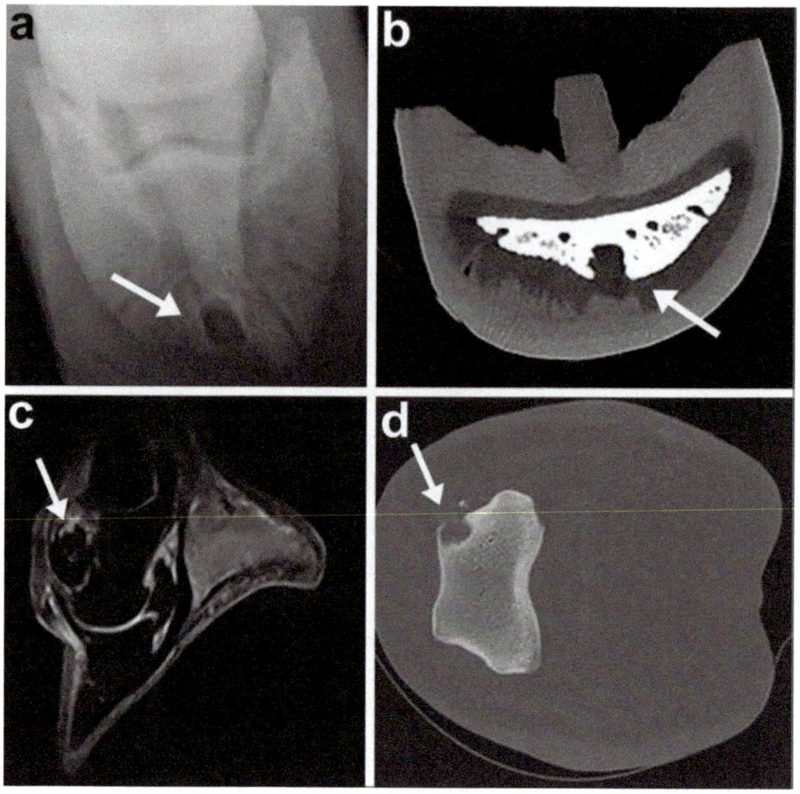


**Figure 10.62.** Intraosseous epidermoid cysts, "keratomas" of the distal and middle phalanx. (a) Digital radiograph with (b, d) CT scan and (c) magnetic resonance imaging (MRI) scan of two horses that exhibited moderate lameness (both horses) and foot soreness (horse of top panels only). (a, b) Prominent well-demarcated intraosseous cystlike radiolucencies circumscribed by sclerotic bone (arrows) are identified within the distal portion of the distal phalanx and (d) dorsal distolateral aspect (arrow) of the middle phalanx, respectively. Sagittal MRI short tau inversion recovery image of the second horse reveals a subcutaneous cystic accumulation (arrow) of dense material (keratin) that communicates with the intraosseous lesion.

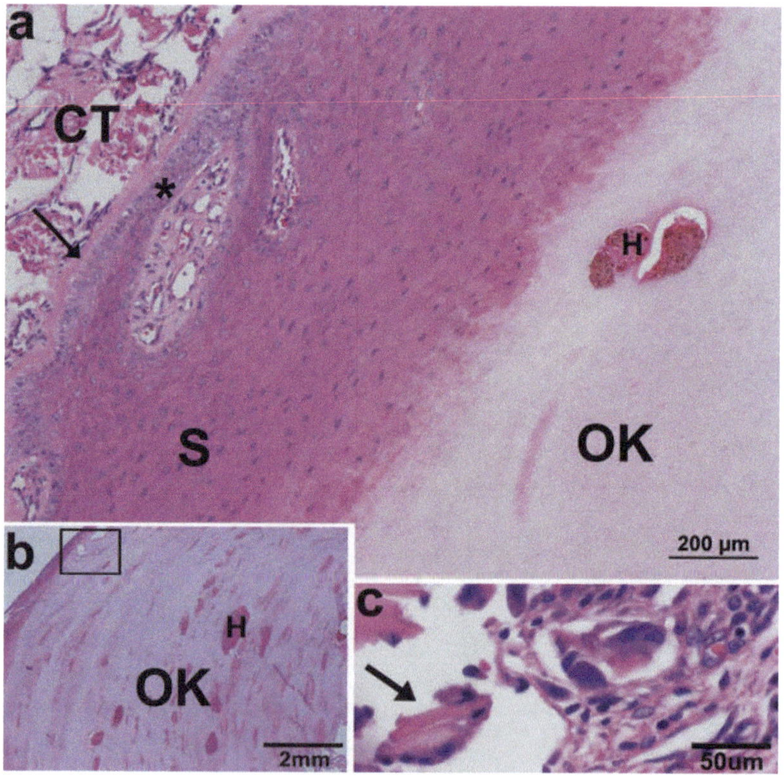


**Figure 10.63.** (a,b) Low and (c) high magnification H&E photomicrographs of the lesion surgically excised from the horse in Figure 10.62c and d show a central accumulation of orthokeratotic keratin (a, b, OK) that contains hemorrhagic foci (a, b, H), and is circumscribed by multiple layers of stratified squamous epithelium (a, S) with a distinct basal cell layer and basement membrane (a, arrow). The structure is surrounded by variably inflamed connective tissue (a, CT). Often, some epidermal structures resembling lamellae of the stratum internum are seen in the periphery of the cyst (a, asterisk), suggesting the potential origin. Pyogranulomatous inflammation is associated with portions of this cyst, with large fragments of keratin phagocytized by multinucleate giant cells (c, arrow). To give size perspective, panel a was magnified from the framed region of panel b.

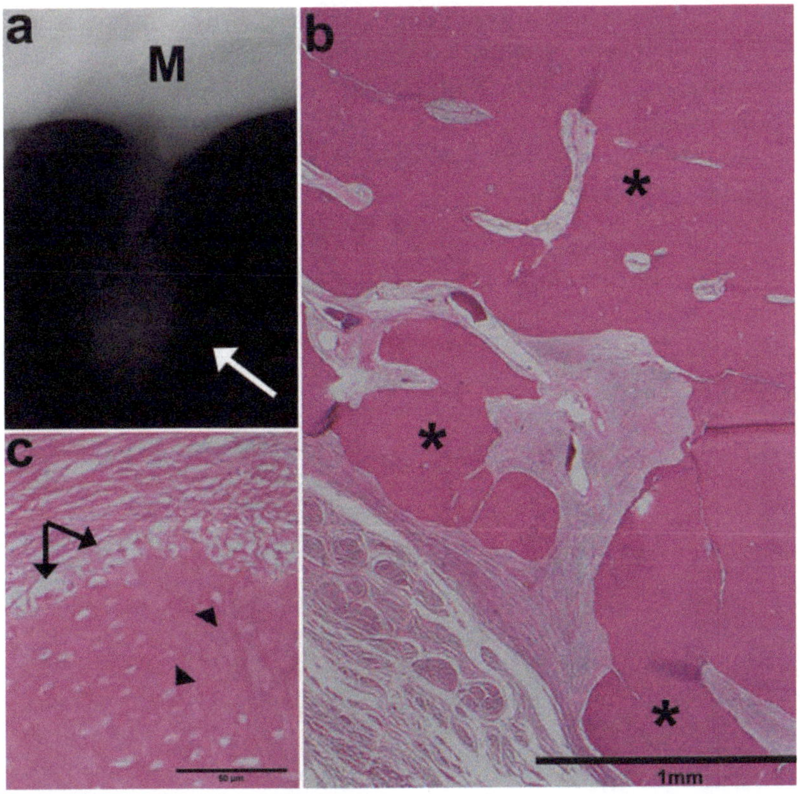


Figure 10.64. Mandibular osteoma in an adult horse with a several year history of a slow-growing (3 cm diameter) mass associated with the mandibular ramus. (a) Plain film radiograph reveals a well-defined mineralized mass (arrow) extending ventrally from the mandibular ramus (M). (b) Low and (c) high magnification H&E photomicrographs of sections from the excised mass show well-demarcated islands of mineralized compact (osteonal) bone (asterisks), encapsulated by fibrous connective tissue. (c) Bone islands are rimmed by a bland population of osteoblasts (arrows). Bone islands contain regularly interspersed osteocyte lacunae (arrowheads) with rare scattered osteoclasts (not shown). Artifact from extensive decalcification resulted in poor cellular detail of osteoblasts and osteocytes.

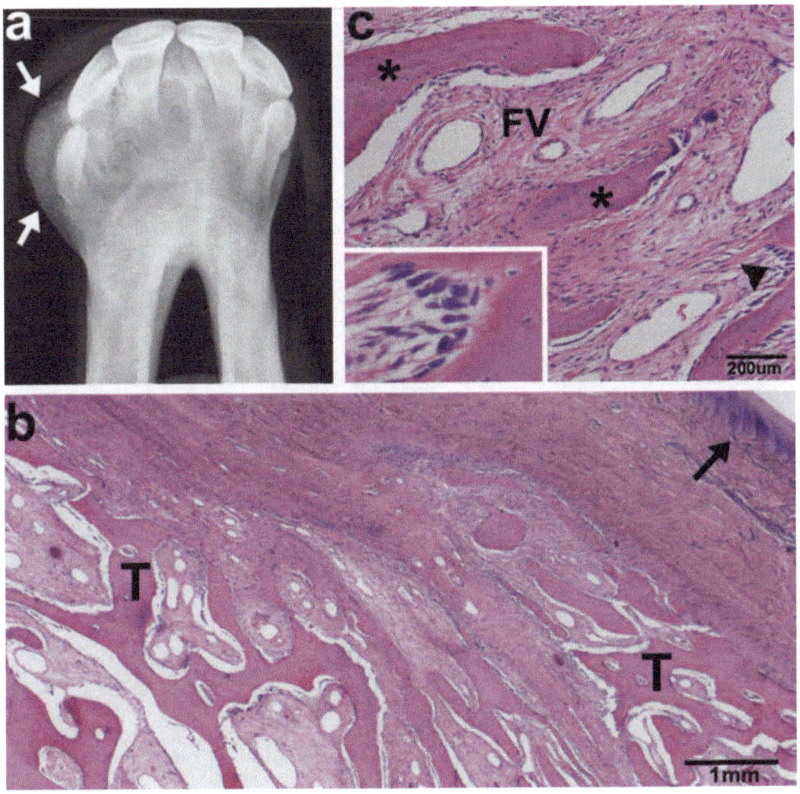


Figure 10.65. Ossifying fibroma in the rostral mandible of 7-month-old filly. (a) Digital radiograph reveals a poorly marginated mass with smooth edges and a trabecular osseous pattern that extends from the rostral edge of the third incisor but does not displace the incisors, consistent with a nonaggressive lesion (arrows). (b) Low and (c) high magnification H&E photomicrographs of sections from the excised mass show an unencapsulated proliferation of anatomizing bone trabeculae (b, T; c, asterisks) interspersed by well-vascularized fibrous connective tissue (c, FV) that elevates the gingival surface (b, arrow). Higher magnification reveals these trabeculae are lined by plump osteoblasts (c, arrow head; c, inset).

Figure 10.66 shows monostotic fibrous dysplasia in the distal radius of an adult horse that was presented with acute forelimb lameness. The lesion resulted in distinct medullary lysis with mild endosteal lysis of the dorsal cortex. Surgical excision of the mass was performed through a dorsal cortical bur ostectomy. The lesion was packed with cancellous bone graft, and the horse recovered uneventfully.

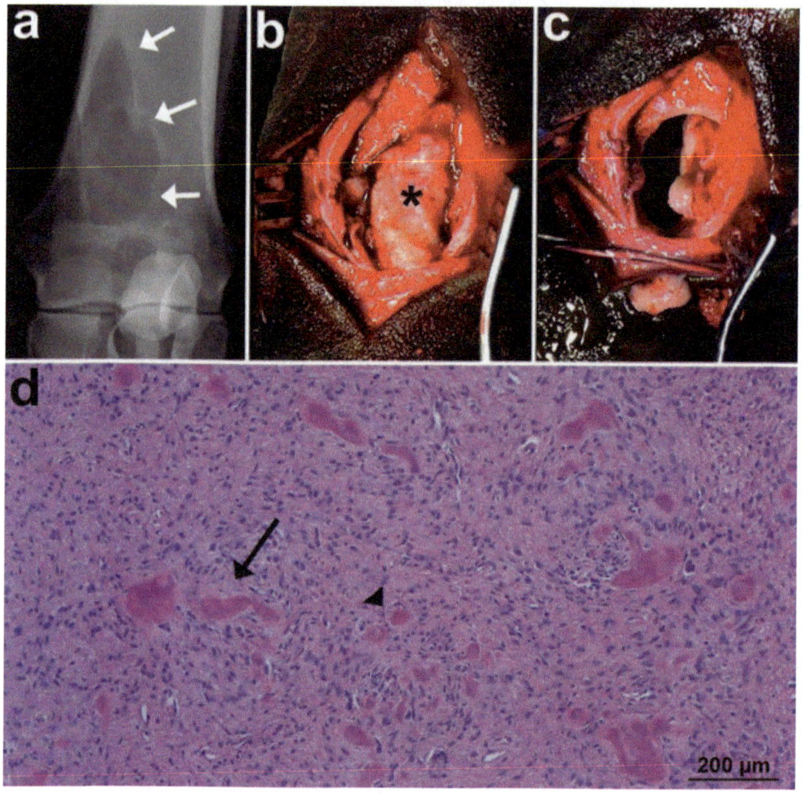


**Figure 10.66.** Horse. (a) Cranial-caudal radiograph shows a well-demarcated radiolucency (arrows) within the medullary cavity of the distal radius with sclerotic margins. (b) Surgery revealed a firm white intramedullary mass (asterisk) with a gritty texture. (c) The mass "shelled out" easily from the surrounding medullary bone; the bony defect was packed with a cancellous bone graft. (d) H&E photomicrograph of a nondecalcified section shows interwoven streams of bland spindle cells embedded within a collagenous stroma that contain mineralized spicules (arrow) and "psammomatous" bodies (arrowhead) of bone not lined by osteoblasts. (Gross photographs courtesy of Dr. D. Richardson, New Bolton Center, University of Pennsylvania.)

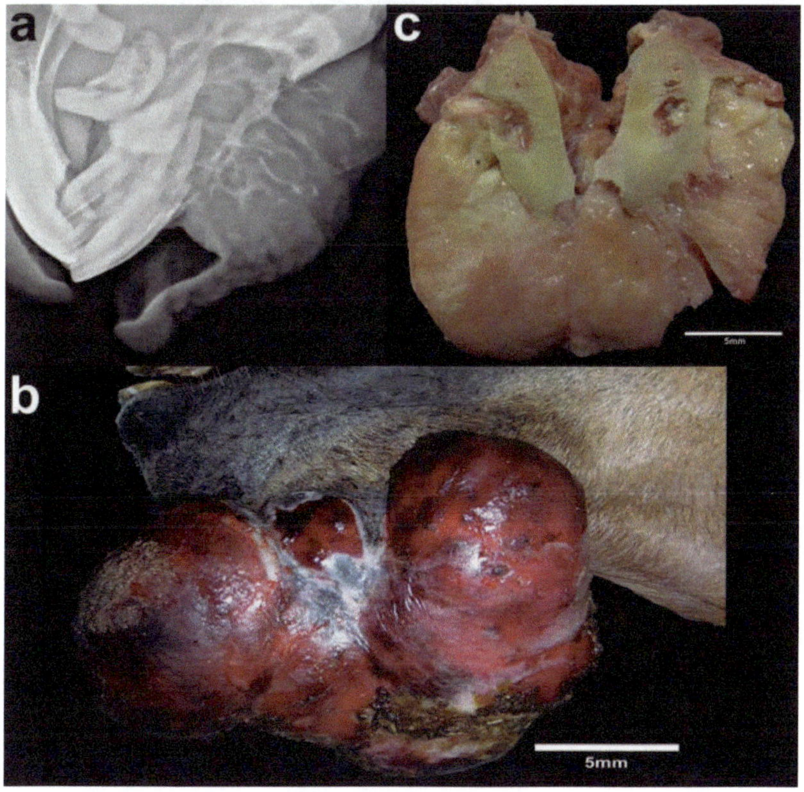


**Figure 10.67.** Desmoid fibroma in a geriatric horse with a history of a rapidly growing mandibular mass. (a) Digital radiograph reveals an exophytic multilobular mass associated with aggressive lysis of the rostral mandibular rami and radiating spicules of bone. (b) The skin over the mass is ulcerated. (c) The transverse section of the rostral mandible reveals a firm, glistening yellow-tan tissue that forms broad fascicular patterns.

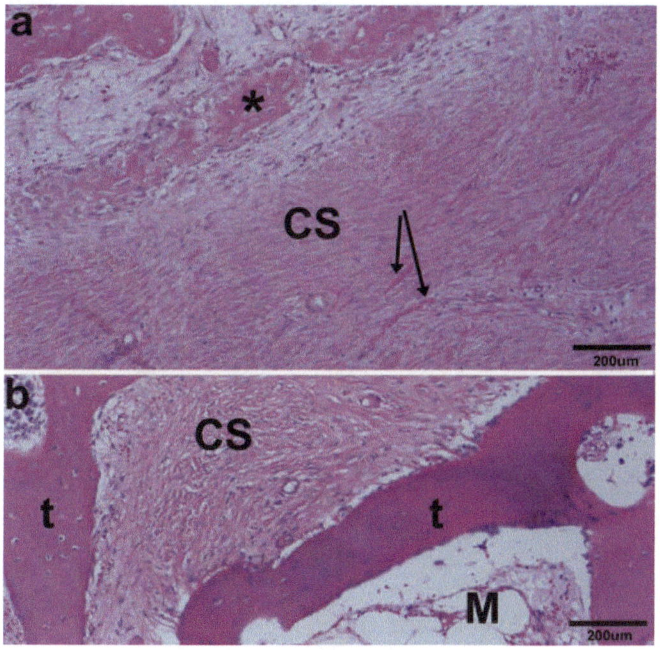


**Figure 10.68.** Horse. Desmoid fibroma. (a,b) H&E photomicrographs of tissue trimmed from the mass in Figure 10.67c show broad interlacing fascicles of a bland spindle cell proliferation embedded within a dense collagenous stroma (CS) that often contain sclerotic "desmoid-like" collagen bundles (a, arrows). The bland spindle cell proliferation extends between and through mandibular bone trabeculae (b, t) and replaces normal medullary fibroadipose tissue (b, M). Within the collagenous stroma are spicules of metaplastic woven bone (a, asterisk).

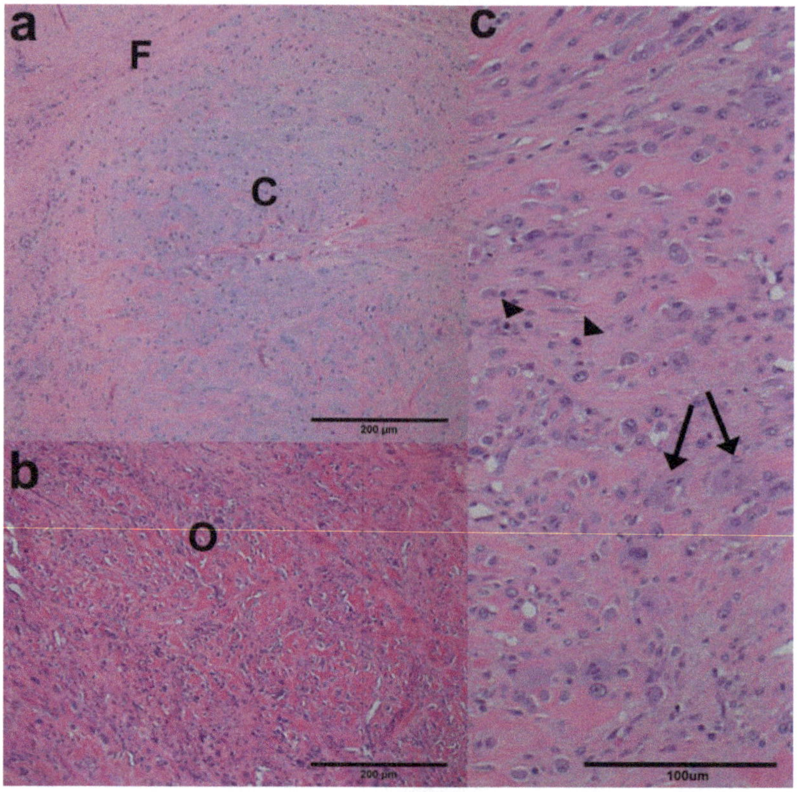


**Figure 10.69.** Extraosseous osteosarcoma in a 17-year-old Welsh-crossbred mare. A subcutaneous mass that was noticed 6 months prior and had progressed to a 5-cm diameter multilobulated growth spreading beneath the skin was excised from the lateral aspect of the right tibia. (a–c) H&E photomicrographs of nondecalcified sections reveal an unencapsulated proliferation of atypical spindle cells demonstrating myxoid, fibrous (a, F), chondroid (a, C), and osseous (b, O) differentiation. (c) Some foci show more pleomorphic plump atypical cells with moderate anisokaryosis and a higher mitotic index (1–2 per ×40 field) (arrowheads). Multinucleate giant (osteoclast-like) cells are scattered throughout the proliferation (arrows).

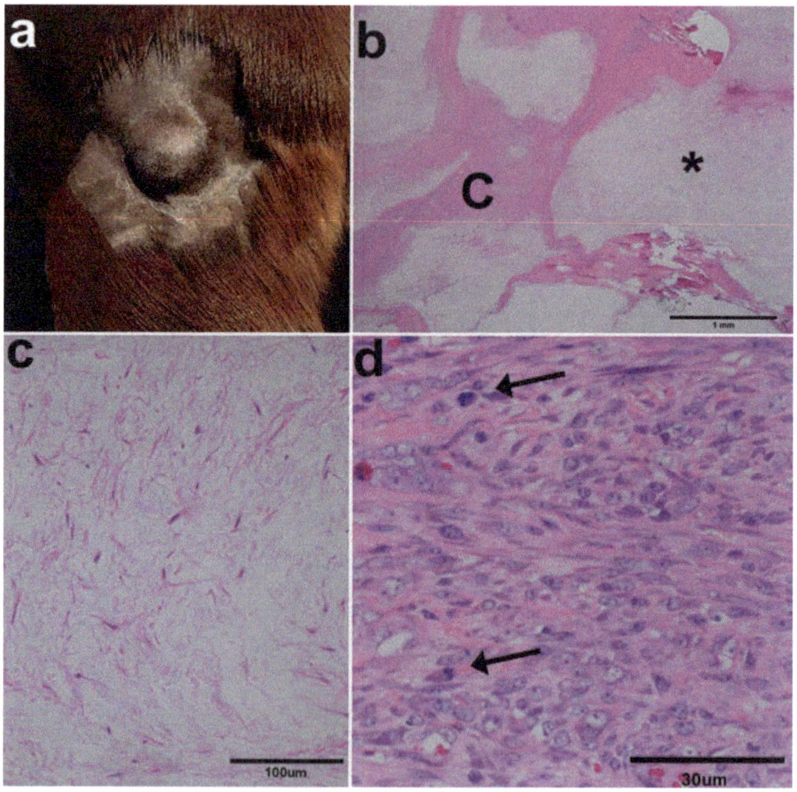


**Figure 10.70.** Synovial cell sarcoma in an adult horse. (a) A subcutaneous mass exhibiting rapid growth was excised from the elbow region. (b) Low and (c,d) high magnification H&E photomicrographs show a poorly circumscribed, unencapsulated, multinodular neoplastic spindle cell proliferation separated into cyst-like cavities (asterisk) by prominent collagenous septae (C). (c) The neoplastic cell morphology varies from paucicellular, loosely interwoven stellate cells embedded in a wispy myxoid matrix with rare mitoses to (d) densely cellular, plump spindle cells (arrows) with a high mitotic index (10 per ×40 field).

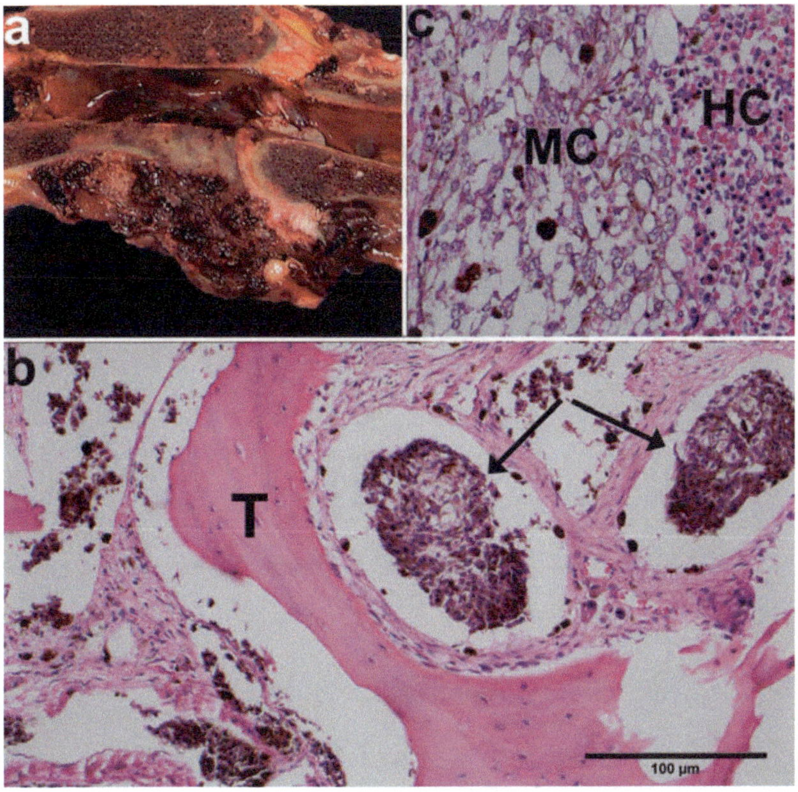


**Figure 10.71.** Metastatic malignant melanoma of the vertebrae from a gray horse with cutaneous and visceral melanomas. (a) Gross photo shows multifocal-coalescing purple black nodules that extend from the ventral aspects of the two vertebral bodies. (b,c) H&E photomicrographs of decalcified sections of infiltrated vertebral bone show sheets and streams of black-pigmented neoplastic melanocytes (b, arrows) that extend into and between trabecular bone spicules (b, T). (c) Collision of neoplastic melanocytes (MC) with hematopoietic precursor cells (HC) is seen within medullary spaces.

## VII. Metabolic bone disease

### *1. Nutritional fibrous osteodystrophy*

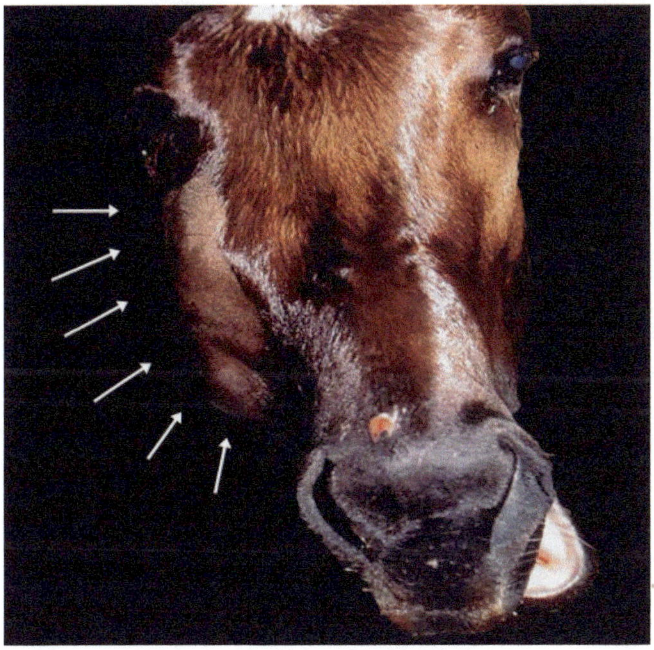

**Figure 10.72.** Nutritional fibrous osteodystrophy, "bran disease," in a horse on a high-phosphorous diet. Gross photo shows marked enlargement of the maxillae, which is most pronounced on the right side (arrows).

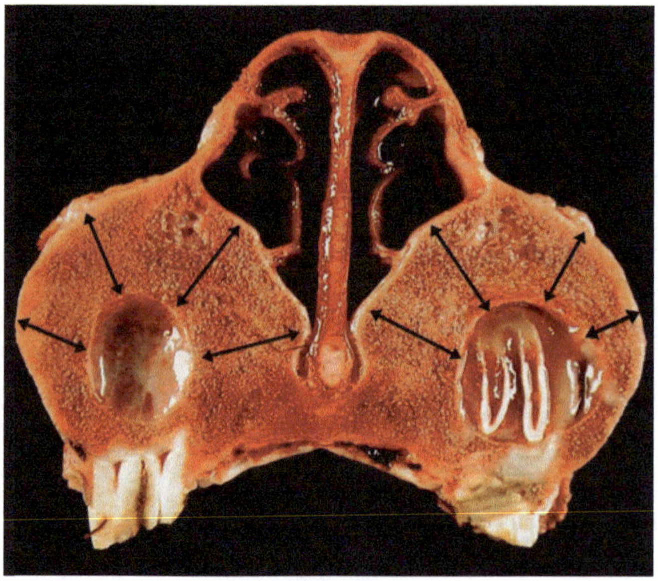

**Figure 10.73.** Horse. Nutritional fibrous osteodystrophy ("bran disease"). Gross photo of a transverse section through the maxillae reveal bilateral enlargement of the periodontal bone due to replacement of mineralized bone by unmineralized trabeculae and fibrous connective tissue (not shown). The bone would be soft and flexible with mechanical manipulation.

## *2. Emaciation with serous atrophy of marrow fat*

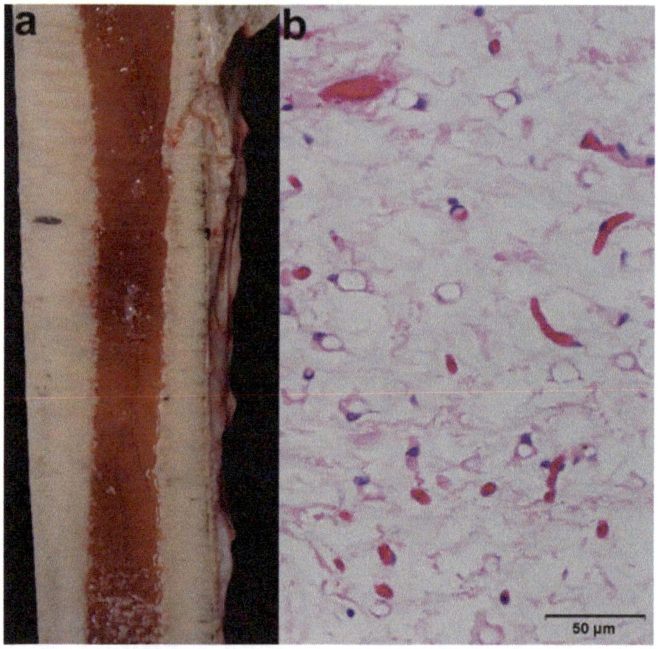


**Figure 10.74.** Emaciation with serous atrophy of marrow fat in a geriatric horse with poor dentition and severe malocclusion. (a) Gross photo shows that normal yellow-white opaque fat of the diaphyseal marrow is replaced by orange-yellow glistening, translucent tissue. Sections of marrow did not float in formalin. (b) H&E photomicrograph of a nondecalcified section of medullary cavity reveals replacement of marrow adipose tissue by collapsed adipocytes admixed with few spindle cells surrounded by a watery pale pink matrix containing scattered capillaries.

## Equine laminitis – Fact sheet

### Definition

A heterogenous disease process affecting the stratum lamellatum of the hoof wall that can result in biomechanical failure of the suspensory apparatus of the distal phalanx

### Incidence

- Second leading cause of death in horses, second to colic
- Associated with individual or combination of predisposing risk factors including:
  - Endocrine/metabolic disease, e.g., Pituitary Pars Intermedia Dysfunction (PPID), hyperinsulinemia, obesity
  - Inflammatory conditions: enterocolitis, metritis/retained fetal membranes, pleuropneumonia, cellulitis, vasculitis, sepsis
  - Ischemic conditions: thromboembolic disease, supporting limb overload

### Range of disease

- Developmental phase (24-48 hour period, "clinically silent")
- Acute-subacute/mild with resolution
- Acute-subacute, severe with progression
- Chronic stable: DP ventral rotation without solar herniation
- Chronic unstable: DP ventral rotation and sinking with solar herniation

### Complications

- Subsolar "toe" abscesses (abscesses can also fistulate through coronary band)
- Circulatory alterations to foot (vascular impingement and regional ischemia), severe pain
- DP osteolysis, solar margin fractures, osteomyelitis, solar herniation

## Equine laminitis – Fact sheet continued

### Gross findings (variable, depending on etiopathogenesis, severity, and chronicity)

- Acute mild
  - Hyperemia of coronary dermal papilla and sublamellar dermis (corium) edema of stratum lamellatum
  - Mild increased thickness of lamellae-corium (average thickness = 5.6 mm front feet and 5.1 mm hind feet for nonlaminitic light breed horses)
- Acute severe
  - Palpable clefting at coronary band with serum exudate or crusting
  - Variably sized hemorrhagic cleft separating hoof wall from lamellar corium with or without visible elongation and distortion of lamellae (regenerative attempts)
  - Subsolar hyperemia/necrosis, DP cortical/medullary hyperemia and medullary edema
- Chronic severe
  - Hoof wall deformities: "founder rings" and distal deviation ("kinking") of proximal horn tubules
  - Lamellar wedge formation with or without hoof wall separation
  - Subsolar hemorrhage, abscesses or necrosis
  - DP remodeling, solar margin fractures, osteomyelitis, gangrenous necrosis

### Microscopic findings (variable, depending on etiopathogenesis, severity, and chronicity)

- Secondary epidermal lamellae: elongation, distortion, necrosis with basement membrane separation
- Primary epidermal lamellae: elongation, keratinized axis displacement, distortion, hyperkeratosis, and separation
- Lamellar wedge: lamellar fusion with hyperplasia/dysplasia/dyskeratosis and hyperkeratosis
- Corium: vasodilation/hyperemia, necrosis +/- thromboemboli, inflammation (neutrophilic, histiocytic to lymphoplasmacytic), fibroplasia to fibrosis
- Distal phalanx: osteoclastic osteolysis and osteoproliferation, bone marrow edema, stromal cell activation, inflammation (neutrophilic, histiocytic, lymphoplasmacytic), necrosis, fracture

## Acknowledgments

Constructed in collaboration with Dr. H. Galantino-Homer, Senior Research Director in Laminitis, Clinical Studies, New Bolton Center, School of Veterinary Medicine, University of Pennsylvania.

## Selected references

Bailey SR, Marr CM, Elliott J. 2004. Current research and theories on the pathogenesis of acute laminitis in the horse. *Vet J* 167(2):129–142.

Carter RA, Engiles JB, Megee SO, Senoo M, Galantino-Homer HL. 2011. Decreased expression of p63, a regulator of epidermal stem cells, in the chronic laminitic equine hoof. *Equine Vet J* 43:543–551.

Collins SN, Pollitt C, Wylie CE, Matiasek K. 2010. Laminitic pain: parallels with pain states in humans and other species. *Vet Clin North Am Equine Pract* 26:643–671.

Eades SC. 2010. Overview of current laminitis research. *Vet Clin North Am Equine Pract* 26(1):51–63.

Engiles JB. 2010. Pathology of the distal phalanx in equine laminitis: more than just skin deep. *Vet Clin North Am Equine Pract* 26:155–165.

Frank N. 2011. Equine metabolic syndrome. *Vet Clin North Am Equine Pract* 27:73–92.

Galantino-Homer HL, Engiles JB. 2012. Insulin resistance and laminitis in broodmares. *J Equine Vet Sci* 32(10):680–688.

Kameya T, Kiryu K, Kaneko M, Satoh H. 1980. Histopathogenesis of thickening of the hoof wall laminae in equine laminitis. *Japanese J Vet Sci* 42:361–371.

Kuwano A, Katayama Y, Yoshihara T, Okada K. 2001. A gross study of lamellar wedge development in equine laminitis. *J Equine Sci* 12:58.

McFarlane D. 2011. Equine pituitary pars intermedia dysfunction. (Special Issue: Endocrine Diseases.) *Vet Clin North Am Equine Pract* 27:1, 93–113.

Wright M, Kidd L, Thorp BH. 1998. Gross, histological and histomorphometric features of the navicular bone and related structures in the horse. *Equine Vet* 30(3):220–234.

Ytrehus B, Carlson CS, Ekman S. 2007. Etiology and pathogenesis of osteochondrosis. *Vet Pathol* 44(4):429–448.

# 11 Diseases of the Endocrine System



*Color Atlas of Equine Pathology*, First Edition. Claus D. Buergelt and Fabio Del Piero.

This chapter covers pathologic changes affecting the pituitary gland, thyroid glands, and adrenal glands. Parathyroids, the endocrine pancreas, and gonads are not included. The latter equine endocrine organs are either very rarely involved in primary pathologic changes (parathyroids, endocrine pancreas) or have been discussed in other chapters (e.g., Chapter 12, "Diseases of the Reproductive Tract"). It should be mentioned that the equine parathyroids are not located anatomically next to the thyroid glands. For their immediate retrieval when performing the necropsy, anatomy textbooks should be consulted before starting the necropsy.

## I. Pituitary gland

Inflammatory changes involving the pituitary gland are very rare and represent either abscesses or secondary involvement from basilar empyema.

Hyperplastic and adenomatous changes in the pars intermedia of the pituitary gland in older horses are responsible for pituitary pars intermedia dysfunction (equine Cushing disease) with clinical manifestations of nonseasonal wavy hair coat, muscle weakness, pendulous abdomen, hyperhydrosis, polydipsia/polyuria, or intermittent episodes of laminitis. These proliferative conditions are due to reduction of dopaminergic effects by the hypothalamus and also may be responsible for insulin resistance. Diagnosis is based on clinical signs and endocrine tests.

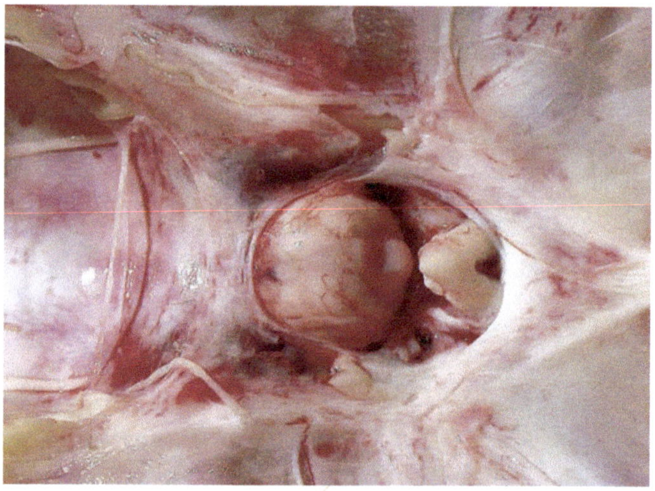

**Figure 11.1.** Horse. Pituitary. Pars Intermedia Adenoma. Pituitary enlargement is clearly visible. The condition leads to Cushing disease.

## II. Thyroid gland

Thyroid hypertrophy and goiter in foals are described in Chapter 2, "Diseases of Foals and Juveniles." Hypothyroidism in foals leads to stunting due to delayed ossification of the skeletal system and to a dull, dry, nonshedding hair coat.

Older horses frequently have small discrete nonfunctional adenomas in the thyroid gland as an incidental finding and without clinical signs. These may measure 1–2 cm in diameter and may be expected in cases of slightly asymmetric thyroid glands at necropsy. Originally thought to be of follicular epithelial origin, they are now classified as C-cell adenomas based on ultrastructural and immunohistochemical findings. Rarely are malignant primary thyroid tumors encountered in the horse.



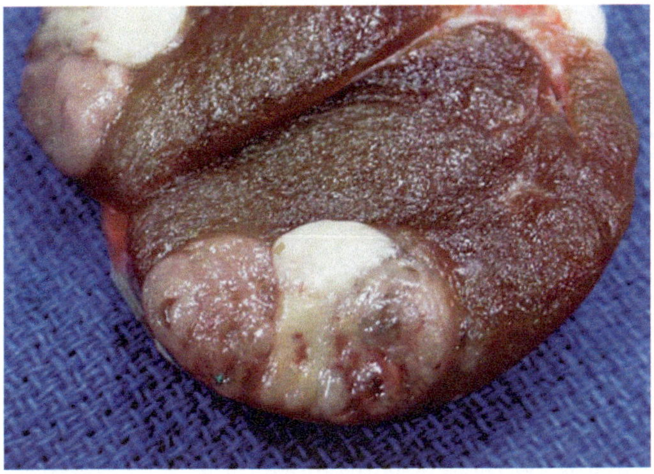

**Figure 11.2.** Horse. Thyroid. Adenoma. This whitish to tan bulging nodule was an incidental finding at necropsy.

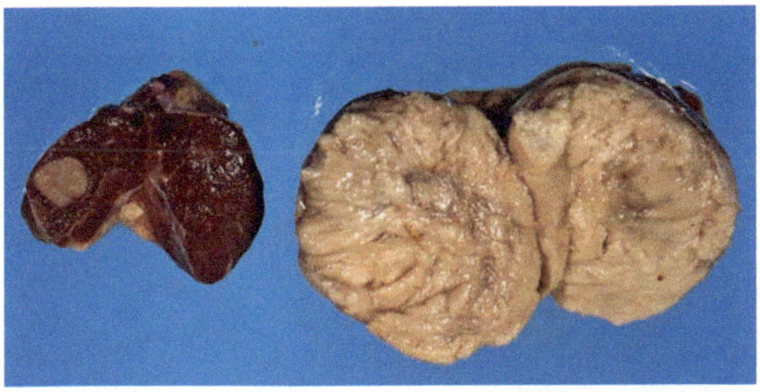

**Figure 11.3.** Horse. Thyroid. Adenoma and Carcinoma. The adenoma on left is small and well delineated. The carcinoma on right is large replacing the normal brown thyroid parenchyma.

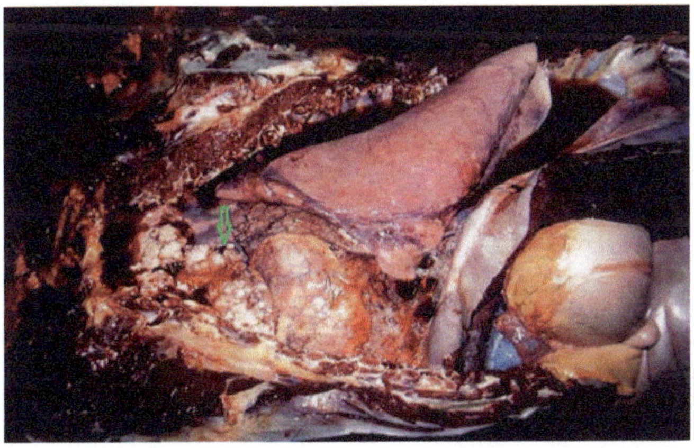

**Figure 11.4.** Horse. Thyroid. Carcinoma with Mediastinal Metastases. Tumor growths are present in the cranial thorax along the mediastinum (arrow). Ectopic thyroid carcinoma is a differential diagnosis.

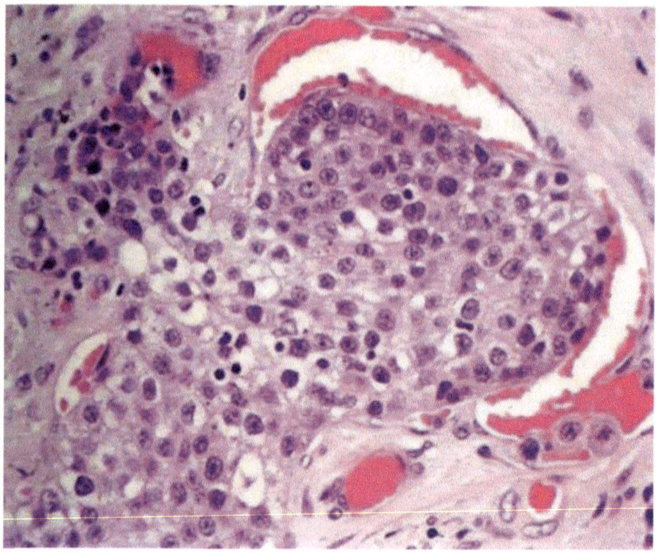

**Figure 11.5.** Horse. Thyroid. Carcinoma. Thyroid C-cells cells have invaded a blood vessel. (H&E)

## III. Adrenal gland

Pathologic changes in the adrenal glands of horses are sporadic and rare. Clinical signs of endocrine dysfunction of either the adrenal cortex or medulla are frequently not correlated with morphologic evidence of pathology. Necrosis and inflammation of the adrenal gland occur as isolated findings, with the exception in septic foals. Aged horses sporadically develop tumors in the cortex or medulla with no clinical signs.

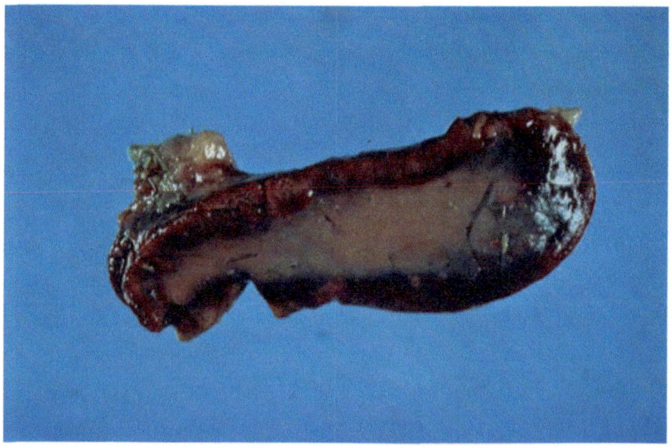

**Figure 11.6.** Horse. Adrenal. Adrenal Cortical Necrosis. The cortex is segmentally marbled due to hemorrhage in necrotic foci. Cortical nodules on the surface are a normal variation of the gross architecture and can be seen in newborn foals and adults, respectively. The cause of the necrosis was not determined.

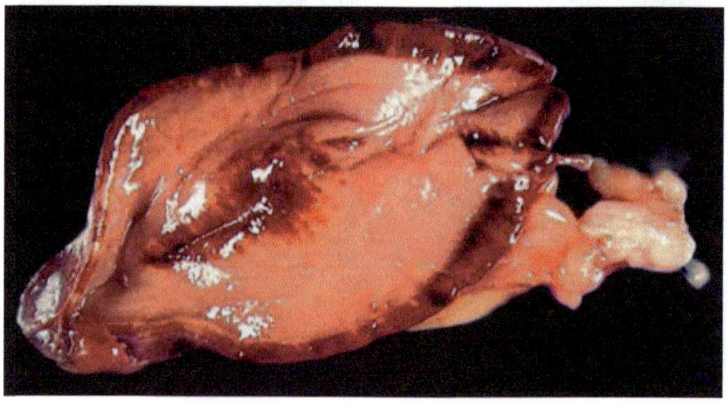

**Figure 11.7.** Horse. Adrenal. Cortical Hemorrhage. Diffuse hemorrhage in the cortex is often apparent in septic foals dying from endotoxic shock and is known as Waterhouse-Friderichsen syndrome when seen in septic children.

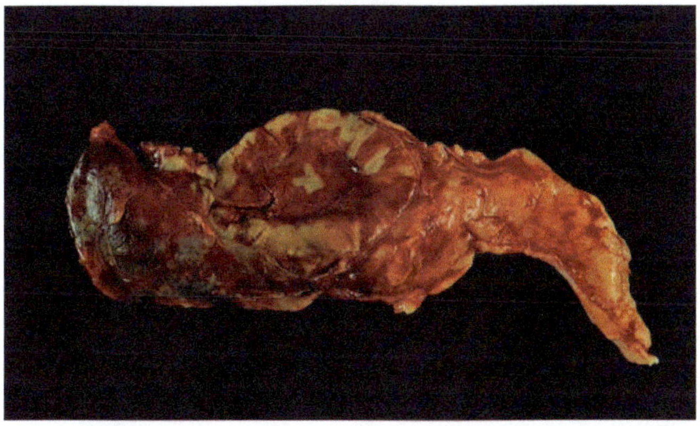

**Figure 11.8.** Horse. Adrenal. Adrenalitis. Multiple yellow nodules in cortex. This Arabian foal died from disseminated nocardiosis that affected both cortex and medulla of the adrenal. *Actinobacillus equuli* is another pathogen to invade the adrenal gland during septicemia.

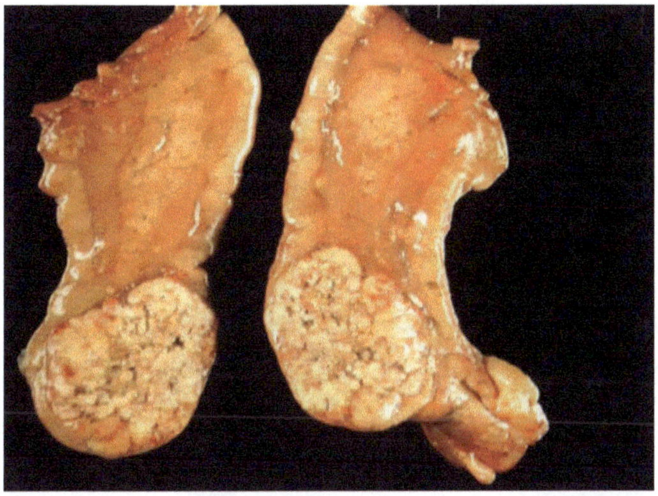

**Figure 11.9.** Horse. Adrenal. Cortical Adenoma. One pole of the adrenal gland contains an elevated yellow growth that felt gritty on cut section suggesting mineralization. Clinical signs of hyperadrenocorticism were not apparent.

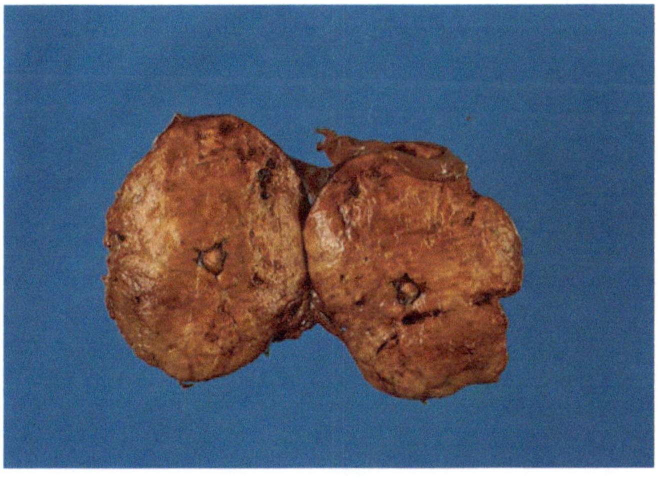

**Figure 11.10.** Horse. Adrenal. Cortical Carcinoma. An irregular pseudo-lobulated yellow mass has distorted the adrenal cortex and replaced the central medulla.

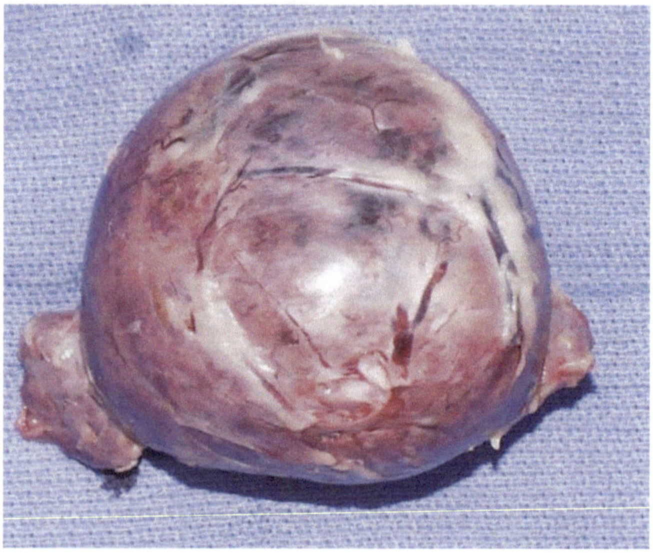

**Figure 11.11.** Horse. Adrenal. Pheochromocytoma. A bulging mass is seen on the surface of an enlarged adrenal gland.

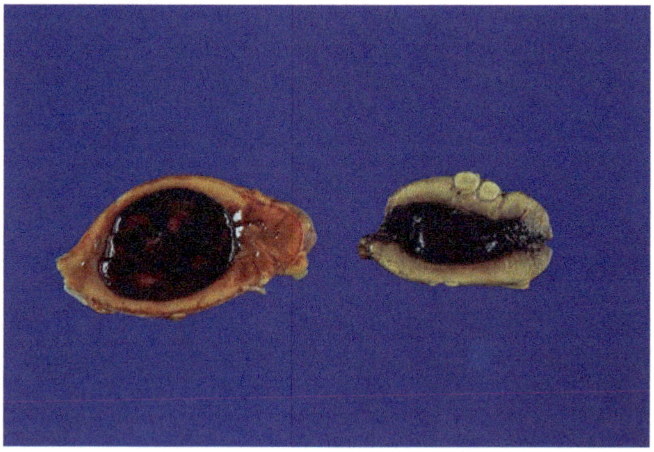

**Figure 11.12.** Horse. Adrenal. Pheochromocytoma. A dark red mass has enlarged the medulla and compressed the cortex. This particular tumor was diagnosed as benign. The tumors may be functional on occasion to produce catecholamines and to exhibit clinical signs of muscle fasciculations, ataxia, and sweating. Pheochromocytomas are usually incidental findings at necropsy. They may occasionally rupture to induce retroperitoneal hemorrhage. Nodules of extracortical hyperplasia are present on right adrenal.

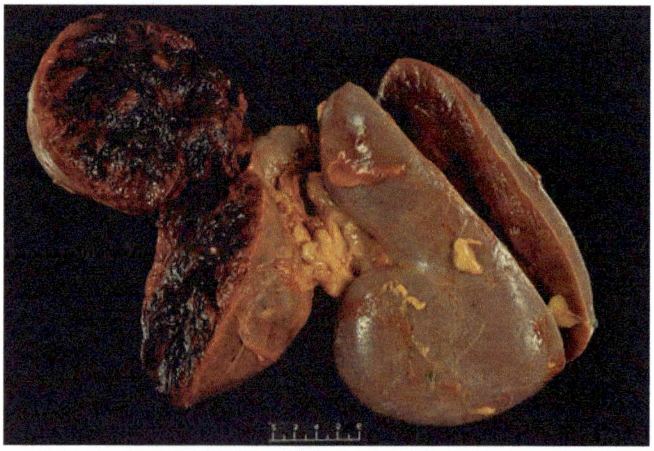

**Figure 11.13.** Horse. Adrenal. Pheochromocytoma. The tumor has enlarged the adrenal on the left as compared with the adjacent kidney. It invades the adrenal cortex and exhibits marked hemorrhage.

The literature contains reports of simultaneously occurring hyperplasia and neoplasia affecting the adrenal medulla (pheochromocytoma), thyroid gland, and pituitary (pars intermedia adenoma) in individual horses resembling human multiple endocrine neoplasia syndrome. One other thought is that these multiple tumors may be coincidental because they are typically found in older horses. On personal observation by one of the authors multiple endocrine tumors were encountered in a 29-year-old Arabian horse with hirsutism that included a pars intermedia pituitary tumor, a bilateral thyroid gland adenoma, a unilateral phaeochromocytoma, and multiple gastrointestinal stromal tumors.

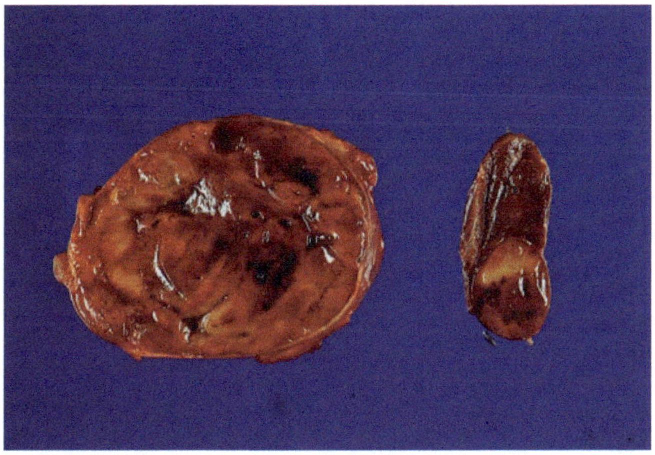

**Figure 11.14.** Horse. Pituitary and Thyroid. Neoplasia. Both the pituitary on the left and the thyroid gland on the right were diagnosed as adenomas on microscopic examination.

## Selected references


Breuhaus BA. 2011. Disorders of the equine thyroid gland. *Vet Clin North Am Equine Pract* 27(1):115–128.

Dalefield RR, Palmer DN. 1994. The frequent occurrence of thyroid tumors in aged horses. *J Comp Pathol* 110(1):57–64.

De Cock HE, MacLachlan NJ. 1999. Simultaneous occurrence of multiple neoplasms and hyperplasia in the adrenal gland and thyroid gland of the horse resembling multiple endocrine neoplasia syndrome: case report and retrospective identification of additional cases. *Vet Pathol* 36(6):633–636.

Germann SE, Ruetten M, Derungs SB, et al. 2006. Multiple endocrine neoplasia-like syndrome in a horse. *Vet Rec* 159:530–532.

Hart KA, Barton MH. 2011. Adrenocorticol insufficiency in horses and foals. *Vet Clin North Am Equine Pract* 27(1):19–34.

Johnson PJ, Goetz TE, Foreman JH, Zachary JF. 1995. Pheochromocytoma in two horses. *J Am Vet Med Assoc* 206(6):837–841.

McCue PM. 2002. Equine Cushing's disease. *Vet Clin North Am Equine Pract* 18(3):533–543.

McFarlane D. 2011. Equine pituitary pars intermedia dysfunction. *Vet Clin North Am Equine Pract* 27(1):93–113.

Miller MA, Pardo ID, Jackson LP, Moore GE, Sojka JE. 2008. Correlation of pituitary histomorphometry with adrenocorticotrophic hormone response to domperidone administration in the diagnosis of equine pituitary pars intermedia dysfunction. *Vet Pathol* 45(1):26–38.

Reilly L, Habecker P, Beech J, Johnston J, Sweeney C, Hamir A. 1994. Pituitary abscess and basilar empyema in 4 horses. *Equine Vet J* 26(5):424–426.

Ueki H, Kowatari Y, Oyamada T, Oikawa T, Yoshikawa H. 2004. Non-functional C-cell adenoma in aged horses. *J Comp Pathol* 131:157–165.

van der Kolk JH, Mars MH, van der Gaag I. 1994. Adrenocortical carcinoma in a 12-year-old mare. *Vet Rec* 134(5):113–115.

van der Kolk JH, Heinrichs M, van Amerongen JD, Stooker RC, in de Wal LJ, van den Ingh TS. 2004. Evaluation of pituitary gland anatomy and histopathologic findings in clinically normal horses and horses and ponies with pituitary pars intermedia adenoma. *Am J Vet Res* 65(12):1701–1707.

# 12 Disease of the Reproductive System

I. Male
  1. Morphology of the normal mature equine testis
  2. Testicular hypoplasia
  3. Testicular degeneration/atrophy
  4. Testicular inflammation
  5. Testicular neoplasia
  6. Accessory male sex organs
  7. External genitalia
  8. Miscellaneous

II. Female (nonpregnant)
  1. Morphology of the normal mature equine ovary
  2. Anomalies
  3. Ovarian cysts
  4. Ovarian inflammation
  5. Ovarian neoplasia
  6. Endometritis
  7. Endometrial biopsy
  8. Uterine neoplasia
  9. External genitalia

III. Female (pregnant)
  1. Placental membranes and umbilicus
  2. Incidental findings associated with the placental membranes
  3. Disturbances of pregnancy

IV. Noninfectious abortion diseases
  1. Fescue grass toxicosis
  2. Mare reproductive loss syndrome

V. Infectious abortion diseases
  1. Equine viral abortions
    a. Equine herpesvirus abortion (EHV)
    b. Equine viral arteritis abortion (EVA)
  2. Equine bacterial abortions
  3. Equine fungal abortions
  4. Abortions caused by microsporidia
  5. Miscellaneous

VI. Choice of samples and diagnostic methods for abortion investigation

*Color Atlas of Equine Pathology*, First Edition. Claus D. Buergelt and Fabio Del Piero.

# I. Male

The male reproductive system in the horse consists of testes and the accessory genital organs that include penis and prepuce. The testes of the sexually mature stallion assume a double complementary function: the production of sperm and the secretion of steroid hormones, mainly testosterone to produce the male phenotype. In domestic animals the testes descend into the scrotum shortly before or after birth and need to remain in this position permanently for regulated optimal spermatogenesis at a temperature lower than that of the body. In the horse, testicular descent is completed at birth or shortly after birth (10–14 days) considering average gestation of 300 days.

## *1. Morphology of the normal mature equine testis*

The stallion testis is enveloped by a protective fibrous tunica albuginea with the epididymis loosely attached to the testis. On cross section, the pigmented testicular parenchyma should bulge indicating functional maturity. It also should present the mediastinum testis as a band of connective tissue passing from pole to pole. The mediastinum testis contains blood vessels, lymphatics, and the rete tubules.

Testicular tissue requires a fixative for optimal preservation of the seminiferous tubules and the interstitium containing the interstitial or Leydig cells. The preferred fixative is Bouin's solution.

The seminiferous tubules containing germ cells and Sertoli cells are extremely sensitive to a variety of exogenous and endogenous adverse influences. Structural integrity and prevention of breakdown of the immunologically protective blood–testis barrier is another point of consideration for certain pathologic immune-deranged processes in the testis.

Sperm development and maturation are complex processes following integrated influences of hormones, nutritional factors, temperature, photoperiod, and genetically determined rate of spermatogenesis (49 days in the stallion).

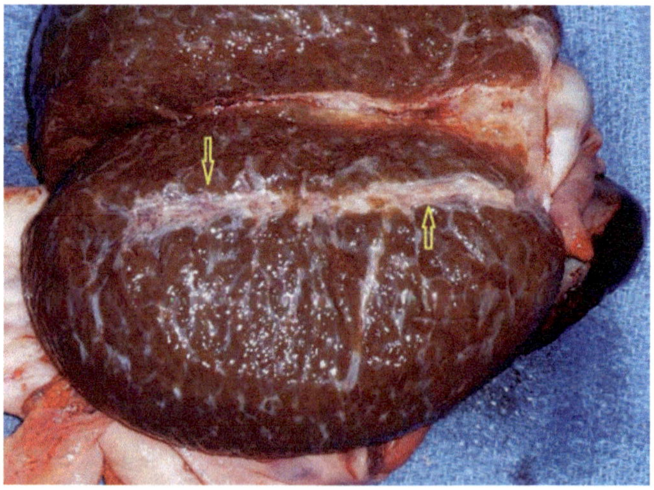

**Figure 12.1.** Horse. Testis. Normal. Sexually Mature Stallion. The cross section shows a slightly bulging red parenchyma and the mediastinum testis as a regular gray band in the center (arrows). The amount of lipopigment wthin the interstitial cells determines the color of the testicular surface. (Courtesy Dr. M. Pozor, University of Florida.)

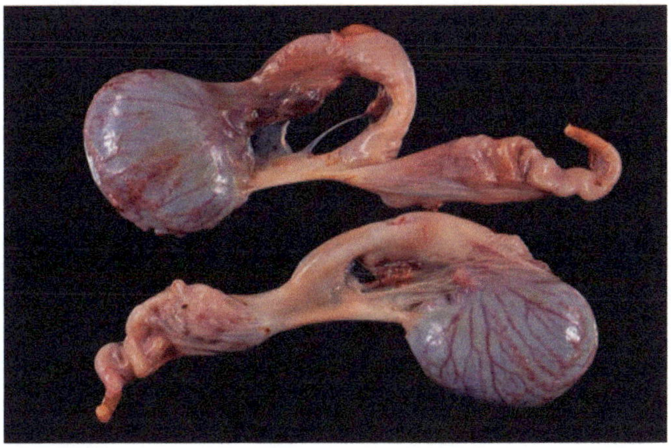

**Figure 12.2.** Horse. Juvenile. Testes and Epididymes. The epididymis normally is loosely attached to the maturing testis.

## *2. Testicular hypoplasia*

Testicular hypoplasia is a pathologic condition at puberty. It needs to be differentiated from testicular atrophy. Cryptorchidism is an example of a condition that leads to testicular hypoplasia. It is the result of failure of testicular descent whereupon one or both testes may be arrested in the abdomen or inguinal ring. Usually testicular descent is completed by the time of birth. Rarely it occurs days after birth.

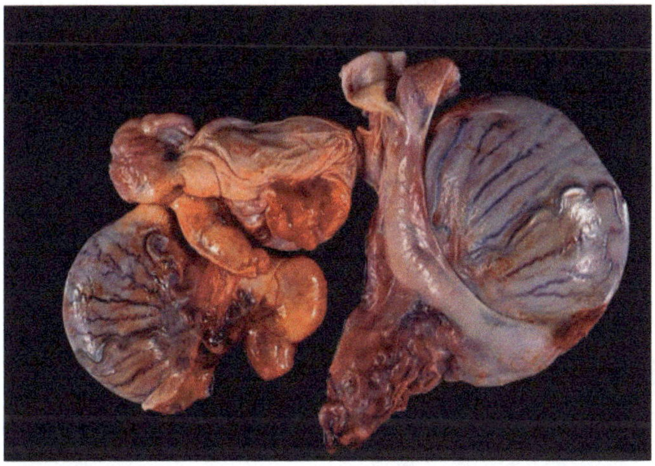

**Figure 12.3.** Horse. Testes. Unilateral Hypoplasia. Cryptorchidism. There is asymmetry in the testicular size with the smaller testis being hypoplastic from failing to descend into the scrotum.

## *3. Testicular degeneration/atrophy*

The seminiferous epithelium is very susceptible to a variety of adverse influences, and injury to the germ cell layers interfering with the spermatogenic cycle frequently induces degeneration with progression to testicular atrophy as end phase of the process.

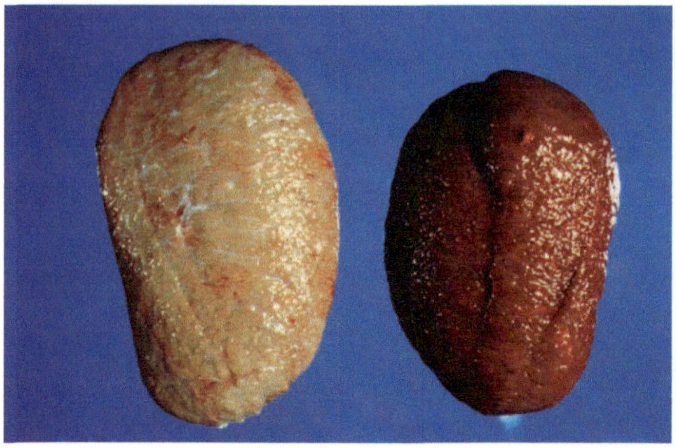

**Figure 12.4.** Horse. Testis. Unilateral Atrophy. The stallion had a unilateral inguinal hernia. The testis on the left is unaffected from the trauma. The testis on the right is small and dark. The red brown color is typical of atrophy. (Courtesy Dr. R. Foster, University of Guelph.)

The literature surprisingly contains very little information about primary testicular degeneration in the horse despite the obvious importance of reproductive health, particularly in breeding stallions. In general, testicular degeneration has a variety of exogenous and endogenous etiologies. It needs to be differentiated from testicular hypoplasia because diffuse, chronic degeneration results also in reduction of testicular size.

### 4. *Testicular inflammation*

Orchitis may start as periorchitis from a preceding, descending peritonitis, or it may ascend from an epididymitis, spread hematogenously, or develop secondary to trauma to the scrotum.

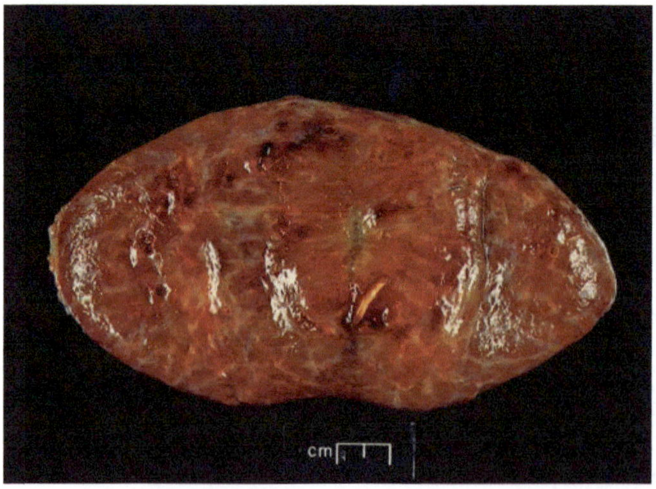


**Figure 12.5.** Horse. Testis. Chronic Verminous Orchitis. The parenchyma has a mottled white appearance indicating fibrosis and does not bulge on cut section. Causes for orchitis in the horse are bacteria such as *Actinobacillus equuli*, *Streptococcus* sp., *Staphylococcus* sp., and parasites such as migrating *Strongylus edentatus* larvae as has been the case in this image. (Reprinted with permission from Color Atlas of Reproductive Pathology of Domestic Animals, Buergelt, Figure 3-41, Page 40, Copyright Elsevier, 1997.)

## 5. Testicular neoplasia

Primary testicular neoplasms affect aged stallions. They are either sex cord (gonadal-stromal) tumors including Leydig cell (interstitial cell) and Sertoli cell tumors, or germ cell tumors to include seminomas and teratomas. Sex cord-stromal tumors are rare with individual case reports in the literature as is the case with mixed germ cell-sex cord-stromal tumors. Cryptorchid testicles in particular should be examined for hidden tumors.

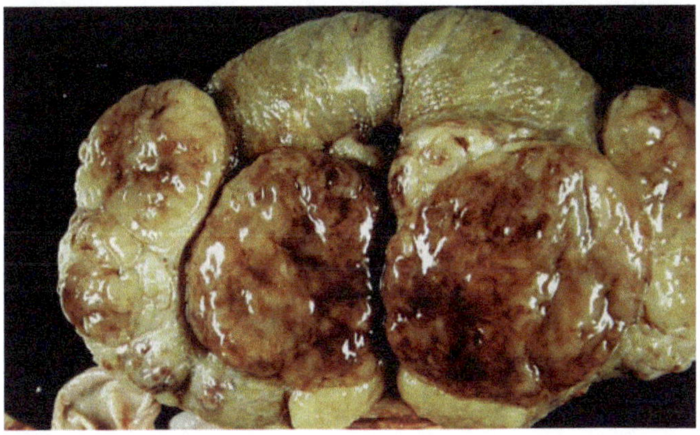

**Figure 12.6.** Horse. Testis. Seminoma. A multilobulated bulging mass has replaced the testicular parenchyma and has caused testicular enlargement. Seminomas are usually unilateral and malignant in horses.

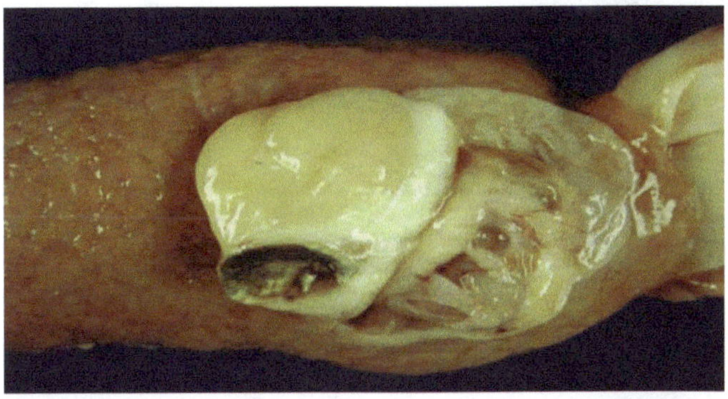

**Figure 12.7.** Horse. Testis. Benign Teratoma. This usually small tumor affects young individuals, deriving from various embryonic germ layers. The tumor may contain visible hair or bone. On occasion it is malignant with local invasion.

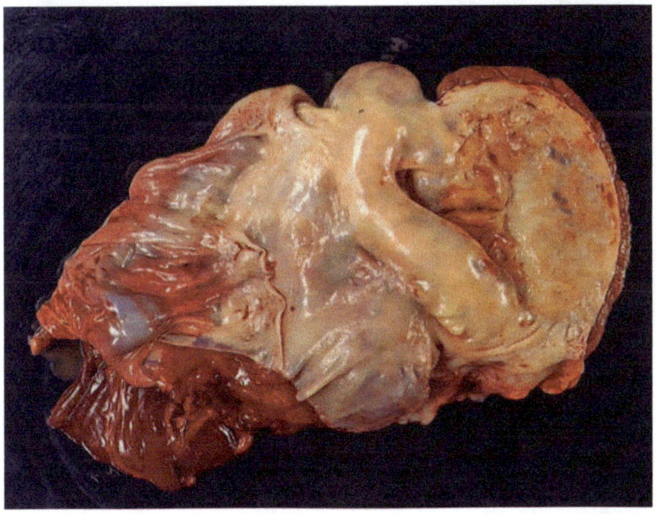

**Figure 12.8.** Horse. Testis. Leiomyosarcoma. This mesenchymal tumor arose from the tunica albuginea and spread into the space between epididymis and vaginal cavity.

## 6. Accessory male sex organs

Seminal Vesiculitis. Gram-negative bacteria such as *Pseudomonas aeruginosa* can be isolated from this uncommon inflammatory disorder.

## 7. External genitalia

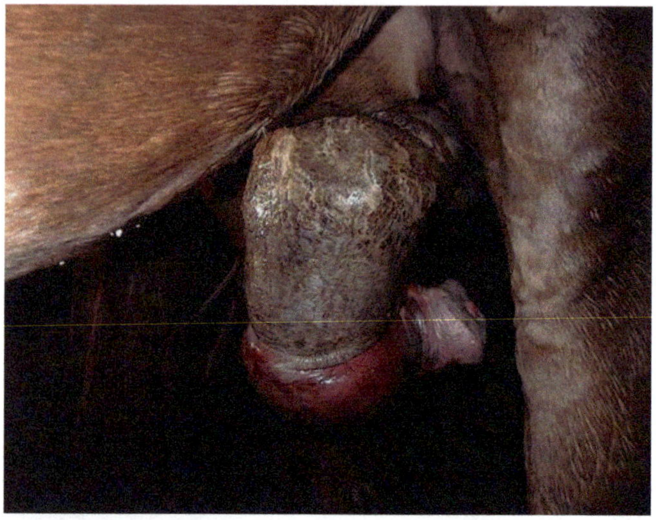

**Figure 12.9.** Horse. Penis. Paraphimosis. This condition is defined as the inability to withdraw the penis into the sheath. The opposite condition, the inability of the penis to extend from the sheath, is defined as phimosis. Paraphimosis occurs congenitally or is acquired after treatment with tranquilizing drugs. Postmortem paraphimosis occurs in conjunction with severe decomposition. (Courtesy Dr. P. Habecker, University of Pennsylvania.)

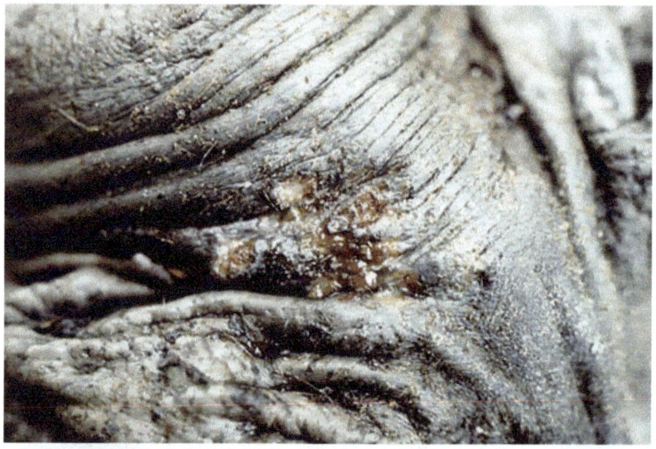

**Figure 12.10.** Horse. Penis. Coital Exanthema. Equine herpesvirus (EHV)-3 causes pustular and ulcerative balanoposthitis. Differential etiologies should include habronemiasis, early squamous cell carcinoma, frostbite, trauma, and infection with *Trypanosoma equiperdum* (equine dourine) in regions where this disease is endemic.

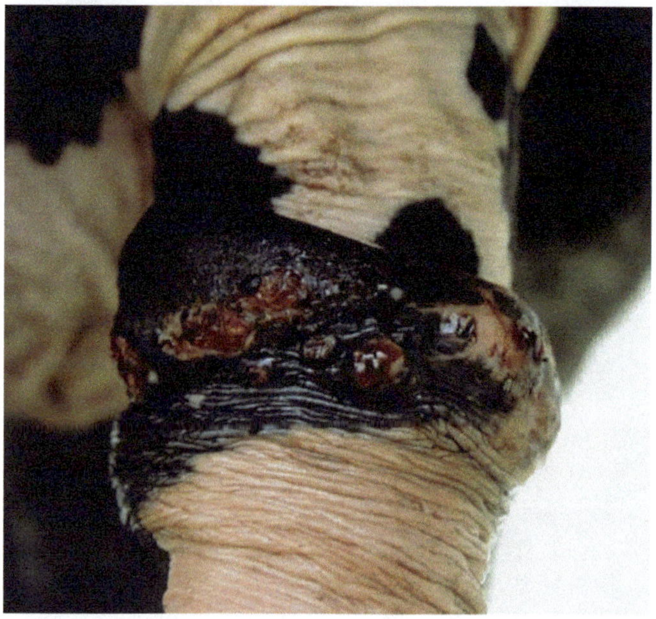

**Figure 12.11.** Horse. Penis. Ulcerative, Pyogranulomatous Balanitis. Habronemiasis. Severe, ulcerative, pyogranulomatous inflammation of the tip of the penis and prepuce (posthitis) can result from infestation of larvae of *Habronema* sp. that have a tissue preference for the urethral process. Immediate differential diagnosis should be squamous cell carcinoma.

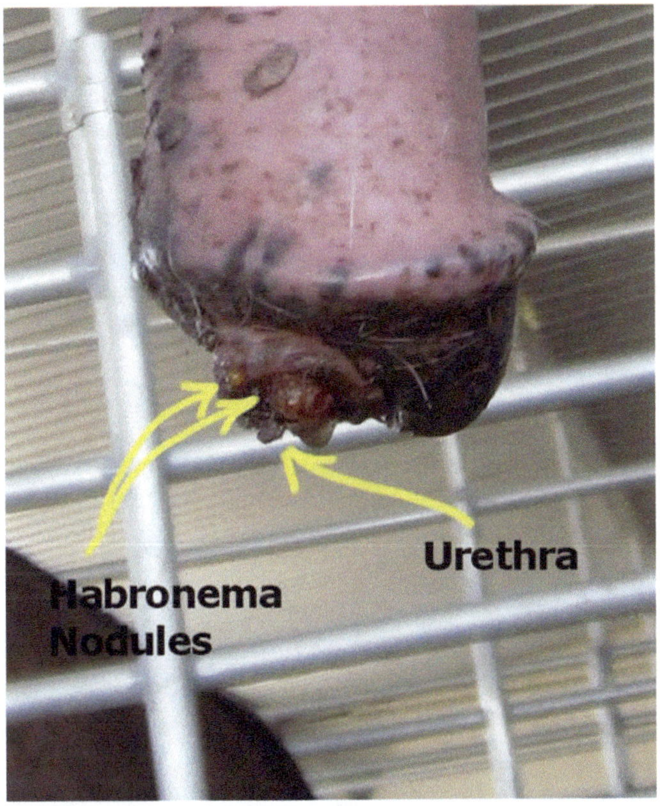


**Figure 12.12.** Horse. Tip of Penis. Habronemiasis. Hebronema larval nodules are present at the urethral orifice, a typical site of deposition. (Courtesy P. Isenbarg, Henderson, NV.)

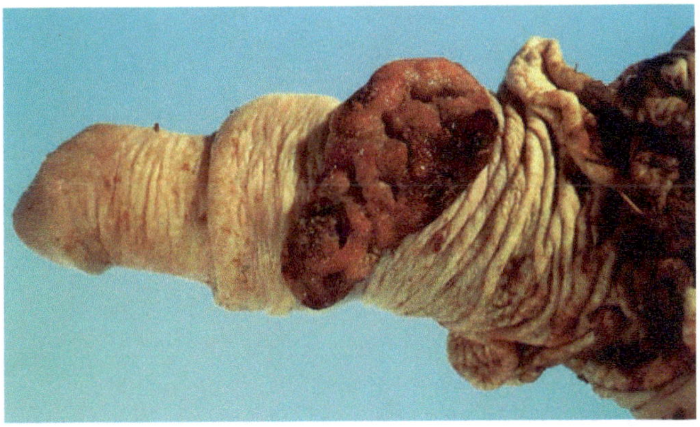

**Figure 12.13.** Horse. Prepuce. Squamous Cell Carcinoma. This neoplasm typically presents as a cauliflower-like ulcerative malodorous growth on the glans penis or prepuce with local invasion and metastasis to regional lymph nodes. Equine papilloma virus has been detected via molecular techniques in equine genital squamous cell carcinomas. Another neoplasm with similar biologic behavior at this penile site is melanoma in aged gray stallions.

## *8. Miscellaneous*

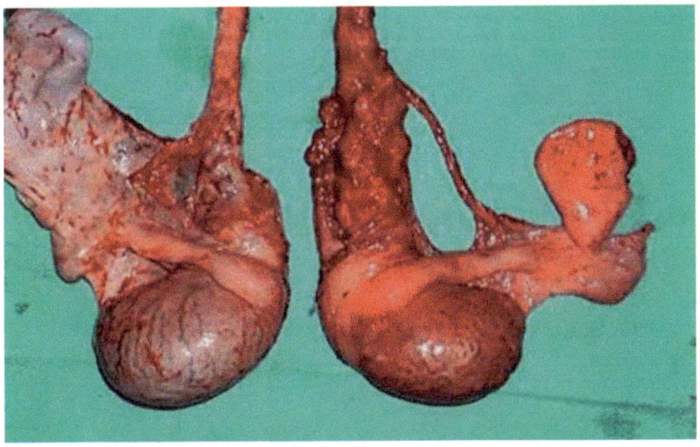

**Figure 12.14.** Horse. Testis. Unilateral Torsion with Ischemic Hemorrhagic Necrosis. This very painful condition is characterized by severe hemorrhagic infarction of the testis and its soft tissues as it twists around its longitudinal axis. The right testis depicted has twisted, with infarction, congestion, and mild atrophy being the principal changes. (Courtesy Dr. A. King, Drost Project, University of Florida.)

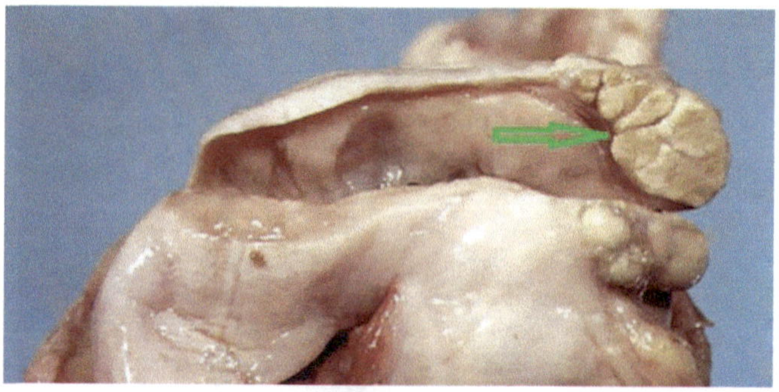

**Figure 12.15.** Horse. Testis. Tunica Albuginea. Ectopic Cortical Adrenal Tissue (arrow). Small discrete nodules on the surface are present.

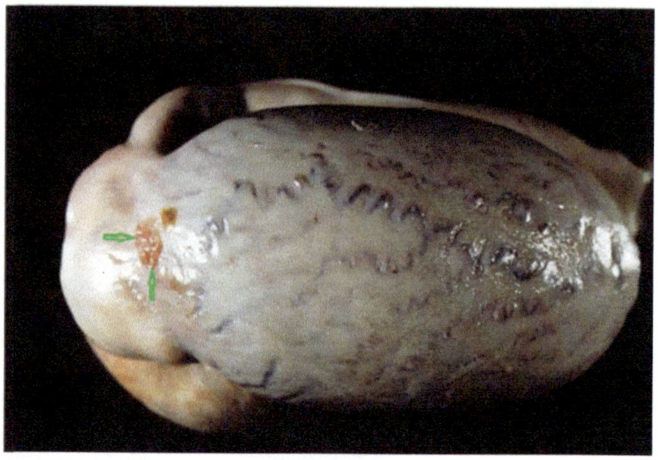

**Figure 12.16.** Horse. Testis. Nodules on Tunica Albuginea. Small discrete nodules on the surface of the gonad and adjacent to the head of the epididymis may be appendix testis (double arrow), a paramesonephric duct vestige.

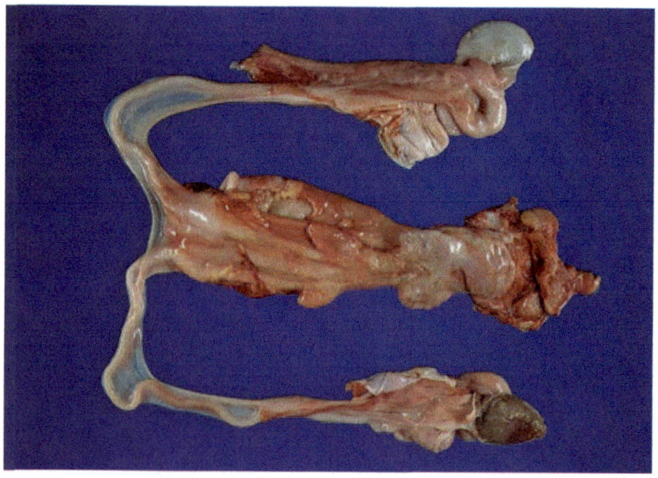

**Figure 12.17.** Horse. Reproductive Tract. Intersex. Intersexes are defined as individuals equivocal as to gender differentiation and phenotype. They are typically sterile and can be appropriately classified according to genotype by sex chromosomal analysis via karyotyping. This reproductive tract has been diagnosed as male pseudohermaphrodite with intra-abdominal testes, epididymes, spermatic cords, and thin tubular structures resembling a juvenile uterus. Externally, prepuce-like and penis-like structures can be expected in equine male intersexes.

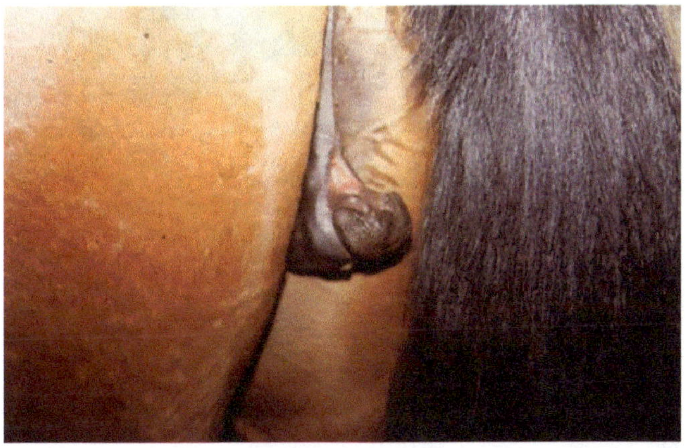

**Figure 12.18.** Horse. External Genitalia. Intersex. Externally, prepuce-like and/or penis-like structures can be expected in equine intersexes.

## II. Female (nonpregnant)

The equine female reproductive tract consists of ovaries, oviducts, uterus, cervix, and vagina representing accessory female sex organs. The function of the ovaries is to produce mature eggs and steroid hormones for the regulation of the reproductive tract in nonpregnant and pregnant conditions. The gametogenic and endocrine functions of the ovary work in a cyclic pattern.

### *1. Morphology of the normal mature equine ovary*

The mare's ovary has unique morphologic and functional features. The medulla is external to the cortex. Ovulation occurs at the site of the ovulation fossa. The Graafian follicles become quite large prior to ovulation measuring up to 6 cm and more in diameter and should not be confused with cystic follicles. The texture of the equine ovary is firm due to a very fibroblastic stroma and should not be mistaken for a mesenchymal tumor during gross and/or microscopic evaluations.

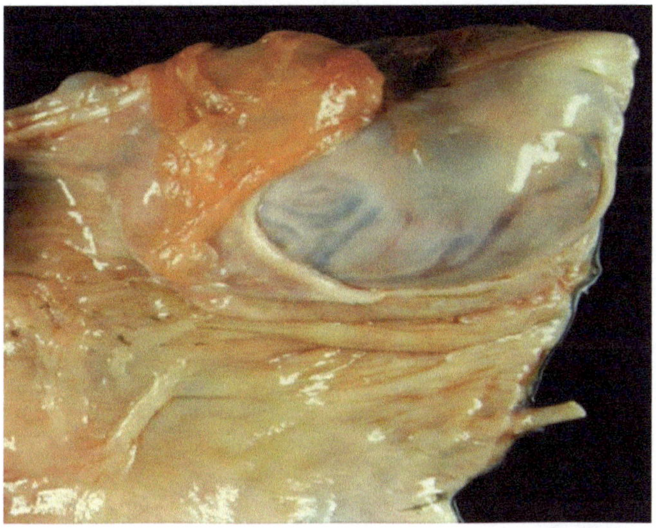

**Figure 12.19.** Horse. Ovary. Normal Configuration. The shape of the ovary is oval with the ovulation fossa being the concave portion adjacent to the fimbriae. The ovary is covered by a fibrous capsule.

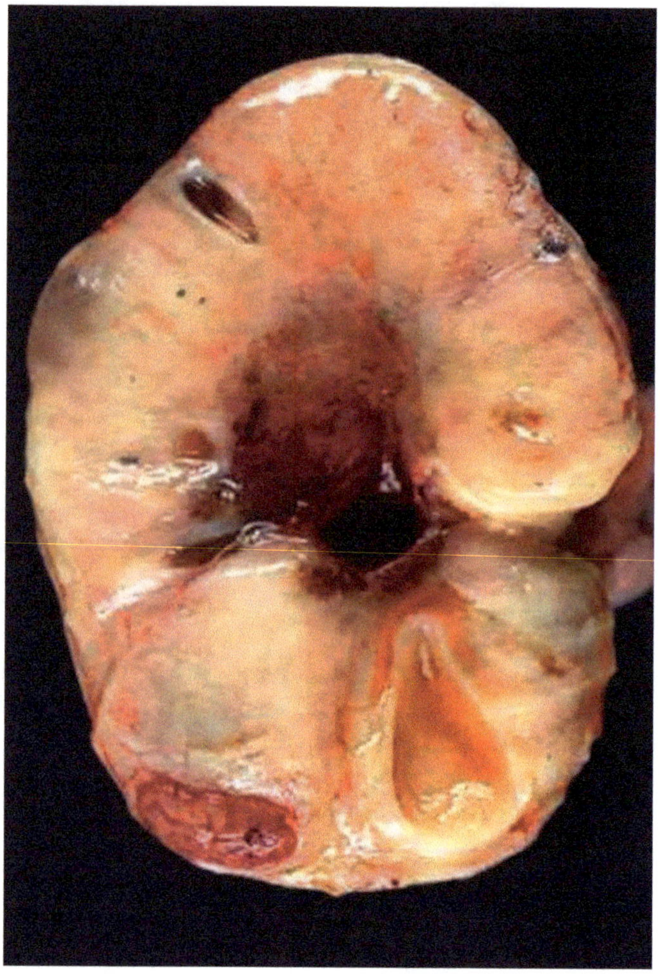

**Figure 12.20.** Horse. Cycling Ovary. On cross section, follicles and a corpus luteum are visible. (Courtesy Dr. J. Roberts, National Zoo, Washington, DC.)

## *2. Anomalies*

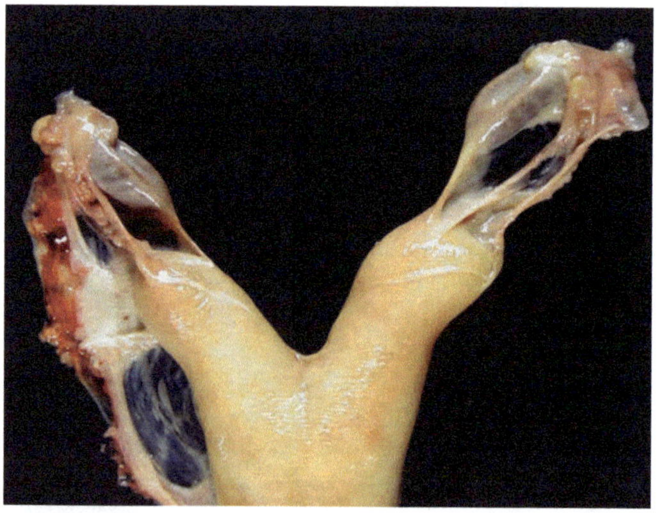

**Figure 12.21.** Horse. Genital Tract. Turner Syndrome. This chromosomal abnormality characterized by an XO karyotype leads to noncycling ovaries and a juvenile female reproductive tract.

X monosomy appears to be a relatively common cytogenetic disorder in mares. Affected animals appear normal externally but with smaller than normal vulva. The uterus is also small, the cervix usually open and flaccid. The ovaries range in size from small to very small. Most XO mares fail to cycle, although some show sporadic or indistinct periods of estrous behavior.

### 3. *Ovarian cysts*

These are either next to the ovary, defined as parovarian cysts and congenital in origin (remnants of the mesonephric ducts or tubules), or intraovarian and depending on the histologic features, also congenital or acquired. Appropriate classification requires histologic examination of cyst lining and wall composition.

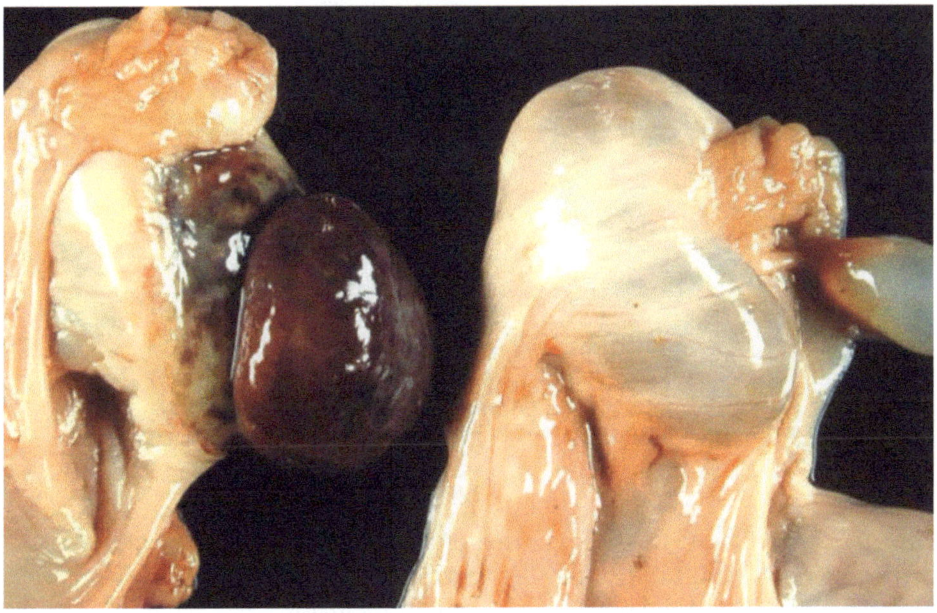

**Figure 12.22** Horse. Left Ovary. Corpus Hemorrhagicum. Hemorrhage occurring into the cavity of the follicle after ovulation produces a corpus hemorrhagicum. Right Ovary. Parovarian Cyst. The cysts are lined by a single layer of cuboidal epithelium and contain clear fluid. About ten morphologic different parovarian and intraovarian cysts may occur. These have to be differentiated by microscopic examination.

### 4. *Ovarian inflammation*

Inflammation of the ovaries is extremely rare in horses. If present, it results from an adjacent peritonitis.

### 5. *Ovarian neoplasia*

Typically in the mare these would be sex cord-stromal tumors known as granulosa cell tumors. The tumors are usually unilateral and benign, and they may reach the size of a grapefruit. They are hormonally active, produce inhibin, estrogens, or androgens, and consequently interfere with the estrous cycle. The contralateral ovary may undergo atrophy. Surgical removal is curative. Germ cell tumors such as dysgerminoma or teratoma are very rare.

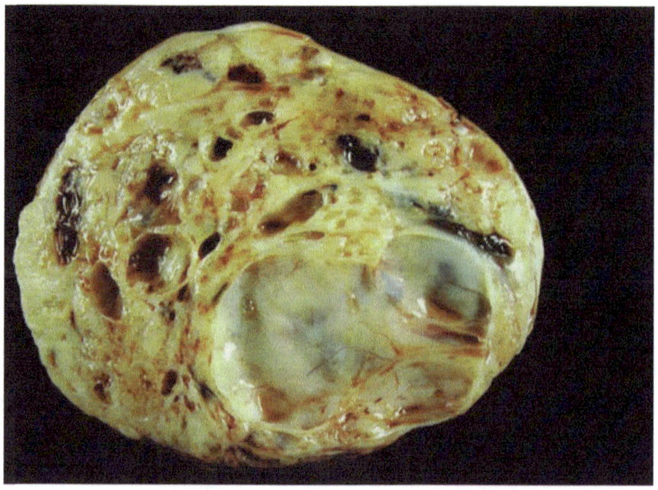

**Figure 12.23.** Horse. Ovary. Granulosa Cell Tumor. The typical appearance on cross section is characterized by multiple cystic spaces separated by dense stromal tissue. Differential diagnoses should consider the infrequent germinal inclusion cyst and cystadenomas.

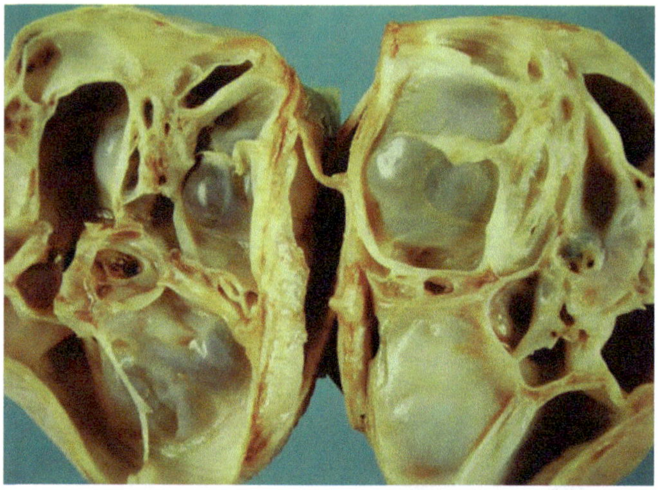

**Figure 12.24.** Horse. Ovary. Cystadenoma. Very rare. This is an example of benign neoplastic intraovarian cysts progressively occupying the entire ovary. (Reprinted with permission from Color Atlas of Reproductive Pathology of Domestic Animals, Buergelt, Figure 9-36, Page 109, Copyright Elsevier, 1997.)

The case was diagnosed as cystadenoma. Cystadenomas are rare, mostly unilateral polycystic tumors that do not metastasize or are not hormonally active. The differential diagnosis is germinal inclusion cysts when peritoneal cells become entrapped in the ovary after ovulation to fill with fluid and to expand within the ovary.

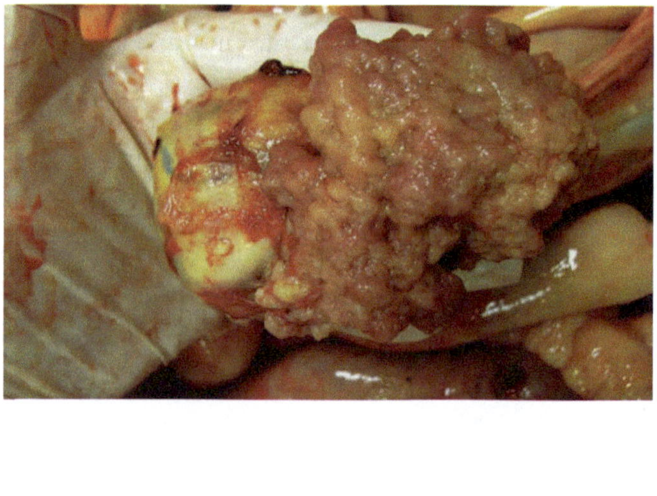

**Figure 12.25.** Horse. Ovary. Papillary Carcinoma of Ovulation Fossa. This shaggy tumor arose from the surface epithelial cells of the ovary. Its occurrence is extremely unique in the horse. (Courtesy Dr. P. Habecker, University of Pennsylvania.)

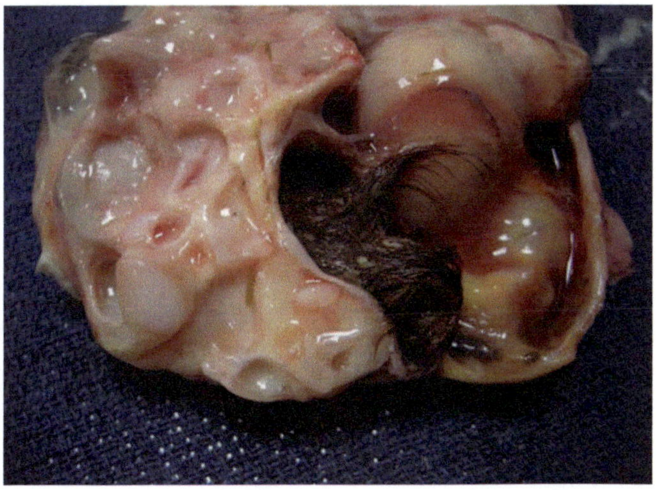

**Figure 12.26.** Horse. Ovary. Benign Teratoma. On cross section an encapsulated cystic growth contains packaged hair in the center. This type of usually benign tumor is composed of multiple tissues foreign to the organ in which they arise.

## 6. *Endometritis*

The main function of the uterus is to provide a protective environment for the gamete and conceptus in the case of pregnancy. The uterus is a target organ for ovarian hormones and responds to hormones secreted by the ovary. The uterus is susceptible to bacteria and fungi that may induce inflammation at the endometrial and myometrial level and possibly progress into pyometra. EHV-1 and equine arteritis virus are able to induce endometrial vasculitis and thrombosis, lesions that are among the triggering factors of abortion caused by these viruses.

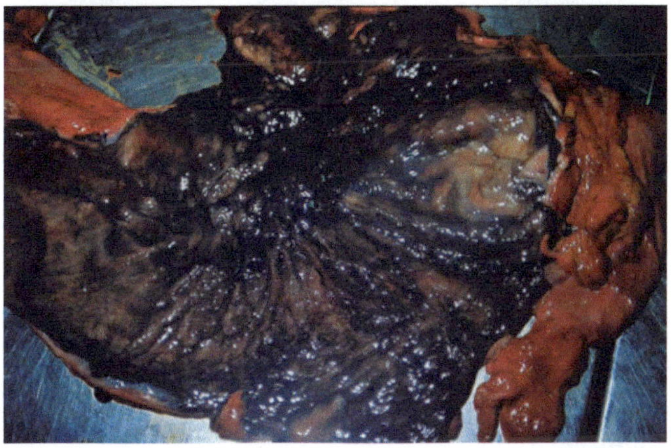

**Figure 12.27.** Horse. Uterus. Necrotizing Endometritis. Pseudomelanosis. The endometrium is thickened and covered by a fibrinous exudate mixed with necrotic tissue. The exudate can be of milky appearance in case of *Tylorella equigenitalis* (Contagious Equine Metritis [CEM]) infection, a reportable disease.

## 7. *Endometrial biopsy*

The endometrial biopsy is considered a tool to assess reproductive health in the mare and to assess the mare's ability to carry a conceptus to term. There are several grading schemes with the grading system established by Robert Kenney the most widely used. The results of the biopsy should be integrated into other findings by ancillary tests such as microbiology and the mare's history.

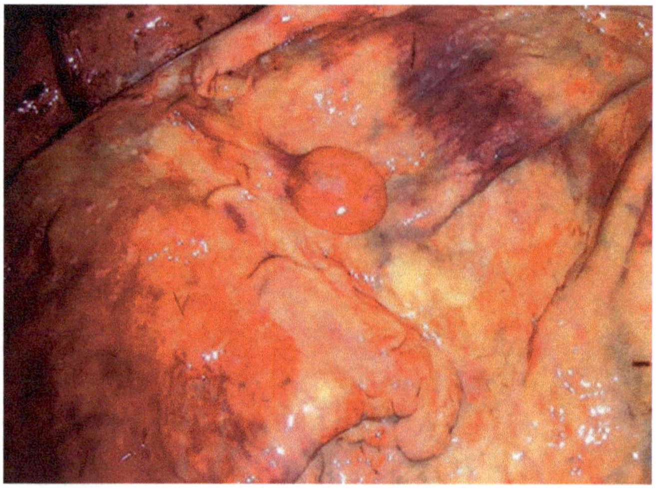

**Figure 12.28.** Horse. Uterus. Lymphatic Cyst. These result from the obstruction of the lymphatic flow in lymphatic vessels of the uterine wall creating lymphatic lacunae. They are grossly visible as pedunculated or sessile distensions containing clear fluid and protruding into the uterine lumen. They are also present on the serosal surface of the uterus.

### *8. Uterine neoplasia*

Primary tumors of the uterus of the mare are extremely rare and may be mesenchymal in origin such as leiomyoma. Lymphoma may occur as a rare secondary tumor.

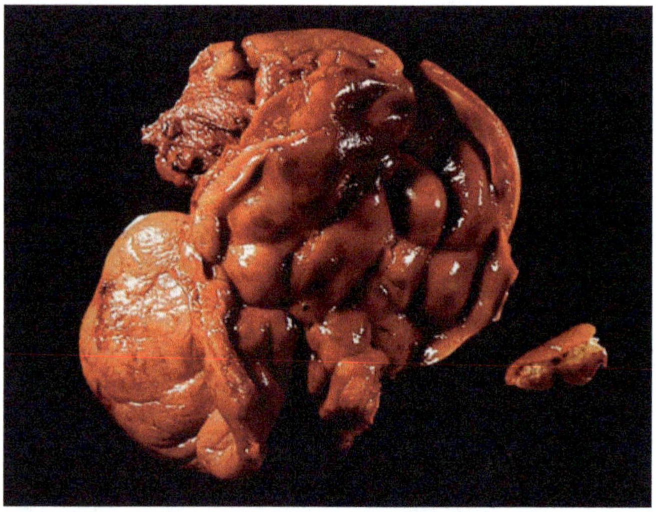

**Figure 12.29.** Horse. Uterus. Lymphoma. Tan nodular tissue proliferations elevate the endometrium.

### *9. External genitalia*

EHV-3 (coital exanthema) may produce a mild pustular and erosive to ulcerative vulvovaginits. Bacteria in combination with trauma also cause vulvovaginitis.

Tumors of the vulva may be melanomas or squamous cell carcinomas.

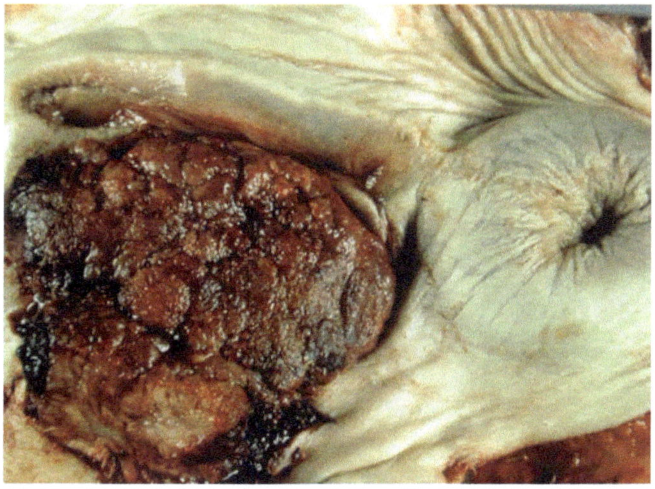

**Figure 12.30.** Horse. Vulva. Squamous Cell Carcinoma. This condition is the female counterpart of penile or peripenile squamous cell carcinoma. (Reprinted with permission from Color Atlas of Reproductive Pathology in Domestic Animals, Buergelt, Figure 11-22, Page 139, Copyright Elsevier, 1997.)

## III. Female (pregnant)

### *1. Placental membranes and umbilicus*

To understand pathogenic aspects of pregnancy and pregnancy disturbances, the concept of placentation needs introduction. The placenta as a diverse temporary organ facilitates mechanical protection and nutrition of the developing conceptus. It is involved in nutrient, gas, and waste product exchange at the maternal–fetal interface. In addition, the placenta produces enzymes, prostaglandins, and cytokines such as $\gamma$ interferon necessary for the attachment and viability of the fetus. The placenta also produces transient hormones such as progesterone to maintain pregnancy.

Placentas are anatomically classified at the gross and microscopic level, the latter on the basis of proximity of the fetal circulation to that of the mother. In the mare placentation is classified at the gross level as diffuse and at the microscopic level as epitheliochorial. The fetus is surrounded by two sets of placental membranes separated by two cavities filled with defined amounts of fluid from fetal excretions (fetal urine within the allantois cavity) and secretions (oral and lung fluid) within the amniotic cavity. The outer fetal membrane is the chorioallantois with the chorionic surface resting against the uterine endometrium. The second membrane is the amnioallantois enveloping the fetus. Fetal membranes are usually expelled within 30 minutes after parturition; retained placental membranes result in serious conditions of metritis, endotoxemia, and laminitis. Maternal connection of the fetus is through the umbilical cord.

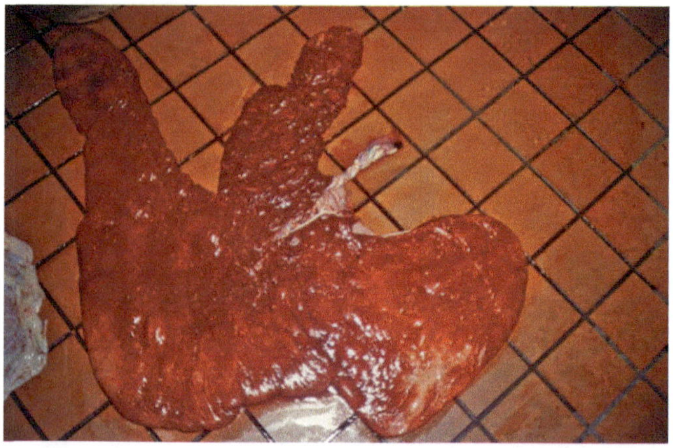

**Figure 12.31.** Horse. Chorioallantois. Normal Surface. The chorionic surface has a velvety red surface as the result of a rich circulation within the microcotyledons. It follows the shape of the pregnant uterus, reflecting the uterine body and the pregnant and the nonpregnant horn.

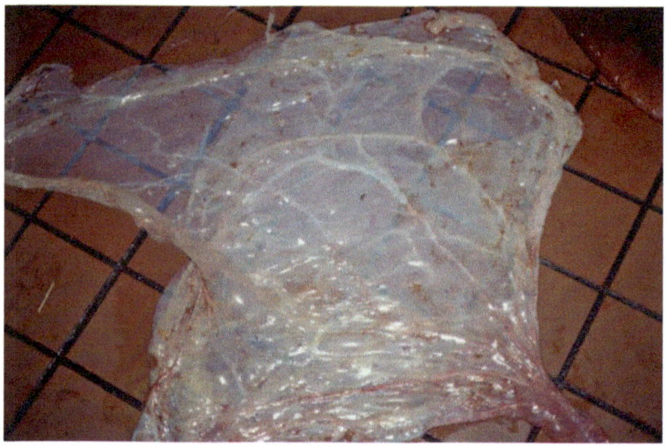

**Figure 12.32.** Horse. Amnioallantois. Normal Surface. The amnion is a thin, white, smooth, semitranslucent membrane containing coiled muscular arteries. Increase in tortuosity may indicate amnion expansion during body pregnancy. These vessels are normally prominently coiled in donkeys, hinnies, and mules.

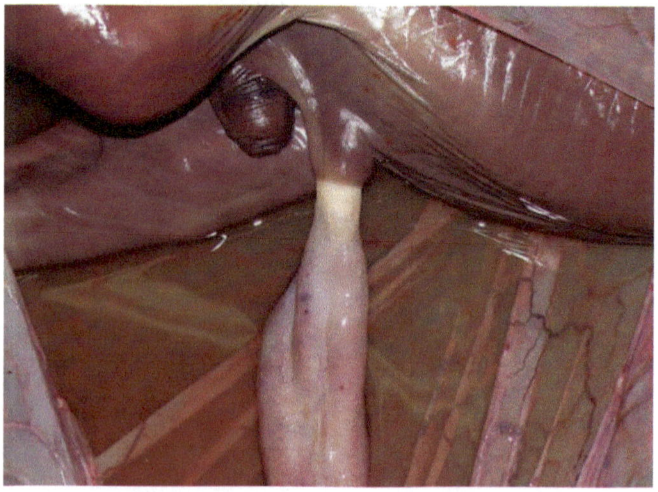

**Figure 12.33.** Fetus. Umbilical Cord. Normal. Attachment of the fetus to the fetal membranes is through the umbilicus. In the region covered by the amnionic portion, the umbilicus contains the urachus, two arteries, and one fused vein; in the region covered by the chorion, it contains the urachus, yolk-sac remnants, two arteries, and two veins. (Courtesy Dr. J. Roberts, National Zoo, Washington, DC.)

## 2. *Incidental findings associated with the placental membranes*



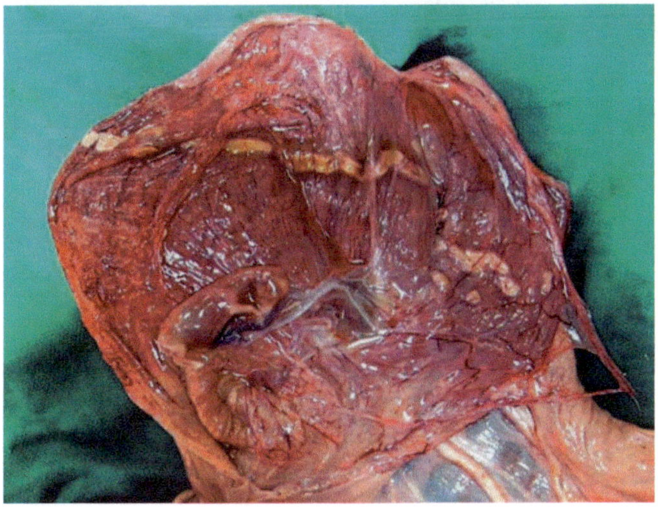

**Figure 12.34.** Horse. Endometrium. Endometrial Cups. Raised circular structures on the endometrial surface of the caudal portion of the uterus develop between days 40 and 100 of gestation and involute thereafter. The cups are composed of trophoblasts enveloping endometrial glands and are of fetal origin. They produce equine chorionic gonadotropin involved in maintaining pregnancy during this period of gestation. A 60-day fetus is present.

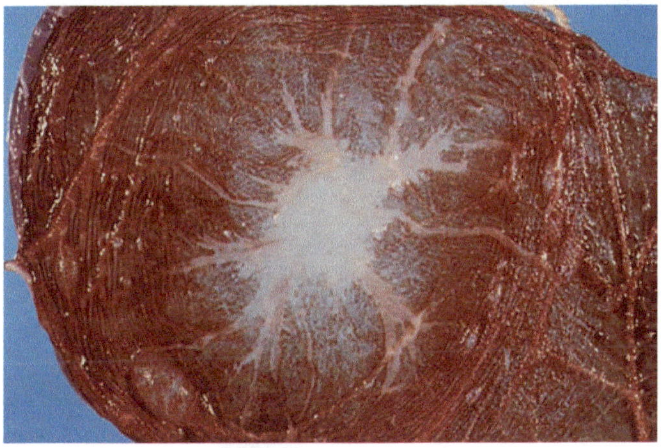

**Figure 12.35.** Horse. Chorion. Cervical Star. This starlike configuration of the chorion at the cervical location indicates absence of microcotyledons as the chorion rests against the inner cervix. It should not be confused with villous atrophy associated with placental insufficiency.

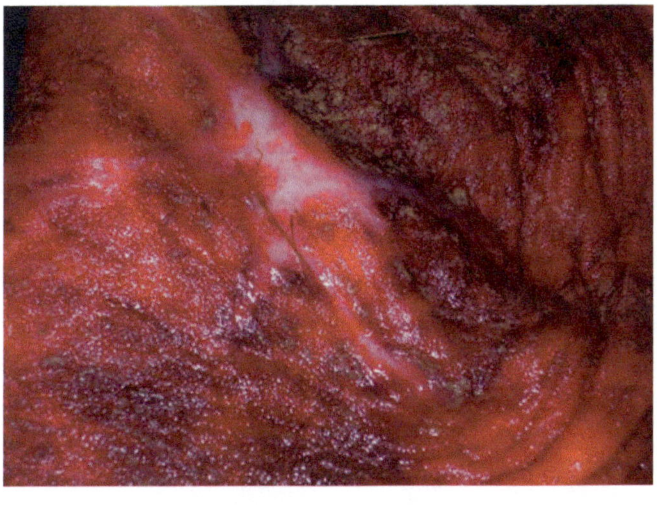

**Figure 12.36.** Horse. Chorion. Mineralization. Calcium is deposited in a network of white spots. The significance of mineralization in equine placental membranes is not well understood. Portions of the cervical star are visible in the center of the image.

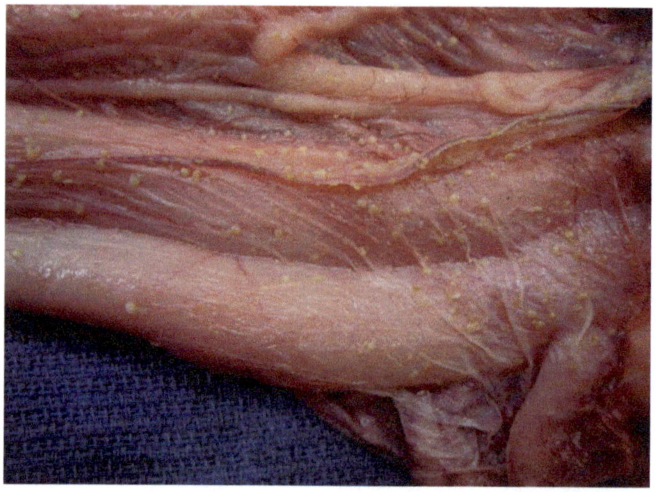

**Figure 12.37.** Horse. Amnion and Umbilical Cord. Amniotic Plaques (Amniotic Pustules). The focal, tan elevations represent plaques, foci of epithelial squamous cell metaplasia. They should not be confused with mycotic lesions. They may occasionally mineralize. There is also evidence of edema of the amniotic stroma.

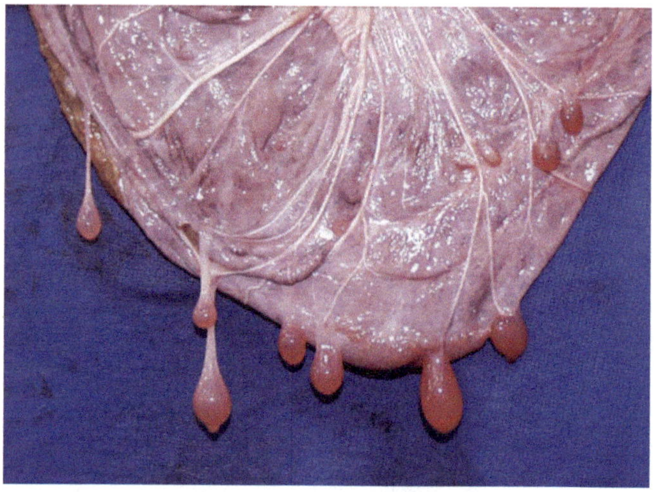

**Figure 12.38.** Horse. Allantois. Vesicles, Cysts, and Pouches. These small pedunculated outgrowths are filled with fluid and epithelial debris. Likewise fluid-filled sessile pouches may develop. It is thought that these structures are degenerating endometrial cups enfolded by chorioallantoic tissue.

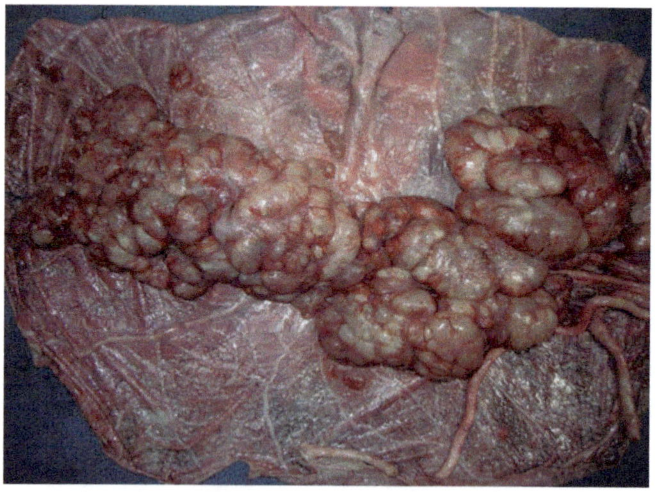

**Figure 12.39.** Horse. Allantois. Adenomatous Hyperplasia. Tumor-like nodules, present near the umbilical stalk or elsewhere, are the result of proliferating fluid-filled gland-like allantoic epithelial structures into the allantoic stroma. It has been associated with chronic placentitis, as in this case.

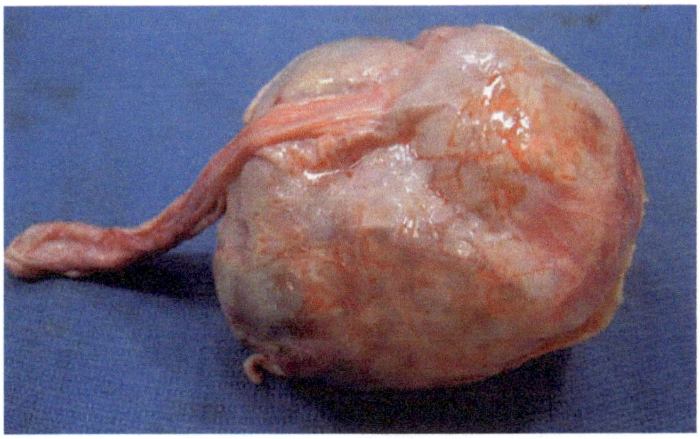

**Figure 12.40.** Fetus. Umbilical Cord. Yolk Sac Remnant. Globoid round ossified variably sized (1–15 cm in diameter) structures are typically attached to the umbilicus by a vesicular stalk. The structures have a smooth surface, a thin, crepitating wall, and are hollow when opened. They are incidental findings , but this one was 15 cm in diameter and associated with dystocia. It mimics an incomplete twin.

### *3. Disturbances of pregnancy*

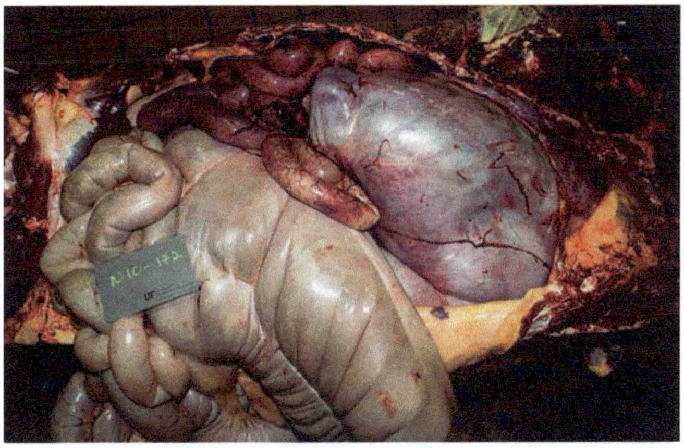

**Figure 12.41.** Horse. Abdomen. Uterine Torsion. The pregnant horn twisted along its longitudinal axis is congested. When not corrected immediately, such a condition leads due to ischemia, even rupture of the uterine wall and demise of the fetus in utero.

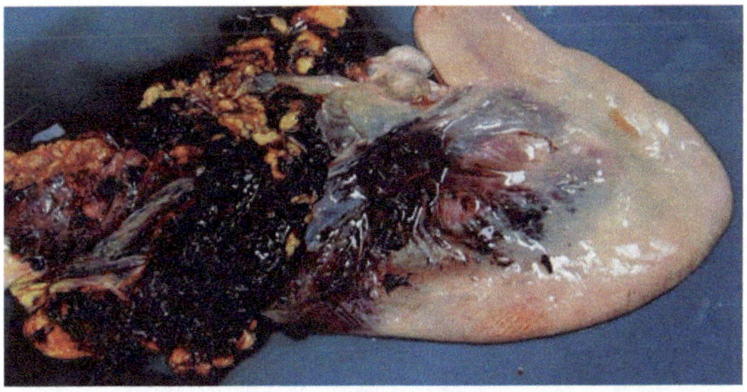

**Figure 12.42.** Horse. Uterus. Rupture of Uterine Artery. Sudden exsanguination into the wall of the uterus, broad ligament, and abdomen results from rupture of a weakened middle uterine artery during term gestation. Older mares having given birth to several foals are affected. Age-associated degenerative changes in the vessel wall predispose to aneurysmal dissection.

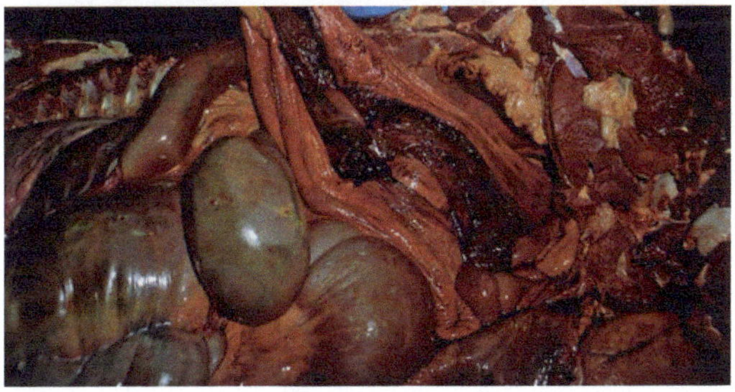

**Figure 12.43.** Horse. Uterus. Laceration after Parturition. A long tear is present in one of the horns.

Other causes interfering with pregnancy are hydroallantois and hydramnion.

## IV. Noninfectious abortion diseases

Noninfectious causes of abortion are sometimes difficult to determine. In this category, established causes in the mare include placental insufficiency as to microcotyledonary function, premature placental separation, twinning, umbilical cord length abnormalities, fescue grass toxicosis, and environmental contamination by an overpopulation of eastern tent caterpillars (*Malacosoma americanum*).

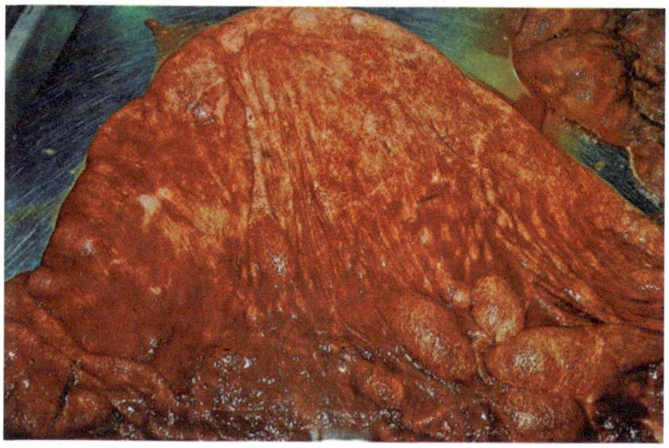

**Figure 12.44.** Horse. Chorion. Atrophy of Villi. Extensive loss of microcotyledons on the chorionic surface results in placental dysfunction and inhibition of fetal growth. It may be associated with cysts and endometrial fibrosis in the mare, body pregnancy, or twinning where the two chorionic surfaces are in contact. Villous atrophy is grossly characterized as pallor of the chorionic surface.

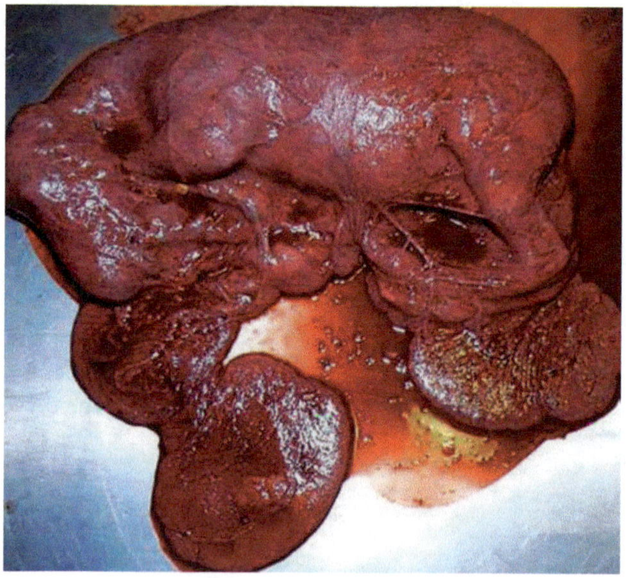

**Figure 12.45.** Fetus. Chorion. "Red Bag." The separated chorion failed to evert to the allantoic surface when passed though the birth canal. Premature separation of the chorion may be responsible. Predisposing factors to consider are EHV-1 endometrial vasculitis, placentitis, systemic illness, drug administration, and fetal death in utero. (Courtesy Dr. J. Roberts, National Zoo, Washington, DC.)

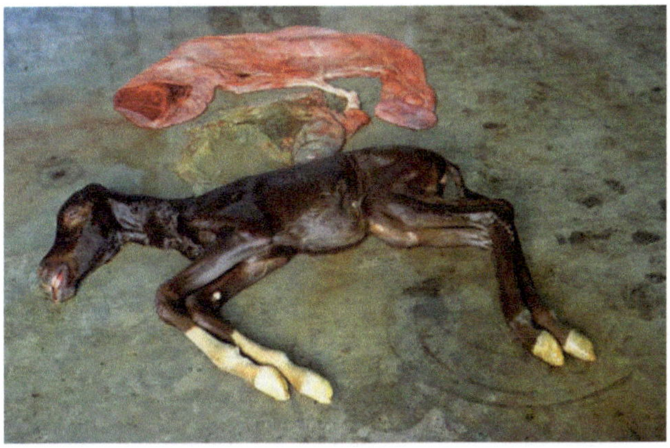

**Figure 12.46.** Fetus. Fetal Membranes. Hypoplasia. The size of the chorion and amnion is reduced leading to placental insufficiency, in utero death, and abortion. Meconium staining caused by fetal diarrhea is also present.

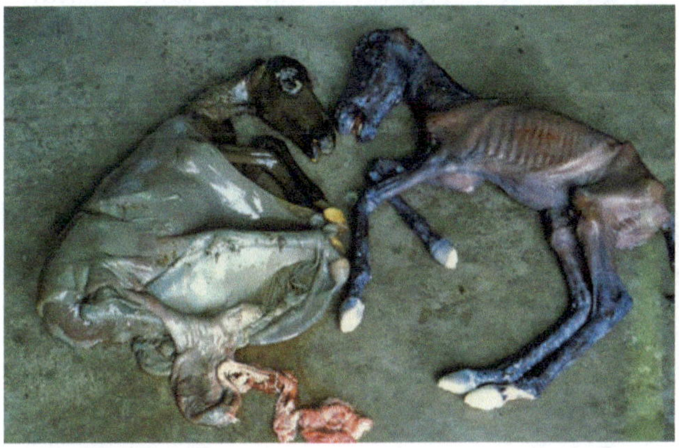

**Figure 12.47.** Fetal Bodies. Abortion from Twinning. The fetus on the left underwent in utero death and decomposition from umbilical cord strangulation.

Advanced twin pregnancy results in abortion and was the most common cause of noninfectious abortions before the event of iatrogenic blastocyst squeezing for the elimination of one twin. Carrying dizygotic twins results in fetal death and abortion in up to 29% of aborted fetal accessions at 8–9 months of gestation. It has been hypothesized that insufficient chorionic placentation is responsible for the death of one or both twins in utero. The close apposition of twins in utero leads to a circumscribed avillous area that may be extensive enough for placental insufficiency. But also decrease of the overall combined placental weight may contribute to insufficient placental function. It has been suggested that weighing the placenta postpartum is an objective estimate of the health of the fetal placental unit. The combined placental weight of the chorioallantois and amnioallantois is normally 10% of the foal's birth weight with the normal placental weight in Thoroughbreds ranging between 4 kg and 8 kg.

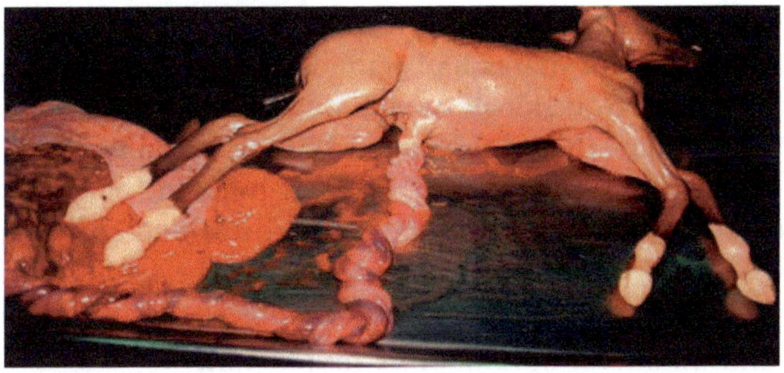

**Figure 12.48.** Fetus. Umbilical Cord. Excessive Twisting. Excessive length, pathologic torsion with edema and hemorrhage.

The umbilical cord normally contains a certain set of twists. If too numerous they may lead to fetal death in an over-lengthy umbilical cord (more than 45 cm in Thoroughbreds). Normal cord length in Thoroughbreds is 40–45 cm. Thickening from edema and umbilical vascular thrombosis or hemorrhage are circumstantial indicators for a pathologically twisted umbilical cord. The torsion generally involves the amniotic portion of the cord, less frequently the allantoic portion, and occasionally both.

### *1. Fescue grass toxicosis*

An important cause of amnionic edema has been reported in pregnant mares grazing on fascue grass pastures being contaminated by the fungal endophyte *Neotyphodium* (formerly *Acremonium) coenophialum*). The endophyte produces the toxic ergot alkaloid ergovaline that causes dysmaturity in foals and infrequent abortions. Ergovaline blocks prolactin, which is important for corpus luteum maintenance and milk production in the lactating mare. Mares are agalactic with minimal colostrum production. Foals die from suffocation within a thickened edematous amnion.

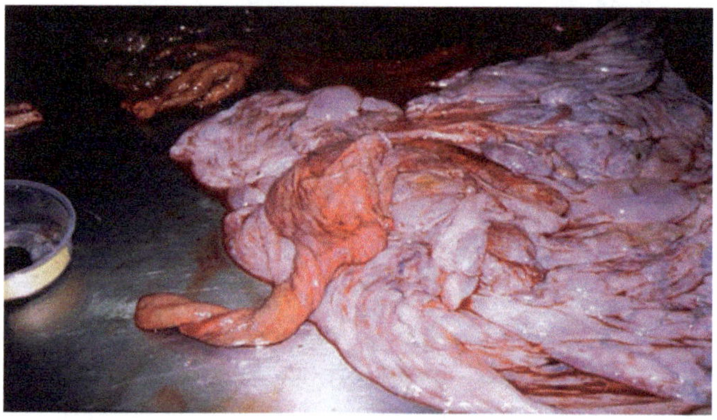

**Figure 12.49.** Horse. Amnion. Edema. Fluid is thickening the amniotic stroma. (Courtesy Dr. J. Roberts, National Zoo, Washington, DC.)

Thickening of placental membranes by edema is indicative of circulatory failure resulting from a variety of causes.

### *2. Mare reproductive loss syndrome*

A combination of unusual weather conditions, excessive blossoming of wild cherry trees (principal food source for caterpillars) and an overpopulation of eastern tent caterpillars (*Malacosoma americana*) lead to explosion of equine abortion in Kentucky between 2001 and 2002. Foals were aborted in early and late term pregnancies. Consistent findings in late term aborted fetuses were funisitis (funicular omphalophlebitis) and amnionitis. Extensive investigation into the causative circumstances and many experiments led to the incrimination of caterpillar setae responsible for the abortions. Caterpillars ingested by pregnant mares had setae hair migrating through the intestinal wall and hematogenously reaching the umbilicus and placental membranes to induce the observed pathologic changes and subsequent abortions. The setae breaching the intestinal mucosal barrier wall became contaminated by gastrointestinal β nonhemolytic *Streptococcus* sp. and *Actinobacillus* sp. to carry those hematogenously to the fetus resulting in fetal septicemia and death. Other pathologic lesions in adult animals included pericarditis and unilateral ophthalmitis (hyphema).

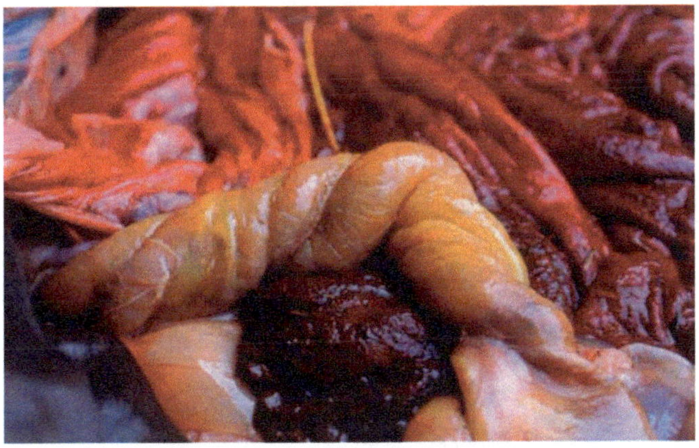

**Figure 12.50.** Fetus. Umbilical Cord. Amniotic Portion. Funisitis. Mare Reproductive Loss Syndrome (MRLS). The cord is edematous and yellowish discolored. (Courtesy Dr. J. Roberts, National Zoo, Washington, DC.)

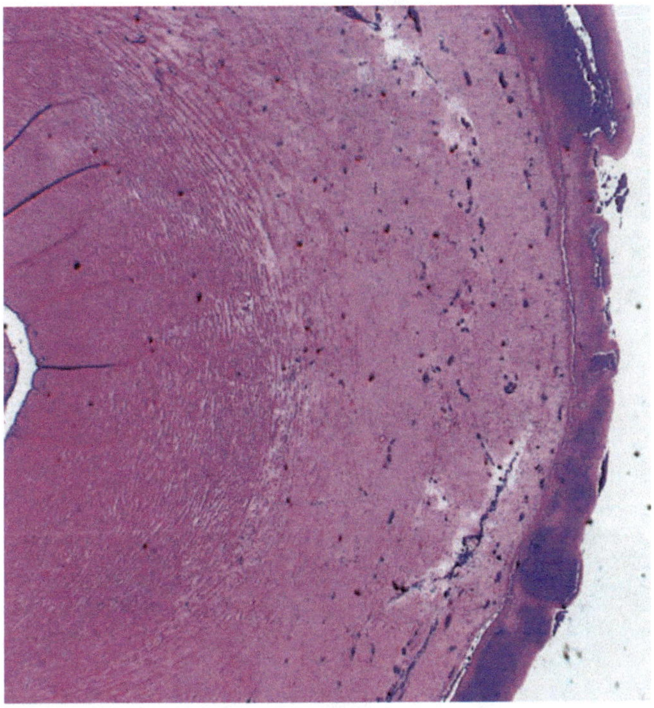

**Figure 12.51.** Fetus. Umbilical Cord. Fibrinonecrotic Funisitis. MRLS. Microscopic changes include fibrin, neutrophils, and bacterial colonies on the surface of the umbilicus. (H&E) (Courtesy Dr. M. Sebastian, University of Kentucky.)

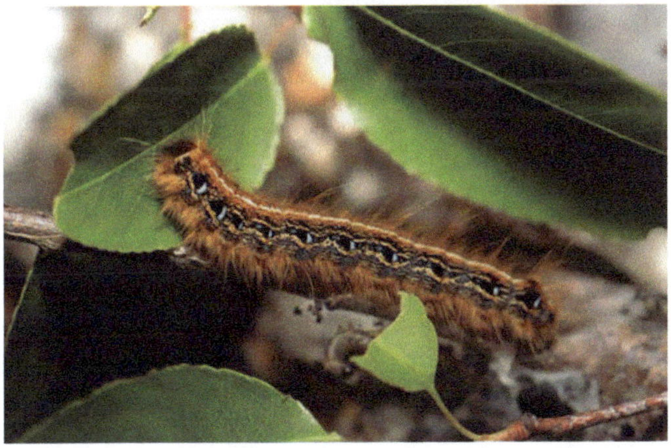

**Figure 12.52.** Eastern Tent Caterpillar (*Melacosoma americana*). Setae on the surface when ingested and digested by the pregnant mare penetrate through the intestinal wall carrying microorganisms with them during the migration. (Courtesy Dr. J. Roberts, National Zoo, Washington, DC.)

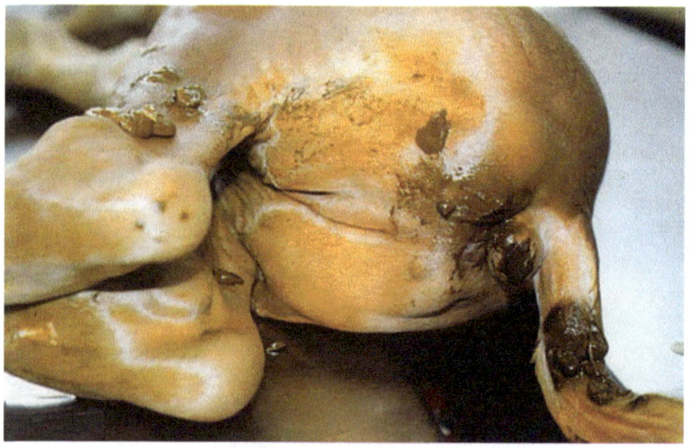

**Figure 12.53.** Fetus. Body. Fetal Stress Syndrome/Fetal Diarrhea. The tail and hind legs of this term fetus are pasted with soft meconium. Normally meconium is passed within a few hours after birth. Hypoxia and/or stress stimulate in utero fetal defecation into the amniotic cavity.

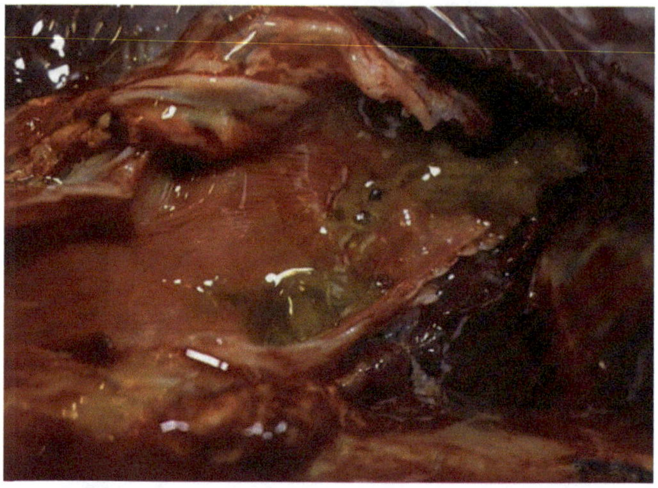

**Figure 12.54.** Fetus. Trachea. Meconium Aspiration.

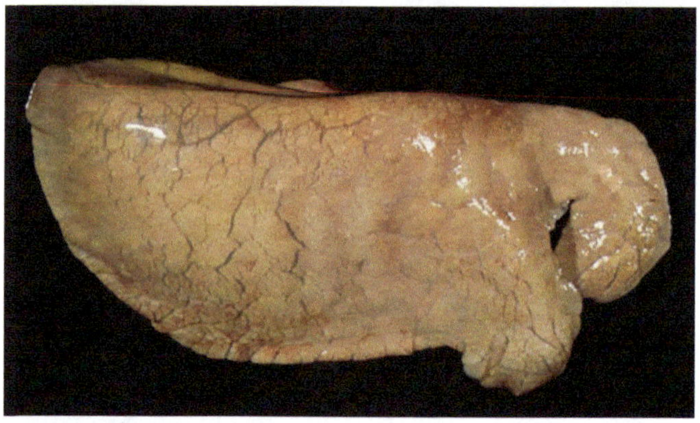

**Figure 12.55.** Fetus. Lung. Meconium Aspiration. The lung is diffusely yellowish with expanded interlobular septa, suggesting aspiration of amniotic fluid containing meconium. (Courtesy Dr. P. Habecker, University of Pennsylvania.)

Fetal stress syndrome is characterized by respiratory failure resulting from aspirated meconium that inhibits phagocytosis by macrophages and stimulates respiratory bursts in alveolar macrophages. The stressed fetus voids within the amniotic cavity and aspirates the meconium. Sterile granulomatous pneumonia may also occur.

## V. Infectious abortion diseases

Abortigenic agents in the mare are viruses, bacteria, protozoa, and fungi. Portals of entry are twofold with the ascending route the major modality for bacteria and fungi and the hematogenous transplacental route for viruses and some bacteria such as *Leptospira* sp. Abortions ensue secondary to fetal death in utero whether it is due to lesions in the pregnant uterus (viral arteritis virus and herpesvirus), placental membranes (bacteria and fungi), or fetus (herpesvirus and some bacteria).

In principle, infectious causes of abortion are more common than noninfectious. Up to 60% of abortions in horses are caused by infectious agents.

Surveys found viral infection in 23% of the aborted foals submitted, bacterial agents in 24%, and fungal infection in 2% of the cases.

### 1. *Equine viral abortions*

#### *a. Equine herpesvirus abortion (EHV)*

Abortion resulting from EHV-1 (occasionally type 4) usually occurs during the ninth or tenth month of pregnancy. Fetal death does not occur until the onset of abortion; the expelled foal is therefore well preserved, with little autolysis. Infected foals may be born alive but are weak and die shortly after parturition from pneumonia. The mare usually shows no signs of clinical illness at the time of abortion. The incidence of abortion may reach up to 90% in unvaccinated pregnant brood mares on the farm. Necrosis and inflammation may affect multiple organs of the infected fetus including lung, liver, adrenal glands, thymus, lymph nodes, and spleen. Newborns infected in utero mainly present necrotizing bronchiolitis with viral inclusions. Lesions in EHV-4 infected aborted fetuses are milder and inclusions are less frequent than with EHV-1 infection. There is evidence of splenic and thymus necrosis as well as of interstitial pneumonia with EHV-4. The examination of lung, liver, thymus, spleen, and adrenal glands is paramount for the histologic diagnosis and antigen detection of abortigenic equine herpesviruses. The infected mare may develop a placental vasculitis in utero and infarction of microcotyledons of the chorion.

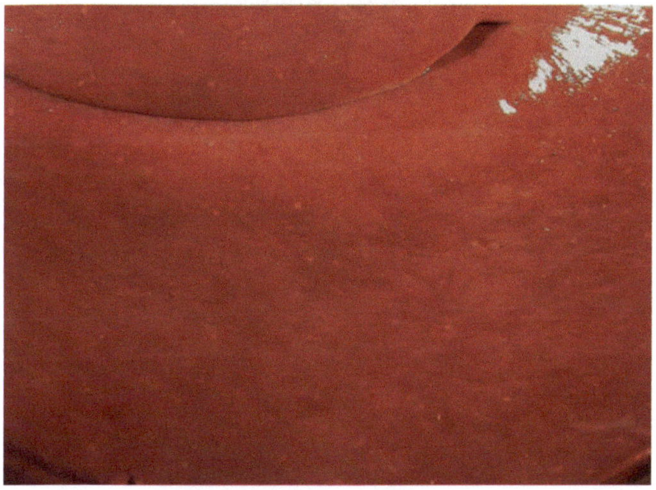

**Figure 12.56.** Fetus. Liver. Abortion. Multifocal Necrosis. EHV-1. Small tan foci of necrosis are present.

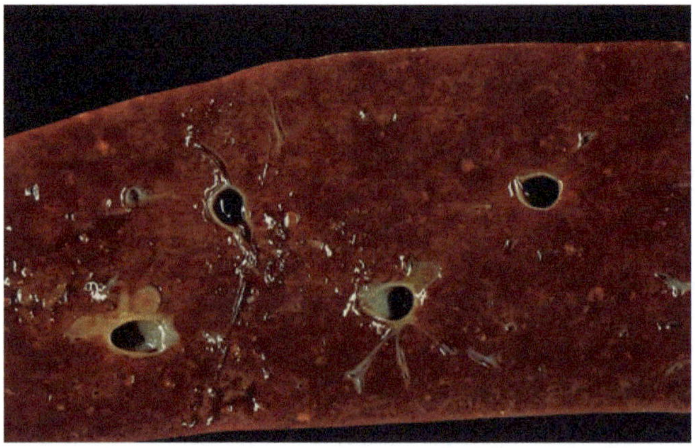

**Figure 12.57.** Fetus. Liver. Abortion. Multifocal Necrosis. EHV-1. Small tan foci of necrosis are present on cross section.

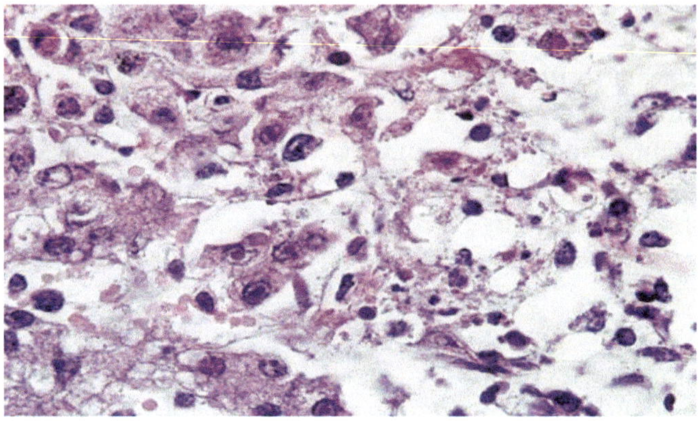

**Figure 12.58.** Fetus. Liver. Necrosis with Intranuclear Viral Inclusion Bodies. EVH-1. Microscopically, focal necrosis with eosinophilic intranuclear viral inclusion bodies in hepatocytes at the periphery of the necrotic foci can be utilized for the specific diagnosis of EHV-1 and EHV-4 infection. Inclusion bodies can also be detected within nuclei of thymic epithelium, splenic reticular cells, bronchiolar epithelial cells, adrenal cortex, and rarely in the chorionic trophoblast. They are mainly present in the lung of newborn foals. (H&E)

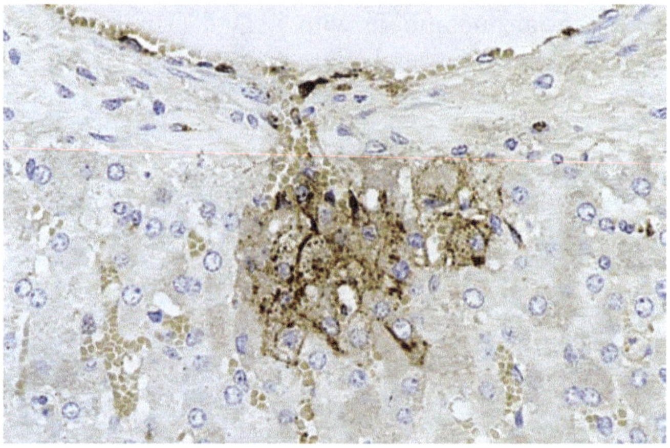

**Figure 12.59.** Fetus. Liver. EHV-1. Indirect immunohistochemistry demonstrates how the virus progressively infects the venular and sinusoidal endothelium and eventually the hepatocytes. (IHC)

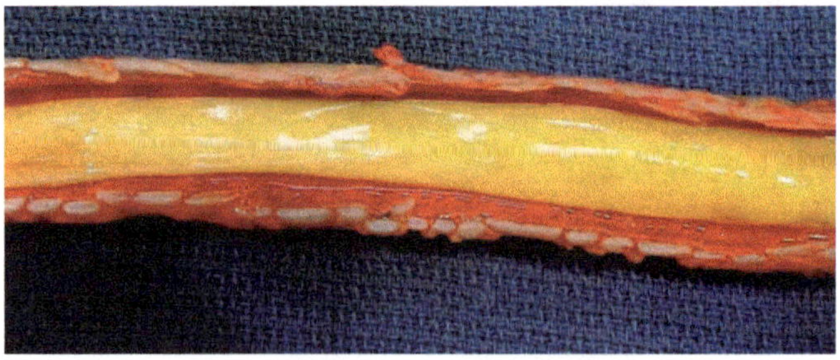

**Figure 12.60.** Fetus. Trachea. Fibrin Cast. EHV-1. A yellow rope-like fibrin cast fills the lumen of an opened trachea. This lesion is highly diagnostic for EHV-1 infection.

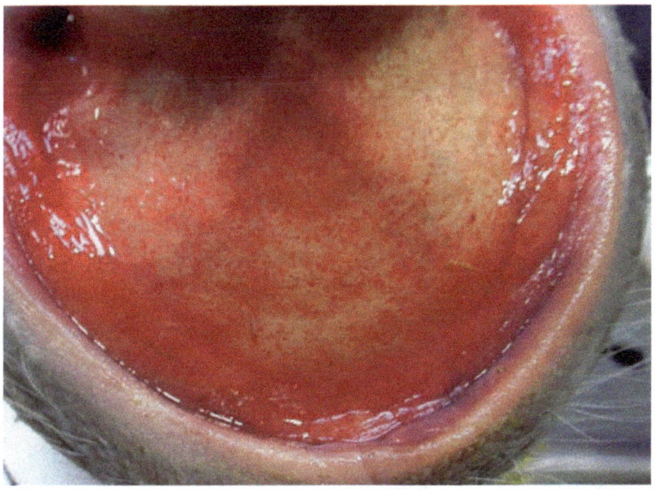

**Figure 12.61.** Fetus. Oral Mucosa. Petechiae. EHV-1.

Other diagnostic techniques for EHV-1 infection are viral isolation and polymerase chain reaction (PCR).

## Pathologic findings of equine herpesvirus abortion – Fact sheet

**Definition:** Infectious herpesvirus type 1 (type 4) leading to in utero death and abortion during term gestation in pregnant mares.

**Incidence:** Ubiquitous, highly contagious agent causing multiple abortions on farm

### Gross findings

- Focal necrosis in liver
- Edema and petechiation of lung
- Fibrin casts in lumen of terminal trachea at bifurcation

### Microscopic findings

- Multifocal necrosis and mild inflammation in liver, lung, adrenal glands, thymus, spleen, lymph nodes, and chorioallantois
- Intranuclear eosinophilic viral inclusion bodies in multiple organs of aborted foal.

### Diagnostic tests

- Viral isolation (VI)
- Fluorescent antibody (FA)
- Indirect immunohistochemistry (IHC)

### Prevention

- Vaccination
- Separation of unaffected horses via quarantine

*b. Equine viral arteritis abortion (EVA)*

The causal virus belongs to the family of *Arteriviridae*. It is transmitted via aerosol or genital routes. Persistently infected stallions harboring the virus within the vesicular glands and shedding the virus into the germ plasma of the semen are reservoirs of the virus. Fetuses are often expelled without clinical signs exhibited by the mare. Abortion occurs as a result of endometrial vasculitis and thrombosis leading to premature separation of the chorion and fetal ischemia. The fetus may become viremic, but histologic changes in the placenta and fetus are rare. Viral antigen can be sporadically detected in the arcadian chorionic trophoblast and chorionic mesenchymal cells.

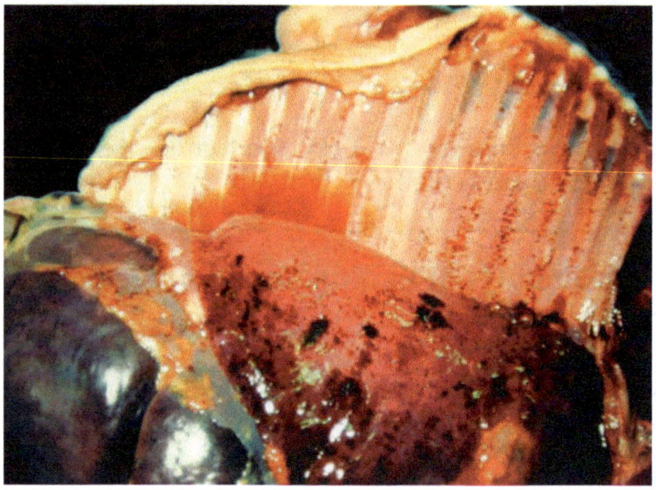

**Figure 12.62.** Fetus. Body Cavities. Petechiae and Hemorrhage. Equine Viral Arteritis (EVA) Abortion. (Reprinted with permission from Color Atlas of Reproductive Pathology of Domestic Animals, Buergelt, Figure 17-5, Page 71, Copyright Elsevier, 1997.)

Abortions occur sporadically. Aborted fetuses have varying amounts of serosanguinous fluid in the body cavities. There may be rib impressions in the lung. Lesions in the fetus are occasionally detected in the lung as perivascular lymphocytic infiltrates. Vasculitis may be sporadically present in the chorion. Pauciviral infections or virologically negative fetuses are a frequent event.

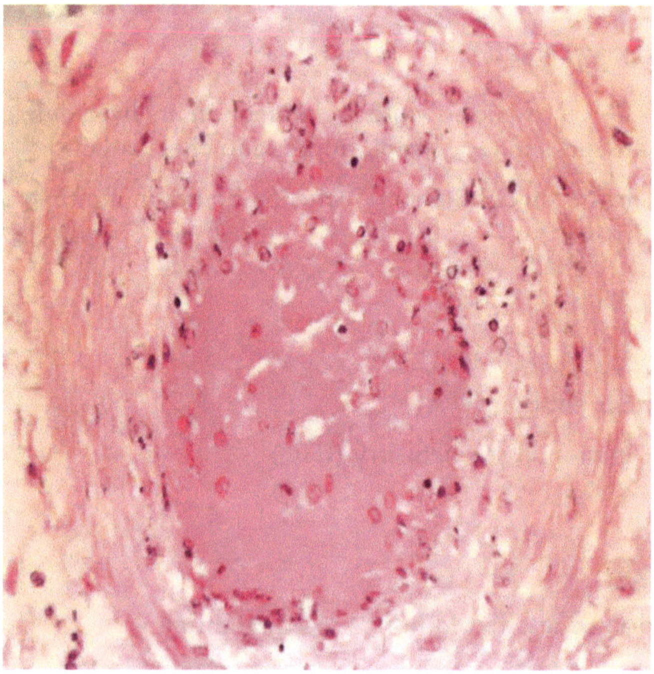

**Figure 12.63.** Fetus. Vessel. Chorionic Vasculitis. Equine Viral Arteritis. The chorionic vessel contains a thrombus and its wall is infiltrated by karyorrhectic lymphocytes. (H&E)

The diagnosis of EVA abortion can be made via virus isolation in permissive equine fetal renal cell lines, chorion indirect immunohistochemistry, PCR on brain, liver, spleen, heart, and placenta, and serum neutralization serology demonstrating seroconversion in the mare. The organs of the fetus to collect for diagnosis are chorion, lung, liver, thymus, spleen, and adrenal gland at least.

Differential diagnoses should include noninfectious and infectious viral (EHV-1) and bacterial abortion causes.

Both equine infectious anemia virus (EIA) and equine influenza virus are reported to have abortigenic properties.

## 2. Equine bacterial abortions

Equine fetuses can become infected from a primary bacterial source in the placental membranes ascending from the mare's vagina and cervix. Gram-positive and gram-negative bacteria can be isolated from the placenta with *Streptococcus equi* subsp. *zooepidemicus* representing the largest contingent. *Crossiella equi* and *Amycolatopsis* sp., a presumptive new species of nocardioform bacteria, are emerging as important abortigenic pathogens. *Mycobacterium avium* subsp *avium* has also been incriminated as cause for equine abortion as have been *Corynebacterium pseudotuberculosis*, *Dermatophilus congolensis*, *Bartonella henselae*, and others. A hematogenous route of placentitis due to salmonellosis or leptospirosis occurs less frequently.

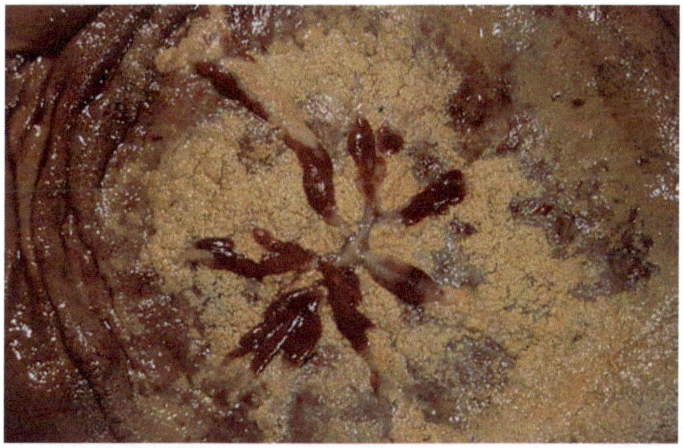

**Figure 12.64.** Horse. Chorion. Fibrinonecrotic Placentitis. Ascending. The chorionic surface is characterized by fibrin and hemorrhage. It is thickened and leathery indicating chronicity. *Streptococcus* sp. was isolated.

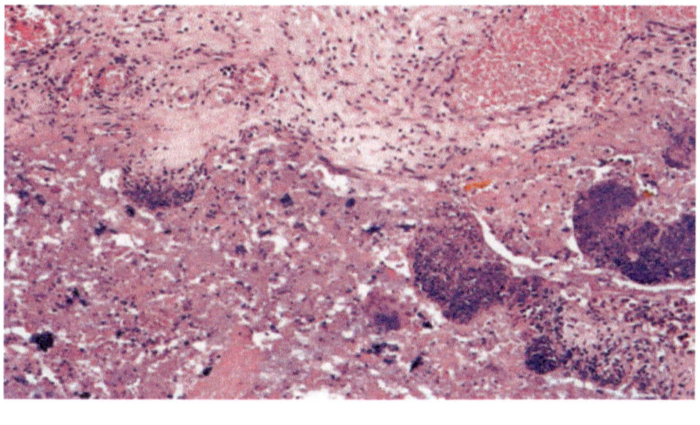

**Figure 12.65.** Horse. Chorion. Fibrinonecrotic Placentitis. The chorionic surface is covered by fibrin, degenerated neutrophils into which embedded are bacteria and mineral deposits. (H&E)

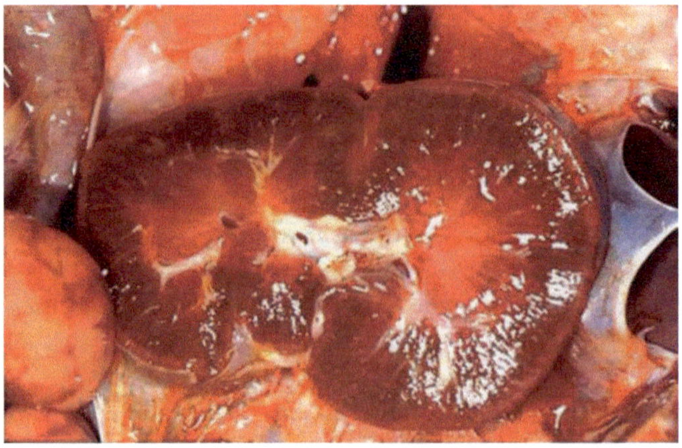

**Figure 12.66.** Fetus. Kidney. Interstitial Nephritis. Leptospirosis. The kidney on cross section reveals minute white foci and white streaks within the cortex and medulla in a term fetus. *Leptospira interrogans* serogroup *pomona* was identified as the associated etiologic agent. Foals may be aborted between 3 and 11 months of gestation. (Courtesy Dr. J. Roberts, National Zoo, Washington, DC.)

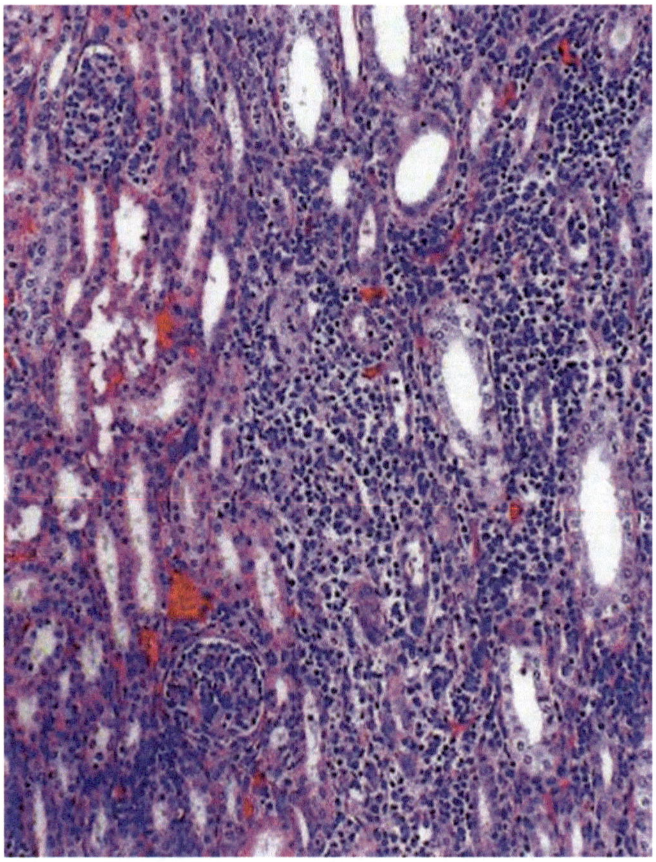

**Figure 12.67.** Fetus. Kidney. Nonsuppurative Interstitial Nephritis. Leptospirosis. Microscopically, the renal interstitium contains an inflammatory infiltrate of lymphocytes. (H&E) (Courtesy Dr. J. Roberts, National Zoo, Washington, DC.)

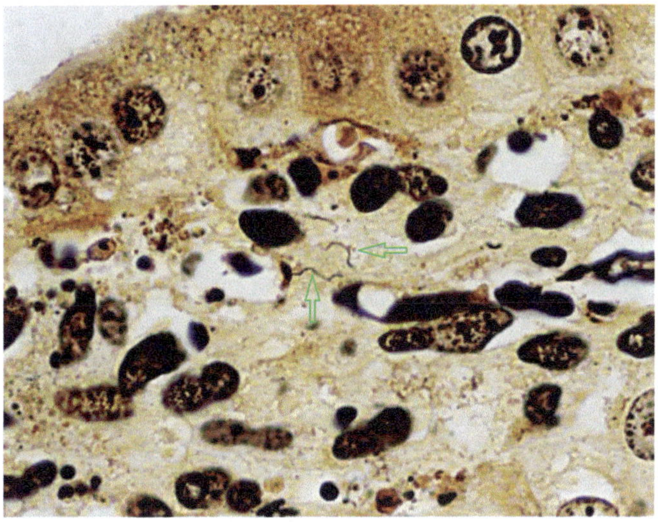

**Figure 12.68.** Fetus. Chorion. Intralesional Spirochetes. Leptospirosis. Foci of lymphocytes may be present. Organisms are outlined in the subtrophoblastic interstitium by silver positive stain (arrows). (Warthin-Stary)

Pneumonia, giant cell hepatopathy, multifocal chorionitis, and myocarditis are additional microscopic findings in fetuses with leptospirosis.

Nocardioform placentitis, with its location at the base of the chorionic body, is an atypical type of placentitis, caused by a group of similar organisms with similar features (gram-positive, nonacid fast, filamentous, aerobic). Nocardioform organsims have been classified as *Crossiella equi* and *Amycolatopsis* sp. PCR on placental tissue detects either species.

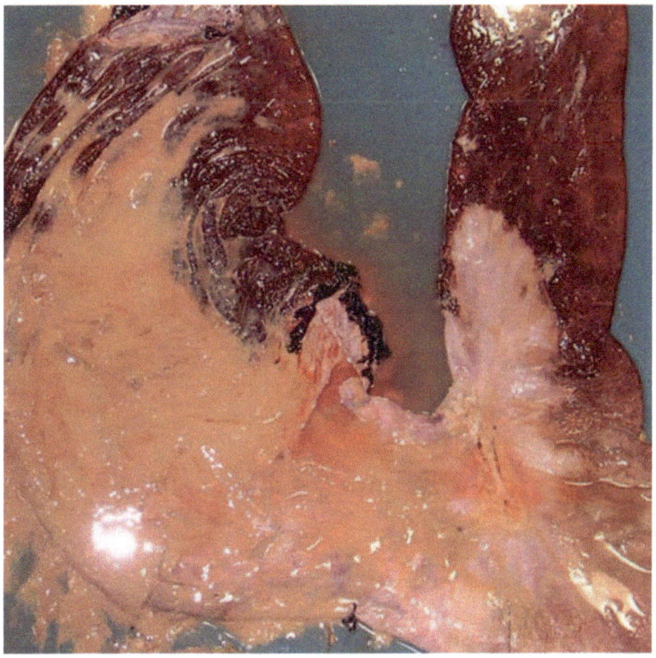

**Figure 12.69.** Horse. Chorion. Exudative Placentitis. Equine Nocardioform Placentitis. Most of the tan, thick exudate is present over the body part of the chorion, but it also extends into both horn segments. *Crossiella equi* was isolated.

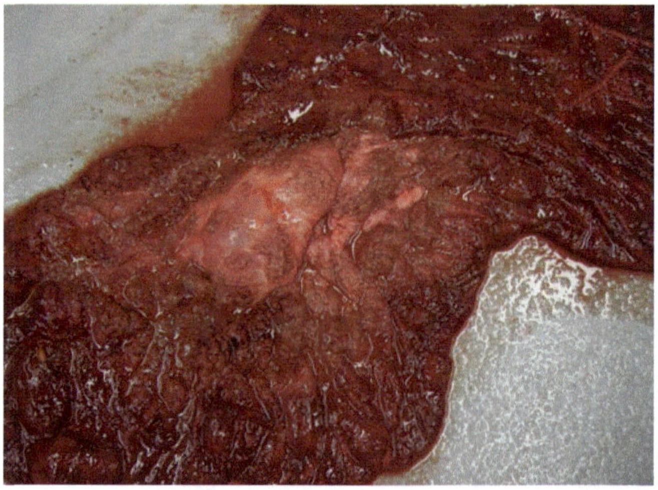

**Figure 12.70.** Horse. Chorion. Exudative Placentitis. Equine Nocardioform Placentitis. The chorionic body portion at the junction of the horns is covered by a pale brown, thick exudate in the periphery which when washed away reveals an avillous center. The location of the placentitis over the body part of the placenta is an important hallmark for its recognition as nocardioform. (Courtesy Dr. N. Williams, University of Kentucky.)

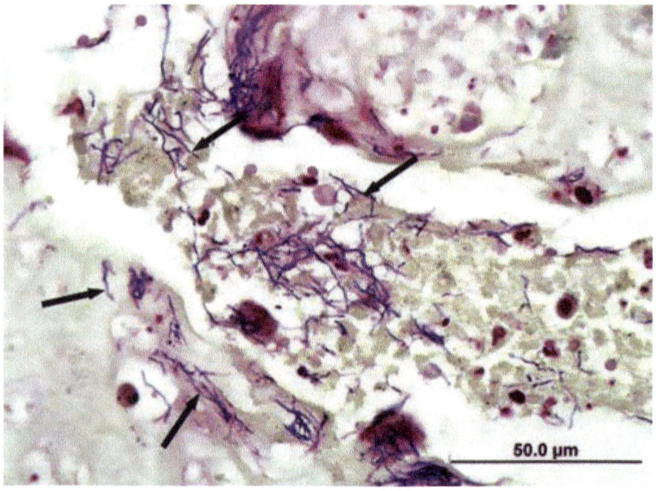


**Figure 12.71.** Horse. Chorion. Intralesional Bacilli. Equine Nocardioform Placentitis. Microscopically, filamentous, branching, gram-positive nocardioform bacilli (*Amycolatopsis* sp) could be demonstrated within the exudate (arrows). (Brown & Brenn stain) (Reprinted with the permission of the Journal of the American Veterinary Medical Association.)

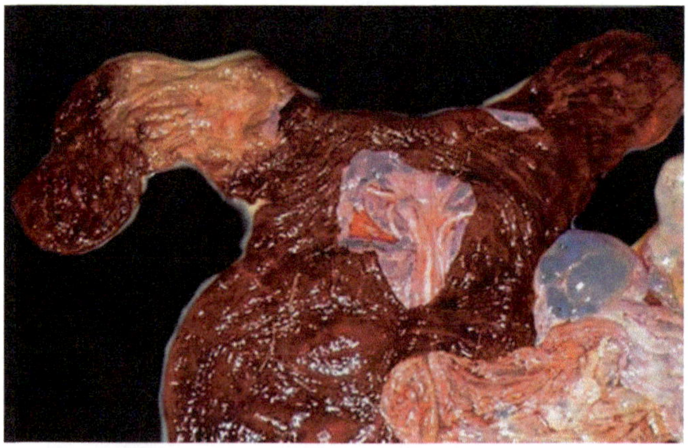

**Figure 12.72.** Horse. Chorion. Focal Necropurulent Placentitis. The tip of one horn is covered by a focal tan exudate. *Mycobacterium avium* subsp. *avium* was isolated.

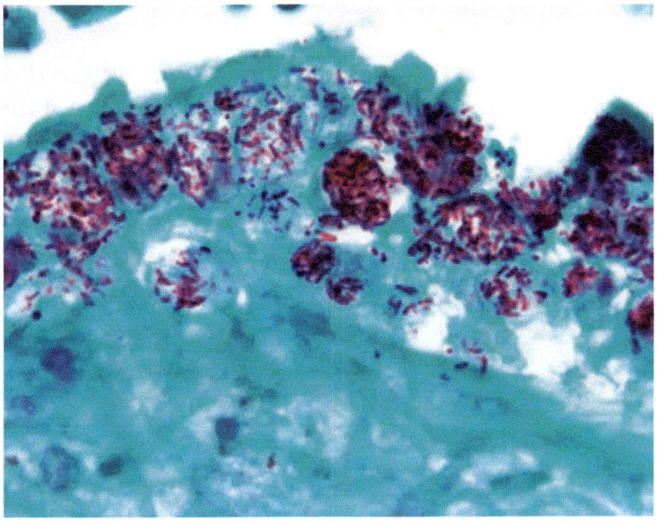

**Figure 12.73.** Horse. Chorion. Mycobacterial Placentitis. Intralesional acid-fast bacilli. *Mycobacterium avium* subsp. *avium* was isolated. (Acid-fast stain) (Courtesy Dr. J. Roberts, National Zoo, Washington, DC.)

### Reported bacterial pathogens of equine abortions

- *Escherichia coli*
- *Streptococcus equi* subsp. *zooepidemicus*
- *Staphylococcus aureus*
- *Leptospira interrogans* serogroup *pomona*
- *Myobacterium avium* subsp. *avium*
- *Actinobacillus equuli*
- *Amycolatopsis* sp.
- *Crossiella equi*
- *Coynebacterium pseudotuberculosis*
- *Salmonella enterica*
- *Actinomyces* sp.
- *Bartonella henselae*
- *Borrelia parkeri*
- *Serratia marcescens*
- *Rhodococcus equi*
- *Klebsiella pneumonia*
- *Chlamydophila* sp. (Europe)
- *Dermatophilus congolensis*
- *Brucella abortus*

### 3. Equine fungal abortions

*Aspergillus* sp., *Mucor* sp., *Histoplasma capsulatum*, and *Candida* have been isolated from mycotic placentitis cases. Mycotic abortions are rare in horses. Route of placentitis is ascending and starts at the cervical star and placental body segment. Hyphae may be found in the placenta, and fetal liver, lung, or stomach contents.

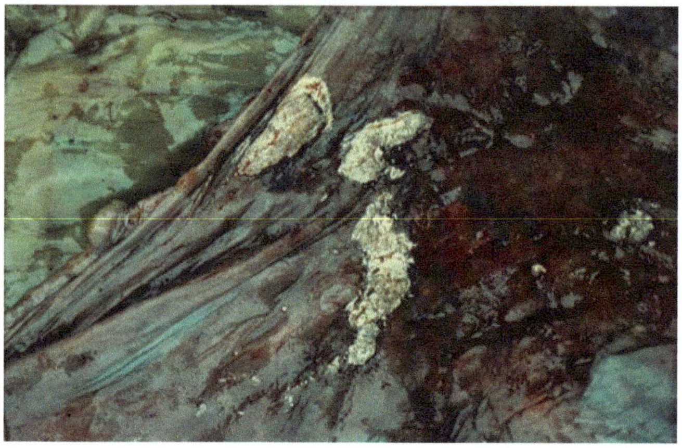

**Figure 12.74.** Horse. Amnion. Caseous Fungal Placentitis. A multifocal dry caseous exudate is embedded close to a red area of the amniotic surface. A fungal agent was identified but not further specified.

### 4. Abortions caused by microsporidia

*Encephalitozoon cuniculi* was identified in a 90-day-old aborted fetus. On gross examination one yellow plaque was noticed in the abdominal skin. The skin plaque was diagnosed as lymphohistiocytic dermatitis. Microscopic examination of placental membranes and umbilicus revealed vasculitis in the chorion, amnion, and umbilical cord. The clusters of intralesional coccoid organisms were identified as gram-positive organisms via Machiavelli stain. PCR was positive for *Encephalitozoon cuniculi* genotype III (dog genotype). Genetic and molecular studies suggest that the *E. cuniculi* is more related to fungi than protozoa.

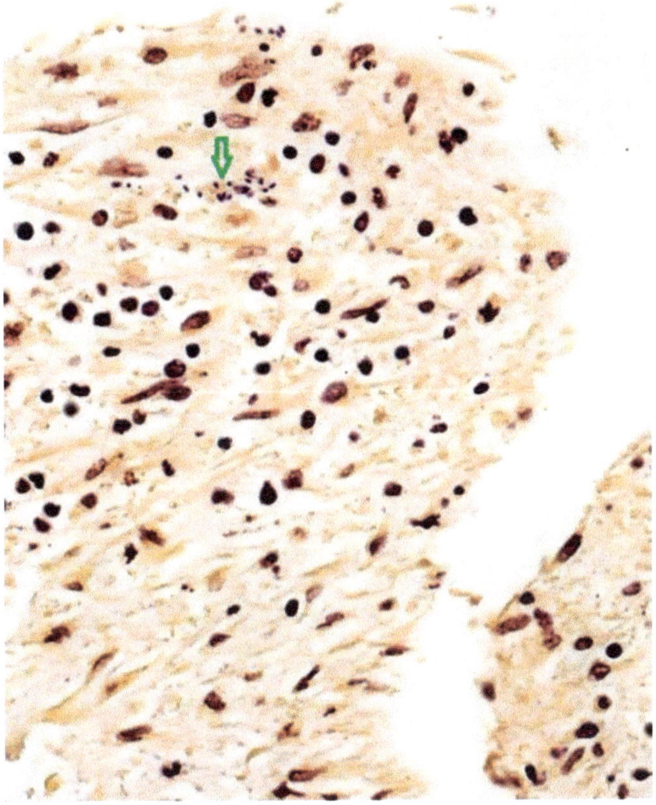

Figure 12.75. Horse. Chorion. Lymphocytic Chorionitis. There is evidence of a mild lymphocytic stromal inflammation with intralesional gram-positive clusters of coccoid organisms (arrow) identified as *E. cuniculi*. (Brown & Brenn) (Courtesy Dr. T. Heskett, Kissimmee, FL.)

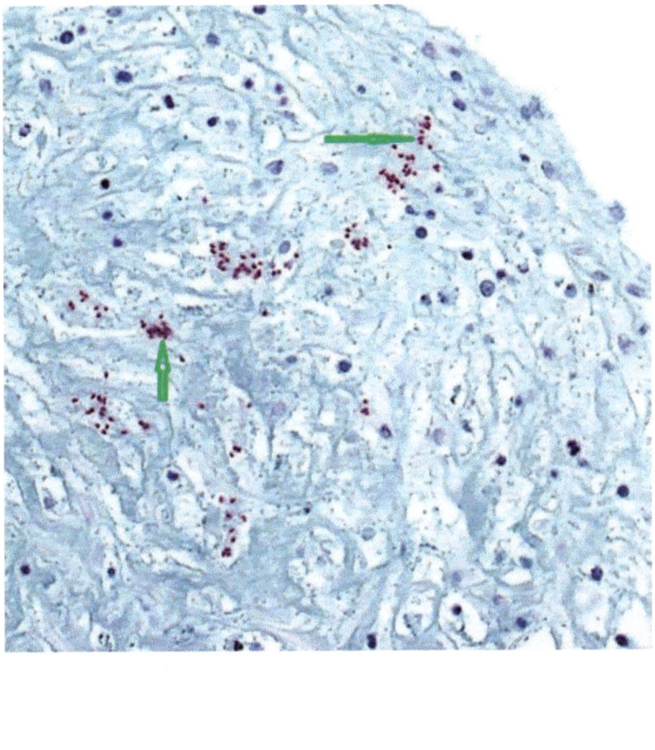

Figure 12.76. Horse. Chorion. Intralesional *Encephalitozoon* sp. A Macchiavello stain highlights intralesional red microsporidia spores (arrows). (Macchiavello) (Courtesy Dr. T. Heskett, Kissimmee, FL.)

## 5. Miscellaneous

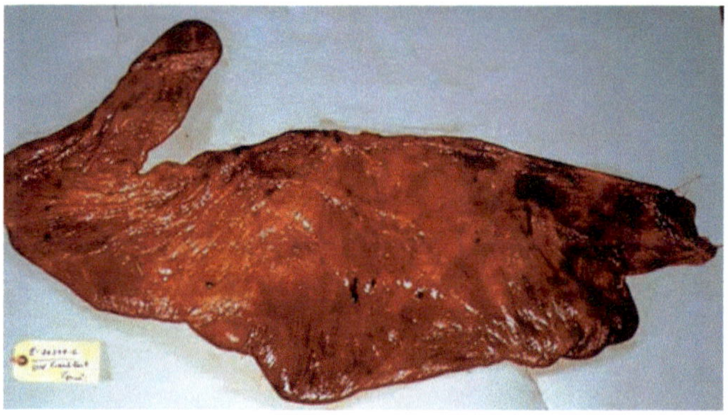

**Figure 12.77.** Horse. Chorioallantois. Single Horn. It exhibits only one horn. On occasion the expelled chorioallantois may display three horns.

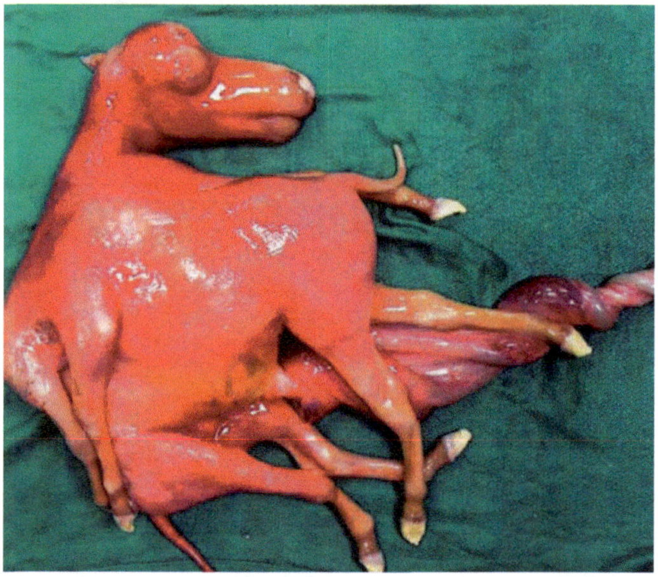

**Figure 12.78.** Fetus. *Dipygus parasiticus*. Attached to the thorax are two posterior body portions with two sets of pelvis and hind extremities.

## VI. Choice of samples and diagnostic methods for abortion investigation

### Sample submissions

- Entire fetus
- Placental membranes and umbilical cord
- Blood from dam and fetus
- Bodily fluids

### Tests for abortigenic diseases

- Necropsy
- Histopathology
- Placental impression smears
- Microbiology
- Virology
- Toxicology
- Fluorescent microscopy
- Immunohistochemistry
- Molecular biology
- Serology
- Pooling of samples

A complete necropsy should be performed on the fetus regardless of post-mortem condition. Samples for histology should be taken from main fetal tissues, placental membranes, and umbilical cord. Recommended diagnostic laboratory procedures are described elsewhere.

## Selected references

Arnold CE, Thompson PM, Slovis NM, Bain FT. 2008. Periparturient hemorrhage in mares: 73 cases (1998–2005). *J Am Vet Med Assoc* 232(9):1345–1351.

Buergelt, Claus D. 1997. *Color Atlas of Reproductive Pathology of Domestic Animals*. St. Louis: Mosby.

Cummins C, Carrington S, Fitzpatrick E, Duggan V. 2008. Ascending placentitis in the mare: a review. *Ir Vet J* 61(5):307–313.

Donahue JM, Williams NM. 2000. Emergent causes of placentitis and abortion. *Vet Clin North Am Equine Pract* 16(3):443–456.

Erol S, Sells SF, Williams NM, et al. 2012. An investigation of a recent outbreak of nocardioform placentitis caused abortions in horses. *Vet Microbiol* 158(3–4):425–430.

Njaa, Bradley L. 2012. *Kirkbride's Diagnosis of Abortion and Neonatal Loss in Animals*. 4th ed. Ames: Wiley-Blackwell.

Scase T, Brandt S, Kainzbauer C, et al. 2010. Equus caballus papillomavirus-2 (EcPV-2): an infectious cause for equine genital cancer? *Equine Vet J* 42(8):738–745.

Schumacher J. 1999. Testicular neoplasia of horses: an underreported condition. *Equine Vet J* 32(4):270–272.

Sebastian MM, Bernard WV, Riddle TW, Latimer CR, Fitzgerald TD, Harrison LR. 2008. REVIEW Paper: Mare Reproductive Loss Syndrome. *Vet Pathol* 45(5): 710–722.

Smith KC, Blunden AS, Whitwell KE, Dunn KA, Wales AD. 2003. A survey of equine abortion, stillbirth and neonatal death in the UK from 1988-1997. *Equine Vet J* 35(5):496–501.

Szeged L, Hotel H, Sachsen K. 2005. High prevalence of chlamydial (*Chlamydophila psittaci*) infection in fetal membranes of aborted equine fetuses. *Vet Res Commun* 29(Suppl 1):37–49.

Williams NM, Bryant UK. 2011. Periparturient arterial rupture in mares: a postmortem study. Available at www.j-evs.com/.

# 13 Diseases of the Skin (Integument)

**Contributed by Pamela Eve Ginn and Julia A. Conway**

I. Congenital and hereditary disorders
   1. Dermatosparaxis
   2. Epidermolysis bullosa
II. Disorders of epidermal differentiation
   1. Coronary band disease
   2. Linear alopecia
   3. Seborrhea
III. Disorders of pigmentation
   1. Leukotrichia and leukoderma
   2. Vitiligo
IV. Physiochemical and actinic injury to the skin
   1. Actinic dermatitis
   2. Photosensitization
   3. Photoactivated vasculitis
V. Immune-mediated dermatoses
   1. Hypersensitivity dermatoses
      a. Atopy
      b. Culicoides hypersensitivity
      c. Urticaria/angioedema
   2. Autoimmune dermatoses
      a. Bullous pemphigoid
      b. Pemphigus foliaceus
      c. Lupus erythematosus
   3. Other immune-mediated dermatoses
      a. Alopecia areata
      b. Amyloidosis
VI. Helminthic diseases of the skin
   1. Habronemiasis
   2. Onchocerca
VII. Viral diseases of skin
   1. Equine papillomaviral infection
   2. Poxvirus infection
      a. Molluscum contagiosum
      b. Equine poxvirus
VIII. Bacterial diseases of the skin
   1. Dermatophilosis
   2. Botryomycosis
   3. Fistulous withers and poll evil

*Color Atlas of Equine Pathology*, First Edition. Claus D. Buergelt and Fabio Del Piero.

IX. Fungal diseases of skin
  1. Dermatophytosis
  2. Phaeohyphomycosis
  3. Sporotrichosis
  4. Epizootic lymphangitis
  5. Zygomycosis
X. Oomycete diseases of the skin: pythiosis
XI. Protozoal diseases of the skin
  1. Leishmaniasis
  2. Besnoitiosis
XII. Ectoparasites: Mange
XIII. Miscellaneous skin disorders
  1. Canker
  2. Chronic progressive lymphedema
  3. Cushing syndrome
  4. Drug eruption
  5. Erythema multiforme
  6. Eosinophilic granuloma
  7. Exuberant granulation tissue
  8. Follicular cyst
  9. Lightning
  10. Multisystemic eosinophilic epitheliotropic disease
  11. Pastern dermatitis
  12. Toxic epidermal necrolysis
  13. Systemic sterile granulomatous disease
  14. Envenomation
XIV. Neoplasia of the skin
  1. Squamous cell carcinoma
  2. Sarcoid
  3. Cutaneous lymphoma
  4. Hemangioma/hemangiosarcoma
  5. Melanoma
  6. Peripheral nerve sheath tumor
  7. Papilloma
  8. Mast cell tumor
  9. Basal cell tumor
  10. Myoma
  11. Fibroma/Fibrosarcoma
  12. Mammary gland neoplasia

# I. Congenital and hereditary disorders

## 1. Dermatosparaxis

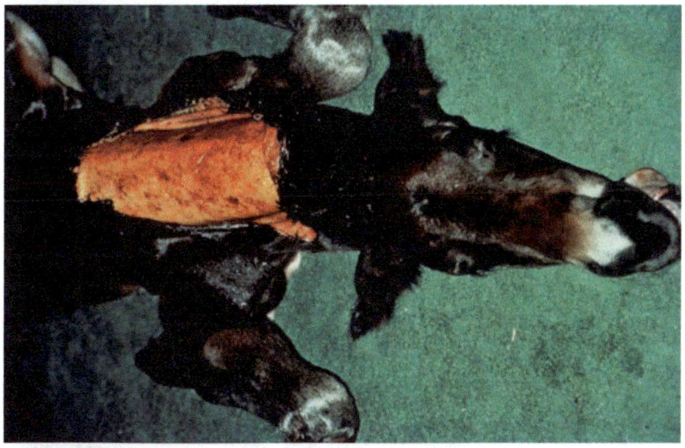

**Figure 13.1.** Foal. Neck and Withers. Dermatosparaxis. A large tear is evident in the skin of the neck and dorsal thorax. Differential diagnosis: epitheliogenesis imperfecta.

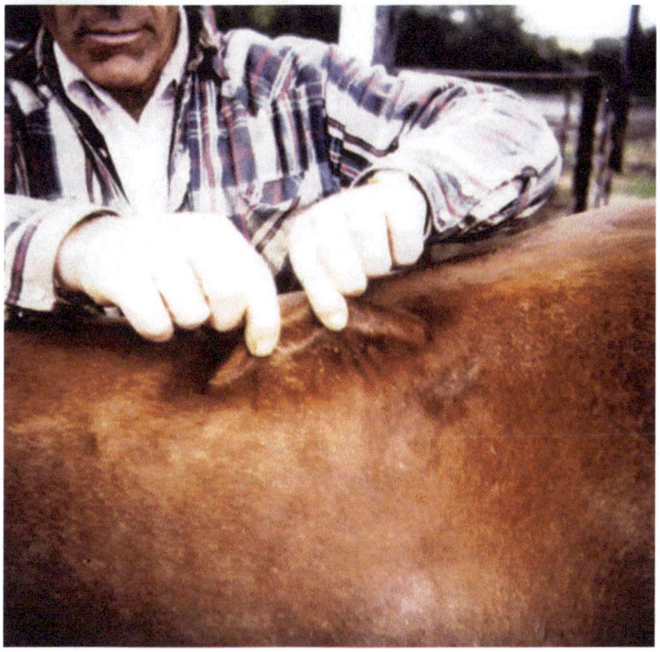

**Figure 13.2.** Horse. Dorsal Back. Cutaneous Asthenia. Note the loose, hyperextensive areas of skin. Minor trauma easily damages skin of affected animals. (Courtesy Dr. E.G. Clark, Calgary, Canada.)

Cutaneous asthenia (dermatosparaxis) is considered an inherited autosomal recessive congenital condition resulting in faulty assembly of collagen, the major structural protein in the dermis. The condition is seen in the American Quarter horse and rarely in other breeds. It is characterized by loose, hyperextensible, and unusually fragile skin that is torn by minor trauma. Animals appear normal at birth but develop skin wounds by 6–12 months of age. Tears in the skin may be preceded by hematomas or seromas. The affected skin may be palpably thin, very stretchy, and velvety. The patches of thinned, hyperextensible, fragile skin are often sunken below the surface of surrounding, normal skin. The legs, shoulders, and saddle areas are most often affected. The diagnosis is usually made by clinical lesions and breed association. Microscopically, collagen fibers may be smaller and sparser, and the dermis may be thin compared with normal skin.

## 2. *Epidermolysis bullosa*

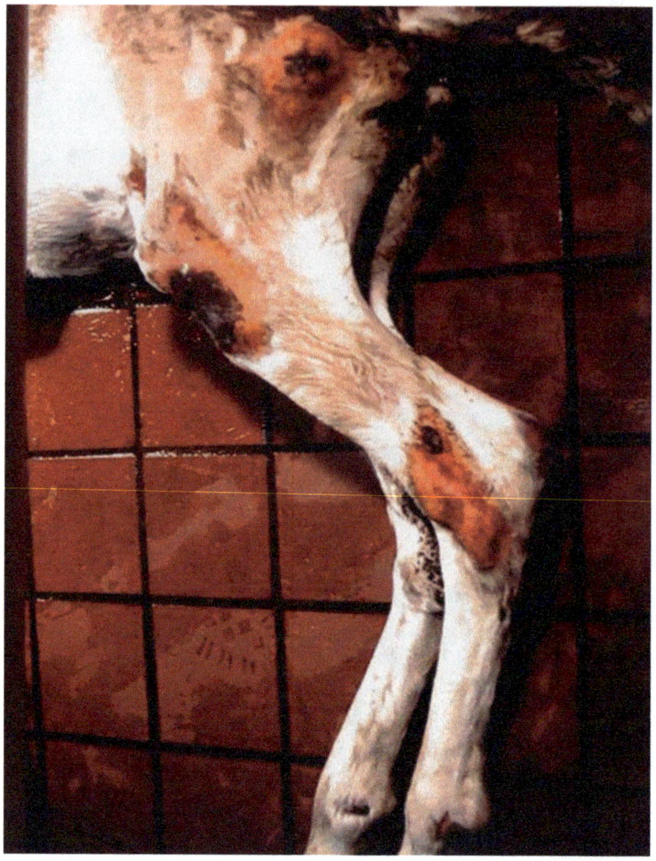

**Figure 13.3.** Foal. Epidermolysis Bullosa. Ulcers overlying the point of the hip, stifle, and lateral hock.

Epidermolysis bullosa (EB) refers to a rare group of hereditary and congenital diseases caused by defects in the structural proteins in the basement membrane zone that result in weakening of the dermal epidermal junction. The pathogenesis of the different forms are not completely studied in the horse, but in other species that have been studied document mutations in genes that lead to defective formation of keratin intermediate filaments or anchoring proteins such as collagen types VII and XVII, laminin, plectin, and integrins.

Foals may appear normal at birth but quickly develop subepidermal vesicles and bullae that eventuate into extensive sharply demarcated regions of ulceration. Areas of the body subject to friction or minor trauma such as the tongue, oral mucosa, and pressure points over bony prominences are most often affected. Foals may slough the entire hoof capsule.

EB is most often seen in draft horses but has also been documented in other types of horses. Expression of the condition can be variable due to the different subtypes of EB, but there is no cure for the condition, and extensive ulcerations can lead to euthanasia.

## II. Disorders of epidermal differentiation

### *1. Coronary band disease*

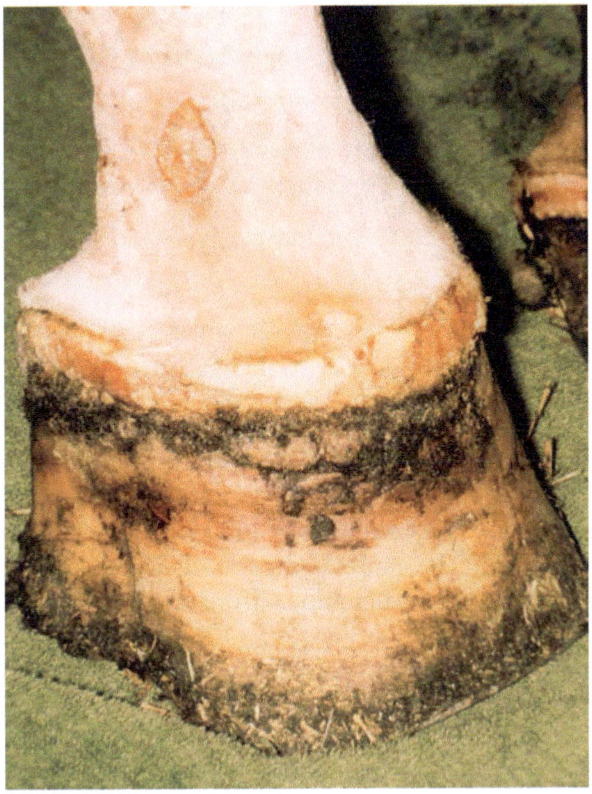

**Figure 13.4.** Horse. Coronary Band. Ulcerative Coronitis. Ulcerative lesions on the coronary band. (Courtesy of Dr. E.G. Clark, Calgary, Canada.)

The coronary band region of the foot can be involved in a number of different more widespread cutaneous or systemic disease processes. Lesions of the coronary band can be proliferative, hyperkeratotic, vesicular, ulcerative, or necrotizing. Conditions to consider when faced with coronary band lesions are pemphigus foliaceus, vasculitis, vesicular stomatitis, multisystemic epitheliotropic disease, sarcoidosis, vitamin A deficiency, selenium toxicity, hepatocutaneous syndrome, dermatophilosis, dermatophytosis, or coronary band dysplasia, to name a few.

Differentiating between these conditions depends on evaluation of a complete history and physical examination, concurrent cutaneous lesions, evidence of systemic disease, biopsy interpretation, and tissue culture and sometimes response to therapy. A few examples of conditions primarily affecting the coronary band are discussed here.

Coronary band dysplasia (coronary band dystrophy) is a condition of the horse characterized clinically by extensive crusting, proliferation, and hyperkeratosis and often exudation of coronary bands. Although most affected horses are not lame, chronic lesions can lead to hoof wall deformities that can lead to fissuring and cracking of the hoof wall and eventual lameness. The condition is symmetric.

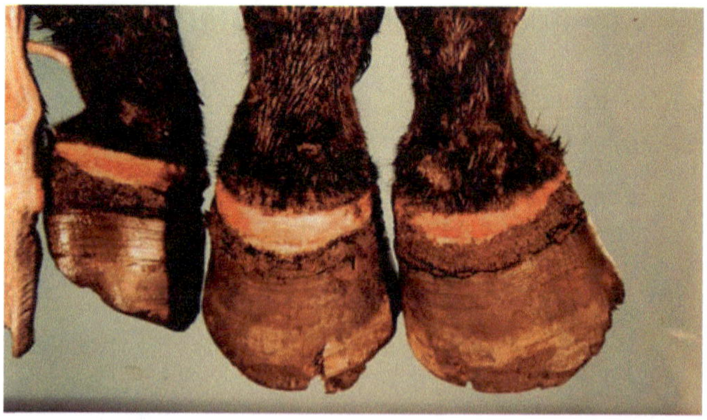

**Figure 13.5.** Horse. Hooves. Selenium Toxicosis. Coronary Band Ulcers. Cracking and brittle hooves that slough from the coronary band, exposing the sensitive laminae.

Histologically, the lesions are characterized by marked epidermal papillary hyperplasia and parakeratotic hyperkeratosis. Suppurative to eosinophilic inflammation and pustule formation and epidermal dysplasia have been reported. Most cases are reported in draft breeds, but clear breed dispositions are not well established. The cause of the lesions is not known and has been speculated to be a type of cornification disorder.

Selenium is a metalloid that acts as an antioxidant and also competes with sulfur in the formation of some proteins such as keratin. Chronic exposure to sublethal doses of selenium occurs in horses and other ungulates feeding on plants that accumulate selenium from the selenium rich soil found in Utah, Colorado, Montana, South and North Dakota, Wyoming, Arizona, Kansas, and Nebraska. Soil in parts of many other countries may be high in selenium as well. Chronic selenium ingestion leads to weight loss and alopecia and hoof wall deformities consisting of rings and grooves and possible sloughing of the hoof wall. Lameness is common. Cutaneous lesions are characterized histologically by atrophic, hyperkeratotic hair follicles.

## 2. *Linear alopecia*

Linear alopecia is a rare cutaneous condition occurring most often in young Quarter horses. It is characterized clinically by one or more vertically oriented 2- to 10-mm-wide and from 3 cm to 1 m in length linear areas of alopecia with variable crusting and scaling. The lines of alopecia are most often noted on the neck, shoulder, or thorax. The cause is unknown but speculated to be a form of an immune-mediated attack on follicles or a manifestation of keratinocyte-altered cytokine production that incites inflammation. The diagnosis is made by histologic examination of the affected regions that reveals a lymphocytic to lymphohistiocytic to granulomatous mural folliculitis with giant cells. Follicular destruction may occur. The condition is usually asymptomatic and most often permanent.

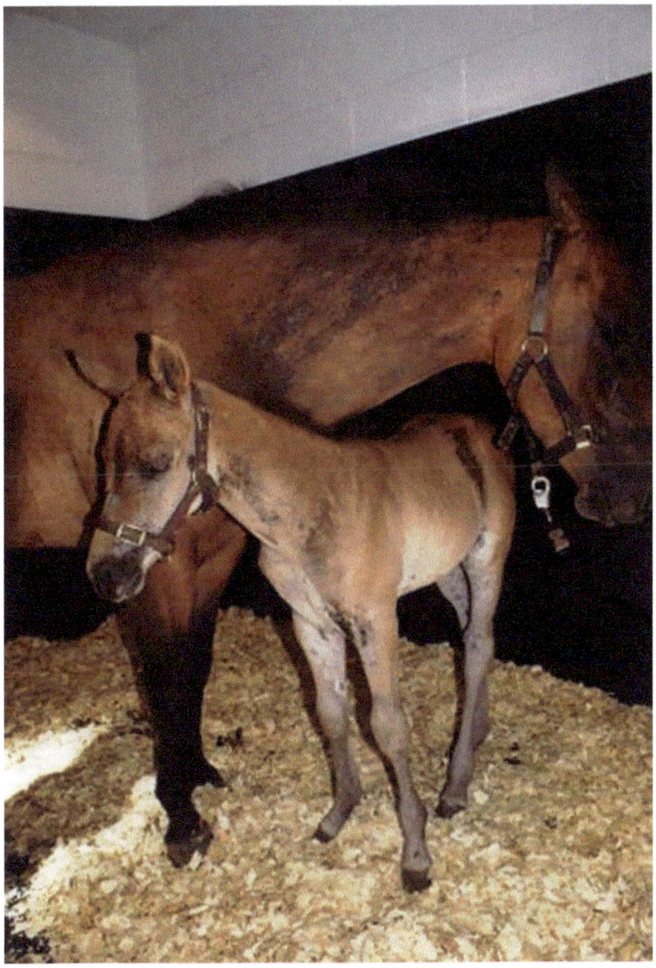

**Figure 13.6.** Mare and Foal. Whole Body. Linear Alopecia. Linear alopecia and linear crusting affecting both animals. mare and foal. (Courtesy Dr. E.G. Clark, Calgary, Canada.)

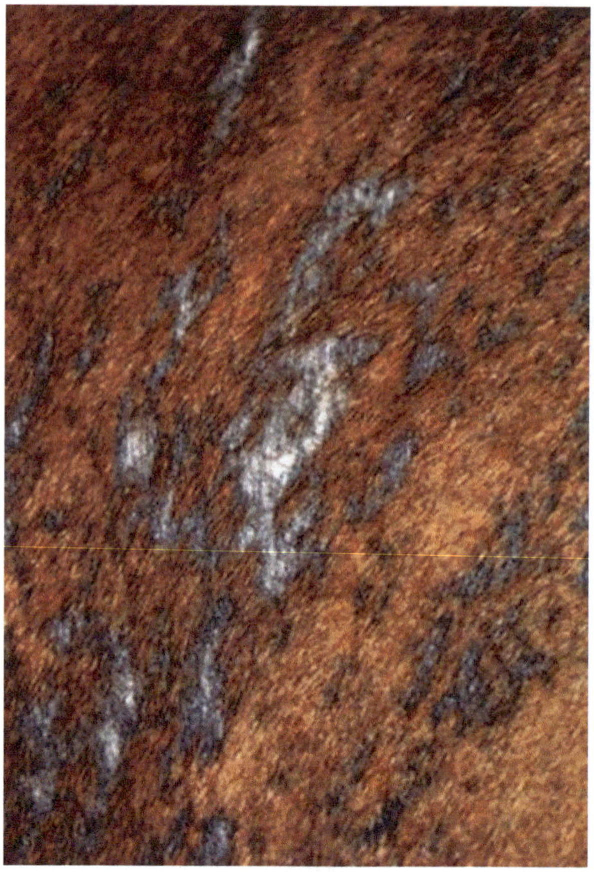

**Figure 13.7.** Horse. Lateral Neck. Linear Alopecia. Vertical bands of alopecia and crusting. Scars should be considered as a differential diagnosis. (Courtesy Dr. E.G. Clark, Calgary, Canada.)

### *3. Seborrhea*

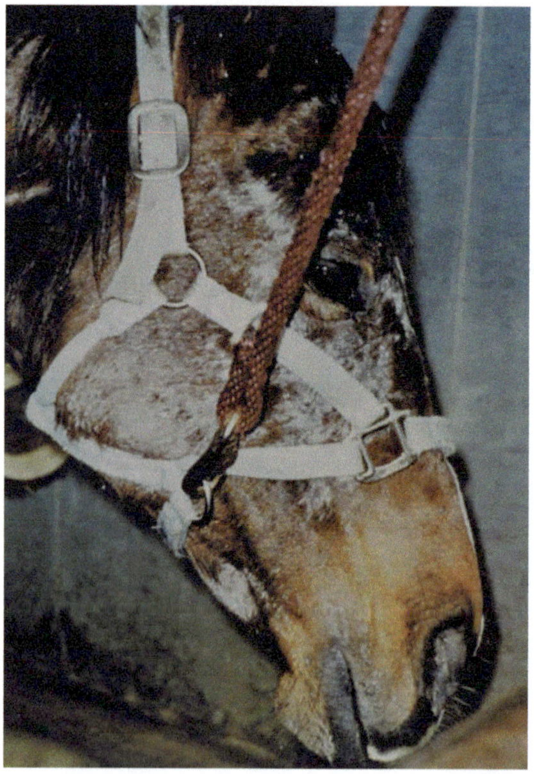

**Figure 13.8.** Horse. Head. Seborrhea. Note large areas of alopecia and white scales. (Courtesy Dr. E.G. Clark, Calgary, Canada.)

Seborrhea is a disorder of cornification leading to scaling and crusting. It occurs in the horse most often secondary to other inflammatory, nutritional, or infectious conditions of the skin or in conjunction with systemic disease. In many cases, a specific cause cannot be identified. In the horse, seborrhea most often occurs in the mane and tail or anterior surface of the rear cannon bone region (cannon keratosis) and leads to excessive production of white scale and variable degrees of alopecia. In some cases, seborrhea can affect large areas of the body. Histologically, there is acanthosis and hyperkeratosis with variable degrees of inflammation.

## III. Disorders of pigmentation

### *1. Leukotrichia and leukoderma*

Acquired loss of pigment of the hair (leukotrichia) or skin (leukoderma) can occur secondary to trauma such as burns, freezing, inflammation, or immunologic attack on either melanocytes or cells containing melanin. Exposure to compounds (found in some rubber objects) that inhibit melanogenesis can also lead to depigmentation in areas of contact. The skin and hair may be affected independently or in concert, depending on the underlying cause. Leukotrichia can occur in various patterns such as spots (spotted leukotrichia) or lines (reticulated leukotrichia). The condition can wax and wane or be permanent.

### *2. Vitiligo*

Vitiligo refers to an acquired form of depigmentation of the skin that may be due to antimelanocyte antibodies or other mechanisms that disrupt melanin formation.

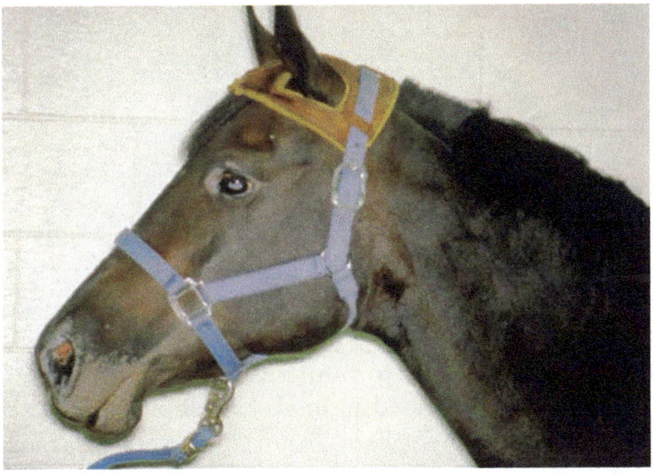

**Figure 13.9.** Horse. Head and Neck. Fading Arabian Syndrome. Color fading of hair of head and neck. (Courtesy Dr. E.G. Clark, Calgary, Canada.)

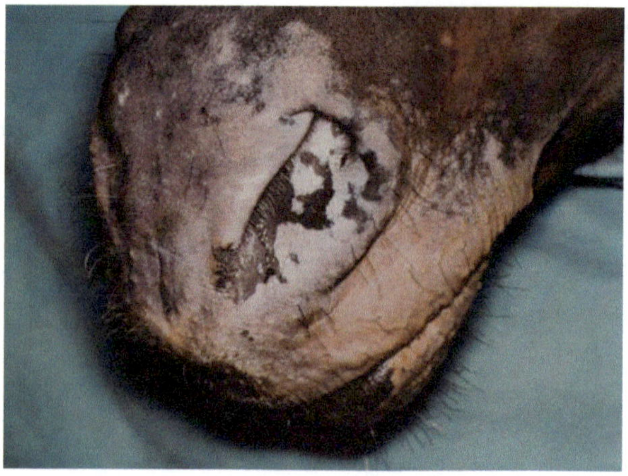

**Figure 13.10.** Horse. Muzzle. Chronic Cheilitis. Fading Arabian Syndrome. Depigmentation of the lips and muzzle. (Courtesy Dr. E.G. Clark, Calgary, Canada.)

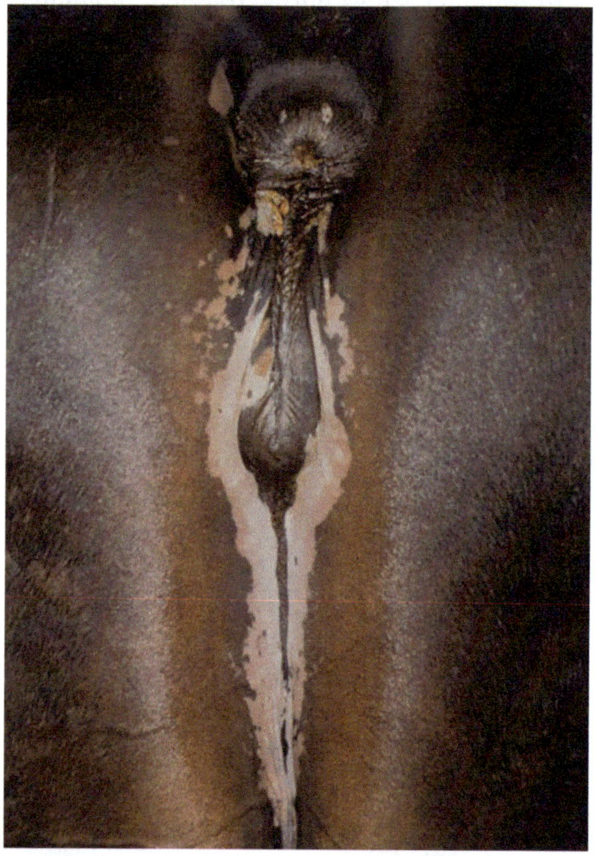

**Figure 13.11.** Horse. Perivulvar Region. Fading Arabian Syndrome. Perivulvar depigmentation. (Courtesy Dr. E.G. Clark, Calgary, Canada.)

Fading Arabian syndrome is a form of vitiligo in young horses, frequently less than 2 years of age. Affected animals develop the characteristic pale, depigmented macules seen in vitiligo, around the eyes, lips, muzzle, hooves, anus, and genitalia.

## IV. Physiochemical and actinic injury to the skin

### *1. Actinic dermatitis*

Ultraviolet radiation damages skin. Lightly pigmented and sparsely haired skin is most vulnerable to absorption of ultraviolet radiation, but other factors such as altitude, latitude, ozone layer, and smog can also influence the degree of radiation reaching the skin. The nose, eyelids, and genital areas of the horse are most often affected, but any lightly pigmented, nonhaired region of skin is susceptible. Ultraviolet radiation stimulates light-absorbing molecules in the skin leading to energy production from electron transfer and free radical production that damage DNA, enzymes, and other cellular proteins. Damaged nucleoproteins can lead to cell death or mutations that can lead to preneoplastic changes and potential development of squamous cell carcinomas or hemangiosarcomas of the skin. Acute lesions are recognized as burns and are characterized by erythema, edema, and possible bullae formation. Chronic exposure leads to gross lesions of alopecia, scaling, and crusting that correspond to epidermal hyperplasia, hyperkeratosis, and erosions. The epidermis over time will become dysplastic and may eventuate into a squamous cell carcinoma. Dermal lesions include congestion, fibrosis, and buildup of collagen and elastin fibers. Dermal hemangiomas and hemangiosarcomas may also develop.

### *2. Photosensitization*

Photosensitization dermatitis occurs when photodynamic agents are deposited in skin that is subsequently exposed to sunlight. Lesions occur on poorly haired, lightly pigmented, sun-exposed skin. This anatomic distribution is key to establishing the cause of the lesions. There are several types of photosensitization. In primary, or type 1, photosensitization, the horse ingests plants or drugs that contain photoreactive agents that are deposited in the skin.

In type 2 photosensitization, animals are born with an inability to properly metabolize erythrocyte breakdown products, and the photoreactive hematoporphyrins are deposited in the skin. This type has not been reported in the horse.

Type 3 photosensitization occurs in horses with hepatocellular damage or biliary obstruction that impairs the excretion of the photoreactive chlorophyll catabolite, phylloerythrin.

Type 4 photosensitization is reserved for poorly understood cases of photosensitivity in which no pathogenesis can be defined.

Finally, some cases of photosensitization occur after contact with photosensitizing agents, and in these cases, lesions are limited to areas of potential contact such as muzzle, extremities, or ventrum.

Cutaneous lesions of photosensitization are similar regardless of the cause. Initial gross lesions consist of erythema and edema that can progress to vesicle formation and ulcers with exudation and tissue necrosis. Histologically, the changes correspond to the initial gross lesions and include subepidermal vesicle formation, coagulative necrosis of the epidermis and dermis with edema, and fibrinoid degeneration of the vasculature. The tissue sloughs, and pruritus is often a feature. Clinical differentials include chemical or thermal burns and other vesicular and necrotizing conditions of the skin. A careful consideration of the sites affected, exposure to plants or other potential sources of photodynamic agents, and evaluation of liver function is usually needed to determine the cause of the photosensitizing dermatitis.

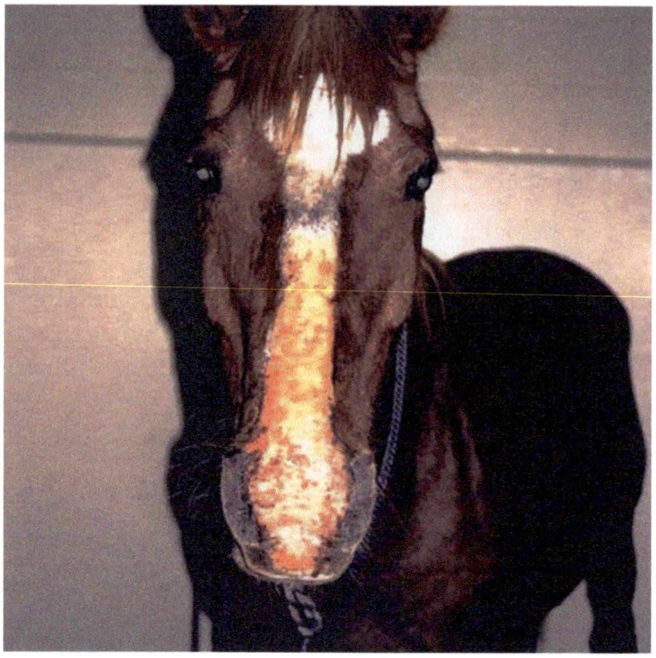

**Figure 13.12.** Horse. Head. Focal Erythematous, Exudative, Ulcerative Dermatitis. Photosensitization. Nonpigmented skin is affected. (Reprinted from *Illustrated Guide to Equine Diseases,* Sameeth M. Abutarbus, Figure 5-61a, Page 302, Wiley-Blackwell, 2009.)

### 3. *Photoactivated vasculitis*

Photoactivated vasculitis occurs in horses and affects white-haired extremities. The pathogenesis of this condition is not clearly defined. Horses have normal liver function and no history of ingestion or cutaneous exposure to photoreactive agents. Not all white-haired extremities are affected, and protection from sunlight does not always lead to resolution of the lesions. Lesions are found on lower extremities and are characterized by erythema, edema and serum exudation. Erosions and ulcers may form. Histologically, there is a vasculitis of the superficial dermal vascular plexus and epidermal erosion or ulceration and dermal edema with mild hemorrhage. In chronic cases, the epidermis becomes hyperplastic and hyperkeratotic.

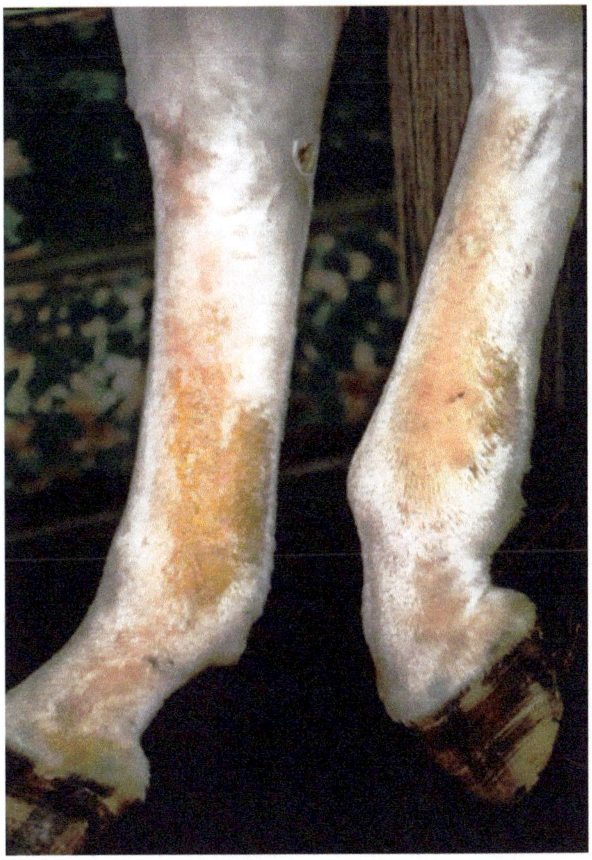

**Figure 13.13.** Horse. Distal Hind Limbs. Focal Exudative Dermatitis. Equine Photoactivated Vasculitis. There is evidence of alopecia, erythema, and serum exudation on lower portion of legs. (Courtesy Dr. E.G. Clark, Calgary, Canada.)

# V. Immune-mediated dermatoses

## *1. Hypersensitivity dermatoses*

### *a. Atopy*

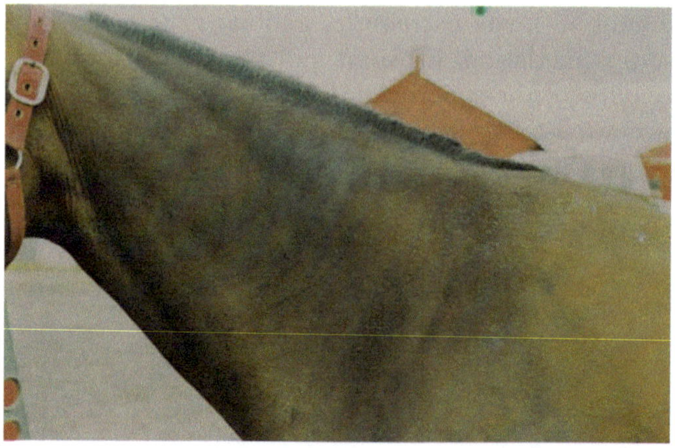

**Figure 13.14.** Horse. Neck. Atopy. Areas of hyperpigmentation. (Courtesy Dr. E.G. Clark, Calgary, Canada.)

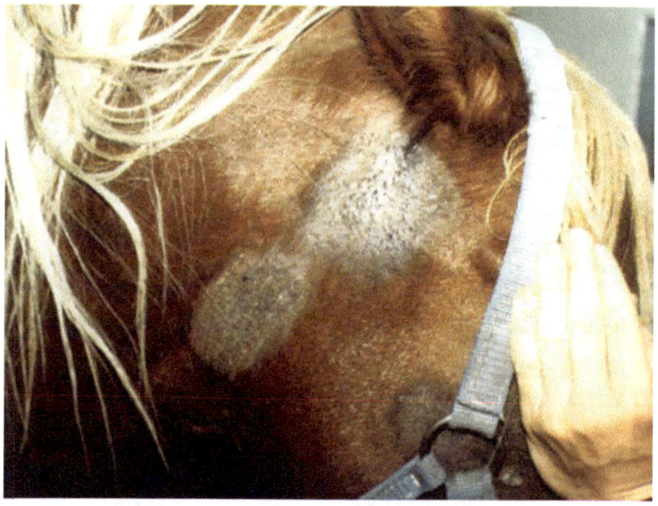

**Figure 13.15.** Horse. Back of Head. Atopy. Areas of excoriation. (Courtesy Dr. E.G. Clark, Calgary, Canada.)

Atopy is a genetically based enhanced or exaggerated immunoglobulin E–mediated immune response (allergic response) to inhaled or transepidermal environmental antigens. It most often manifests as pruritus. Clinical lesions are usually the result of self-trauma and include alopecia, hyperpigmentation, and excoriations. The condition manifests as recurrent urticaria in some horses. The face, ears, legs, and ventrum are the areas most often affected. The mane and tail may also be affected. Microscopically, there is a nonspecific perivascular dermatitis with variable numbers of lymphocytes, histiocytes, and eosinophils. In some horses, there may be an eosinophilic folliculitis or the presence of eosinophilic granulomas. The major differentials are insect and food allergy.

## b. *Culicoides hypersensitivity*

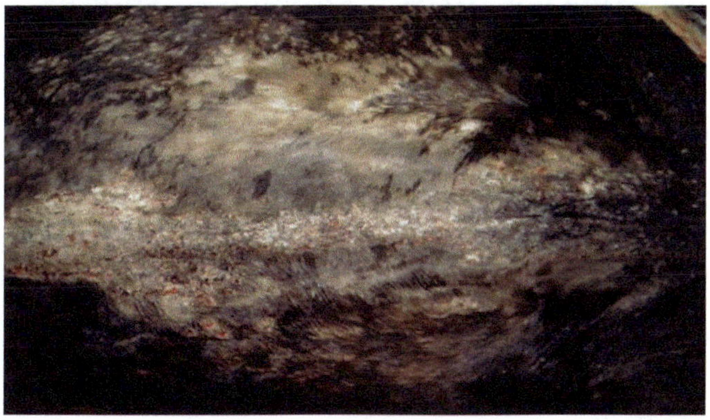

**Figure 13.16.** Horse. Skin over Abdomen. Culicoides Hypersensitivity. Alopecia, crusting, and scaling of the ventral midline.

Culicoides hypersensitivity results in severe pruritus, focal alopecia, and self-mutilation. Gross lesions vary from papules, nodules to erosions, crusts, and alopecia.

### Culicoides hypersensitivity – Fact sheet

#### Definition

- Most common allergic dermatosis of horses
- Intensely *pruritic*
- Hypersensitivity to salivary antigens of *Culicoides* gnats (also known as biting midges, punkies, no-see-ums)
- Combined hypersensitivity reaction; type 1 (immediate and late phase) and type 4 (delayed type)
- Gnats usually feed on mane, belly, and tail
- Also referred to as sweet itch, Queensland itch, muck itch, summer itch, summer eczema, summer fungus
- *Culicoides* sp. implicated as vectors for *Onchocerca cervicalis*

#### Incidence

- Very common
- Occurs worldwide
- Age of onset approximately 1–4 years
- Seasonal: spring and summer
- Often more severe each year
- May occur year-round, especially in tropical and subtropical climates

## Culicoides hypersensitivity – Pathologic features

### Gross findings

- Multifocal papules that may cause hair to stand erect
- Secondary lesions include alopecia, broken hairs, crusting, and scaling
- Lesions often on the head, neck, withers, tail, and ventral midline but vary depending on species of *Culicoides* involved
- May cause depigmentation

### Microscopic findings

- Superficial and/or deep perivascular dermatitis, usually eosinophilic and edematous
- Possible lymphocytes and mast cells
- Possible spongiosis, hyperkeratosis, and acanthosis
- Sterile eosinophilic folliculitis may be seen in conjunction with hypersensitivity reactions
- Possible ulcerations

### Differential diagnosis

- Ectoparasitism
- Other hypersensitivity dermatoses

*c. Urticaria/Angioedema*

Thought to be due to a type 1 hypersensitivity reaction with numerous proposed etiologies, including (but not limited to) drugs, arthropod bites/stings, contact allergens, and temperature extremes. These lesions are often pruritic.

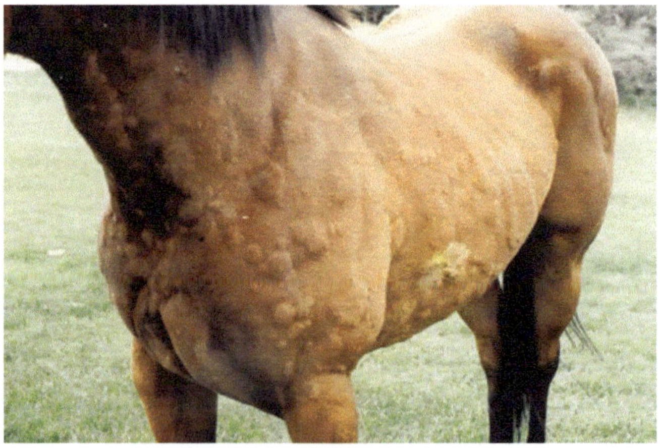

**Figure 13.17.** Horse. Whole Body. Dermal Edema, Multifocal. Urticaria (Hives). Multifocal to coalescing, swelling, and edema of the dermis. (Courtesy Dr. E.G. Clark, Calgary, Canada.)

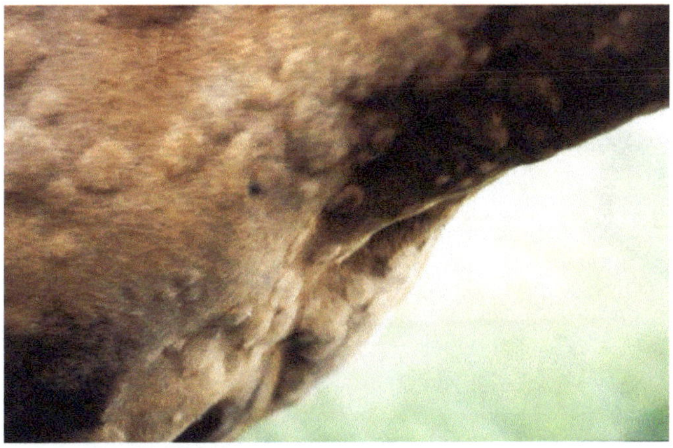

**Figure 13.18.** Horse. Neck. Dermal Edema. Urticaria, Multifocal (Hives). Multifocal swelling. (Courtesy Dr. E.G. Clark, Calgary, Canada.)

## *2. Autoimmune dermatoses*

*a. Bullous pemphigoid*

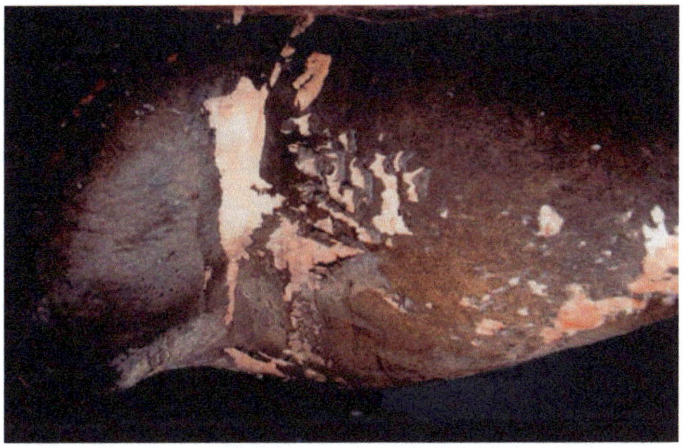

**Figure 13.19.** Horse. Body. Ulcerative Dermatitis, Multifocal. Bullous Pemphigoid. Severe, multifocal ulceration, secondary to ruptured vesicles and bullae present around the lateral flank and abdomen.

Bullous pemphigoid is an autoimmune disease, with antibodies directed against hemidesmosomal proteins that anchor the cells of the stratum basale to the extracellular matrix. Vesicles and bullae develop that progress to ulceration, in which the entire epidermis lifts off the dermis. Crusting is frequently present. Lesions in horses are often generalized with both cutaneous and mucocutaneous sites affected; however, sloughing of the oral mucosa in particular is often marked.

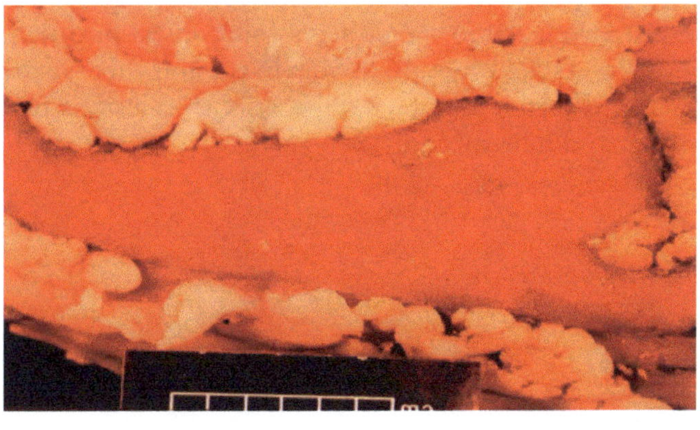

**Figure 13.20.** Horse. Nonglandular Stomach. Ulcerative Gastritis. Bullous Pemphigoid. Extensive, coalescing ulceration of the squamous cell lining.

### *b. Pemphigus foliaceus*

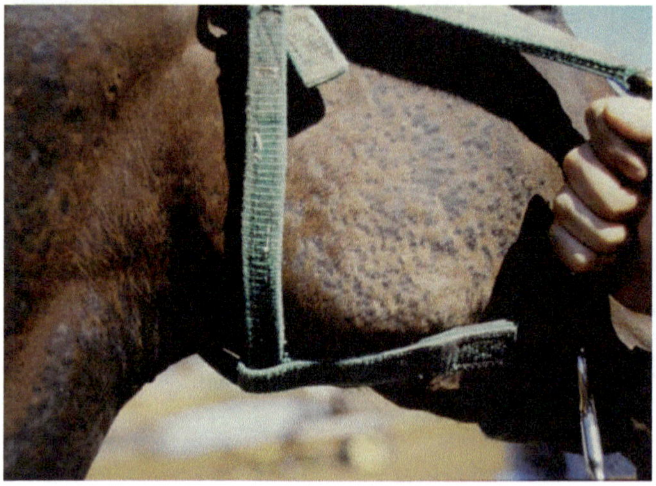

**Figure 13.21.** Horse. Head. Vesicular and Pustular Dermatitis, Multifocal. Pemphigus Foliaceus. Severe annular crusting and alopecia on the face.

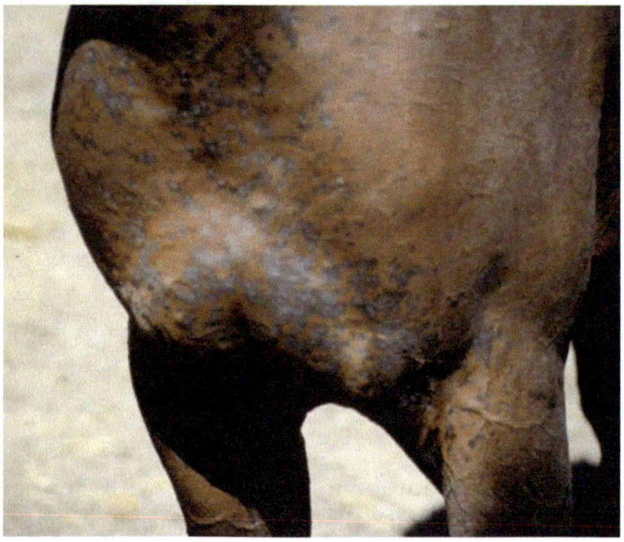

**Figure 13.22.** Horse. Pectoral Region. Vesicular and Pustular Dermatitis, Multifocal. Pemphigus Foliaceus. Numerous pustules with annular areas of crusting and alopecia on chest.

Gross lesions may range from pustules to vesicles, bullae, erosions, and/or ulcers. Appaloosas and Thoroughbreds are predisposed. Pemphigus foliaceus is the most common autoimmune dermatosis in the horse; it begins on the face, ventrum, or legs and may become generalized within a few months. Although the primary lesion of pemphigus foliaceus is pustular and vesiculobullous, these lesions are often very short lived, and there is progression to crusts, erosions, and (often annular) alopecia. Other lesions include matted hair coat, scaling, and hair tufting.

*c. Lupus erythematosus*

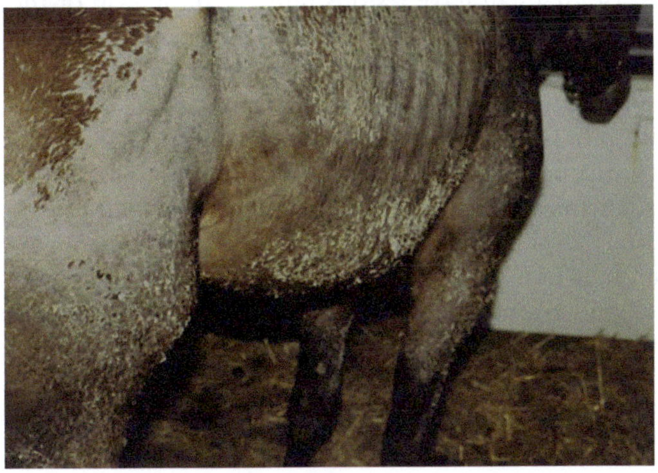

**Figure 13.23.** Horse. Body. Exfoliative Dermatitis. Systemic Lupus Erythematous (SLE). Note the extensive alopecia, scaling, and depigmentation. (Courtesy Dr. E.G. Clark, Calgary, Canada.)

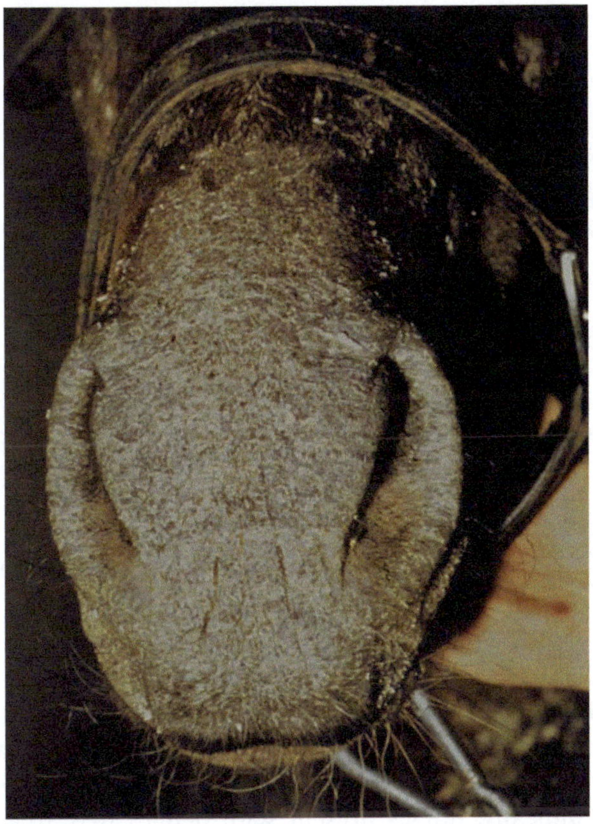

**Figure 13.24.** Horse. Nose and Muzzle. Exfoliative Dermatitis. SLE. Severe scaling. (Courtesy Dr. E.G. Clark, Calgary, Canada.)

Lupus erythematosus in the horse is a rare and incompletely defined immune-mediated disease that can have lesions limited to the skin or the skin can be involved as part of the systemic condition. The lesions are exacerbated by sunlight. Cutaneous lesions in either condition are most often characterized by patchy alopecia, scaling, and leukoderma of the face, neck, and trunk. Depigmentation of the periocular region, lips, and nostrils is common. Cases of systemic lupus erythematosus may also have lymphedema, weight loss, polyarthritis, anemia, uveitis, thrombocytopenia, or a variety of other conditions indicating systemic disease. The diagnosis of cutaneous lupus is based on biopsy findings of a lymphocytic hydropic interface dermatitis with basal cell apoptosis and pigmentary incontinence and possible areas of basement membrane thickening.

### 3. Other immune-mediated dermatoses

#### a. Alopecia areata

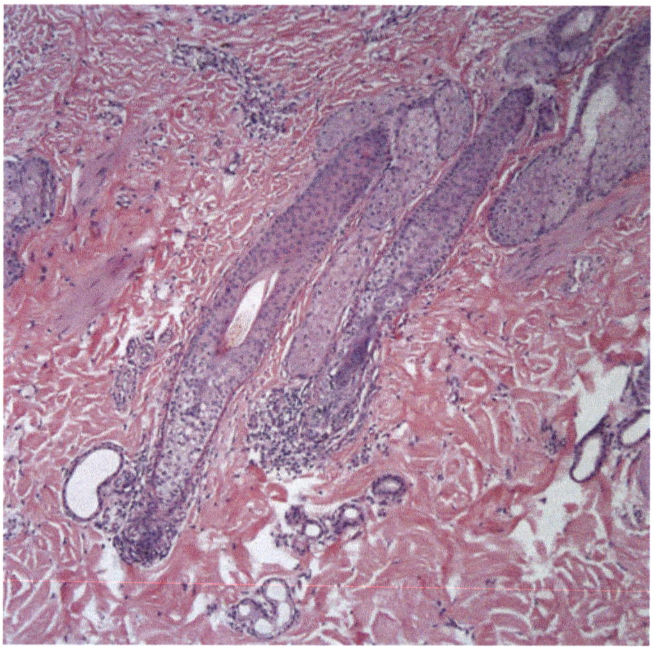

**Figure 13.25.** Horse. Skin. Lymphocytic Mural Folliculitis. Alopecia Areata. Aggregates of lymphocytes surround hair bulbs. The lymphocytic infiltration of anagen hair bulbs is often associated with apoptosis of the developing follicular epithelial cells in outer root sheath and matrix. (H&E)

This disorder is an uncommon cause of alopecia in the horse that is the result of a T lymphocyte mediated attack on the bulb region of anagen (growing follicles). Autoantibodies against follicular antigens have been demonstrated in the horse. Clinically, horses present with demarcated areas of partial to complete hair loss affecting the trunk, head, mane, or tail. Alopecia can be extensive and is sometimes associated with depigmentation. The lesions are usually smooth, often hyperpigmented, and have no clinical evidence of inflammation or pruritus. There are no clear breed, age, or sex predispositions. In chronic cases, inflammation may be absent and histologic changes are limited to small telogen follicles or mild peribulbar fibrosis. The condition can wax and wane or be permanent.

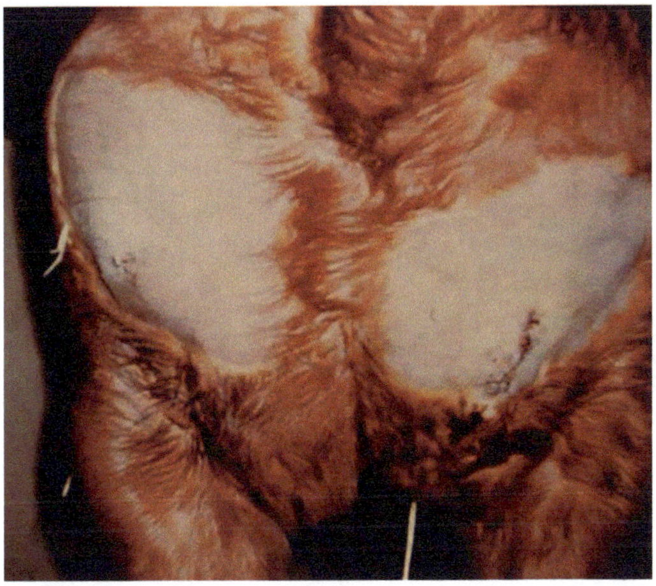

**Figure 13.26.** Horse. Chest. Plaques of Alopecia and Leukoderma. Amyloidosis. Large areas of nodular expansion of the skin of the pectoral region of the horse.

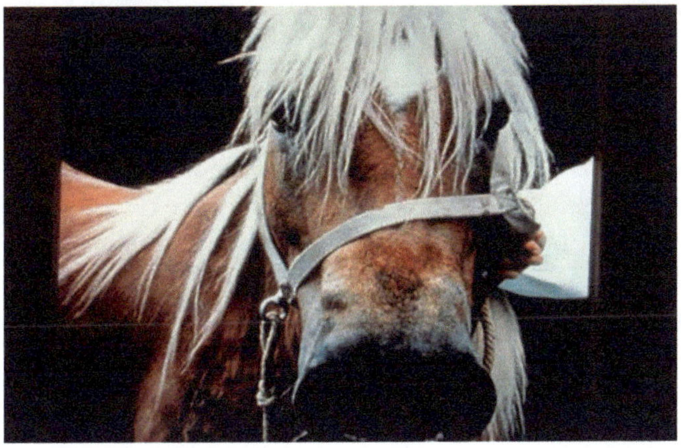

**Figure 13.27.** Horse. Head. Rhinomegaly with Ulcerative Dermatitis. Amyloidosis. The nasal portion of the head has a swollen appearance. Differential diagnosis: nutritional fibrous osteodystrophy (bran disease).

Cutaneous amyloidosis in the horse is characterized clinically by papules, nodules, or plaques most often found on the head, neck, shoulder, or pectoral region. The lesions are not associated with systemic disease and are most often asymptomatic, although some horses with cutaneous amyloidosis may have also have deposits of amyloid in the upper respiratory tract and regional nodes. Lesions vary from 0.5 to 10 cm in diameter and are usually covered by normal skin. The amyloid present has been determined to be AL amyloid derived from immunoglobulin light chains. Clinical differentials include other cases of nodular dermal lesions in the horse such as eosinophilic granulomas, granulomatous inflammation of infectious etiology, or neoplasms.

# VI. Helminthic diseases of the skin

## *1. Habronemiasis*

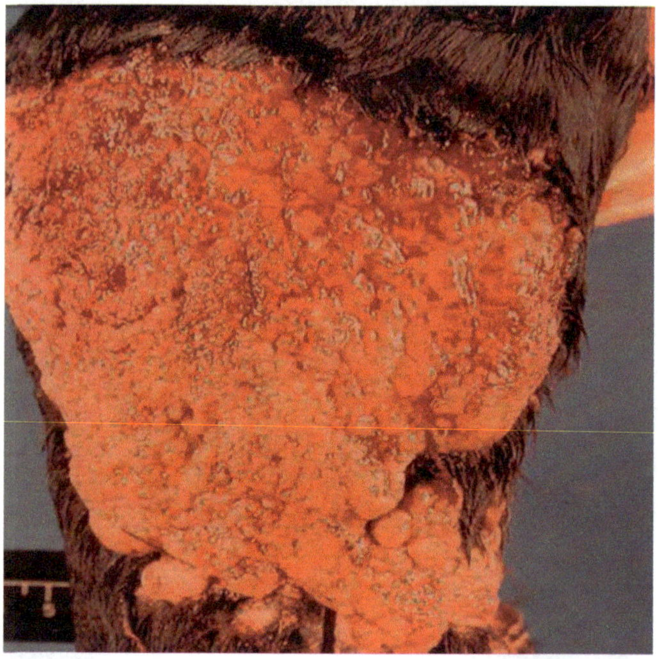

**Figure 13.28.** Horse. Leg. Granular Ulcerative Dermatitis. Cutaneous Habronemiasis (summer sores). An exophytic granular tissue with alopecia is present.

The lesion is considered to be a hypersensitivity reaction to dead and/or dying larvae and develops in areas of moisture such as the genitalia, periocular region, or in preexisting wounds. The nematodes are transmitted by flies that are drawn to areas of moisture or trauma, with eventual aberrant deposition and dermal migration of these larval gastric spiruid nematodes (*Habronema majus* [*microstoma*], *H. muscae*, and *H. megastoma*). Habronemiasis frequently induces pruritic gross lesions that include single to multiple ulcerative granulomas that rapidly progress and on cut section may contain numerous small caseous to gritty yellow granules (similar in appearance to the "kunkers" seen in pythiosis, but without the typical branching pattern). Differential diagnoses for cutaneous habronemiasis include exuberant granulation tissue, pythiosis, bacterial or fungal granulomas, sarcoids, and squamous cell carcinoma. *Habronema* is a common secondary infection, especially in ulcerated lesions.

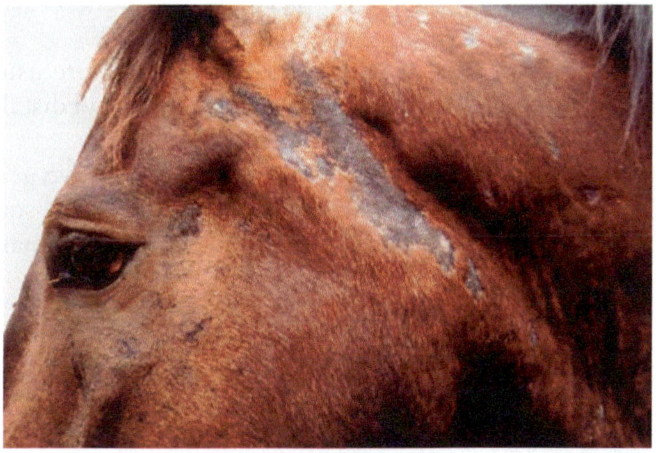

**Figure 13.29.** Horse. Head. Focal Alopecia and Depigmentation. Microfilarial Dermatitis. Cutaneous Onchocerciasis. Alopecia, scaling, and crusting around the face, head, and mane.

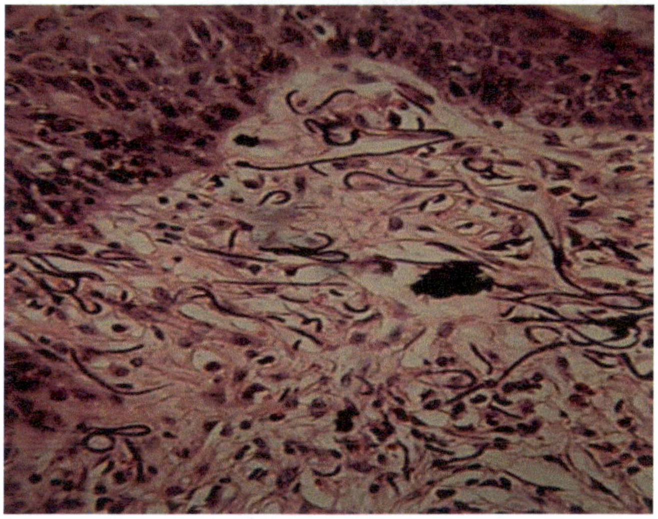

**Figure 13.30.** Horse. Skin. Microfilarial Dermatitis. Cutaneous Onchocerciasis. Numerous microfilariae are present in the superficial dermis. There is little inflammation. Microfilariae can be present in the skin of nonclinical horses as well. (H&E)

Onchocerciasis is a common nonseasonal cause of scaling, alopecia, depigmentation, and pruritus primarily of the ventral midline, neck, and face/periorbital region caused by the filariid nematode parasite, *Onchocerca cervicalis*. The thorax, abdomen, and medial aspects of the forelimbs may also be involved. Adult nematodes are primarily located in the subcutis, tendons, and ligaments (primarily the ligamentum nuchae) and produce microfilaria that migrate through the dermis. The dead and/or dying microfilaria induce an inflammatory response and are responsible for the lesions. The number of microfilaria do not correlate with the severity of lesions; some horses with microfilaria have no clinical signs. *Onchocerca cervicalis* is primarily transmitted by *Culicoides* sp. Differential diagnoses for ventral midline dermatitis include dermatophytosis, *Culicoides* hypersensitivity, and horn fly bites. However, horn fly bites often affect the majority of the horses in a group, whereas both *Culicoides* hypersensitivity and onchocerciasis are sporadic diseases.

# VII. Viral diseases of skin

## *1. Equine papillomaviral infection*

Horses affected by this species-specific papillomavirus 1 are usually young. Lesions typically develop on muzzles, lips, ears, eyelids, and distal limb. They spontaneously regress.

Horses with papillomavirus 2 are older and typically have genital lesions that often do not spontaneously regress and may evolve into squamous cell carcinoma. Papillomavirus-associated squamous cell carcinomas have been reported in nongenital lesions as well.

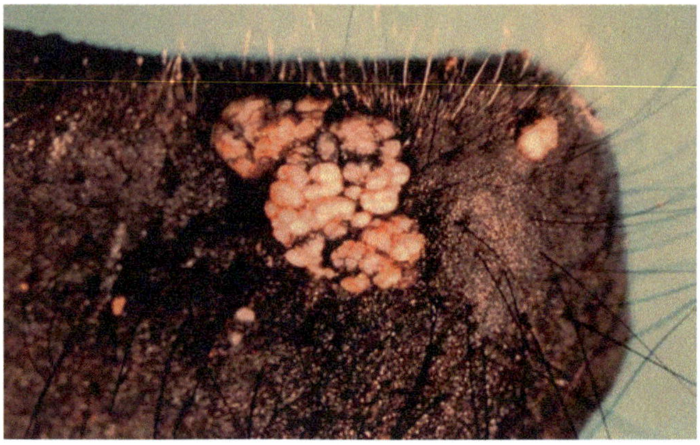

**Figure 13.31.** Horse. Nose. Proliferative Nodular Dermatitis. Raised, confluent clusters of warts are present.

The role of papilloma virus in the development of sarcoid and aural flat warts is discussed in Chapter 14, "Diseases of the Eye and Ear."

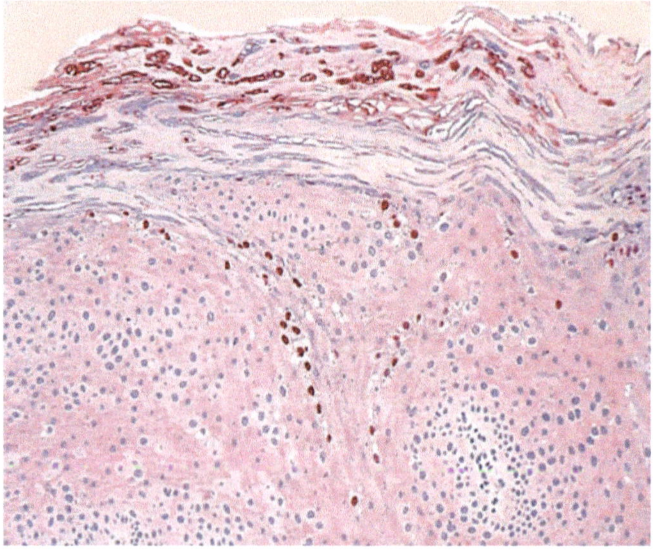

**Figure 13.32.** Horse. Skin. Viral Papillomatosis. Indirect immunohistochemistry identifies the intranuclear papillomavirus antigen distribution and reveals that the virus, starting from basal cells, tends to concentrate within the more superficial and keratinized layers favoring transmission of the infection. (IHC)

## 2. Poxvirus infection



### a. *Molluscum contagiosum*

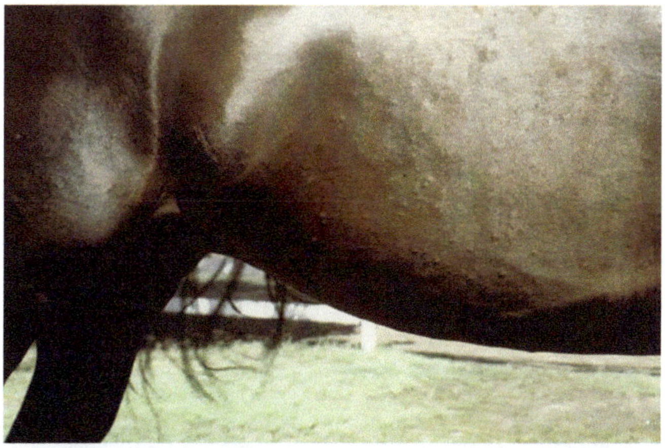

**Figure 13.33.** Horse. Skin. Body. Papular Dermatitis. Molluscum Contagiosum. Shallow papules induced by a poxvirus (*Molluscipoxvirus*) are present in the skin. (Courtesy Dr. E.G. Clark, Calgary, Canada.)

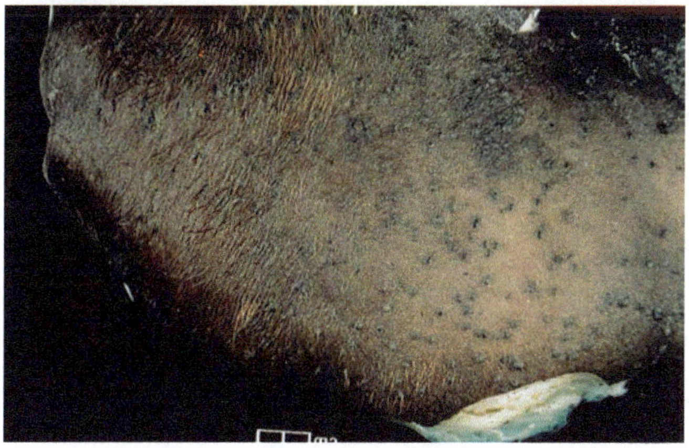

**Figure 13.34.** Horse. Skin. Body. Papular Dermatitis. Molluscum Contagiosum. Multiple small pigmented papules are visible. (Courtesy Dr. E.G. Clark, Calgary, Canada.)

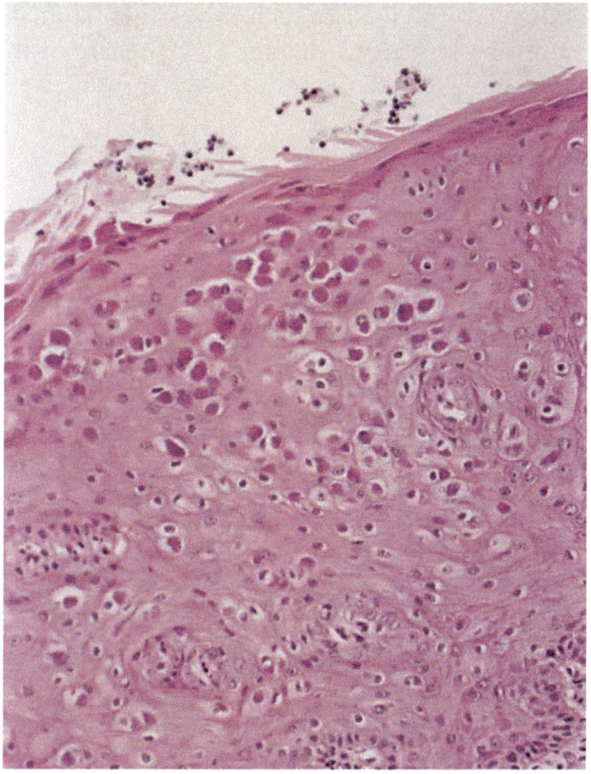

**Figure 13.35.** Horse. Skin. Epidermal Hyperplasia. Molluscum Contagiosum. Well-demarcated foci of epidermal hyperplasia with hypertrophied keratinocytes containing large intracytoplasmic inclusions. Infected keratinocytes exfoliate at the surface. (H&E) (Courtesy Dr. E.G. Clark, Calgary, Canada.)

Equine molluscum contagiosum is a mildly contagious and self-limiting proliferative poxvirus infection thought to be caused by a poxvirus that is very similar to the causal agent of human molluscum contagiosum. The clinical lesions are most often found on the muzzle, prepuce, penis, inguinal, or axillary regions and appear as clusters of smooth white papules that over time become umbilicated and develop a central pore with a caseous plug. In some horses, the lesions become generalized. Histologically, the lesions are characterized by sharply demarcated regions of epidermal hyperplasia with hypertrophied keratinocytes that contain large amphophilic, basophilic intracytoplasmic inclusions referred to as "molluscum bodies." The infected keratinocytes exfoliate from the surface to form a craterlike depression. There is usually no dermal reaction.

*b. Equine poxvirus*

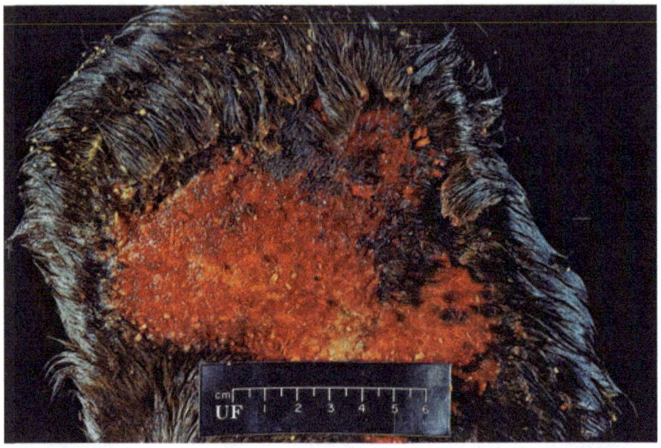


**Figure 13.36.** Horse. Skin of Neck. Exudative Dermatitis. Poxvirus. Erythematous pustules may heal spontaneously.

Other equine cutaneous viral diseases such as vesicular stomatitis and herpes coital exanthema are presented in Chapter 6, "Diseases of the Gastrointestinal Tract," and Chapter 12, "Diseases of the Reproductive Tract."

## VIII. Bacterial diseases of the skin

### 1. *Dermatophilosis*

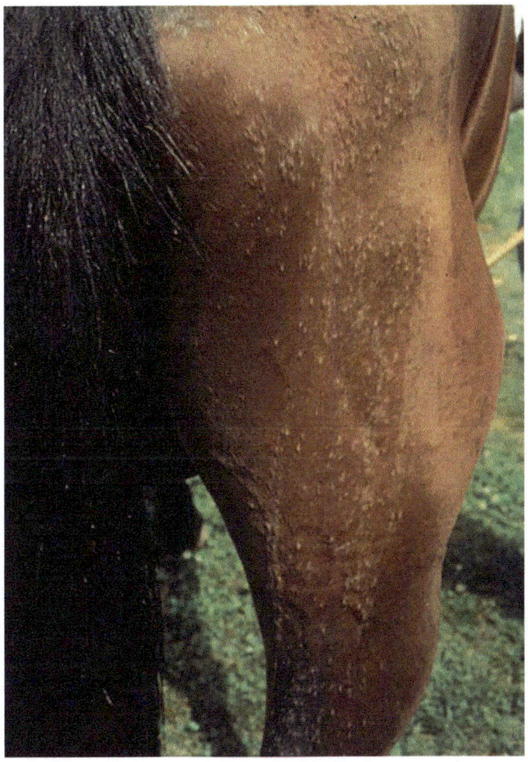

**Figure 13.37.** Horse. Hind Leg. Pustular Epidermatitis. Dermatophilosis. The rump and upper hind leg skin is characterized by papules progressing to pustules.

This pustular and crusting skin infection is caused by *Dermatophilus congolensis*, a gram-positive, partially anaerobic bacterium. Infection is preceded by skin abrasion and moisture. Vectors such as insects play a role in transmission.

Other bacterial skin diseases to consider are staphylococcal and streptococcal organisms responsible for bacterial folliculitis, *Corynebacterium pseudotuberculosis*, and *Actinomyces* sp.

## Dermatophilosis – Fact sheet

### Definition

- Exudative dermatitis caused by *Dermatophilus congolensis*
    - Gram-positive pleomorphic bacteria
- Other names include strawberry foot rot, rain scald, rain rot, lumpy wool

### Incidence

- Common disease, especially during rainy season
- Three factors most important for infection:
    - Chronic carriers (zoospores resist drying and can survive in scabs for years)
    - Moisture, such as rain and sweating
    - Break in skin integrity, such as trauma or ectoparasites (normal healthy skin is resistant to infection)
- No age, breed, or sex predilection

## Dermatophilosis – Pathologic features

### Gross findings

- Multifocal to coalescing exudative dermatitis with dry crusts, scales, tufted papules, pustules, and alopecia that are more painful than pruritic
- Thick "paintbrush" crusts often on the dorsal aspect of the animal, but they may also be on face, sides of neck, flank, distal limb, or generalized
    - Hair easily exfoliates when crusts removed, revealing pink eroded skin
    - Active lesions may contain underlying pockets of purulent material
- Often worse in areas of white skin, and they may be associated with a photodermatitis

## Dermatophilosis – Pathologic features continued

### Microscopic findings

- Thick laminated crusts containing alternating layers of hyperkeratosis and degenerate neutrophils
- Stratum corneum may contain narrow branching bacterial filaments that subdivide longitudinally and transversely forming parallel rows of coccoid zoospores

### Differential diagnosis

- Dermatophytosis
- Bacterial folliculitis
- Pemphigus foliaceus
- Demodicosis

### *2. Botryomycosis*

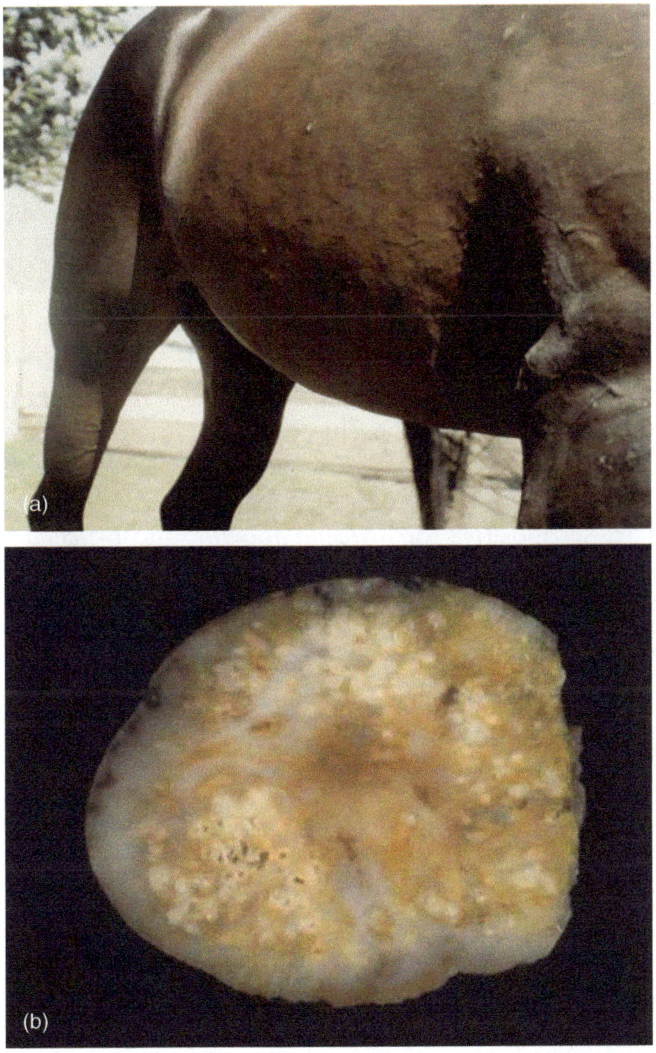


**Figure 13.38.** Horse (a) Body and (b) Cross Section through Nodule. Nodular, Pyogranulomatous Dermatitis. Botryomycosis (bacterial pseudomycetoma). (Courtesy Dr. E.G. Clark, Calgary, Canada.)

Botryomycosis is a relatively uncommon disease in horses that is due to chronic granulomatous bacterial infection. On cut section, nodules contain white to yellow granules. Microscopically these granules correspond to compact colonies of bacteria surrounded by Splendore-Hoeppli material and further surrounded by granulomatous or pyogranulomatous inflammation. Although the pathogenesis is unclear, infection is thought to occur secondary to trauma, immunosuppression, or wound contamination. Grossly lesions are characterized by single to multiple firm nonpruritic nodules, often on the face, limbs, and/or scrotum. The nodules may eventually ulcerate, develop fistulas, and drain purulent material containing yellow granular material. Severe infection has been associated with dysfunction of the pars intermedia. Differential diagnoses include actinomycotic and eumycotic mycetomas, habronemiasis, granulation tissue, and other causes of granulomatous inflammation.

### *3. Fistulous withers and poll evil*

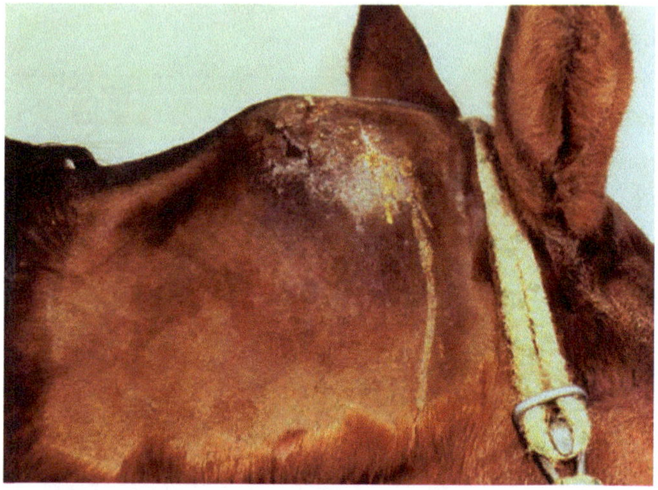

**Figure 13.39.** Horse. Neck. Necrosuppurative Fistulous Bursitis and Focal Dermatitis. Poll Evil. The condition involves the supra-atlantal bursa, whereas fistulous withers affects the supra-spinous bursa. (Courtesy Dr. D. Meuten, North Carolina State University.)

In cases of fistulous withers or poll evil, the bursae over the cranial vertebral spinal processes are filled with a viscid purulent exudate that swells the skin of the neck and opens to the surface of the skin via fistulous tracts.

The nuchal ligament may become involved in the inflammation as well. Some horses are seropositive for *Brucella abortus*, and *Brucella abortus* may be isolated from the fistulous tracts. Other bacteria cultured from the exudate are *Streptococcus* sp., *Staphylococcus aureus*, and *Actinomyces bovis*.

# IX. Fungal diseases of skin

## 1. Dermatophytosis

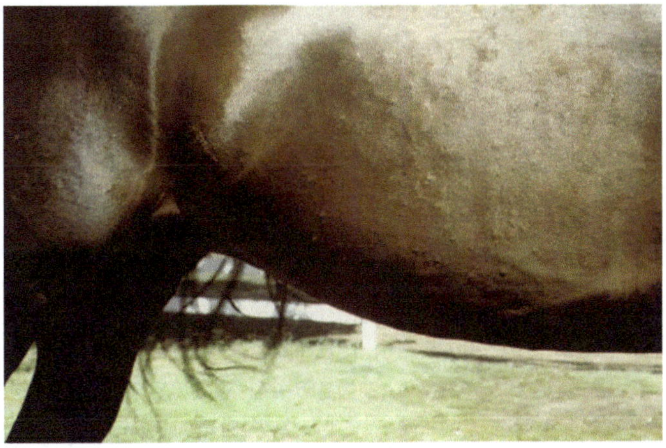

**Figure 13.40.** Horse. Body. Papular Dermatitis. Dermatophytosis (ringworm, girth itch, tinea). Early changes are characterized by papules. (Courtesy Dr. E.G. Clark, Calgary, Canada.)

Dermatophytosis is a common fungal infection in equines caused by a variety of organisms including *Trichophyton equinum* (the most common cause in the horse), *Trichophyton mentagrophytes*, *Microsporum gypseum,* and, less commonly, *Trichophyton verrucosum* and *Microsporum canis.* Young animals are especially susceptible, as are those in high-stress environments (overcrowding, poor sanitation, nutritional). Dermatophytosis is often seasonal, occurring primarily in the wettest seasons (winter in colder regions and summer in hot regions). Because normal skin is relatively resistant, infection often requires skin microtrauma. For this reason, lesions are most commonly located in saddle/tack areas, such as the face, neck, thorax, and girth (the mane and tail are usually unaffected). Occasionally lesions may be present on the caudal aspect of the pastern and rarely on the coronary bands. Grossly, lesions may originate as multiple edematous and tufted papules that quickly progress to patchy annular crusting and scaly areas of alopecia that usually are not pruritic. Scabs can be removed easily, and the underlying epidermis is generally smooth and intact. Transmission occurs via direct contact with infected animals or via fomites. Differential diagnoses include other causes of scaling/crusting dermatoses such as *Dermatophilus congolensis*, bacterial folliculitis, pemphigus foliaceus, and demodicosis.

## 2. Phaeohyphomycosis

Phaeohyphomycosis is caused by a heterogenous group of relatively uncommon, opportunistic mycotic infections whose pigmented (dematiaceous) fungal hyphae contain melanin in their cell walls. Infections are rare in horses and are frequently secondary to trauma. Lesions may be single or multiple, firm, well-circumscribed subcutaneous nodules that are occasionally pigmented. The overlying hair coat ranges from normal to alopecic or ulcerated. Lesions in horses are frequently multiple and may be localized or disseminated over the whole body. There are no known sex, breed, or age predilections. Clinical differential diagnoses for phaeohyphomycosis include melanoma (if nodule is pigmented), granulomas (foreign body, infectious or sterile), or other neoplasms. Histologically, lesions are pyogranulomatous, with intralesional pigmented hyphae. Numerous isolates of fungi have been identified in horses with cutaneous phaeohyphomycosis, and due to the similar histologic appearances between species, culture is required for specific identification.

### 3. Sporotrichosis

Sporotrichosis is an uncommon disease caused by *Sporothrix schenckii*, a ubiquitous dimorphic, saprophytic fungus that occurs most commonly in tropical and temperate zones. In the horse the cutaneous lymphatic form is the most common presentation. Infection occurs via wound inoculation (e.g., wood splinters, thorns, or contaminated claws) and is often limited to the skin, subcutaneous tissue, and associated lymphatics. Lesions usually originate on the distal limbs, presenting as firm round nodules at the point of inoculation, and spread proximally along lymphatics. Lymphatics eventually develop a thickened corded appearance that develops into a series secondary ulcerative and exudative (seropurulent) nodules. These nodules may develop cavitated abscesses that expose underlying skeletal muscle and bone. Histologic findings are characterized by a multifocal to diffuse pyogranulomatous dermatitis and panniculitis. Yeasts have a refractile cell wall, are round to oval to "cigar" shaped, and often few in number, making them difficult to identify on histologic examination. Differential diagnoses include granulomas (due to infectious causes and foreign bodies) as well as neoplasms.

### 4. Epizootic lymphangitis

Caused by *Histoplasma capsulatum* var. *farciminosum*, this disorder usually affects lymphatics to result in ulcerative dermatitis of the extremities. It can appear in any area of trauma. It can be transmitted by flies or fomites. Clinical signs are similar to farcy (*Burkholderia mallei)*, sporotrichosis, and ulcerative lymphangitis caused by *Corynebacterium pseudotuberculosis*.

### 5. Zygomycosis

Zygomycosis refers to infections caused by a wide variety of Zygomycetes, encompassing mucormycosis (*Absidia, Mortierella, Mucor, Rhizomucor, Rhizopus*) and entomophthoromycosis (*Basidiobolus* and *Conidiobolus*). The disease, which is due to ubiquitous saprophytes, occurs most commonly in tropical and subtropical areas.

Zygomycosis is thought to occur secondary to trauma, inhalation, or ingestion. Infections may be systemic, subcutaneous, rhinal, or cerebral. Mucormycosis generally causes widespread disease, often with characteristic angioinvasion, whereas entomophthoromycosis often presents with localized subcutaneous granulomas. Most frequently, zygomycosis in horses is due to basidiobolomycosis (*Basidiobolus ranarum*) and conidiobolomycosis (*Conidiobolus coronatus*). Basidiobolomycosis has a predilection for the head, neck, chest, or lateral trunk; conidiobolomycosis characteristically prefers the nares, nasal mucosa, and surrounding skin.

Gross lesions are often characterized by proliferative, ulcerative, and exudative dermatitis with small yellow "kunkers" or "leeches" of no particular shape. On cut section, edematous granulation tissue is distinctly separated from superficial hemorrhage by yellowish white serpentine material.

Histologically, Zygomycetes are characterized by large (5–20 μm in diameter) fungal hyphae with nonparallel walls that are rarely septate and irregularly branching, often surrounded by Splendore-Hoeppli material. The microscopic lesion includes multifocal to coalescing eosinophilic to pyogranulomatous dermatitis and panniculitis, with central areas of necrosis often containing hyphae. The differential diagnoses for zygomycosis include pythiosis, habronemiasis, foreign body granulomas, granulation tissue, sarcoids, and squamous cell carcinoma.

## X. Oomycete diseases of the skin: pythiosis

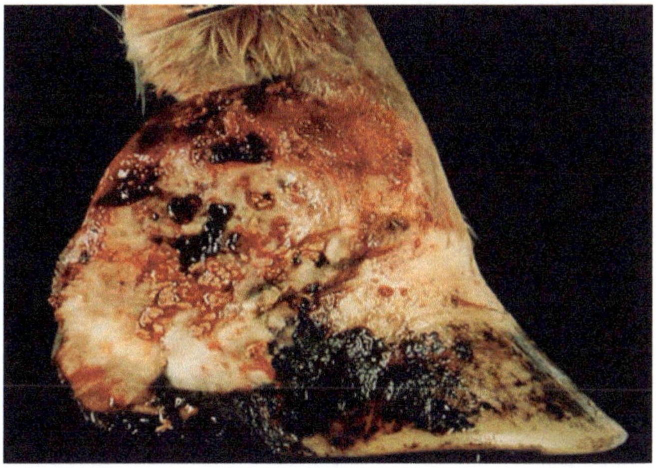

**Figure 13.41.** Horse. Distal Limb. Pyogranulomatous Dermatitis. Pythiosis (Cutaneous Oomycosis). Focally extensive proliferative and exudative dermatitis of the distal limb with yellow "kunkers" or "leeches."

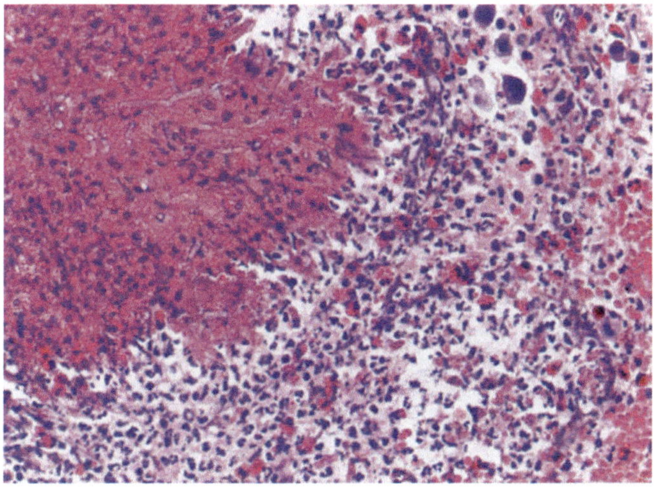

**Figure 13.42.** Horse. Skin over Mandible. Eosinophilic Pyogranulomatous Dermatitis. Phythiosis. A nodular inflammatory infiltrate is composed of degranulating eosinophils, centered on hypereosinophilic degenerated bundles of collagen and surrounded by lymphocytes, neutrophils, epithelioid macrophages, and rare multinucleate giant cells (eosinophilic granuloma also referred to as "kunkers"). Argyrophilic hypha-like structures of the agent can be demonstrated by special silver stains. (H&E)

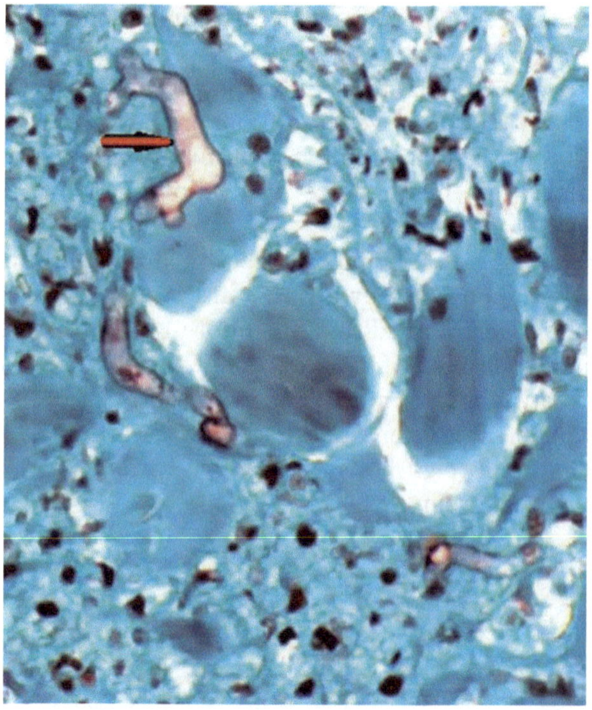

**Figure 13.43.** Horse. Skin. Eosinophilic Pyogranulomatous Dermatitis. Pythiosis. A silver stain shows argyrophilic hypha-like structures (arrow) within the eosinophilic granuloma. Hypha-like structures have nonparallel, often bulging walls, are 3–10 μm in diameter, and are occasionally branching and rarely septate (etiology consistent with *Pythium insidiosum*). (GMS)

*Pythium insidiosum* is an aquatic dimorphic water oomycete that is an opportunistic pathogen reported primarily in tropical and subtropical regions. Infection frequently occurs in sites of trauma and is thought to occur after exposure to stagnant fresh water containing the infective zoospores. Lesions are most common on the distal limbs and ventrum. Although lesions are initially nodular, they quickly progress to ulcerated draining masses. Differentials for the gross appearance of pythiosis include exuberant granulation tissue, sarcoids, cutaneous habronemiasis, squamous cell carcinoma, and basidiobolomycosis.

## XI. Protozoal diseases of the skin

### *1. Leishmaniasis*

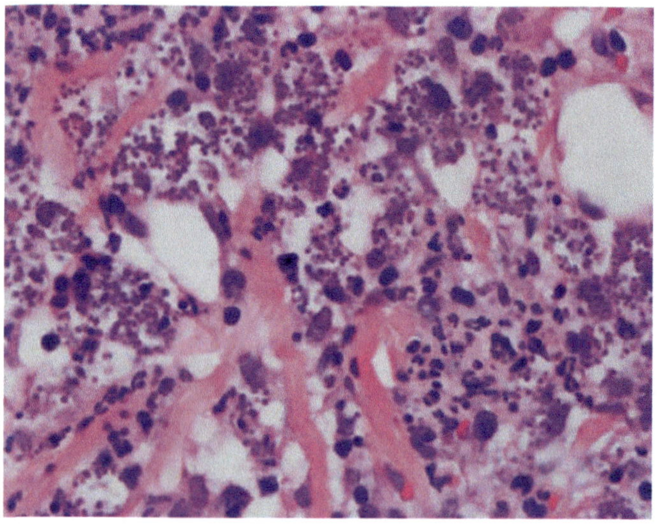

**Figure 13.44.** Horse. Skin. Histiocytic Dermatitis. Leishmaniasis. Numerous intrahistiocytic intracytoplasmic amastigotes are present. (H&E) (Courtesy Dr. M. Calderwood Mays, Gainesville, FL.)

Cutaneous leishmaniasis caused by *Leishmania brasiliensis* or *mexicana* in the New World has been reported on occasions in Floridian horses with a history of being imported from Latin America. The sandfly (*Lutzomyia* sp.) is considered the vector in the New World and perhaps ticks. The head, neck pinna, and legs are typically involved. Skin lesions are characterized by solitary or multiple nodules with a central ulcer. The nodules are histologically composed of granulomas. Specific diagnosis is made by smears, serology (enzyme-linked immunosorbent assay), indirect fluoroscopy, and polymerase chain reaction (PCR). A recent case of autochthonous *Leishmania siamensis* was identified in a Floridian horse in aural skin samples by PCR. The mode of transmission in this case was undetermined. Differential diagnoses should include aural plaque (warts), *Trypanosoma cruzi,* and sarcoid.

## *2. Besnoitiosis*

Caused by *Besnoitia bennetti*, equine besnoitiosis has been rarely observed in North America, where it typically has been reported in donkeys. A recent report described besnoitiosis in donkeys from Pennsylvania. Other donkey cases were diagnosed in the northeastern states, Midwest, and western states of the United States. Gross lesions of chronic dermatitis are described as multifocal small parasitic cysts spread over nares, neck, sclera (pearls), pinnae, and on limbs. Histologically, the protozoal cysts are fairly large, spherical, and packed by bradyzoites.

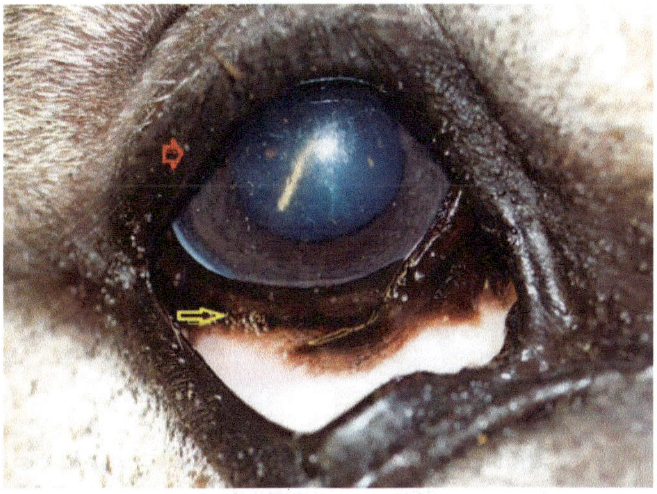

**Figure 13.45.** Donkey. Eye and Eyelid. Papular Dermatitis. Besnoitiosis. The eyelids contain pinpoint papules and protozoal cysts (red arrow) and the sclera "pearls" (yellow arrow). (Courtesy Dr. J. Peters-Kennedy, Cornell University.)

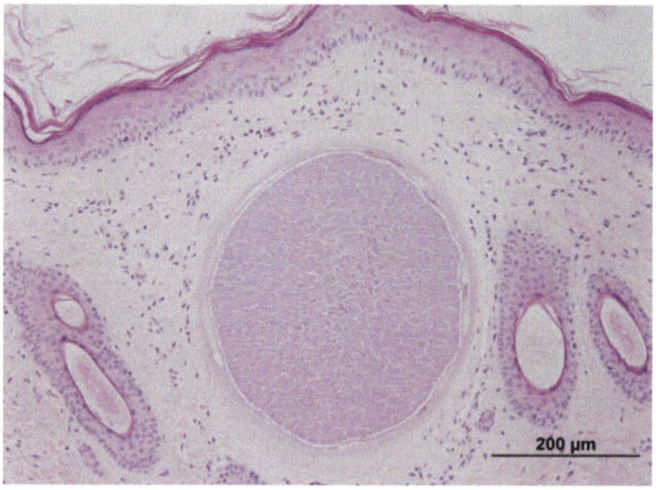


**Figure 13.46.** Donkey. Skin. Lymphocytic Dermatitis. Besnoitiosis. A large protozoal cyst containing bradyzoites is surrounded by minimal dermal inflammation. The cyst wall is prominent and translucent. (H&E) (Courtesy Dr. J. Peters-Kennedy, Cornell University.)

## XII. Ectoparasites: Mange

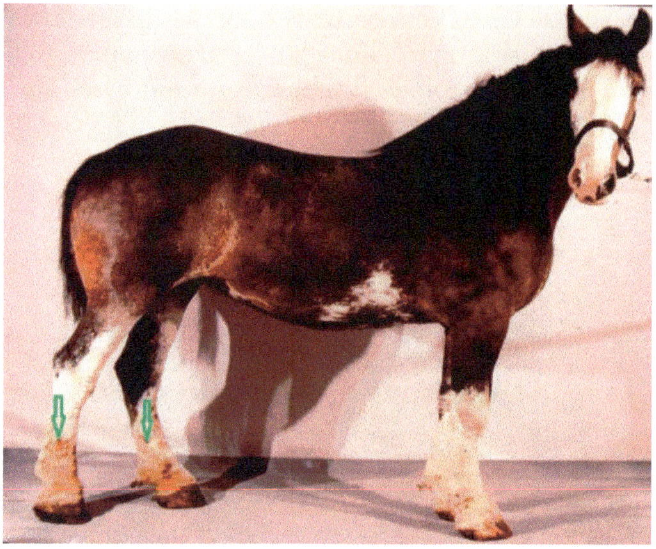

**Figure 13.47.** Horse. Distal Limbs. Ulcerative Dermatitis. Chorioptic Mange. Alopecia, crusting, and ulceration of the distal limbs in a draft horse (arrows).

Four species of mites that cause mange affect horses: *Chorioptes* sp., *Psoroptes* sp., *Sarcoptes* sp., and *Demodex* sp. Pruritus is almost always present and is often associated with mechanical injury or trauma to the skin, and hypersensitivity to mite products. In general the life cycles range from 14 to 28 days and are completed on the host. Clinical signs depend on the mite involved, with the severity of lesions usually reliant on the number of mites affecting the animal. The disease commences with papules, and there are often secondary skin lesions associated with trauma and bacterial infection.

*Chorioptic mange.* Chorioptic mange (leg mange, tail mange) is a potential cause of pruritic dermatitis in horses, especially draft horses and other horses with feathered fetlocks. Lesions from the surface dwelling mites (*Chorioptes equi* or *C. bovis*) are usually present on the lower limbs, and they may progress proximally to the upper limbs, tail, and ventral abdomen. Affected animals have papules, scales, alopecia, excoriations, and crusts, often depending on duration of lesions and level of secondary trauma. Histologic lesions are characterized by an eosinophilic superficial perivascular to interstitial dermatitis with varying degrees of epidermal inflammation and damage. Mites are difficult to demonstrate on histologic examination. Transmission can be via direct or indirect contact. Mite populations are sensitive to host and environmental factors and do not survive for extended periods of time in higher temperatures and arid conditions, making clinical signs most prominent in the colder months.

*Demodectic mange.* The mites causing demodectic mange (follicular mange) are normal inhabitants of the pilosebaceous units of most domestic species. Demodicosis is a rare pruritic follicular dermatosis of equids, with two species of the mite affecting horses. *Demodex caballi* most commonly affects the eyelids and muzzle, whereas *D. equi* can parasitize the whole body but usually originates in the region of the head, neck, and shoulders. As with the other manges, the primary lesion is papular, but nodules, pustules, scaling, and alopecia can be present. Because demodectic mites are normal inhabitants of hair follicles and sebaceous glands, clinical disease is usually present in animals that are immunocompromised, whether it is due to environmental stress, concurrent disease, or administration of glucocorticoids.

*Psoroptic mange.* Psoroptic mange of horses is due to *Psoroptes* sp. mites, which most commonly cause pruritic dermatitis and/or otitis externa. *Psoroptes equi, P. cuniculi, P. natalensis,* and *P. ovis* have all been reported to parasitize the horse. *Psoroptes* sp. do not burrow but live on the skin under crusts and scale, feeding on tissue fluids. Transmission may occur via direct or indirect contact. Clinical signs are extremely variable and may range from asymptomatic to extreme pruritus. Head, base of mane, and tail are commonly affected, but lesions may progress and become generalized. If parasitic otitis externa is present, head shaking, head shyness, and lop-eared carriage may occur. Multiple nonfollicular papules are the primary lesions, which are associated with crusts, excoriations, and alopecia.

*Sarcoptic mange.* Sarcoptic mange due to *Sarcoptes scabiei* var. *equi* is a very rare (eradicated in the United States) reportable disease in horses that causes erythematous macular or papular dermatitis, primarily of the head, ears (edges of the pinnae), neck, progressing to generalized disease. The mites feed on tissue and fluids; the female burrows through the epidermis and lays eggs. The number-one clinical sign of sarcoptic mange is pruritus, considered to be primarily a hypersensitivity reaction to mite irritants and mechanical damage caused by the mites. Transmission of this highly contagious disease is via direct and indirect contact. *Sarcoptes* sp. are found on numerous mammalian hosts, and cross infestations between animals and humans are common. Mites are very difficult to demonstrate on scrapings or histopathologically. However, definitive diagnosis requires identification of the parasite.

*Other ectoparasites.* Ticks, lice, biting flies, mosquitoes, and biting midges (discussed earlier).

## XIII. Miscellaneous skin disorders

### 1. Canker

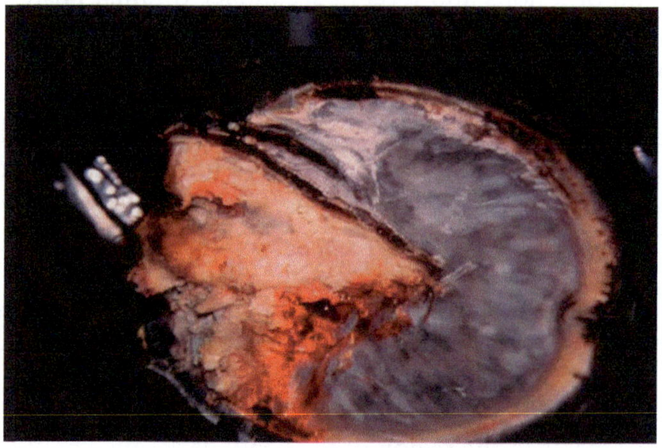

**Figure 13.48.** Horse. Sole. Proliferative Nodular Pododermatitis. Canker. A grayish red brittle vegetative tissue occupies the frog and the sole.

The etiology of this chronic hypertrophy of keratin-producing tissue in the frog and sole of the equine hoof of the hind legs is poorly understood. Draft horses are mainly affected. Intralesional organisms have been demonstrated in the affected areas, especially gram-negative anaerobic bacteria and spirochetes. Recent studies have demonstrated bovine papillomavirus (BPV)-1 and -2 in the lesions.

### 2. Chronic progressive lymphedema

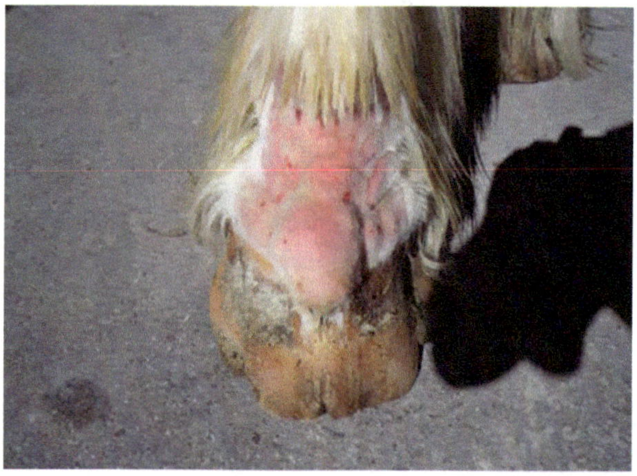

**Figure 13.49.** Horse. Limb. Dermal Fibrosis and Alopecia. Chronic Progressive Lymphedema. The distal limb of this draft horse is disfigured by large nodular areas of dermal fibrosis. (Courtesy P. Hambleton, Ocala, FL.)

Chronic progressive limb edema is a condition found in draft horses characterized by long-standing edema of the distal limbs that progressively leads to ulceration and dermal fibrosis. The pathogenesis is thought to be an inherited disorder of dermal elastin leading to poor support of the limb lymphatics, edema, tissue hypoxia, and eventual nodular dermal fibrosis and epidermal hyperplasia. The condition usually begins by 2–4 years of age and often leads to death secondary to disfigurement and untreatable lameness.

### 3. *Cushing syndrome*

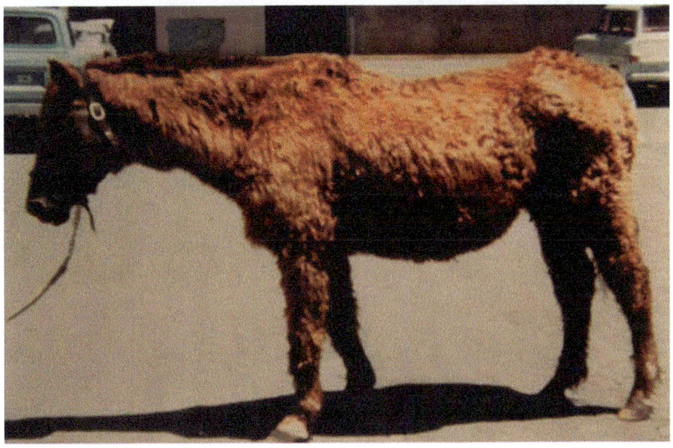

**Figure 13.50.** Horse. Whole Body. Hypertrichosis. Cushing Syndrome. Curly coat from failure of shedding hair.

Hypertrichosis caused by the failure of seasonal shedding (hirsutism), pot belly, and sway back is a common finding in cushingoid horses and is due to a functional pituitary adenoma of the pars intermedia (see Chapter 11, "Diseases of the Endocrine System"). These tumors are frequent incidental findings at necropsy, but they can grow large enough to protrude from the sella turcica, causing compression of the overlying hypothalamus and resultant clinical signs because the hypothalamus is responsible for regulation of cyclic shedding of hair, body temperature, and appetite.

### 4. *Drug eruption*

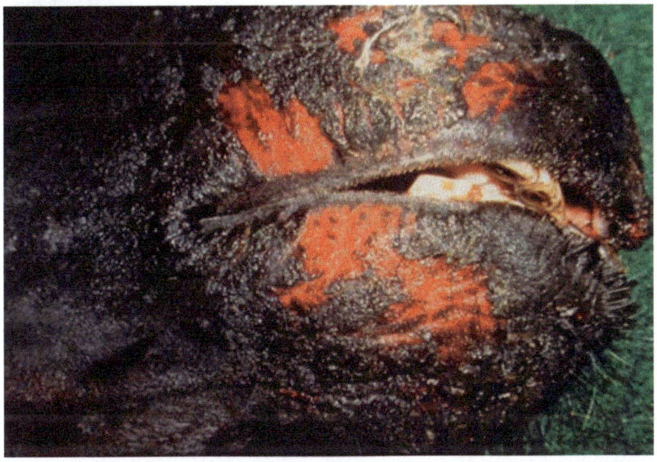

**Figure 13.51.** Horse. Muzzle. Ulcerative Cheilitis. Multifocal to coalescing ulcerations on muzzle.

Drug eruptions are clinically pleomorphic entities that may have almost any clinical appearance. A history of spontaneous occurrence after treatment with drugs such as nonsteroidal anti-inflammatories, sulfonamides, penicillin, biologics, or vaccination is important for the diagnosis and to rule out other causes such as mechanical, infectious, and autoimmune etiologies.

### 5. *Erythema multiforme*

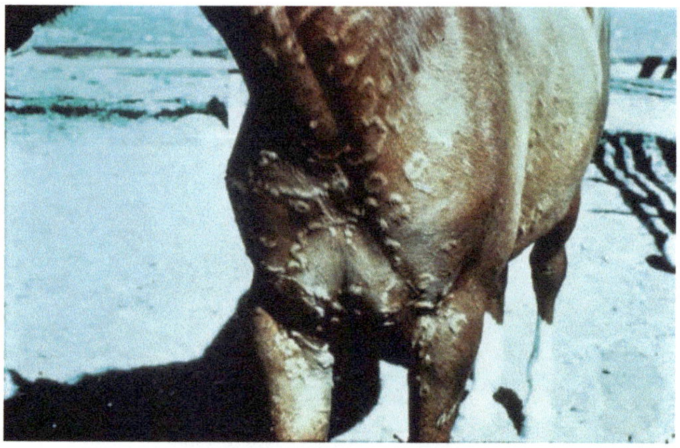

**Figure 13.52.** Horse. Neck and Pectoral Region. Papular Dermatitis with Central Ulcers. Erythema Multiforme. Annular, serpiginous to arciform lesions, often characterized by vesicular or ulcerated central regions surrounded by pale regions and an erythematous peripheral ring that is best visualized in poorly haired areas.

The disorder is often obscure as to etiology and may resolve after several weeks. A recent publication associated equine herpesvirus-5 with the condition.

### 6. *Eosinophilic granuloma*

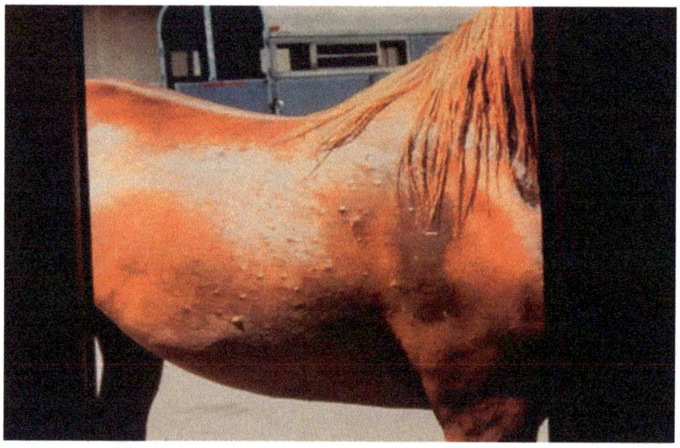

**Figure 13.53.** Horse. Skin. Lateral Thorax. Nodular Dermatitis. Eosinophilic Granulomas (Equine Nodular Necrobiosis). A cluster of nodules is present. Differential diagnoses should include: sterile granulomatosis, erythema multiforme, calcinosis circumscripta, neoplasia.

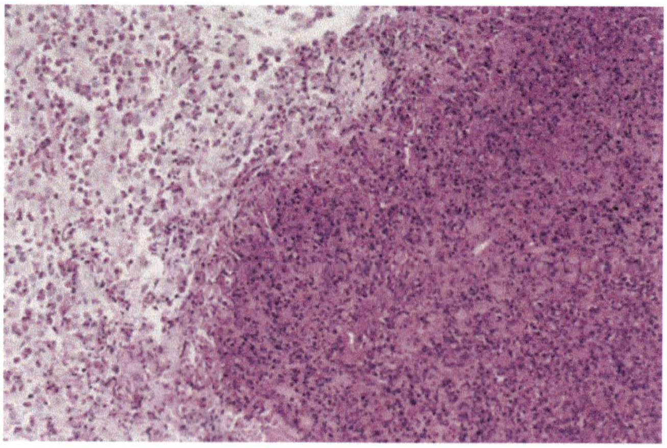

**Figure 13.54.** Horse. Skin. Granulomatous Dermatitis. Eosinophilic Granuloma. Nodular aggregates of degranulated eosinophils and influx of histiocytes and lymphocytes. (H&E) (Courtesy Dr. E.G. Clark, Calgary, Canada.)

Eosinophilic granulomas, also known as nodular necrobiosis or collagenolytic granulomas, are common nodular skin lesions in the horse. The pathogenesis of lesion formation is not known but is speculated to represent a cutaneous response to an allergen such as in atopy or insect bite reactions. Nodules are 0.5–10 cm in diameter and occur over the withers, back, or neck most often. The lesions are usually asymptomatic. Histologically, the nodule corresponds to a collection of degranulated and intact eosinophils accompanied by granulomatous or lymphocytic inflammation in the dermis and subcutis. Some lesions are mineralized.

### *7. Exuberant granulation tissue*

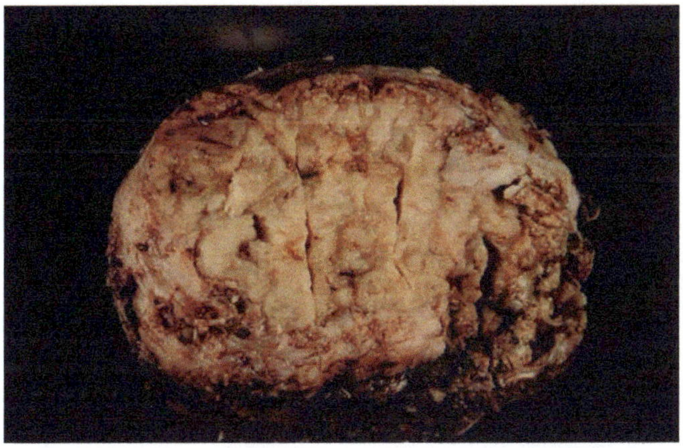

**Figure 13.55.** Horse. Skin. Limb. Dermal Fibrosis. Exuberant Granulation Tissue (Proud Flesh). Cross section. Dense fibrous tissue has proliferated within the dermis and has expanded toward the epidermis. Often the epidermis ulcerates.

These proliferations of well-vascularized, fibrous connective tissue can grow to be quite large. Neoplasia, parasites, and oomycosis are differential diagnoses for exuberant granulation tissue.

### *8. Follicular cyst*

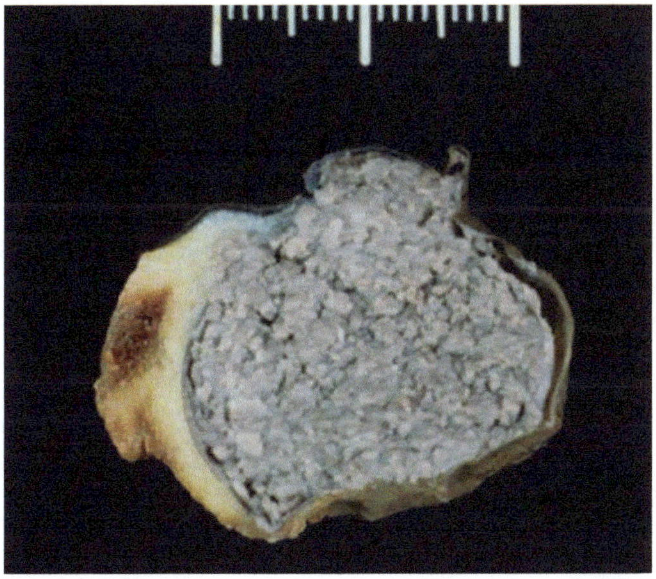

**Figure 13.56.** Horse. Skin. Caseous Dermatitis. Follicular Cyst. Follicular cyst on cross section, containing gray granular, caseous material that on histopathology is lamellar keratin within a cyst wall undergoing epidermal differentiation. (Courtesy Dr. E.G. Clark, Calgary, Canada.)

These uncommon nonneoplastic nodules are found primarily on the head and distal limbs of horses. Follicular cysts are classified into different forms based on the portion of the follicle that they develop from (infundibular, isthmus, matrical, and hybrid). In horses, follicular cysts are typically of the infundibular type.

## 9. Lightning

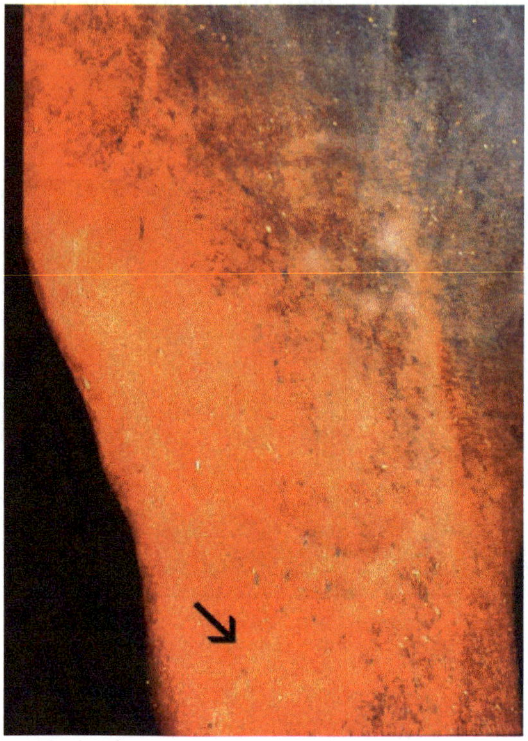

**Figure 13.57.** Horse. Skin. Kinked Hair. Burn Line. A single white line of hair (arrow) is descending distally at the cranial portion of the upper hind leg. (Courtesy Dr. J. Roberts, National Zoo, Washington, DC.)

Lightning is defined as a powerful electric discharge during a thunderstorm reaching a potential of 1 billion volts. The lightning spark can be more than 3 miles long, and charges reach the ground in a leader-like fashion. When the leader charges reach the ground, an immediate exchange between the electric leader charges and the electric ground charges occur, hitting objects in its path. At that time the lightning strike may reach peaks as high as 200,000 amperes.

Lightning is one of the causes of sudden death with sudden death defined here as death of a regularly observed and apparently healthy animal not exhibiting premonitory signs.

The specific diagnosis of lightning is extremely difficult to establish because less than 30% of animals struck by lightning have burn marks on the skin. The situation becomes more clear if a few animals are found dead on the pasture around a tree or close to a fence, usually in the summer after a severe thunderstorm. Rather than looking for burn marks on the dead animal, it is more important to look for circumstantial evidence in the environment of the animal(s): trees with broken bark, closeness of wire fences, posts, undisturbed bedding on which the animal is found dead (absence of signs of struggle), and history of local weather report verifying severe thunderstorms.

Burn marks, when present, appear as lines where there is kinking of hair and deviation of individual burned hair 90 degrees to the length of the visible burn line. The best spots to find burn lines are the medial sites of the legs.

When animals are struck by lightning, electric injuries occur to the skin, cardiovascular, neurologic, and ophthalmic systems. Examples of findings with or without burn lines are subcutaneous hemorrhages, blood roping in trachea, jugular vein distension by excessive blood (venous stasis), splenic rupture, vertebral fractures in unusual locations (e.g., cranial thorax).

## Causes of sudden death in horses – Fact sheet

**Definition:** Death of healthy animal without premonitory signs

### Causes

- Anthrax
- Aortic rupture of stallions
- Basosphenoid bone fracture
- Castor bean toxicity (*Ricinus communis*)
- Envenomation
- Excess selenium
- Gastric rupture
- Gunshot
- Intracarotid injection
- Lightning
- Monensin toxicity
- Rupture of middle uterine artery in mares
- Japanese yew (*Taxus cuspidata*)

### *10. Multisystemic eosinophilic epitheliotropic disease*

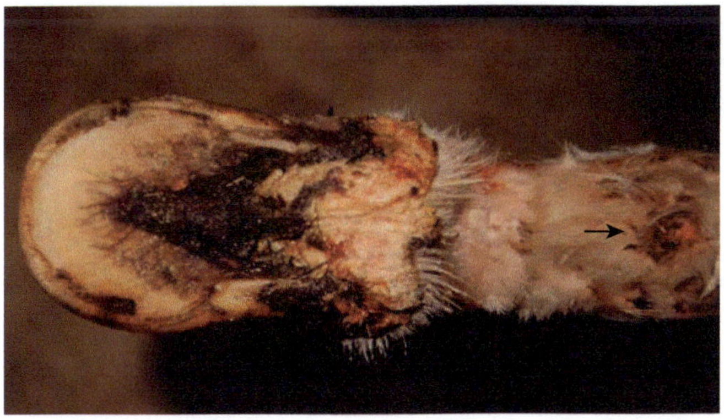

**Figure 13.58.** Horse. Distal Limb. Ulcerative Dermatitis. Multisystemic Eosinophilic Epitheliotropic Disease. Ulcerative changes in the skin are present in the long pastern area (arrow) above the hoof. Diagnosis is made by histology and by the clinical history of systemic disease. The hoof itself developed canker.

Multisystemic eosinophilic epitheliotrophic disease (MEED) is characterized by exfoliative dermatitis leading to ulceration and alopecia. Histologic changes are composed of eosinophilic granulomas. Other organs involved with similar inflammatory lesions are alimentary tract, pancreas, lung, and liver.

### 11. Pastern dermatitis

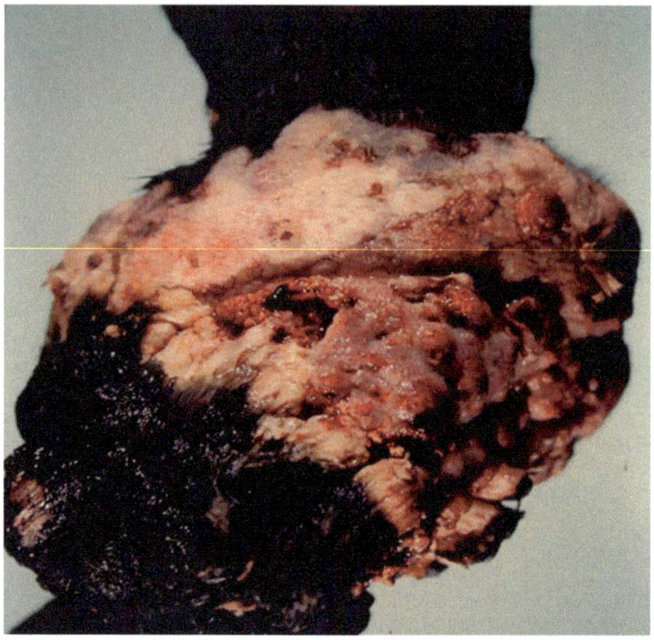

**Figure 13.59.** Horse. Distal Limb. Proliferative Granulomatous Dermatitis. Chronic Pastern Dermatitis. Alopecia with marked nodular fibrous tissue proliferation. Differential diagnoses include exuberant granulation tissue, pythiosis, habronemiasis, and squamous cell carcinoma.

Pastern dermatitis affects the heels of front and hind legs of mainly draft horses. It starts with an odiferous, exudative, ulcerative, crusty dermatitis complicated by mats of moist hair. The chronic disease is characterized by proliferative granulomatous tissue growth mimicking exuberant granulation tissue, pythiosis, habronemiasis, or squamous cell carcinoma.

### 12. Toxic epidermal necrolysis

This skin disorder has morphologic and likely causative similarities to erythema multiforme. It starts with dermal ulcers over the head, body, and legs and progresses to severe epidermal necrosis. Causes may include purpura hemorrhagica, toxic shock syndrome from *Staphylococcus aureus* infection, burns, chemicals, drugs, and bullous diseases.

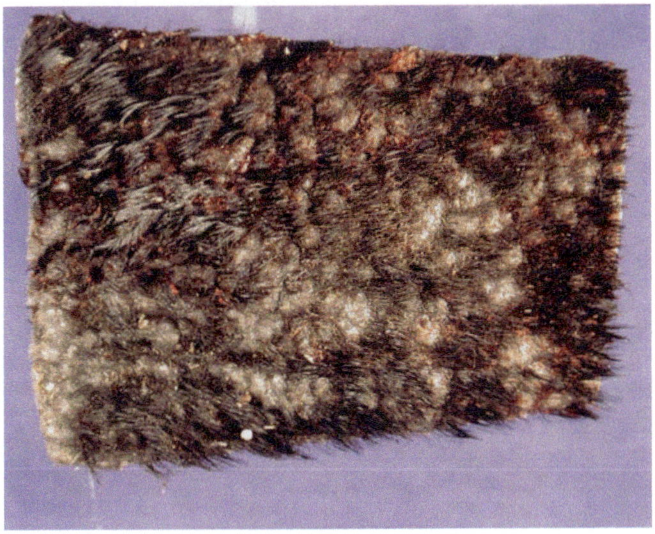

**Figure 13.60.** Horse. Skin. Nodular Granulomatous Dermatitis with Alopecia. Equine Sarcoidosis (Sterile Granulomatosis). Multiple hairless granulomas occupy the skin.

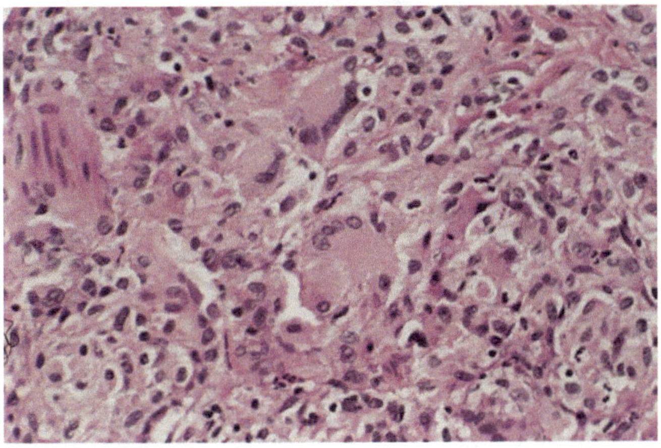

**Figure 13.61.** Horse. Skin. Granulomatous Dermatitis. Equine Sarcoidosis. Sterile Granulomatosis. Cutaneous nodules from Figure 13.60 are characterized by lymphocytes, histiocytes, and multinucleate Langhans giant cells with no organisms demonstrable by special stain or culture. (H&E) (Courtesy Dr. E.G. Clark, Calgary, Canada.)

Systemic granulomatous disease, also known as equine sarcoidosis, is a rare condition characterized by weight loss, generalized exfoliative dermatitis, and granulomatous inflammation of many organ systems. Any age, breed, or sex of horses can be affected, at any time of the year. The condition may have a slow progressive onset or may be rapidly progressive. Horses develop severe scaling of the head that becomes generalized and proliferative. The mane and tail are not affected. Over time, wasting occurs as systemic organs become affected. The condition should not be confused with skin tumors such as sarcoid. A recent publication identified mycobacterial DNA by nested PCR in skin and liver samples of a horse affected by generalized sarcoidosis.

## 14. Envenomation

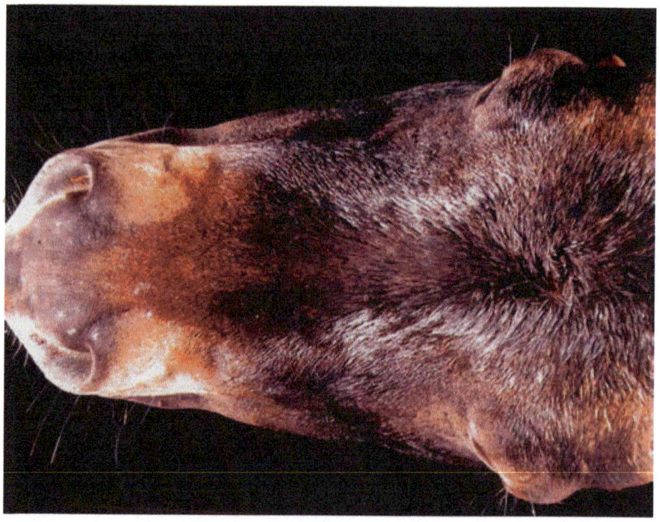

**Figure 13.62.** Horse. Head. Facial Edema. Snake Bite. Marked diffuse facial swelling of the entire head. It will be difficult to find bite marks under this condition. Differential diagnosis should consider nutritional fibrous osteodystrophy (bran disease) and lymphatic drainage obstruction due to neoplasia.

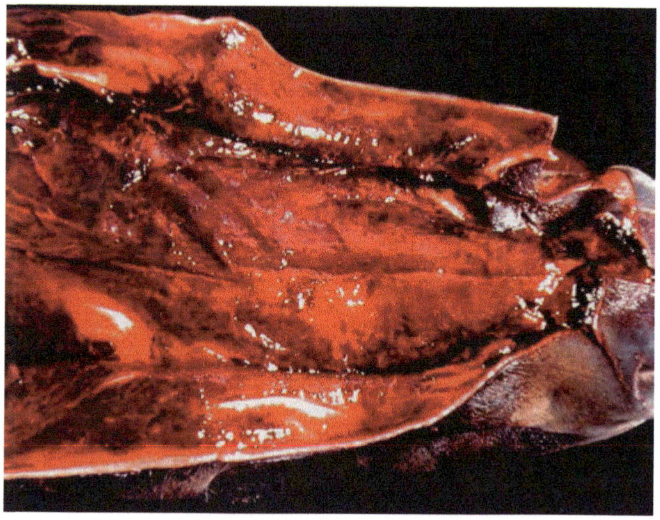

**Figure 13.63.** Horse. Head. Subcutis. Edema and Hemorrhage. Snake Bite. After reflection of the skin, the subcutis is markedly expanded by red, watery fluid.

In the United States, venomous rattlesnakes (Serpentes: *Crotalidae* and water moccasins (Serpentes: *Colubridae*) are largely responsible for snakebites in humans and animals. The bites lead to a local skin reaction and have a low mortality in most species. In horses, rattlesnake bites have been reported with a mortality rate as high as 25% in older horses and even higher in foals, which may die within 48 hours. Bites typically occur to the head and less frequently to the lower legs with head/neck swelling and limb swelling being visible signs following snakebite. Other clinical signs include respiratory distress, colic, atrial fibrillation, and changes in demeanor. Antivenom treatment may provide clinical relief.

# XIV. Neoplasia of the skin

## *1. Squamous cell carcinoma*

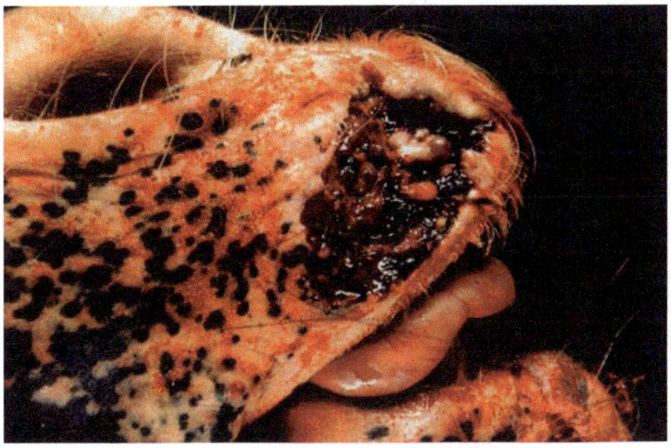

**Figure 13.64.** Horse. Muzzle. Squamous Cell Carcinoma. An ulcerated, necrotic, proliferative mass in an area of decreased pigmentation.

Squamous cell carcinoma (SCC) is an invasive neoplasm composed of malignant epithelial cells exhibiting varying degrees of squamous differentiation. SCC in situ refers to malignant keratinocytes that remain within the epidermis, without breaching the basement membrane underlying the basal layer. With the exception of sarcoids, SCC is the most common cutaneous neoplasm in the horse. Squamous cell carcinoma tends to be locally invasive, rarely metastasizing. When metastases do occur, it is primarily to local lymph nodes. SCCs often occur in skin that has undergone actinic damage and therefore anything that increases overall exposure to ultraviolet light (e.g., increased age, decreased pigmentation, sparsely haired regions, and increased altitude) increases the prevalence of the neoplasm.

Gross findings are variably sized, variably demarcated, firm, white nodular masses that are often red, ulcerated, and necrotic. Frequently, especially when associated with the eye or external genitalia, lesions may be raised, proliferative, and cauliflower-like.

The p53 tumor suppressor gene is overexpressed in equine SCC, and exposure to UV light has been associated with overexpression of the p53 protein, resulting from mutations of the p53 tumor suppressor gene. Recent findings suggest a relationship between infection with equine papillomavirus (EPV)-2 and the development of penile SCC. Genetic factors and exposure to carcinogens, such as smegma, are associated with the occurrence of SCCs. There has been empirical evidence associating the development of SCC at sites of chronic inflammation and burn scars.

## Squamous cell carcinoma – Fact sheet

**Definition:** Malignant neoplasm of epithelial cells exhibiting varying degrees of squamous differentiation.

### Incidence

- Second most common cutaneous neoplasm (increased risk with increased age).
- Occurs frequently in skin that has actinic damage.
- Increased occurrence in areas of decreased pigmentation and sparsely haired regions.
- Belgian, Clydesdale, Shire, Appaloosas, Paints, Pintos, Quarter horses, and Thoroughbreds predisposed, especially with increased exposure to UV radiation.
- Can arise in burn scars, nonhealing wounds, or chronically infected skin.

## Squamous cell carcinoma – Pathologic features

### Gross findings

- Proliferative, variably sized, firm, nodular, cauliflower-like masses
- Frequently ulcerated and necrotic

### Microscopic findings

- Nests, islands, cords and trabeculae of malignant epithelial cells exhibiting varying degrees of keratinization
- Prominent intercellular bridging (desmosomes)
- Possibly keratin pearls
- Possibly desmoplasia
- Frequently associated with solar elastosis
- May be preceded by solar keratosis and/or carcinoma in situ
- May be associated with severe inflammation

### Differential diagnosis

- Equine sarcoid
- Granulation tissue
- Habronemiasis
- Pythiosis

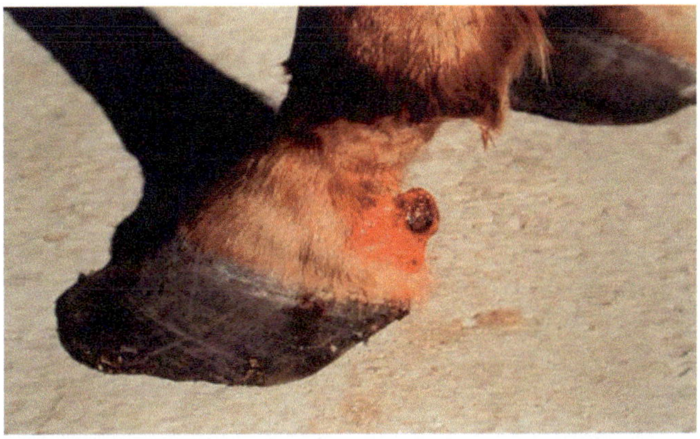

**Figure 13.65.** Horse. Heel Bulb. Fibroblastic Sarcoid. Fibrous, fleshy and ulcerated nodule that often resembles granulation tissue.

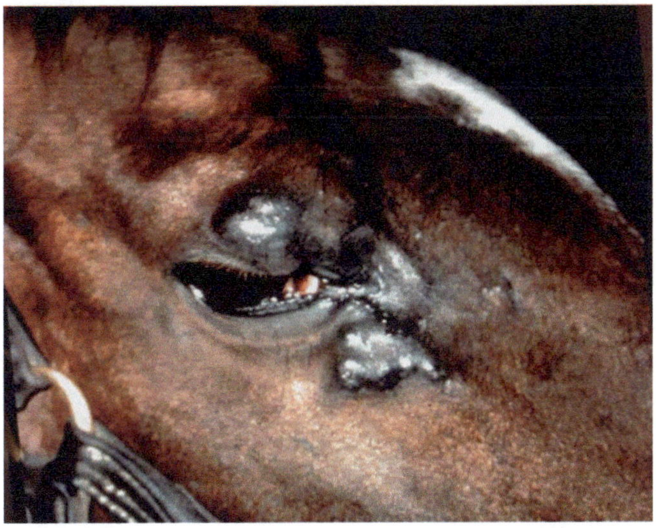

**Figure 13.66.** Horse. Periocular Skin. Nodular Sarcoid. Multiple to coalescing, firm nodular lesions in the region of the medial canthus and palpebra superior. Differential diagnosis: melanoma.

Sarcoids are the most common cutaneous neoplasms of equids, occurring in horses, mules, donkeys, and zebras. They are nonmetastatic, locally aggressive fibroblastic skin tumors that are considered biphasic, containing both epidermal and dermal components. Although they have not been shown to be transmissible via direct contact, sarcoids are associated with a nonproductive infection with bovine papillomavirus (BPV) types 1 and 2. Based on gross appearance, tumors are separated into categories that include verrucous, fibroblastic, nodular, mixed, and occult. Sarcoid lesions may be single or multiple and can appear at any age, although young horses are most commonly affected. Sarcoids are most frequently found on the ventral abdomen, legs, neck, and head (most commonly ear, eye, and commissure of the mouth). Tumors frequently recur after surgical excision. Sarcoids often develop in areas of previous trauma.

Sarcoids are associated with a nonproductive infection with BPV-1 and -2. Sarcoids express BPV-1 and BPV-2 major transforming protein E5, which may contribute to viral persistence via downregulation of MHC class I. Signal transduction via the binding of E5 to the β receptor of platelet-derived growth factor (PDGF) results in an intracellular growth stimulatory signal.

Several factors are potentially associated with the development of a sarcoid including exposure to virus, genetic predisposition and trauma.

Although the mode of transmission has not been definitively identified, there has been a suggestion that spread may be associated with exposure to insects, fomites, and/or mechanical trauma (e.g., biting, rubbing).

## Sarcoid – Fact sheet

### Definition

- Most common cutaneous neoplasm of equids
- Nonmetastatic, locally aggressive, biphasic, fibroblastic skin tumors
- Associated with a nonproductive infection with bovine papillomavirus types 1 and 2

### Incidence

- Occurs in horses, mules, donkeys, and zebras
- Occur most commonly in young horses
- Appaloosas, Arabians, Paints, and Quarter horses have an increased incidence
- Standardbreds have a decreased incidence
- Frequently sarcoids are found on the ventral abdomen, legs, neck, and head (most commonly ear, eye, and commissure of the mouth)
- Lesions may be single or multiple

## Sarcoids – Pathologic features

### Gross findings

- Four different categories:
  - Occult form: Flat to slightly thickened, with alopecia and slightly roughened surface
  - Verrucous: Small (<6 cm), wartlike, sessile or pedunculated mass, with variable alopecia and a dry, roughened to horny surface
  - Fibroblastic: Fibrous and fleshy, variably sized nodules that may be ulcerated
  - Mixed type: Transition of verrucous and fibroblastic sarcoids
  - Nodular: Firm, well-circumscribed nodules with a normal-appearing or alopecic overlying epidermis

### Microscopic findings

- Biphasic: Dermal and epidermal components
- Epidermis: Rete ridges that extend into the underlying dermal proliferation. Epidermis is often ulcerated

## Sarcoids – Pathologic features continued

- Dermis: Proliferation of neoplastic fibroblasts arranged in streams and whorls
- At the dermal–epidermal junction, neoplastic cells often orient perpendicular to the basement membrane ("picket fence")

**Differential diagnosis**

- Granulation tissue
- Peripheral nerve sheath tumor
- Squamous cell carcinoma
- Habronemiasis
- Pythiosis
- Papilloma
- Fibroma/fibrosarcoma

### *3. Cutaneous lymphoma*

Cutaneous lymphoma is a relatively rare neoplasm of the horse that arises from lymphocytes. The two forms of cutaneous lymphoma are nonepitheliotropic and epitheliotropic (mycosis fungoides). In the horse, nonepitheliotropic lymphoma is the most common form of cutaneous lymphoma and is generally a T-cell-rich B-cell lymphoma (formerly referred to as equine cutaneous histiolymphocytic lymphosarcoma). The current supposition is that the B lymphocytes (CD79a+) are the neoplastic cells, which produce cytokines that signal the infiltration of reactive immune T lymphocytes (CD3+), in addition to other leukocytes. The mixed nature of the cell population can cause these tumors to be occasionally misdiagnosed as inflammation. This neoplasm presents as multiple dermal and subcutaneous nodular masses that often appear to follow lymphatics. Differential diagnoses for the gross lesions of nonepitheliotropic lymphoma include urticaria, drug eruptions, collagenolytic granulomas, and pseudolymphoma.

Epitheliotropic lymphoma (mycosis fungoides) is a neoplasm of T-cell origin and in horses presents as an exfoliative dermatitis, with scaling, crusting, and alopecia. Pruritus, nodules, and ulceration in this form of lymphoma are variable.

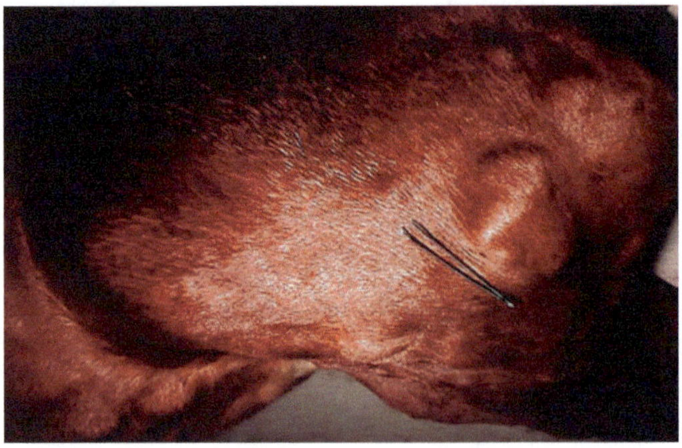

**Figure 13.67.** Horse. Skin. Hind Leg. Cutaneous Lymphoma. The cutaneous nodules may become quite large.

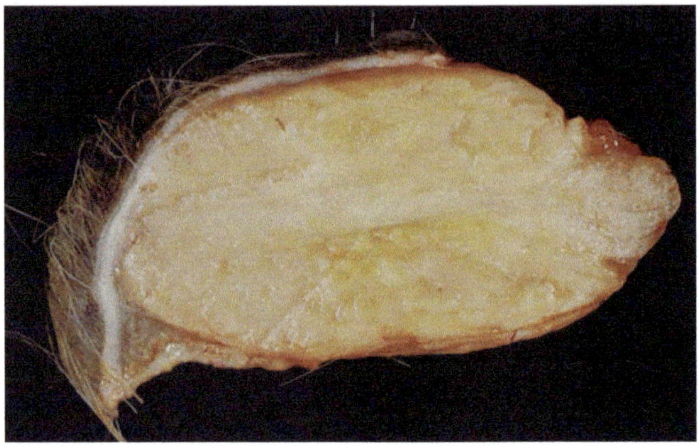

**Figure 13.68.** Horse. Skin. Cutaneous Lymphoma. On cross section the nodule is white, lobulated, and bulges the epidermis. (Courtesy Dr. E.G. Clark, Calgary, Canada.)

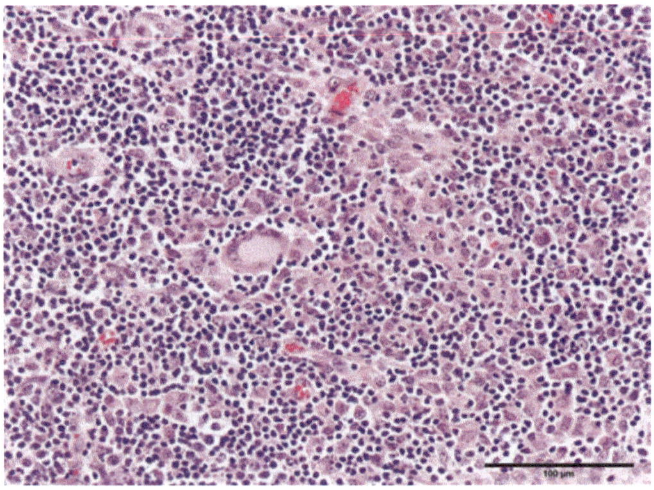

**Figure 13.69.** Horse. Skin. Cutaneous Lymphoma. Aggregates of small to medium-sized hyperchromatic lymphocytes are interspersed with lesser numbers of histiocytes, epithelioid type macrophages, plasma cells, and multinucleate giant cells. Mitotic figures are rare. (H&E) (Courtesy Dr. M. Law, North Carolina State University.)

### 4. *Hemangioma/Hemangiosarcoma*

Hemangiomas and hemangiosarcomas are uncommon cutaneous neoplasms in the horse arising from endothelial cells. These neoplasms can occur at any age and have no sex or breed predilection. However, congenital hemangiomas have been reported, with increased incidence in Arabian horses. These neoplasms can occur anywhere, but hemangiomas most commonly affect the distal limbs, whereas hemangiosarcomas most commonly affect the head, neck, trunk, and proximal limbs. Differential diagnosis is cutaneous angiomatosis.

### 5. *Melanoma*

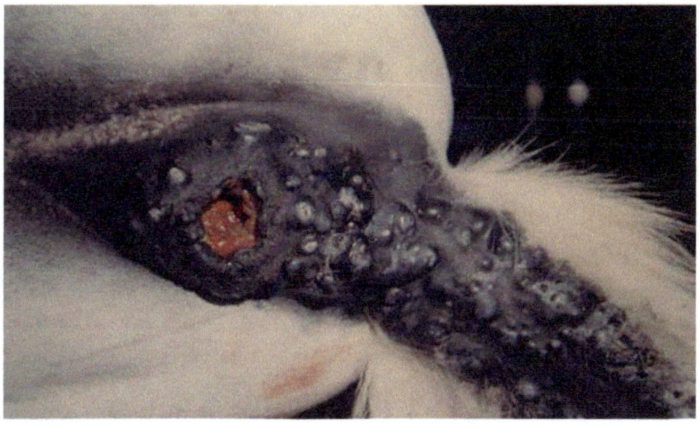

**Figure 13.70.** Horse. Ventral Tail and Perianal Region. Melanoma. Multiple black nodules in the perianal region and ventral aspect of the tail.

Melanomas derive from melanocytes. In horses, melanomas occur most commonly in older gray horses, with preferred sites that include the tail and perineum. Other locations that may be affected include the eyelid, parotid region, lips, and genitalia. Behavior and growth rates of melanomas are variable; they slowly metastasize to regional lymph nodes. Congenital melanomas (nevus) are rare but may occur. There has been no correlation between UV light exposure and the development of melanoma in horses as is the case in humans.

### 6. *Peripheral nerve sheath tumors*

Peripheral nerve sheath tumors (schwannoma, perineural fibroblastoma, neurofibroma, neurilemmoma) are rare neoplasms of the horse arising from Schwann cells and/or perineural cells. These neoplasms usually occur in adult animals and are generally well circumscribed, solitary, semi-firm to firm, slow-growing nodules that can occur anywhere. The overlying epidermis is frequently normal but may become alopecic or ulcerated. There is no breed or sex predilection. The etiology of these neoplasms is not known. Histologically, spindle-shaped cells form interlacing fascicles, bundles, palisades, and whorls. (Examples of PNST are presented in Chapter 3.)

## 7. Papilloma

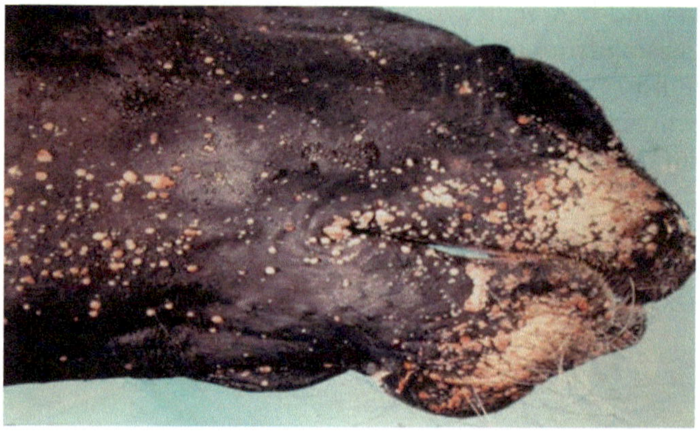

**Figure 13.71.** Horse. Face and Muzzle. Papillomatosis. Multifocal to coalescing small smooth white proliferative papules on the face and muzzle.

Papillomas may appear as pedunculated, exophytic, frondlike projections composed of keratin. These lesions are most common on the muzzle, nose, lips, periocular region, distal limbs, genitalia, mammary glands, and lateral aspect of the pinnae (aural plaques are thought to be a form of papilloma) caused by species specific papovaviruses. Lesions generally occur in young animals (although they can occur in adults) and are often self-limiting, regressing as the foal's immune system develops. Although these lesions are often cosmetic problems, there has been a recent suggestion of a correlation between papillomavirus infection and the development of SCC of the penis. Differential diagnosis for these lesions include verrucous equine sarcoids. (Examples of papilloma are also presented in this chapter in Section VII, "Viral Diseases of Skin.")

## 8. Mast cell tumor

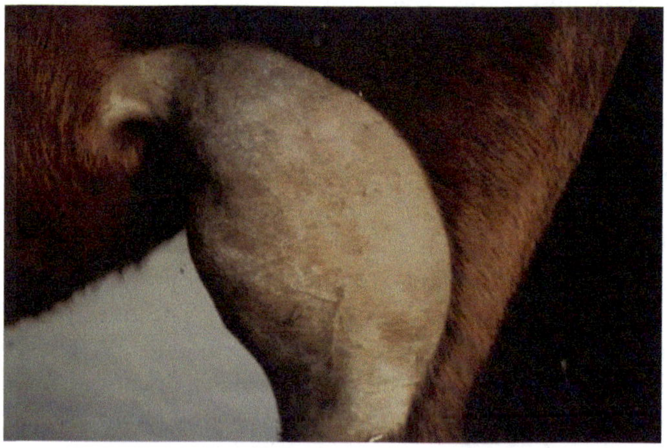

**Figure 13.72.** Horse. Hind Limb. Dermal Nodule. Mastocytosis (Mast Cell Tumor). A slightly raised nodule is present just below the left stifle. (Courtesy Dr. E.G. Clark, Calgary, Canada.)

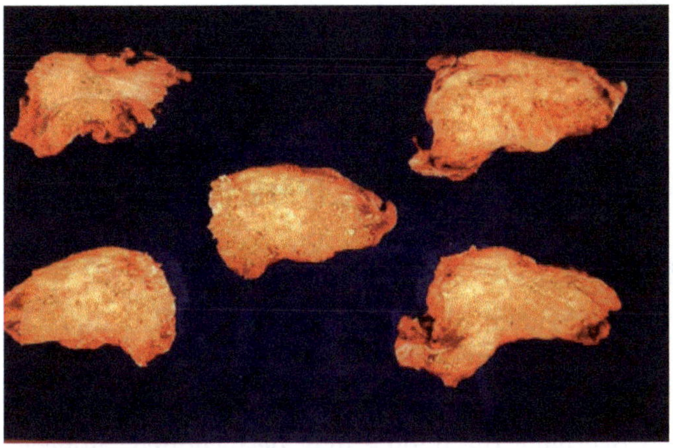

**Figure 13.73.** Horse. Unencapsulated Expensile Dermal Nodule. Cutaneous Mast Cell Tumor. On cross section multifocal mineralization within tumor tissue is extensive.

## Mast cell tumor – Fact sheet

### Definition

- Benign neoplasm arising from mast cells
- Occasionally referred to as mastocytoma or cutaneous mastocytosis
- Nonpainful, nonpruritic
- Usually slow-growing
- Unclear if equine mast cell tumors are truly neoplastic or hyperplastic lesions
- May spontaneously resolve

### Incidence

- Relatively uncommon
- No breed predisposition
- Male horses have increased incidence
- Affects all ages

## Mast cell tumor – Pathologic features

### Gross findings

- Present as individual or multiple, firm, raised nodules most commonly on the trunk, neck, head, or limbs. Lesions of the head, often affect nostrils, lips, and periorbital areas
- The skin overlying the nodule may be ulcerated, alopecic, or have increased pigmentation
- Otherwise healthy foals may develop multicentric, widespread, waxing and waning mast cell tumors that resemble urticaria pigmentosa (maculopapular cutaneous mastocytosis) of humans
- Mineralization can occur

### Microscopic findings

- Unencapsulated, variably demarcated mass composed of sheets and coalescing nodules of well-differentiated mast cells that often have poorly staining intracytoplasmic granules
- Special stains such as Giemsa and Toluidine blue may help accentuate metachromatic granules present
- Mitoses are rare
- Eosinophils are frequently present in very large numbers scattered throughout the mass and often forming variably sized aggregates
- Eosinophils may outnumber mast cells
- Aggregates of degranulated eosinophils and necrosis may be surrounded by eosinophils and histiocytes, and possibly fibrosis.
- Possibly collagen degeneration
- Possibly dystrophic mineralization

### Differential diagnoses

- Histologic differential diagnoses
  - Cutaneous habronemiasis
  - Equine nodular collagenolytic granuloma
  - Pythiosis

### 9. Basal cell tumor

Basal cell tumors are exceedingly rare benign neoplasms in the horse that presumably arise from the stratum basale and have no obvious breed or sex predilection. The most common locations in the horse are the face, neck, trunk, and distal limb. Grossly, lesions are often well-circumscribed, firm, solitary rounded nodules with the overlying skin exhibiting a spectrum of appearance, ranging from normal to alopecic, ulcerated or hyperpigmented.

Basal cell tumors may resemble sarcoids, melanomas, or even SCCs grossly. The correlation between UV light exposure and the development of basal cell tumors in humans has not been demonstrated in horses. Histologically, these neoplasms are composed of proliferations of basaloid cells, with numerous subtypes that include solid, ribbon, trabecular, spindle, granular, adenoid, and basosquamous. Numerous subtypes often found within a single neoplasm are not prognostically significant.

### 10. Myoma

Leiomyomas are generally solitary, small, well-circumscribed dermal masses composed of interlacing and intersecting bundles of smooth muscle fibers that arise from erector pili muscles, cutaneous blood vessels, or specialized muscles of the genital skin. Cell nuclei are elongate and have characteristic blunt ends, hence the moniker "cigar-shaped nuclei." These neoplasms are exceedingly rare in the horse and the cause is unknown.

### 11. Fibroma/Fibrosarcoma

Fibromas (benign) and fibrosarcomas (malignant) are neoplasms arising from fibroblasts, either in the dermis or subcutis, and are relatively rare neoplasms in the horse. Both of these neoplasms generally occur in adult animals with no apparent breed or sex predilection. In both cases, lesions are usually solitary, firm, and fairly well-circumscribed (fibrosarcomas may be less well circumscribed). The overlying skin may be normal, alopecic, hyperpigmented, or ulcerated. Both of these types of tumors may occur anywhere, but fibromas are most commonly found on the legs, neck, and periocular region, whereas fibrosarcomas are most commonly found on the legs, trunk, and eyelid. Microscopically, fibromas are well-circumscribed, unencapsulated dermal or subcutaneous nodules composed of whorls of interlacing and intersecting bundles of fibroblasts admixed with variably abundant collagen. Fibrosarcomas are microscopically very similar to fibromas; however, they may exhibit greater pleomorphism, have an increased mitotic rate, and variable amounts of collagen. Histopathologically, these tumors can easily be confused with sarcoids, especially when the overlying epidermis is ulcerated and the characteristic epidermal component of a sarcoid is absent. Additionally, in small biopsies, differentiation between fibromas/fibrosarcomas from reactive granulation tissue can occasionally pose a challenge.

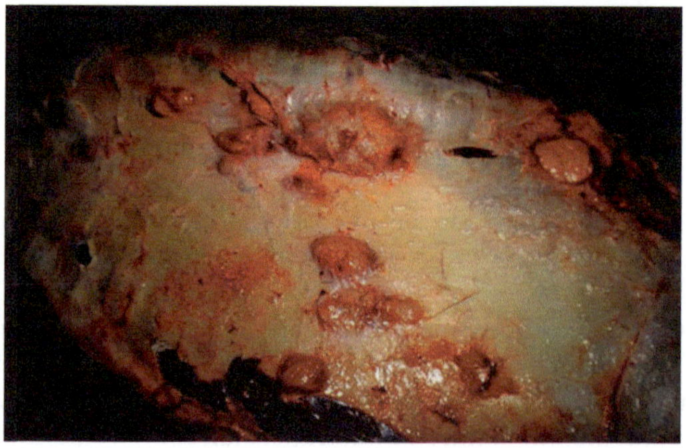

**Figure 13.74.** Horse. Subcutis. Trunk. Fibrosarcoma. Multiple firm nodules in the subcutis were diagnosed as anaplastic fibrosarcoma. Differential diagnosis: cutaneous lymphoma.

## *12. Mammary gland neoplasia*

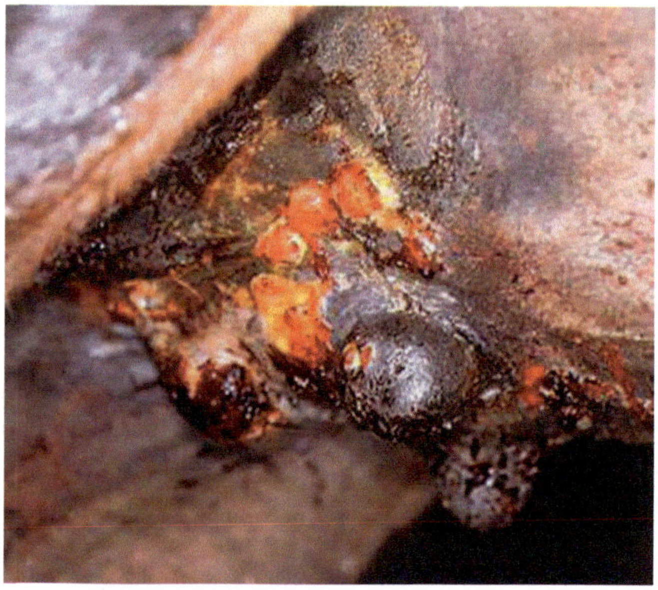

**Figure 13.75.** Horse. Mammary Gland. Adenocarcinoma. Multiple ulcerative nodules are associated with the mammary gland. Papillary ductal carcinoma was the microscopic diagnosis. (Courtesy Dr. J. Roberts, National Zoo, Washington, DC.)

The equine mammary gland appears to be rather resistant to pathologic changes. There are only individual case reports of mastitis or primary tumors in the literature.

Neoplasms of the mammary gland are either adenocarcinomas or ductal papillary adenocarcinomas, and they are extremely uncommon. Clinical signs are asymmetry and firm swelling of the gland with ulceration of the skin.

## Selected references

Brandt S, Schoster A, Tober R, et al. 2011. Consistent detection of bovine papillomavirus in lesions, intact skin and peripheral blood mononuclear cells of horses affected by hoof canker. *Equine Vet J* 43(2):202–209.

Cohen N, Carter GK, McMullan WC. 1992. Fistulous withers in horses: 24 cases (1984–1990). *J Am Vet Med Assoc* 201(1):121–124.

Dickinson CE, Traub-Dargatz JL, Dargatz DA, Bennet DG, Knight AP. 1996. Rattlesnake venom poisoning in horses: 32 cases (1973–1993). *J Am Vet Med Assoc* 208(11):1966–1970.

Herder V, Barsnick R, Walliser U, et al. 2012. Equid herpesvirus 5-associated dermatitis in a horse: resembling herpes-associated erythema multiforme. *Vet Microbiol* 155:420–424.

Langdon Fielding C, Pusterla N, Magdesian KG, Higgins JC, Meier CA. 2011. Rattlesnake envenomation in horses: 58 cases (1992–2009). *J Am Vet Med Assoc* 238(5):631–635.

McCue PM, Wilson WD. 1989. Equine mastitis – a review of 28 cases. *Equine Vet J* 21(5):351–353.

Nagamin CM, Castro F, Buchanan B, Schumacher J, Craig LE. 2005. Proliferative pododermatitis (canker) with intralesional spirochetes in three horses. *J Vet Diag Invest* 17(3):269–271.

Ness SL, Peters-Kennedy J, Schares G, et al. 2012. Investigation of an outbreak of besnoitiosis in donkeys in northeastern Pennsylvania. *J Am Vet Med Assoc* 240(11):1329–1337.

Oliveira-Filho JP, Monteiro LN, Delfiol DJ, et al. 2012. Mycobacterium DNA detection in liver and skin of a horse with generalized sarcoidosis. *J Vet Diag Invest* 24(3):596–600.

Petersen AD, Schott H. 2005. Cutaneous markers of disorders affecting adult horses. *Clinical Techniques in Equine Practice* 4(4):324–338.

Repass GP, McClintock SA, Canfield PJ, Watson GF. 1996. Papillary ductal adenocarcinoma in the mammary glands of horses. *Vet Rec* 138(21):518–519.

Reuss SM, Dunbar M, Calderwood-Mays MB, et al. 2012. Autochthonous *Leishmania siamensis* in a horse, Florida, USA [letter]. *Emerg Infect Dis.* Centers for Disease Control and Prevention Web site. http://wwwnc.cdc.gov/eid/article/18/9/12-0184_article.htm.

Scott DW, Miller WH Jr. *Equine Dermatology*. St. Louis, MO: Saunders; 2003.

Vandenabeele SI, White SD, Affolter VK, Kass PH, Ihrke PJ. 2004. Pemphigus foliaceus in the horse: a retrospective study of 20 cases. *Vet Dermatol* 15(6): 381–388.

# 14 Diseases of the Eye and Ear

**Contributed by Ingeborg Maria Langohr**

I. Eyes
   1. Congenital ocular diseases
   2. Degenerative ocular diseases
   3. Inflammatory ocular diseases
   4. Neoplastic ocular diseases

II. Ears
   1. Inflammatory otic diseases
   2. Nonneoplastic and neoplastic proliferative otic diseases

*Color Atlas of Equine Pathology*, First Edition. Claus D. Buergelt and Fabio Del Piero.

# I. Eyes

As instinctive prey animals, horses are very dependent on vision, with a total visual field of almost 350 degrees. Ocular health is therefore critical to the well-being of horses, which have particularly large and prominent eyes, making them prone to injury. Whereas many ocular diseases have the potential to heal if detected early and treated adequately, they can just as easily progress to irreversible vision loss. This chapter summarizes both congenital and acquired inflammatory, degenerative, and neoplastic ocular diseases that affect the horse.

## 1. *Congenital ocular diseases*

Ocular anomalies usually affect multiple structures, reflecting the stepwise embryology and interdependence of the various parts of the developing eye.

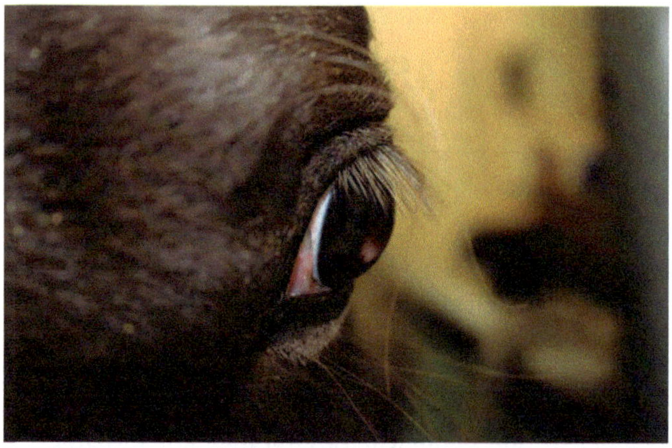

**Figure 14.1.** Horse. Eye. Cornea Globosa. Horses with this alteration have a globular corneal contour with a protruding cornea and a deep anterior chamber. (Courtesy Comparative Ophthalmology Service, Michigan State University, East Lansing, MI.)

Cornea globosa can be seen in addition to multiple other anterior segment anomalies such as cataract, lens luxation, and iris hypoplasia as part of the multiple congenital ocular anomalies (MCOA) syndrome described in Silver-Colored Rocky Mountain horses, Kentucky Mountain saddle horses, Icelandic horses, Miniature horses, Morgan horses, and Shetland ponies.

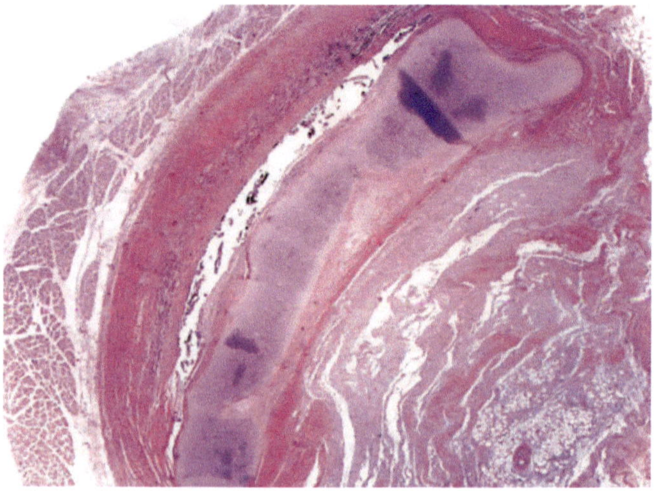

**Figure 14.2.** Fetus. Eye. Severe Microphthalmia. No internal structures, such as lens and retina, are apparent in this malformed globe that consists solely of a scleral sheet and some pigmentary differentiation, typical of persistence of the primary optic vesicle. The adjacent plate of cartilage is likely derived from the third eyelid analog. (H&E)

*Entropion* and *Ectropion*. Inversion of the eyelid margin (*entropion*) may occur as a primary condition or may be secondary to enophthalmos associated with microphthalmos and prematurity or dysmaturity. It generally affects the lower eyelid, but in Miniature horses it may affect the upper eyelid only. Eversion of the eyelid margin (*ectropion*), rarely congenital, is more often secondary to scarring of the eyelids resulting from trauma or burns.

*Aniridia* and *Iridal hypoplasia*. Complete absence of the iris (*aniridia*) is a rare congenital anomaly that is usually bilateral. Underdevelopment and thinning of the iris (*iridal hypoplasia*) is, in contrast, relatively common in Appaloosas and eyes with heterochromia iridis. The thin iris stroma may balloon into the anterior chamber from the higher pressure in the posterior chamber.

*Retinal dysplasia* is an uncommon developmental lesion characterized histologically by retinal folds and rosettes. It may occur in association with other ocular anomalies in animals with anterior segment dysgenesis. *Retinal detachments* are generally secondary to posterior segment inflammation in equine recurrent uveitis (ERU), head trauma, perforating globe wounds, and tumors. Nonetheless, they may also be congenital, possibly associated with other ocular abnormalities.

## 2. Degenerative ocular diseases

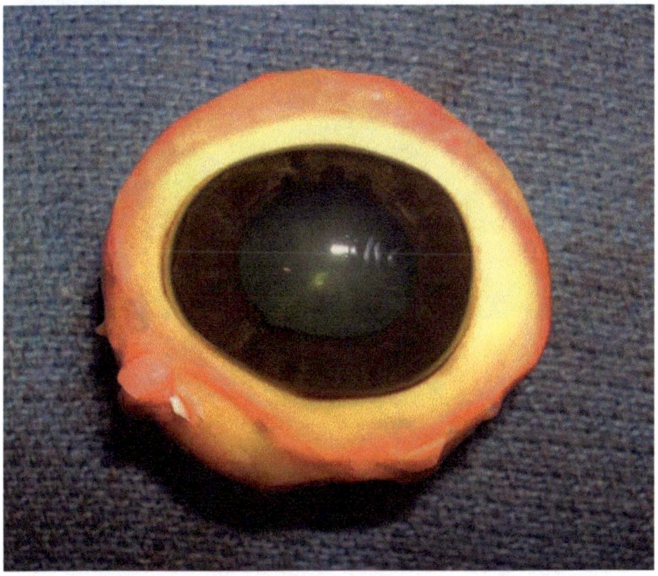

**Figure 14.3.** Foal. Eye. Icterus. Neonatal Isoerythrolysis. The conjunctiva is one of the first tissues to change color as bilirubin levels rise in diseases that lead to jaundice.

*Atrophia* and *phthisis bulbi*. These terms refer to shrunken eyes at, respectively, the advanced and end stage of severe ophthalmitis, most commonly seen in association with corneal perforation. When ocular structures have still some recognizable orientation, the alteration is more properly termed *atrophia bulbi*. The *phthisic eye* is structurally more disorganized, with barely any recognizable content.

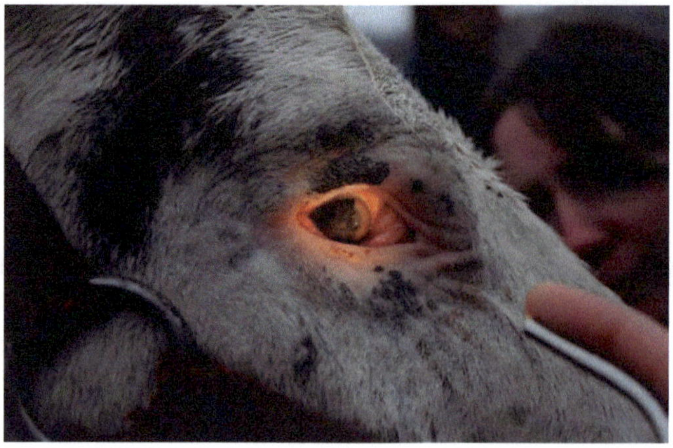

**Figure 14.4.** Horse. Eye. Phthisis Bulbi. Clinically, this condition is characterized by a shrunken globe within a normal sized orbit following severe trauma. The third eyelid is prominent. (Courtesy Comparative Ophthalmology Service, Michigan State University, East Lansing, MI.)

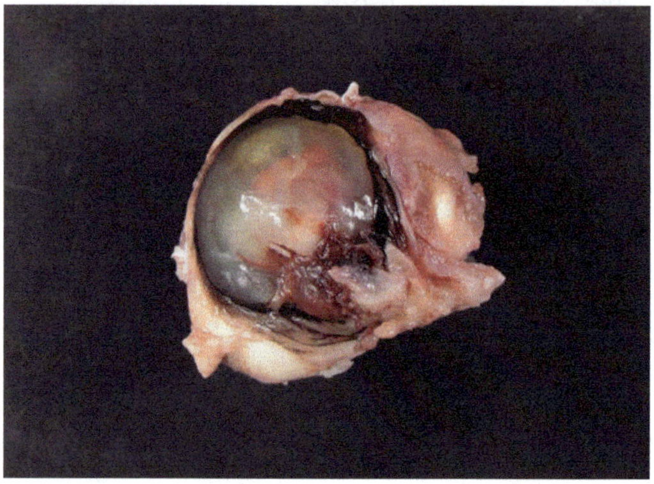

**Figure 14.5.** Horse. Eye. Atrophia Bulbi. This horse had previous trauma to this eye. Ophthalmologic exam revealed enophthalmos, corneal laceration near the medial canthus, and a shrunken globe. A stick was found lodged between the medial canthus and the globe.

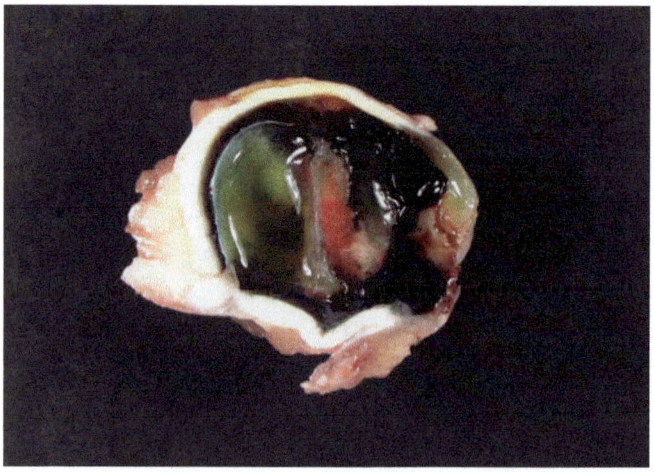

**Figure 14.6.** Horse. Eye. Atrophia Bulbi (same as in Figure 14.5). On cut section, the globe is shrunken and distorted, but the internal structures are still partially recognizable. There is lens rupture and complete retinal detachment. Lenticular capsular and retinal fragments are surrounded by granulating fibrosis, hemorrhage, and inflammation. The limbus and sclera are focally perforated, with prolapse of the anterior uveal tract through the defect in the fibrous tunic.

*Cataract.* Lenticular opacity is a common sequela to uveitis, either as a result of uveal adhesions to the lens surface, altered aqueous flow with lenticular malnutrition, exposure to injurious inflammatory by-products, or stagnation of the aqueous humor in postinflammatory glaucoma. It is also a frequent congenital ocular defect in foals.

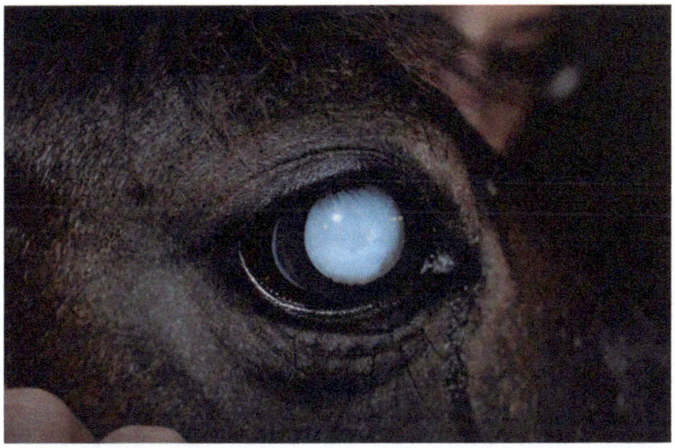

**Figure 14.7.** Foal. Eye. Cataract. The late immature cataract affecting more than 90% of the lens of both eyes of this animal and the absence of any other sign of ocular disease suggested a congenital inherited rather than an acquired condition. (Courtesy Comparative Ophthalmology Service, Michigan State University, East Lansing, MI.)

*Prolapse or herniation of orbital fat.* This is a rare condition that may be associated with weakened episcleral fascia or trauma. The resulting lobular subconjunctival masses can mimic neoplasms, from which they can be easily differentiated through cytologic or histologic evaluations.

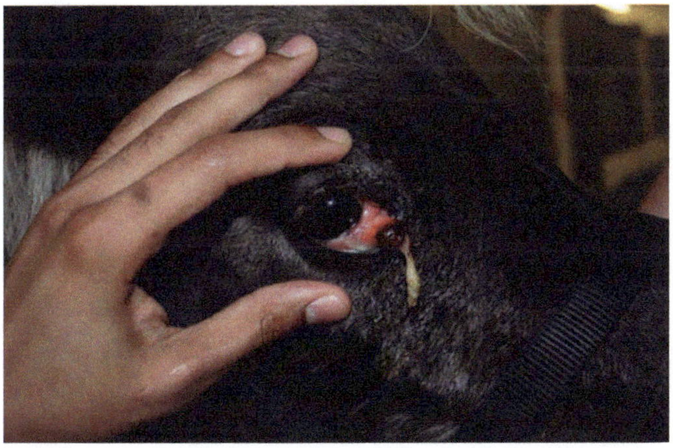

**Figure 14.8.** Horse. Eye. Partial Prolapse of the Extraorbital Fat Pad. The prolapse involves the third eyelid and is complicated by secondary bacterial infection. (Courtesy Comparative Ophthalmology Service, Michigan State University, East Lansing, MI.)

*Glaucoma*. Once thought to be a very rare disease in horses, glaucoma has emerged as a relatively frequent, underdiagnosed condition in this species. Clinical claims that affected horses all have had previous bouts of uveitis are often difficult to substantiate by histologic assessment. Most horses with glaucoma have no histologic explanation for the development of this disease. Elevation of intraocular pressure in such cases may be due to obstruction of alternative uveal routes of aqueous outflow through the ciliary muscle interstitium into the suprachoroidal space and sclera.

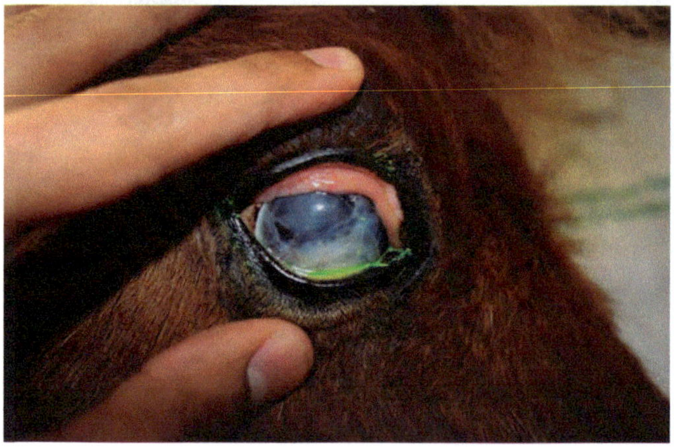

**Figure 14.9.** Horse. Eye. Haab's Striae. The numerous white linear streaks in the cornea of this horse with glaucoma represent breaks in the Descemet's membrane. They are the result of corneal stretching due to enlargement of the glaucomatous globe (buphthalmos). Note also the concurrent presence of circumlimbal corneal neovascularization affecting approximately 50% of its circumference. (Courtesy Comparative Ophthalmology Service, Michigan State University, East Lansing, MI.)

*Senile changes*. Aged horses present a number of minor degenerative ocular alterations that, if extensive, may culminate in vision deficit.

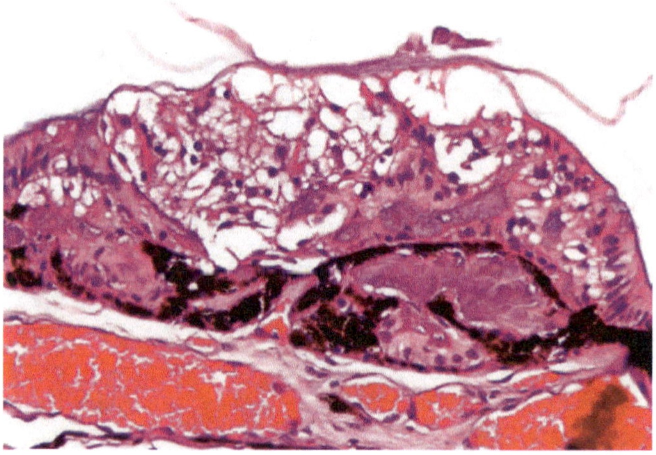

**Figure 14.10.** Horse. Eye. Retina. Degeneration. Peripheral retinal degeneration is a finding related to old age characterized by neurosensory retinal degeneration with pigmentary changes. Additionally, the aged horse can have chorioretinal scars in the fundus, most commonly in the nontapetal region, which may represent the sequela of subclinical equine herpesvirus-1 infection. (H&E)

### 3. *Inflammatory ocular diseases*

*Orbital cellulitis* forms in response to infectious agents introduced into the orbit via a penetrating wound, a migrating foreign body, or an inflammatory focus in an adjacent location (e.g., sinusitis and tooth root abscess). Only rarely does uncontrolled endophthalmitis spread through the sclera into the orbit because the sclera is generally an effective barrier to leukocytes and infectious agents.

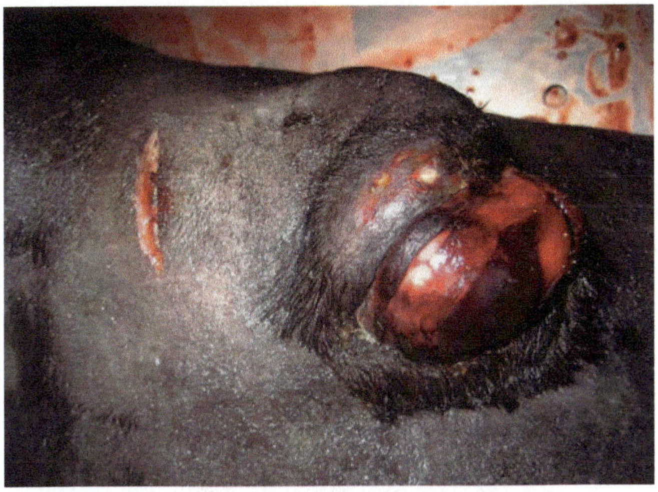

**Figure 14.11.** Horse. Eye. Severe Facial and Orbital Cellulitis. The severe unilateral swelling of the supraorbital fossa, exophthalmos, and hyphema in this horse were associated with an oral fistula. Similar lesions may also occur as the result of injuries of the orbital region on the racetrack, in trailers, or on the pasture, by rearing and hitting stall ceilings, or from kicks by other horses.

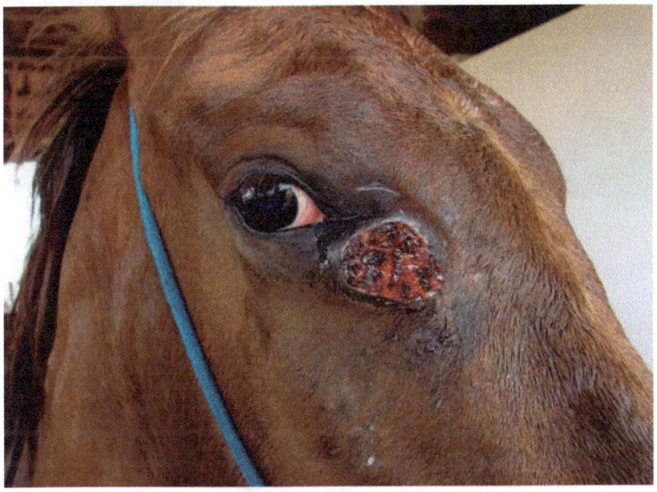

**Figure 14.12.** Horse. Face. Cutaneous Habronemiasis. The medial canthus is one of the preferred areas for aberrantly migrating larvae of *Habronema muscae*, *H. majus,* and *Draschia megastoma* to develop ulcerative lesions that expose granulation tissue containing eosinophilic granulomas. (Courtesy Dr. Rafael A. Fighera, Santa Maria, RS, Brazil.)

*Corneal ulceration.* Loss of corneal epithelium has a number of causes such as physical and chemical trauma and bacterial or fungal infection. Bacteria and fungi are generally secondary. Ulcers may heal, may persist as nonprogressive lesion, or may progress to involve more of the stroma, with the possibility of eventually leading to corneal perforation.

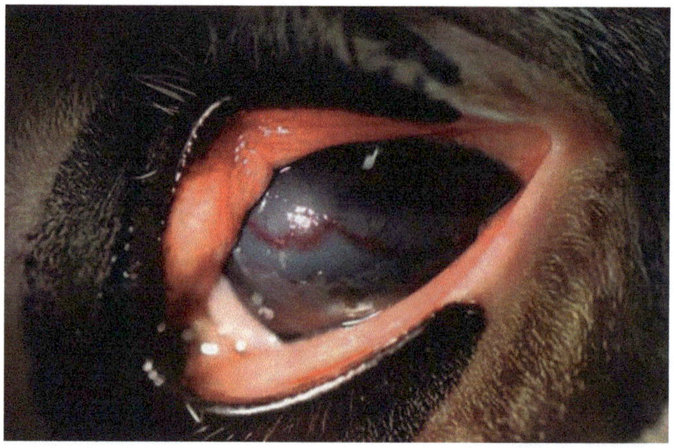

**Figure 14.13.** Horse. Eye. Cornea. Superficial Corneal Ulceration and Band Keratopathy. The nonadherent loose epithelium at the inferior ulcer margin is characteristic of a persistent or indolent ulcer. Additionally, there is also mild diffuse corneal edema and neovascularization. (Courtesy Comparative Ophthalmology Service, Michigan State University, East Lansing, MI.)

Band keratopathy represents a nonspecific degenerative process characterized by a horizontal white band of superficial stromal or basal laminar mineralization of the cornea observed in a number of ocular diseases.

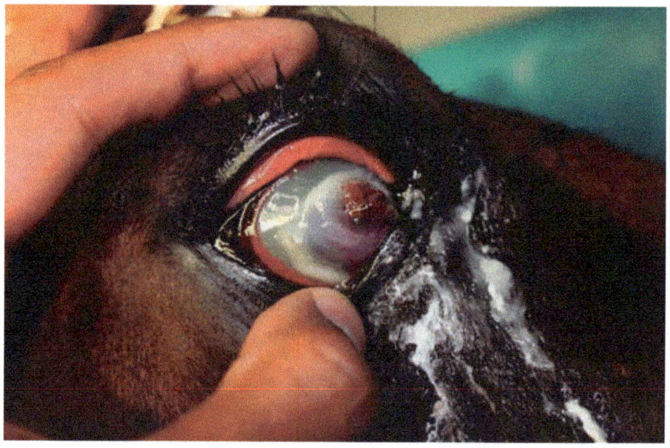

**Figure 14.14.** Horse. Eye. Cornea. Corneal Ulceration. It progresses in this globe to keratomalacia (liquefactive necrosis) and later to corneal rupture with iris prolapse. (Courtesy Comparative Ophthalmology Service, Michigan State University, East Lansing, MI.)

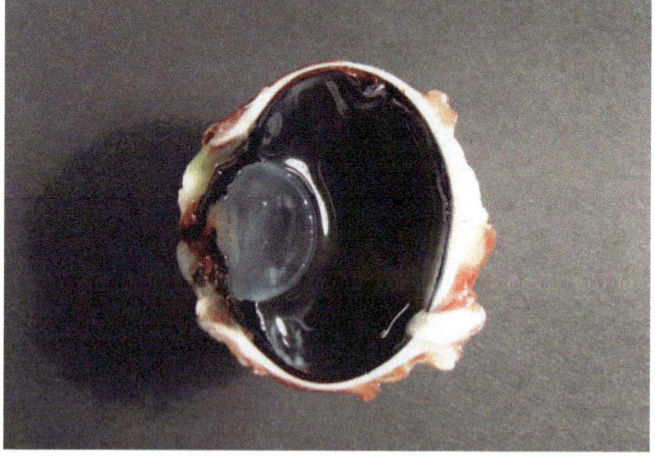

**Figure 14.15.** Horse. Eye. Iris Prolapse (same as in Figure 14.14). On cut surface, the iris is prolapsed through the central corneal defect, accompanied by secondary anterior uveitis.

*Equine mycotic keratitis.* This important ocular disease is thought to be a complication of chronic antibiotic and/or steroid administration for traumatic corneal ulceration. *Aspergillus* is the most frequent isolate, but other fungi of the conjunctival flora, such as *Penicillium*, *Alternaria*, and *Cladosporium*, can be seen in association with this lesion as well.

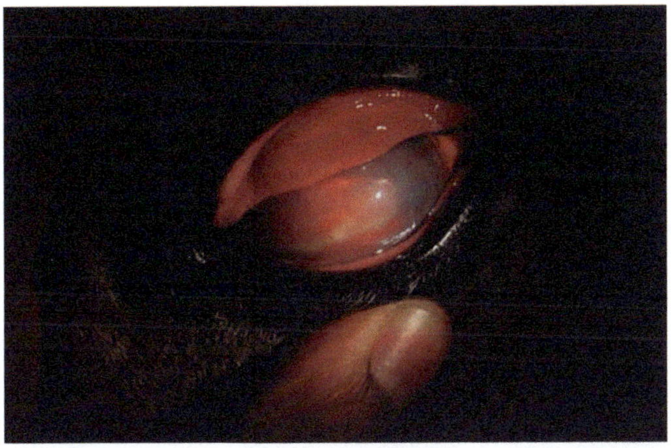

**Figure 14.16.** Horse. Eye. Mycotic Keratitis. Peripheral corneal fibrosis and neovascularization are associated with an extensive central inflammatory cellular infiltrate. Such a lesion is often chronic and deep, with healing of the overlying stroma and epithelium, creating a deep-seated stromal "abscess." In many cases, this is the only location in which the fungi can be found, which is an important consideration in the diagnosis of this disease. (Courtesy Comparative Ophthalmology Service, Michigan State University, East Lansing, MI.)

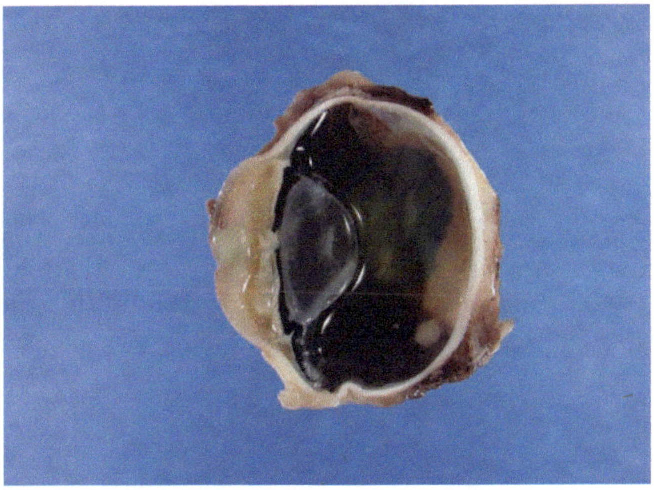

**Figure 14.17.** Horse. Eye. Mycotic Keratitis and Anterior Uveitis. Although very rare, the inflammation within the anterior and posterior chambers in the eye of this horse most likely arose from extension of the corneal lesion. Fungal hyphae were identified in the deep cornea and in a separated fragment of the Descemet's membrane within the anterior chamber.

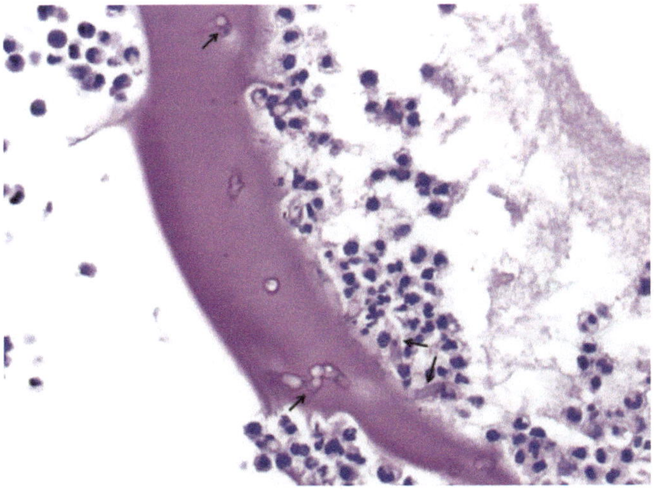

**Figure 14.18.** Horse. Eye. Mycotic Keratitis. The histologic lesion is a distinctive deep stromal suppurative keratitis adjacent to the Descemet's membrane, associated with intralesional fungi (arrows). (Periodic Acid Schiff (PAS))

*Suppurative uveitis* generally reflects a bacterial pathogenesis such as in neonatal septicemias.

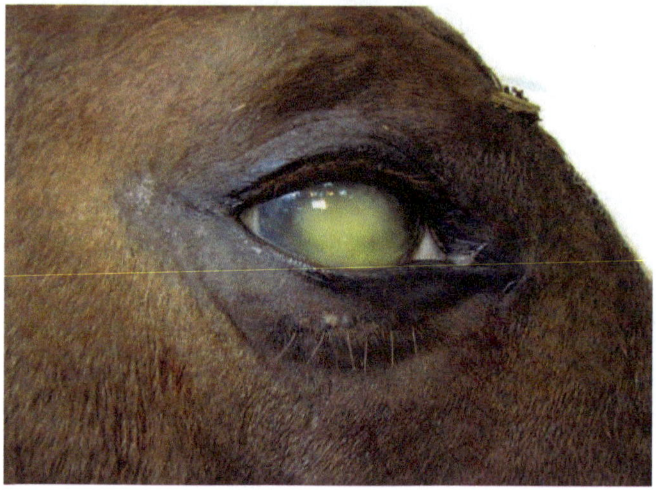

**Figure 14.19.** Foal. Eye. Suppurative Anterior Uveitis. Systemic *Rhodococcus equi* infection. The pupil of this septic foal is completely obscured by marked suppurative inflammatory exudate in the anterior chamber. The exudate may settle ventrally, an alteration referred to clinically as "hypopyon."

*Equine recurrent uveitis.* It is assumed that this disease has an immune-mediated pathogenesis, with epidemiologic evidence that cross-reaction between leptospiral and intraocular antigens plays an important role. As the name implies, the disease is clinically characterized by recurrent episodes of intractable uveitis.

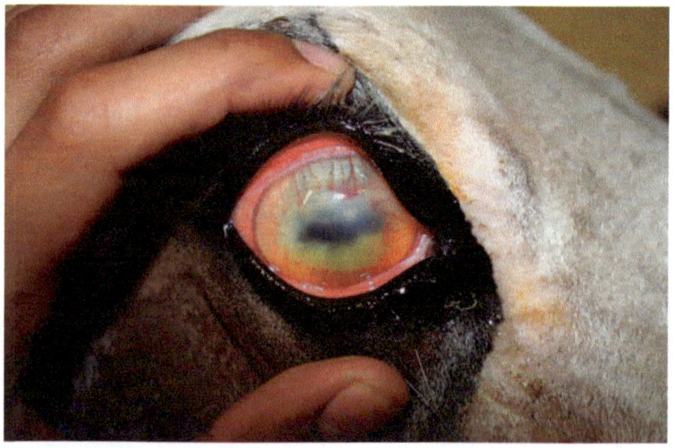

**Figure 14.20.** Horse. Eye. Equine Recurrent Uveitis. This horse had a waxing and waning history of anterior uveitis. Mild conjunctival hyperemia and corneal edema with 360-degree neovascularization, accompanied by marked aqueous flare and hypopyon, are the illustrated pathologic features. (Courtesy Comparative Ophthalmology Service, Michigan State University.)

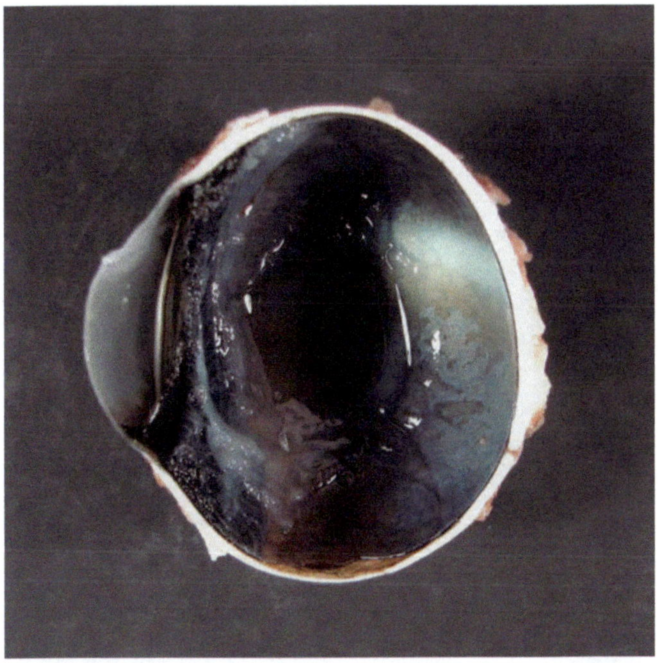

**Figure 14.21.** Horse. Eye. Equine Recurrent Uveitis. This horse was being treated for this condition for 5 years. When secondary glaucoma developed in the eye, it was enucleated. A thin membrane is tightly adhered to the ciliary body.

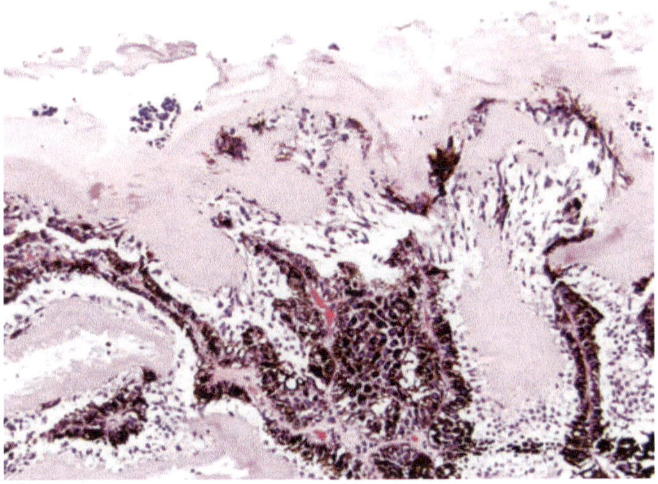

**Figure 14.22.** Horse. Eye. Equine Recurrent Uveitis. Histologically, a thick hyaline membrane of amyloid-like material covering the inner nonpigmented ciliary epithelium is a characteristic feature of this disease. Additionally in such a case, there are perivascular accumulations of lymphocytes and plasma cells within the iris and ciliary body and occasionally within the choroid. No infectious agent is seen. (H&E)

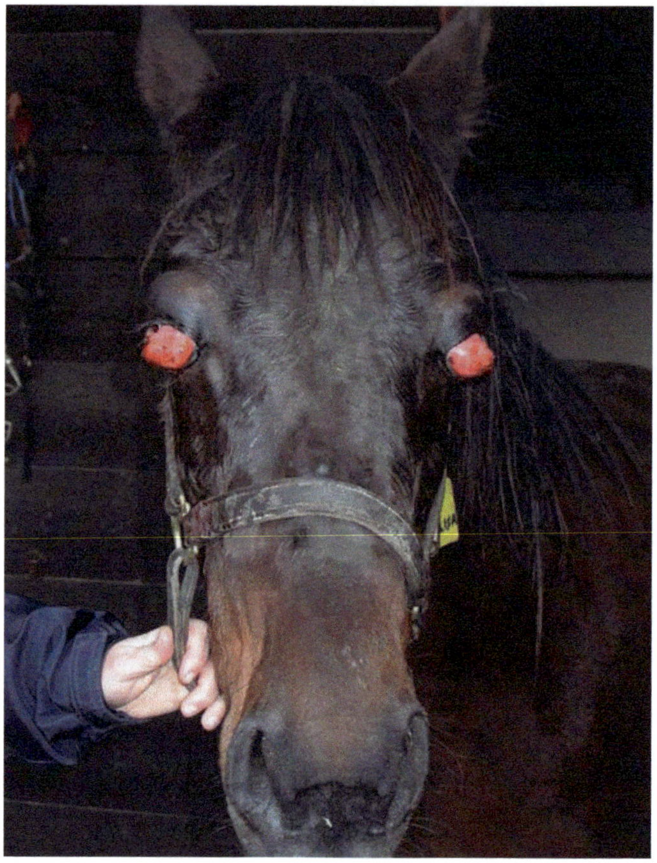

**Figure 14.23.** Horse. Head. Bilateral Conjunctival Pseudotumors. These pink, smooth, secondarily ulcerated conjunctival masses that clinically resemble neoplasms are histologically composed of a predominantly lymphocytic inflammatory cell infiltrate. An immune-mediated pathogenesis is suspected. Reported cases are primarily unilateral and with a predilection for the perilimbal region. (Courtesy Dr. Roberta Rossi, Pinerolo, Turin, Italy.)

### *4. Neoplastic ocular diseases*

The eye can be the site of a variety of primary and metastatic neoplasms, but only a few are of sufficient importance to justify discussion.

*Squamous cell carcinoma.* This neoplasm affects the sunlight-exposed, nonpigmented epithelium of the limbic bulbar conjunctiva, the third eyelid and the other eyelids, most commonly in horses with white, gray-white, or palomino hair colors and increased exposure to ultraviolet radiation. Consequently, neoplasm prevalence is correlated with high altitude and intense sunlight exposure. The neoplasm is preceded by a series of precancerous epithelial changes involving actinic injury and dysplastic repair prior to malignant transformation, giving rise to a temporal sequence of lesions called squamous plaque, squamous papilloma, squamous carcinoma in situ, and invasive squamous cell carcinoma. In the cornea, the tumor can also have a distinctive intrastromal growth pattern with a smooth intact corneal epithelium, in which case it may be misdiagnosed as stromal keratitis.

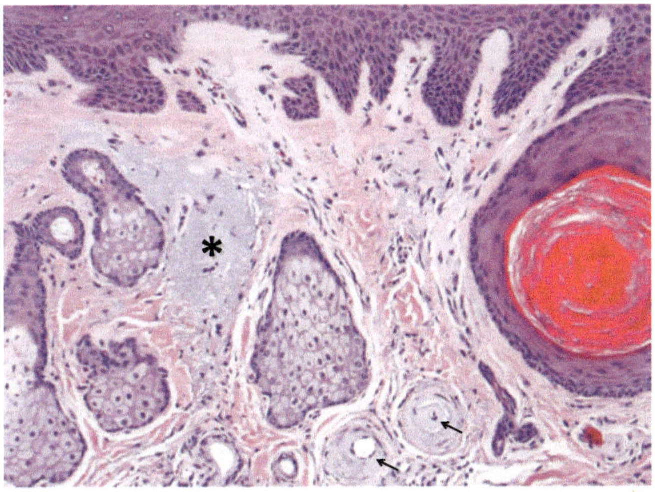


**Figure 14.24.** Horse. Eyelid with Actinic Injury. Irregular epidermal hyperplasia, solar elastosis (asterisk), and vascular sclerosis (arrows) are indications of the underlying ultraviolet-induced damage to the nonpigmented skin that may lead to neoplastic transformation of the lining epithelium. (H&E)

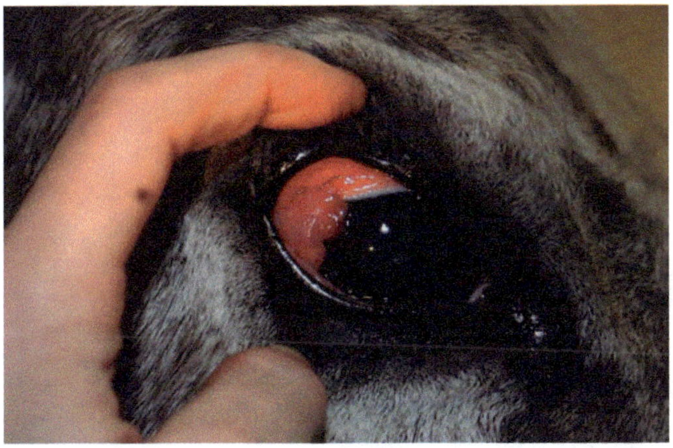

**Figure 14.25.** Horse. Eye. Neoplasia. Limbal Squamous Cell Carcinoma. A pink, fleshy, hyperemic, raised, 2-cm diameter temporal limbal neoplastic mass is present in this eye with mild epiphora. The mass was accompanied by elastosis histologically, providing evidence for solar induced mucosal damage. (Courtesy Comparative Ophthalmology Service, Michigan State University, East Lansing, MI.)

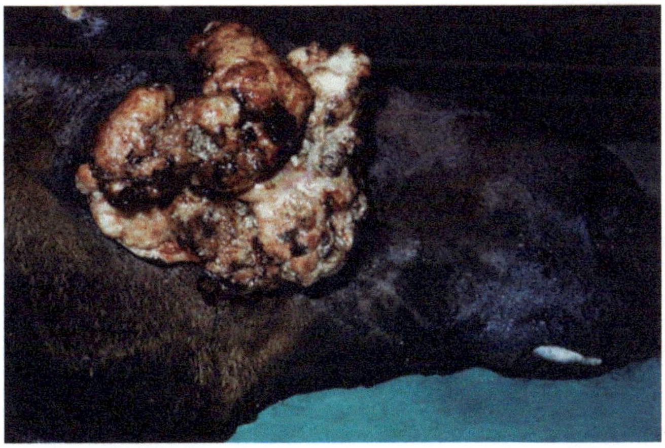

**Figure 14.26.** Horse. Face. Neoplasia. Conjunctival Squamous Cell Carcinoma. This large exophytic tumor is extensively ulcerated and inflamed, with secondary myiasis. Such a neoplasm is able to penetrate the sinuses and eventually metastasize to draining lymph nodes and disseminate into thoracic and abdominal organs. (Courtesy Dr. William W. Carlton, West Lafayette, IN.)

*Melanomas.* Primary melanocytic neoplasms of the eye and ocular adnexa are rare in horses. They may occur in the eyelid of gray horses as part of the generalized melanosis syndrome, or they may occur sporadically in any horse. Melanomas are also rarely encountered within the anterior uvea and conjunctiva.

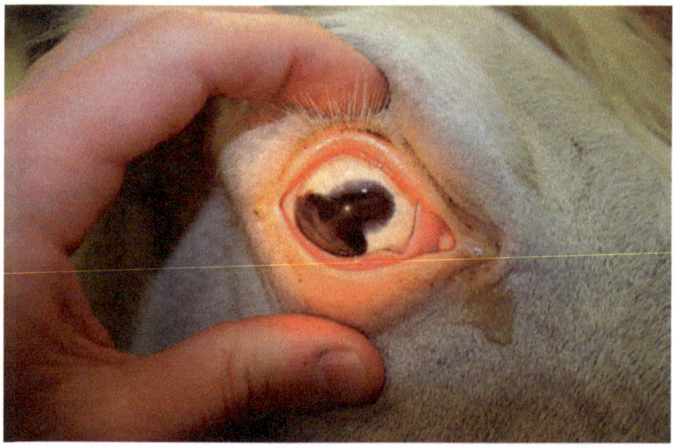

**Figure 14.27.** Horse. Eye. Neoplasia. Intraocular Melanoma. This large dark brown mass with irregular margins protrudes from the iris into the anterior chamber, contacting the cornea and extending into the drainage angle. This horse also had a melanoma in the contralateral eye and in the perineum. Equine intraocular (anterior uveal) melanomas are in general slow-growing, locally infiltrative neoplasms that do not metastasize. (Courtesy Comparative Ophthalmology Service, Michigan State University, East Lansing, MI.)

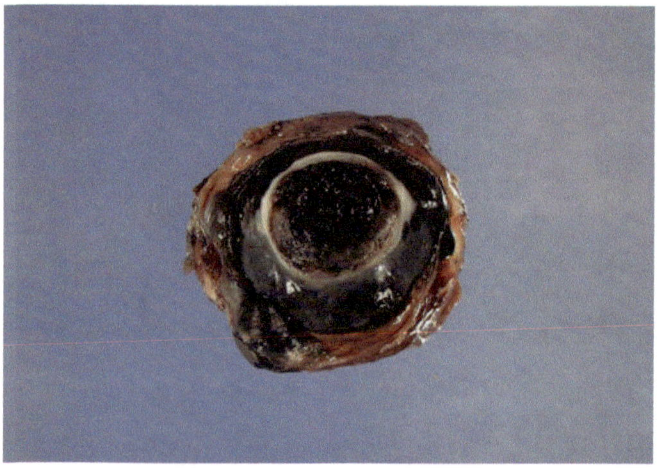

**Figure 14.28.** Horse. Eye. Neoplasia. Intraocular Melanoma. This neoplasm is more aggressive than usual, with extension into the limbus and cornea, leading to extensive central corneal ulceration.

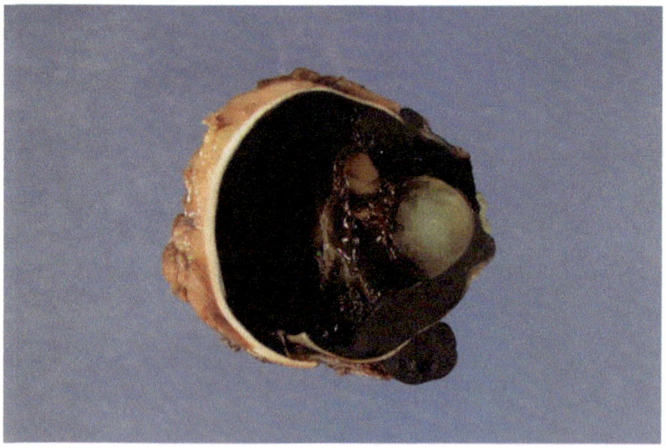

**Figure 14.29.** Horse. Eye. Neoplasia. Intraocular Melanoma (same as in Figure 14.28). The cut surface further illustrates the extensive involvement of the anterior uvea by the melanoma, with extension into the limbus and cornea. Corneal perforation, cataractous change, plasmoid vitreous, and complete retinal detachment were considered secondary to the neoplastic process.

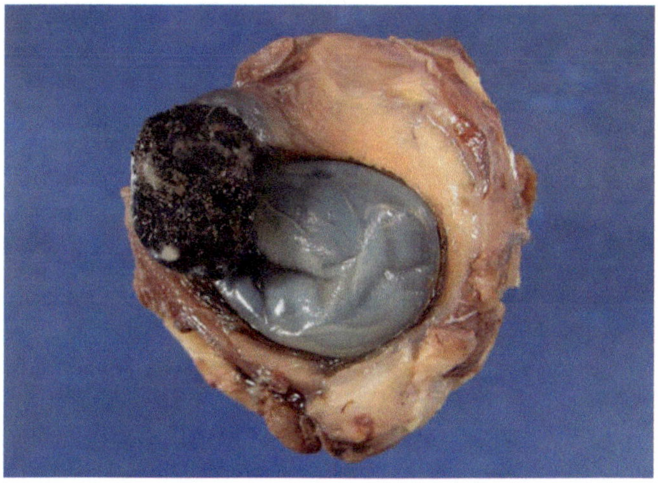

**Figure 14.30.** Horse. Eye. Neoplasia. Limbal Melanoma. The limbus area has a 2.5 cm × 1.5 cm polypoid, heavily black pigmented, well-demarcated, extensively ulcerated mass.

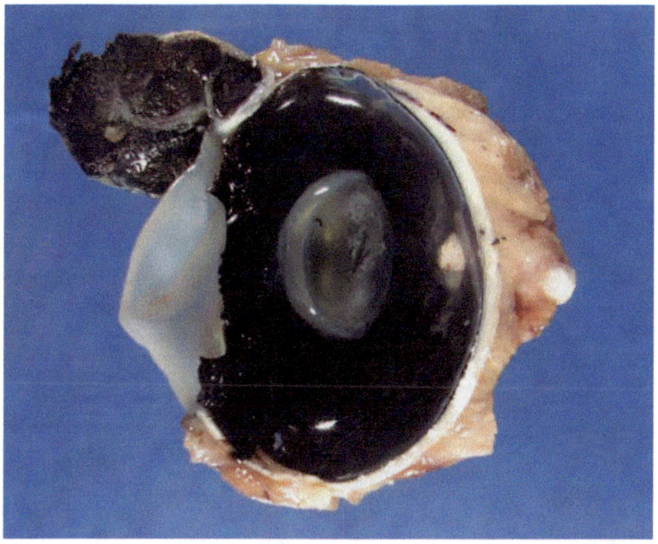

**Figure 14.31.** Horse. Eye. Neoplasia. Limbal Melanoma (same as in Figure 14.30). Cut section reveals a lobulated neoplasm with histologic features of malignancy including anisokaryosis and increased mitotic index.

There are a few reports of locally invasive, histologically malignant conjunctival or epibulbar melanomas in horses. Some limbal melanomas may metastasize to parotid gland or supraorbital lymph nodes.

*Vascular neoplasms.* Most of the published cases have been locally invasive, solid, spindle cell neoplasms of the third eyelid. Horses may also develop hemangiomas and hemangiosarcomas similar to those seen most frequently in dogs.

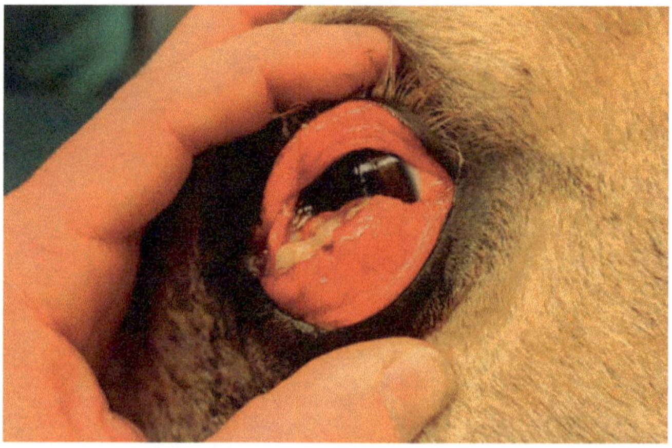

**Figure 14.32.** Horse. Eye. Neoplasia. Hemangiosarcoma with secondary Bacterial Infection. This type of neoplasm arises within the conjunctival lamina propria, most often on the bulbar aspect of the third eyelid near its free margin. (Courtesy Comparative Ophthalmology Service, Michigan State University, East Lansing, MI.)

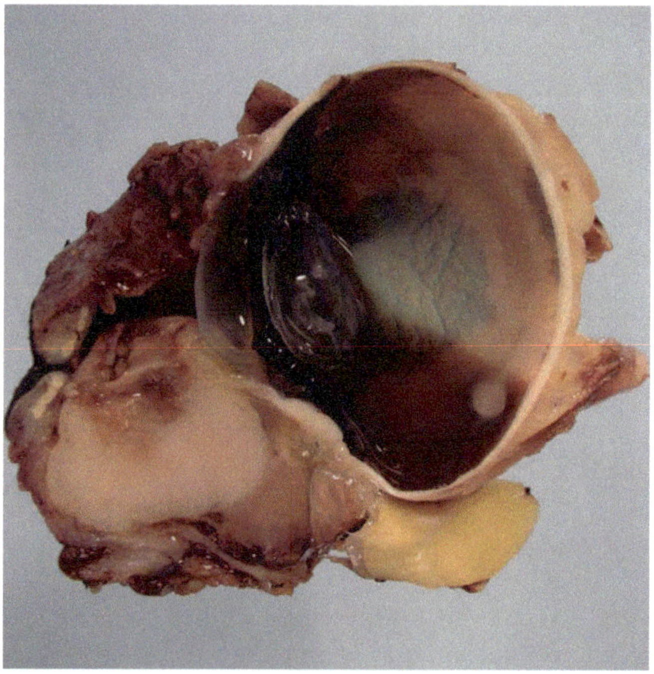

**Figure 14.33.** Horse. Eye. Neoplasia. Hemangiosarcoma with secondary Bacterial Infection (same as in Figure 14.32). On cut surface, the neoplasm is characterized by a superficially ulcerated, solid, fairly well-demarcated, nonencapsulated mass within the subepithelial collagenous connective tissue of the third eyelid.

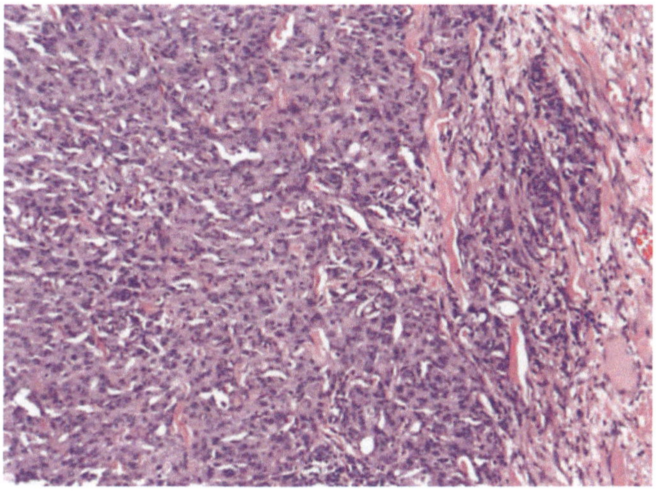

**Figure 14.34.** Horse. Eye. Neoplasia. Hemangiosarcoma. Microscopically, the endothelial cells are occasionally separated to form narrow vascular channels.

These mostly solid hemangiosarcomas may be mistakenly diagnosed histologically as fibrosarcoma by those who are not familiar with this distinctive variant. Immunohistochemical labeling for factor VIII–related antigen or for CD31 may useful to establish the definitive diagnosis.

*Medulloepithelioma.* This uncommon, histologically distinctive neoplasm is often reported in horses as the most frequent primary ocular neoplasm. By definition it is a congenital neoplasm, with clinical recognition delayed for several years. The tumor is found growing into the vitreous body from its origin, the embryonic neurectoderm lining the inner layer of the optic cup anywhere along the ciliary body or retina, and may show differentiation into any of the derivatives of pluripotential tissue: iridociliary epithelium, retina, vitreous, and neuroglia. These neoplasms may also contain foci of muscle, bone, cartilage, and brain tissue (teratoid medulloepithelioma). Metastasis has not been reported.

*Optic nerve glioma.* There are several reports of astrocytoma or undifferentiated glioma affecting the optic disk of horses. Most of these cases are thought to represent proliferation of astrocytes and lipid-laden macrophages as a consequence of optic nerve damage (i.e., proliferative optic neuropathy).

## II. Ears

Horses use their ears to communicate and to detect sounds to avoid danger. Ear diseases in horses are uncommon. Specifically the pinna can be affected by a variety of skin diseases. These include inflammatory, nonneoplastic, and neoplastic conditions, many of which just happen to affect the ear, although some have a predilection for this site. Diseases of the actual middle and inner ear are rare. Horses are more likely to have infection of the guttural pouch, a ventral diverticulum of the auditory tube (for more information on diseases of the guttural pouch, refer to Chapter 4, "Diseases of the Respiratory System").

## 1. Inflammatory otic diseases

*Fly strike*. The stable fly, *Stomoxys calcitrans*, can induce a hypersensitivity reaction on the pinna, as well as on the face and trunk, characterized by pruritic papules and wheals with central hemorrhagic crusts.

*Ear mites*. Horses affected by the spinose ear tick (*Otobius megnini*) may present with droopy and sensitive ears, head shaking and rubbing, and dark waxy discharge.

*Otitis*. In horses, otitis externa is generally caused by ticks or foreign bodies. Middle or inner ear infections can arise as an extension of prolonged otitis externa and of ascending infections from the guttural pouch. A possible sequela of otitis media is thought to be the temporohyoid osteoarthropathy.

## 2. Nonneoplastic and neoplastic proliferative otic diseases

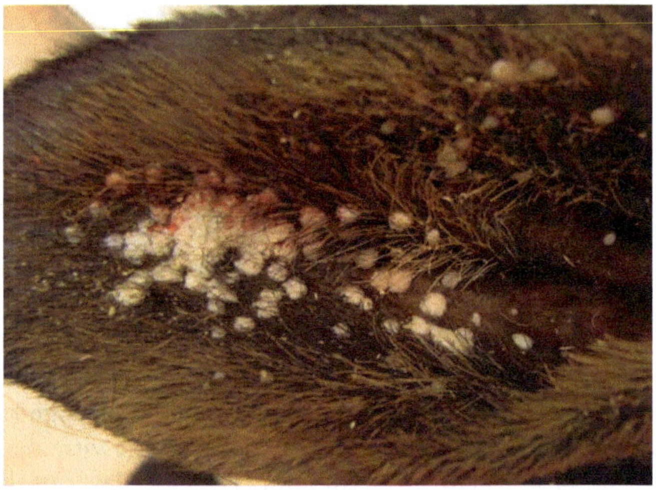

**Figure 14.35.** Horse. Pinna. Aural Plaque. Numerous 3- to 5-mm round, raised, white cutaneous hyperkeratotic plaques cover the inner surface of the ear of this horse. The lesion, which was recently associated with equine papillomavirus 3, is frequently bilateral. The plaques are generally persistent but are usually asymptomatic and therefore considered an incidental finding.

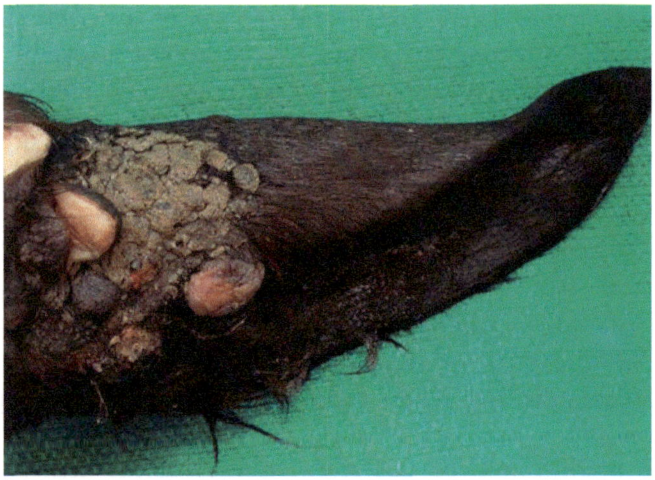

**Figure 14.36.** Horse. Pinna. Sarcoid. This skin neoplasm has a predilection for the head and external ear. It does not, however, differ histologically from the same neoplasm found in other locations.

## Example of eye diseases in specific horse breeds – Fact sheet

### Appaloosa

- Iridal hypoplasia
- Equine recurrent uveitis → Glaucoma
- Squamous cell carcinoma

### Arabian

- Congenital cataract

### Belgian

- Aniridia
- Cataract

### Draft breeds

- Squamous cell carcinoma

### Miniature horse

- Entropion

### Morgan

- Congenital cataract

### Quarter horse

- Limbal dermoid
- Aniridia or iridal hypoplasia
- Congenital cataract
- Squamous cell carcinoma

### Silver or chocolate coat color breeds

- Anterior segment dysgenesis

### Standardbred

- Retinal detachment

### Thoroughbred

- Congenital cataract
- Aniridia
- Entropion

## Selected references


Andersson LS, Axelsson J, Dubielzig RR, Lindgren G, Ekesten B. 2011. Multiple congenital ocular anomalies in Icelandic horses. *BMC Vet Res* 26(7):21.

Brooks DE, Matthews AG. 2007. Equine ophthalmology. In Gelatt KN, ed. *Veterinary Ophthalmology*. 4th ed. Ames, IA: Blackwell:1165–1274.

Crowe MW, Swerczek TW. 1985. Equine congenital defects. *Am J Vet Res* 46(2):353–358.

Cutler TJ. 2002. Ophthalmic findings in the geriatric horse. *Vet Clin North Am Equine Pract* 18(3):545–574.

Cutler TJ. 2004. Corneal epithelial disease. *Vet Clin North Am Equine Pract* 20(2):319–343, vi.

Dubielzig RR, Ketring KL, McLellan GJ, Albert DM. 2010. *Veterinary Ocular Pathology: A Comparative Review*. New York: Saunders Elsevier.

Gaarder JE, Rebhun WC, Ball MA, Patten V, Shin S, Erb H. 1998. Clinical appearances, healing patterns, risk factors, and outcomes of horses with fungal keratitis: 53 cases (1978–1996). *J Am Vet Med Assoc* 213(1):105–112.

Komáromy AM, Rowlan JS, La Croix NC, Mangan BG. 2011. Equine multiple congenital ocular anomalies (MCOA) syndrome in PMEL17 (Silver) mutant ponies: five cases. *Vet Ophthalmol* 14(5):313–320.

Labelle AL, Hamor RE, Townsend WM, et al. 2011. Ophthalmic lesions in neonatal foals evaluated for nonophthalmic disease at referral hospitals. *J Am Vet Med Assoc* 239(4):486–492.

Moore CP, Grevan VL, Champagne ES, Collins BK, Collier LL. 2000. Equine conjunctival pseudotumors. *Vet Ophthalmol* 3(2–3):57–63.

Nell B, Walde I. 2010. Posterior segment diseases. *Equine Vet J Suppl* 37(3):69–79.

Plummer CE, Ramsey DT. 2011. A survey of ocular abnormalities in miniature horses. *Vet Ophthalmol* 14(4):239–243.

Pusterla N, Watson JL, Wilson WD, Affolter VK, Spier SJ. 2003. Cutaneous and ocular habronemiasis in horses: 63 cases (1988–2002). *J Am Vet Med Assoc* 222(7):978–982.

Rebhun WC. 1998. Tumors of the eye and ocular adnexal tissues. *Vet Clin North Am Equine Pract* 14(3):579–606, vii.

Wilcock BP. 2007. Eye and ear. In Maxie MG, ed. *Jubb, Kennedy, and Palmer's Pathology of Domestic Animals*. 5th ed. New York: Saunders Elsevier:459–552.

Wilkie DA. 2010. Equine glaucoma: state of the art. *Equine Vet J Suppl* 37:62–68.

# 15 Diseases of the Hemolymphatic System

With contributions by Donald J. Meuten and Claus D. Buergelt



*Color Atlas of Equine Pathology*, First Edition. Claus D. Buergelt and Fabio Del Piero.

Diseases of the spleen, bone marrow, thymus, and lymph nodes may involve all these organs concurrently or individually. The most important diseases are equine infectious anemia (EIA), lymphoma, strangles, Rhodococcus infection, and red maple toxicity. Two important congenital diseases, severe combined immunodeficiency disease (SCID) and neonatal isoerythrolysis, are also mentioned in Chapter 2, "Diseases of Foals and Juveniles." Hyperplasia is a more common reaction than inflammation in lymph nodes, spleen, and bone marrow, and the gross lesions in each organ are usually subtle. Red bone marrow is more likely due to congestion than erythroid regeneration. Evaluation of blood is a common antemortem technique; bone marrow taken from ribs, sternum, or long bones is usually examined postmortem; and biopsy and/or fine-needle aspiration are usually reserved for peripheral lymph nodes. Regenerative anemia is not reflected in the peripheral blood as it is in other species; therefore do not expect to see increased reticulocytes, increased mean corpuscular volume (MCV), or decreased mean corpuscular hemoglobin concentration (MCHC).

## I. Diseases of the bone marrow

### *1. Severe combined immunodeficiency disease*

SCID is seen primarily in Arabian foals as an autosomal recessive trait. In such animals 25% may be carriers of a gene defect that blocks the development of B and T lymphocytes. The disorder is characterized by severe hypoplasia of primary and secondary lymphoid tissues. Occurrence of this inherited disease has declined in recent years due to selective breeding and genetic testing for the recessive carrier genes. SCID affects both T and B lymphocyte lineages. Opportunistic pathogens (viruses, adenovirus, bacteria, *Cryptosporidium* sp, *Pneumocystis jiroveci* [previously *carinii*], *Candida* sp.) take advantage of the animal's compromised immune function. Colostral antibodies, if adequate, usually protect affected foals for the first 4–6 months of their lives, but when these antibodies are depleted, infectious diseases and death are inevitable. Additional examples of pathologic changes are discussed in Chapter 2, "Diseases of Foals and Juveniles." Pathologic and clinicopathologic findings useful in the diagnosis of SCID include hypogammaglobulinemia, lymphopenia, and hypoplasia of lymphoid organs. By far the most common immunodeficiency in horses is failure of passive transfer of colostral antibodies. Without treatment these foals develop sepsis in joints, bones, lungs, and internal organs resulting in the foal's death. Uncommon immune deficiencies in other breeds of horses include agammaglobulinemia, selective immunoglobulin M (IgM) deficiency, and the fell pony syndrome.

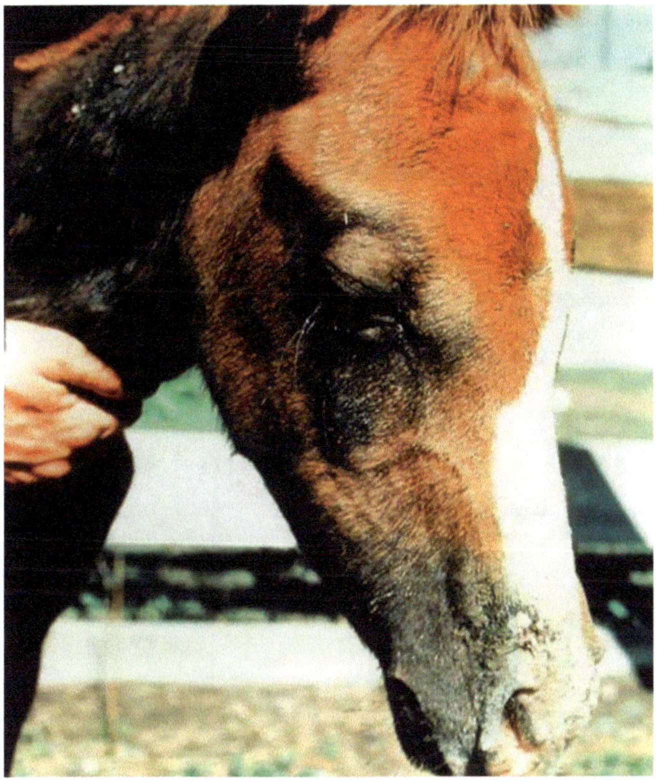

**Figure 15.1.** Arabian Foal. Head. Epiphora and Rhinorhea. SCID. The nostrils are partially occluded by discharge from bronchopneumonia, and there is evidence of ocular discharge from conjunctivitis.

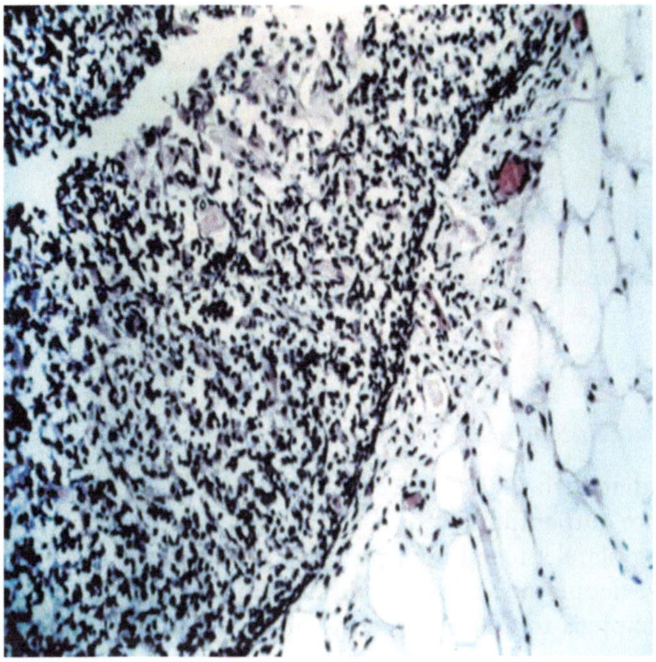

**Figure 15.2.** Arabian Foal. Thymus. Lymphoid Hypoplasia. SCID. Because of severe hypoplasia, the thymus will be small and difficult to identify grossly. Microscopically, it is characterized by a paucity of lymphocytes in cortex and medulla. (H&E) (Courtesy Dr. L. Perryman, Colorado State University.)

## 2. *Myeloid necrosis*

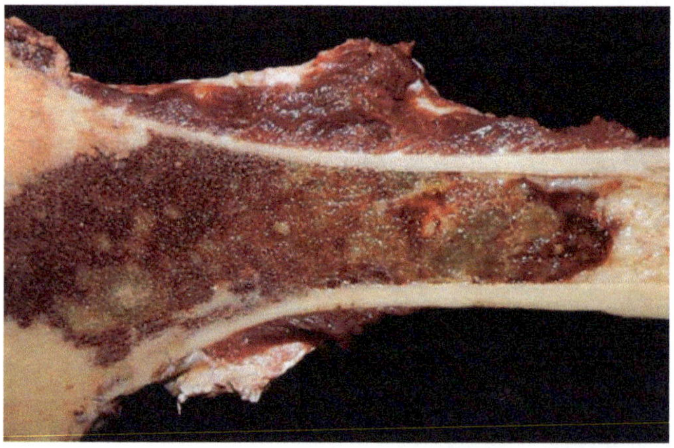

**Figure 15.3.** Horse. Long Bone. Bone Marrow Necrosis. The marrow is of variable but also of multifocal brown discoloration. There was evidence of necrosis and inflammation in the bone marrow as well as intranuclear herpesvirus inclusions in multinucleate inflammatory giant cells. The myeloid necrosis, contributed to the horse's pancytopenia. This was a case of gamma herpesvirus infection with PCR positive for EHV-2 and EHV-5. The horse also had evidence of multinodular pulmonary fibrosis. (Courtesy Dr. J. Roberts, National Zoo, Washington, DC.)

## 3. *Myelodysplasia*

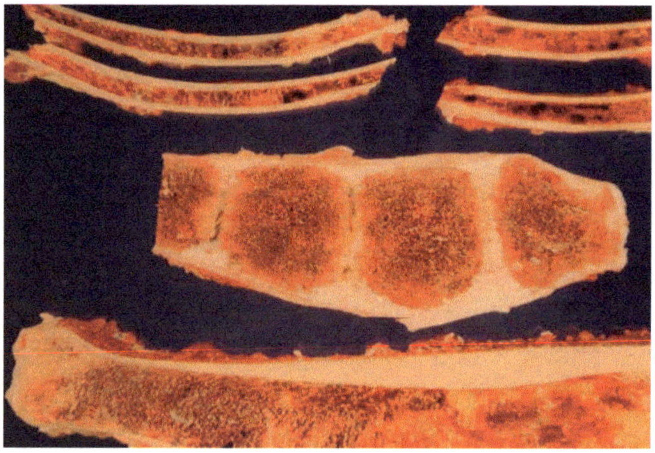

**Figure 15.4.** Horse. Ribs and Sternum. Bone Marrow Hypercellularity. Cross section. The bone marrow of the ribs is abundant and diffusely red due to marked hypercellularity. This was a case of myeloproliferative disorder with hematologic findings of anemia and thrombocytopenia and clinical signs of disseminated hemorrhage. Microscopic evaluation of the bone marrow aspirate revealed megakaryocytic aplasia, dyserythropoiesis, and granulocytic hypoplasia with maturation arrest. The syndrome eventually leads to various forms of overt leukemia.

## 4. *Immune-mediated thrombocytopenia*

Immune-mediated thrombocytopenia (ITP) The disorder is either primary, resulting from autoantibodies directed against bone marrow megakaryocyte or circulating platelet membrane antigens, or secondary to a variety of infectious agents, neoplasms, and/or drug administration that typically provide circulating haptens to adhere to megakaryocyte or platelet membranes and induce an immune-mediated destruction. Antibodies are usually directed against platelets and not megakaryocytes, and only platelets are decreased in the peripheral blood. There is no simple and accurate test for ITP. If platelet counts remain low and disseminated intravascular coagulation (DIC) is ruled out, then ITP is a likely cause. Numerous megakaryocytes, especially if they are regenerative with active thrombocytopenia in a horse that does not have DIC, are most likely due to ITP. Petechiae and thrombocytopenia are seen in a few horses postinfection with *S. equi*. The syndrome is referred to as purpura hemorrhagica, and the thrombocytopenia is most likely due to immune-mediated mechanisms. Clinical signs of severe thrombocytopenia include epistaxis and petechiae in the skin and oral, nasal, and vaginal mucous membranes. Thrombocytopenia is defined as a platelet count less than 90,000/μL in affected horses; however, most horses with immune-mediated thrombocytopenia have counts of less than 20,000/μL. Bleeding is not usually due to thrombocytopenia unless the counts are 10,000/μL or less. The most common causes of thrombocytopenia are DIC and poor venipuncture technique, such that tissue thromboplastin has been released. Thrombocytopenia due to tickborne diseases is common in dogs, suspected in horses but rarely proven. Snap tests used in dogs are used in horses. Positivity implies antibodies are present, and exposure occurred, but not that the disease is present or that antigen is present.

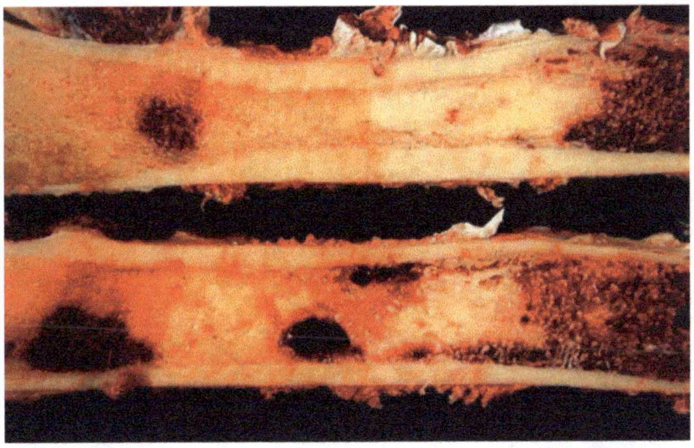

**Figure 15.5.** Horse. Bone Marrow. Hypercellularity. Immune-Mediated Thrombocytopenia. There are only a few areas of active bone marrow left. Most has been displaced by adipose tissue. Megakaryocytes are absent microscopically, and therefore the antibodies were most likely directed against megakaryocytes. All other cell lines were unaffected.

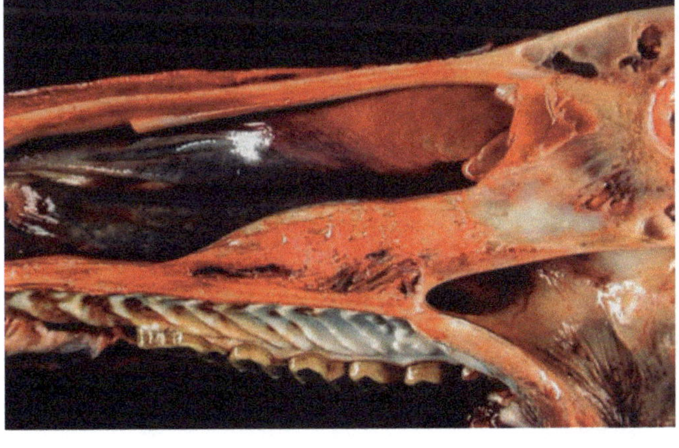

**Figure 15.6.** Horse. Head. Midsagittal Section. Turbinate Hemorrhage. Immune-Mediated Thrombocytopenia. The turbinates are reddened by severe acute hemorrhage.

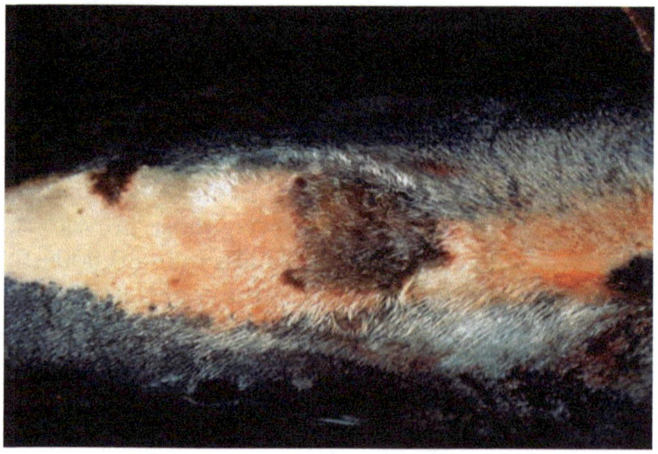

**Figure 15.7.** Horse. Head. Frontal Bones. Acute Dermal Hemorrhage. Immune-Mediated Thrombocytopenia. The skin over the nose and frontal bones is characterized by petechiae and hemorrhage.

### *5. Neoplasia*

The primary tumors involving the bone marrow of horses include stage 5 lymphoma and acute lymphoid leukemia. Other tumors such as multiple myeloma (plasma cell tumor of the marrow) have been seen in horses, but these are rare.

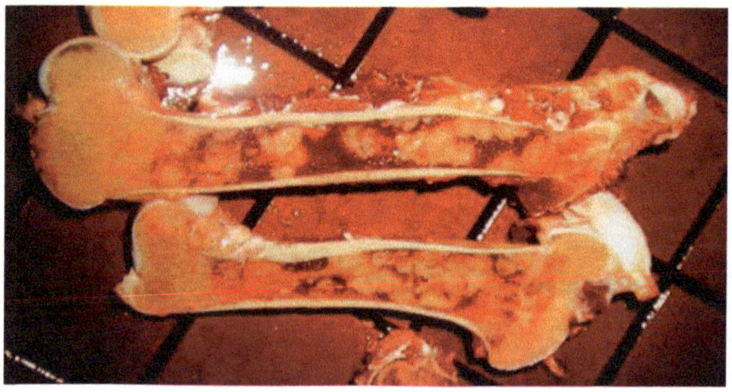

**Figure 15.8.** Horse. Long Bone. Bone Marrow. Acute Lymphocytic Leukemia. Lymphoid leukemia is diagnosed when the tumor begins in the marrow and may spread to liver, spleen, and other peripheral tissues. Most of the marrow has been displaced by an off-white multifocal to coalescing neoplastic tissue.

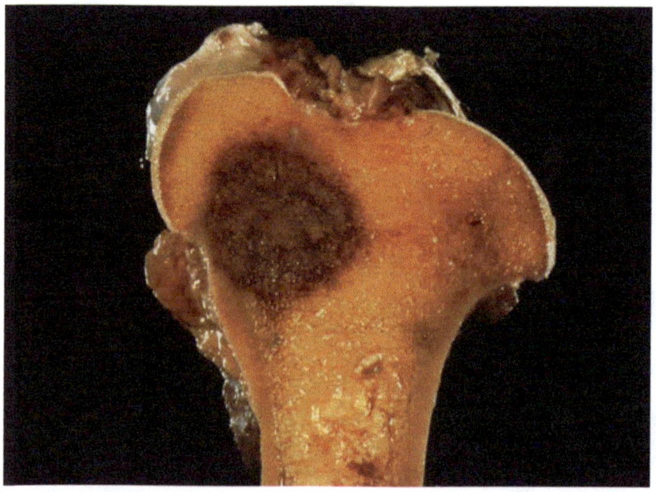

**Figure 15.9.** Horse. Long Bone. Bone Marrow. Myeloma. The cut surface of long bone has a discrete circular gray region that was diagnosed as myeloma. This is a rare tumor in horses. It is associated with marked hyperproteinemia and monoclonal gammopathy. (Courtesy P. Stromberg, Ohio State University.)

### 6. *Bone marrow biopsy*

Sampling bone marrow in the horse, ante- or postmortem, is done infrequently. If only one cell line is abnormally decreased or increased, the etiology is usually outside of the bone marrow, and therefore examination of marrow elements is not needed once the cause is established. When two or more hematopoietic cell lines are affected, then examination of the bone marrow is indicated and may help establish the cause. Bone marrow examination is warranted for any of the following: (1) two or more hematopoietic cell lines are decreased, (2) leukemia is suspected, and/or (3) there is an unexplained decrease or increase in hematopoietic cells.

## II. Diseases of circulating blood cells

### 1. *Immune-mediated hemolytic anemia*

#### *a. Isoerythrolysis of the newborn*

This condition affecting red blood cells is described in Chapter 2, "Diseases of Foals and Juveniles."

#### *b. Autoimmune hemolytic anemia*

This condition is better referred to as immune-mediated hemolytic anemia (IMHA) because the cause is only rarely due to autoantibodies directed against red blood cell antigens. Most cases have antibodies and/or complement nonspecifically attached to the surface of red blood cells often due to a hapten that has altered the red blood cell antigens in such a way that they are considered foreign to the immune system, or the antibody is directed against an antigen attached to the red blood cells. The hapten is usually not known, but some known causes are penicillin, *Clostridium perfringens* myositis of the cervical region, and red blood cell parasites. In most cases the hemolysis is extravascular due to phagocytosis of red blood cells coated with IgG by macrophages in the spleen and liver. Therefore, the urine and kidneys are not discolored red brown. Intravascular hemolysis is usually associated with IgM and complement attachment. With either mechanism there often is moderate to severe anemia and prominent hepatosplenomegaly.

Autoagglutination is uncommon but diagnostic when present. Spherocytosis is difficult to recognize in the horse because central pallor of red blood cells is not a normal feature. Coombs positivity is associated with IMHA but is also seen in other diseases. A positive Coombs test means there is antibody and/or complement attached to red blood cells. However, this can happen nonspecifically; it does not guarantee IMHA is present, and it does not differentiate autoimmune from immune-mediated unless direct and indirect tests are performed. The Coombs test, like any test, can also be falsely negative for several reasons and IMHA is present.

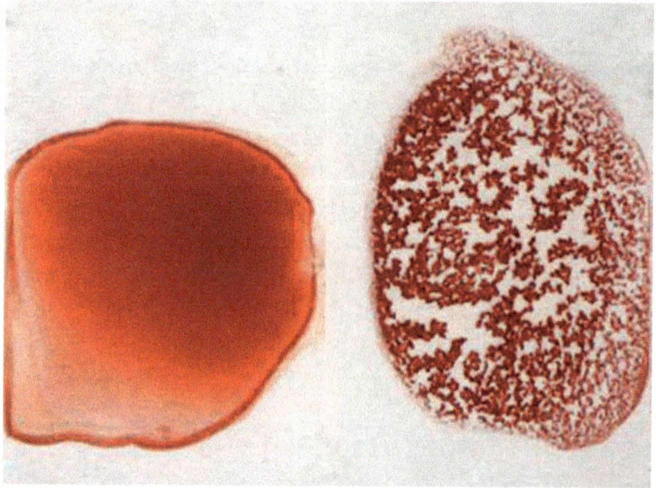

**Figure 15.10.** Horse. Blood Smear. IMHA. Blood is agglutinating spontaneously on a glass slide, to right; normal to left.

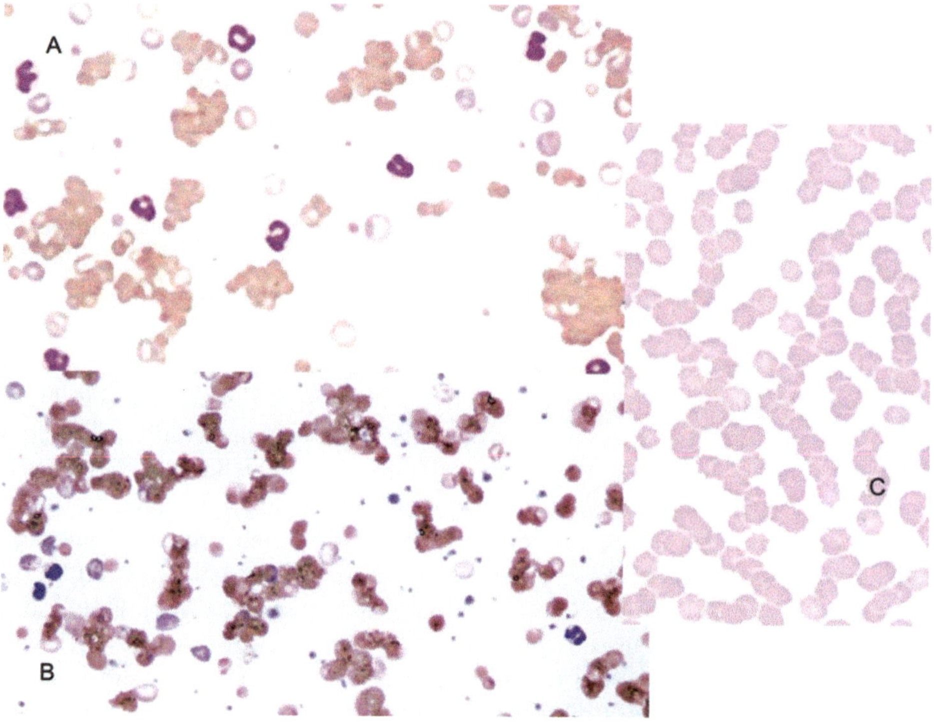


**Figure 15.11.** Blood Smear. IMHA. Light microscopic agglutination is evidenced by red blood cells adhered together in irregularly sized and organized clusters or morulae (left). Rouleaux is common in the horse and differentiated from agglutination by red blood cells arranged in a linear fashion, like a stack of coins (right). It does not mean a specific disease is present because it can be seen in normal horses and horses with increased serum protein.

## 2. *Infections*

Infectious agents targeting equine red blood cells are *Trypanosoma* sp. (*T. evansi*), protozoa (*Babesia* sp.), bacteria (*Clostridium perfringens*), or viruses (equine lentivirus). *Babesia equi* or *B. caballi* are the causative agents for equine piroplasmosis. Equine lentivirus is the etiology of equine infectious anemia (EIA). Trypanosomiasis is exotic to the Northern Hemisphere and involves *Trypanosoma evansi* (Surra) as it affects circulating blood cells.

*a. Equine infectious anemia*

EIA is considered one of the most important infectious diseases of equines. The agent has a worldwide distribution; however, the prevalence of EIA has largely declined in North America due primarily to the rigorous testing required for selling or trading horses or moving them across state lines. EIA is caused by an arthropod-borne lentivirus of the family *Retroviridae* that induces a cyclic immune-mediated hemolytic anemia with disseminated petechial hemorrhage and edema. The virus absorbs to erythrocytes leading to hemolysis. Hemolysis occurs both extravascularly and intravascularly. Some aspects of anemia are due to the immune response (IgM, IgG, complement activation) causing lysis of erythrocytes. Tissue macrophages, typically those in the spleen, account for most of virus replication. The virus replicates less than 1% in circulating monocytes. Despite the low viral burden in circulating monocytes, hematophagous flies, particularly the horsefly (genus *Tabanus*), are responsible for transmission of the disease. Mechanical transmission by blood-contaminated grooming equipment, shared syringes, and needles and nasogastric tubes is also possible. Vertical transmission of the virus occurs transplacentally, leading to abortion. Foals may be born with or without antibody. If the mare is positive, the foal serum should be checked before colostrum intake to determine if no antibodies are present in foal as the virus did not cross the placenta. The official test for EIA diagnosis is the agar gel immunodiffusion test performed in certified diagnostic laboratories. STAT test now is available. EIA is a reportable disease.

Three different clinical forms of EIA are distinguished: acute, subacute, and chronic.

i. Acute form of EIA. This form is characterized by fever, icterus, and anemia within a week of infection and frequently results in a high mortality rate. There is a decrease in the number of red blood cells, white blood cells (marked lymphopenia), and platelets. Dependent edema and petechial hemorrhages are common gross findings together with splenomegaly, hepatomegaly, and lymphadenopathy. Extensive necrosis of lymphocytes and renal tubular necrosis are typical microscopic findings. The microscopic liver lesions of focal infiltrations of lymphocytes are indicators of an immune response to viral antigens.

ii. Subacute form of EIA. In this form of the disease, pathologic lesions are similar to the acute form, but survival is possible. Hyperplasia of lymphocytes should be expected.

iii. Chronic form of EIA. The chronic form is encountered most frequently. It leads to generalized activation of the resident phagocytic system in several organs. Horses are typically emaciated and have an enlarged spleen and liver due to monocyte-macrophage ("reticuloendothelial") hyperplasia. There also is liver hemosiderosis. Viral antigen-antibody-C3 form circulating immune-complexes that may deposit in glomeruli causing a progressive glomerulonephritis and eventual renal failure. Neurologic leukoencephalitis occurs occasionally in horses infected with EIA.

Asymptomatic carrier, with positive AGID test but no clinical signs, is probably the most common way the disease is encountered today.

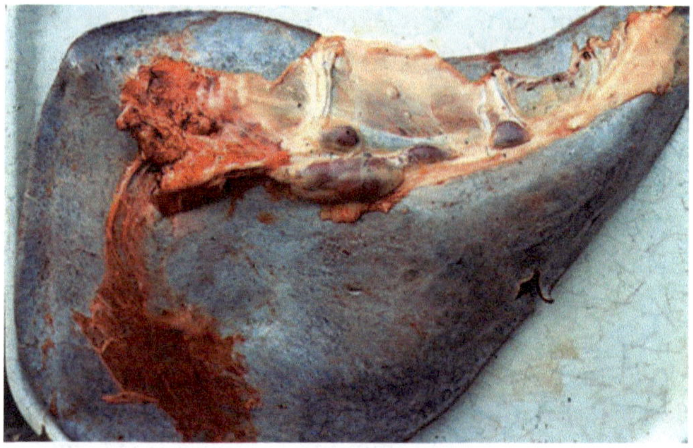

**Figure 15.12.** Horse. Spleen. Splenomegaly and Lymphadenomegaly. Chronic EIA. Spleen with lienal vein thrombosis. There is hilus lymphadenomegaly due to hemosiderosis and lymphoid hyperplasia. (Courtesy Dr. J. King, Cornell University.)

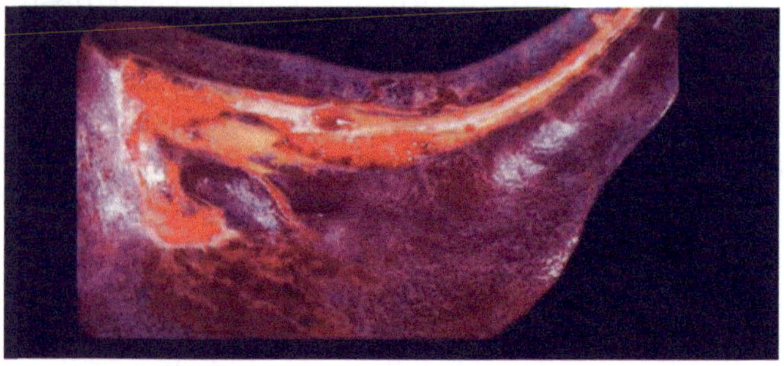

**Figure 15.13.** Horse. Spleen. Splenomegaly. Chronic EIA. "Blackberry jam" appearance due to hyperemia, hemosiderosis, and lymphoid hyperplasia. (Courtesy Dr. Cho, Louisiana State University, Noah's Arkive, University of Georgia.)

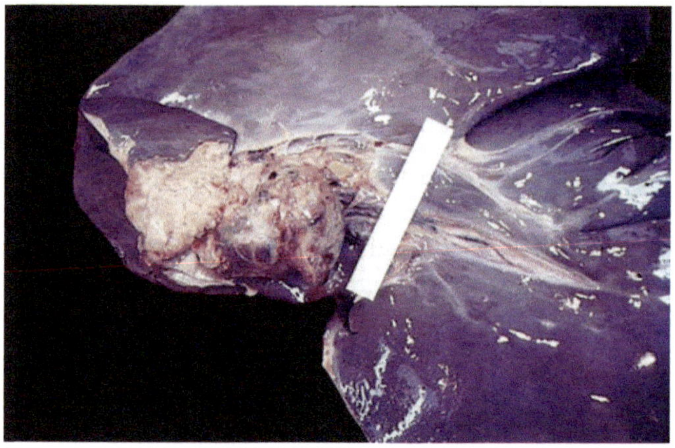

**Figure 15.14.** Horse. Liver. Hepatomegaly and Lymphadenomegaly. Chronic EIA. Hepatomegaly, discoloration, and lymphadenomegaly due to hepatitis, hemosiderosis, and lymphoid hyperplasia. (Courtesy Dr. J, King, Cornell University.)

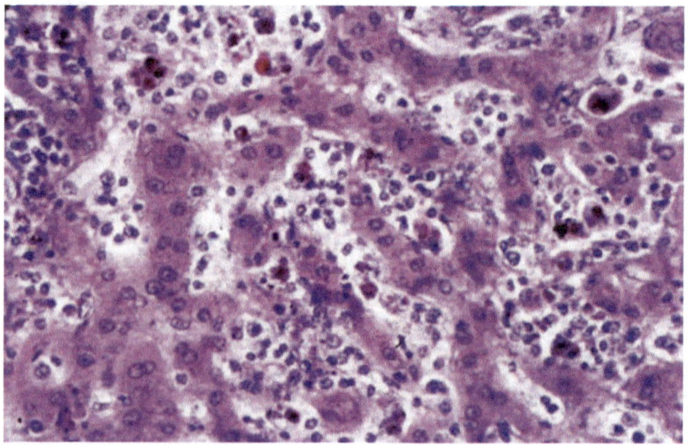

**Figure 15.15.** Horse. Liver. Multifocal Intrahepatic Lymphocytic Aggregates. Chronic EIA. A microscopic hall mark for EIA infection are clusters of lymphocytes within liver sinusoids. (H&E) (Courtesy Dr. J. King, Cornell University.)

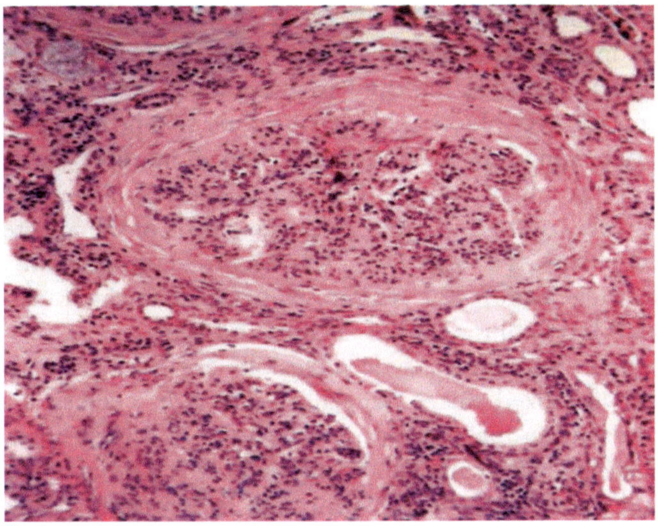

**Figure 15.16.** Horse. Kidney. Membranoproliferative Glomerulitis. Chronic EIA. Immune-complex glomerulopathy characterized by thickening of Bowman capsule and capillary loops (proliferative glomerulitis). (H&E) (Courtesy Dr. J. King, Cornell University.)

## Equine infectious anemia – Fact sheet

**Definition:** Vector-borne lentiviral infection with global distribution causing an immune-mediated cyclic hemolytic anemia

### Transmission

- Hematophagous flies (family *Tabanidae*)
- Mechanical
- Colostrum
- Transplacental

### Clinical forms

- Acute
- Subacute
- Chronic

**Diagnosis:** Agar gel immunodiffusion (AGID)

### Gross pathology

- Emaciation
- Anemia
- Thrombocytopenia
- Splenomegaly
- Hepatomegaly
- Lymphadenopathy

### Microscopic pathology

- Multifocal lymphocytic hepatitis
- Membranoproliferative glomerulitis
- Lymphocytic leukoencephalitis

### *b. Equine piroplasmosis*

The infection in equids is caused by *Babesia equi* or *B. caballi*. The tick-transmitted hemoparasites multiply in red blood cells via binary fission. Merozoites invade red blood cells and become trophozoites. Trophozoites divide into two round to oval or pear-shaped merozoites. Intravascular hemolysis is the result of rupturing of infected erythrocytes. Extravascular hemolysis may also occur and is due to phagocytosis of the infected red blood cells by macrophages. Ticks such as *Dermacentor, Amblyomma,* or *Boophilus* and others are vectors for transmission. Mechanical transmission may also occur via blood-contaminated needles and syringes.

Teardrop-shape intraerythrocytic inclusions are formed by the parasites. These can be visualized microscopically on Wright-Giemsa stained blood films and are useful in making a rapid diagnosis in acutely infected animals with clinical disease. Polymerase chain reaction (PCR) analysis is the preferred method for species identification and is a more sensitive diagnostic test compared with microscopic evaluation of blood films, particularly in chronically infected or subclinically infected carrier animals.

Peracute, acute, subacute, and chronic forms of the disease can occur. Infected horses develop fever, pendent edema, anemia, thrombocytopenia, icterus, splenomegaly, hepatomegaly, and red-brown urine from hemoglobinuria if the hemolysis is intravascular. Pathologic changes in addition to icterus and anemia include hemoglobinuric nephrosis, hepatomegaly from hemosiderosis, myeloid hyperplasia, and lymphadenopathy. The spleen is actively involved in eliminating hemoparasites. Differential diagnoses for affected animals in the United States include EIA, purpura hemorrhagica, and red maple toxicity.

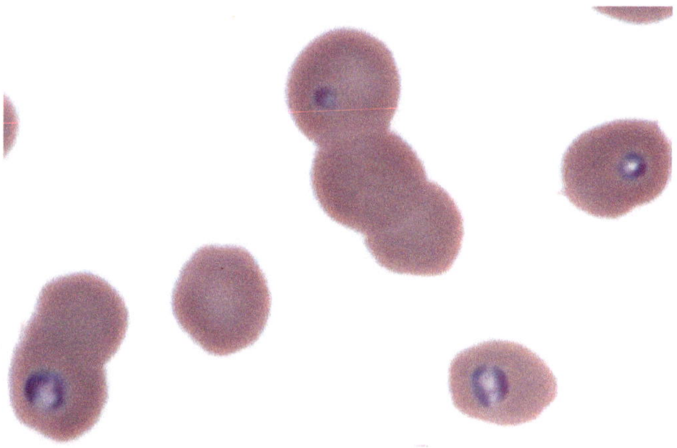

**Figure 15.17.** Horse. Blood Smear. Red Blood Cells. *B. equi* Hemoparasites. Infected erythrocytes contain merozoites. (Wright-Giemsa) (Courtesy Dr. J. Harvey, University of Florida.)

i. Granulocytic anaplasmosis. The disease is caused by the rickettsia agent *Anaplasma phagocytophilum* (formerly *Ehrlichia equi*) and is of low mortality. Ticks (*Ixodes* spp) are vectors for transmission. The horse is considered an aberrant host. The hemoparasite affects horses older than 3 years and causes fever, limb edema, mucosal petechiation, and hemorrhage. A vasculitis is observed histologically in multiple sites of the subcutis. Hematologic findings include leukopenia, anemia, and thrombocytopenia, and in acute cases, cytoplasmic inclusions (morulae) are observed in circulating neutrophils in blood films.

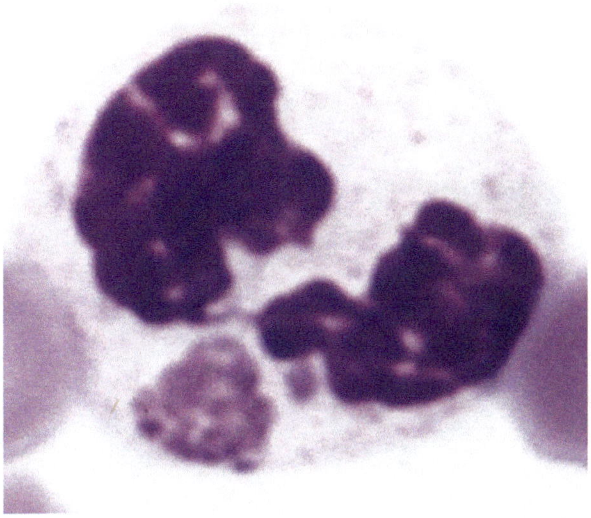

**Figure 15.18.** Horse. Blood Smear. Neutrophil. Granulocytic Anaplasmosis. Morula inclusion in cytoplasm of granulocyte. (Wright-Giemsa) (Courtesy Dr. J. Harvey, University of Florida.)

### *3. Toxicities*

Toxins causing lysis of red blood cells include lead, red maple leaves, onions, and other compounds that cause oxidant damage to the hemoglobin molecule of the erythrocyte. Onion or red maple leaf toxicities induce intravascular hemolytic anemia associated with Heinz body formation. Heinz bodies are aggregates of denatured hemoglobin resulting from oxidant damage to the sulfhydryl groups of the molecule. Heinz bodies are best identified as small dark blue inclusions in or on erythrocytes if they are stained with new methylene blue. However, with Wright-Giemsa or Diff-Quik they are difficult to see and often are missed because they form indistinct pale inclusions that protrude along the erythrocyte membrane. Today, red maple leaf is one on the most common toxicities in horses, and it causes moderate to life-threatening anemia, icterus, and brown to tan mucous membranes from methemoglobin, splenomegaly, and red-brown urine from hemoglobinuria. It is often lethal. Plasma during the hemolytic event may be pink, the MCHC is increased (artifact of free hemoglobin), and gradually the plasma and the patient become icteric. Heinz bodies should be searched for in all suspected cases. The PCV is decreased to variable degrees depending on the severity of the hemolysis. There often is a history of a recent storm; it is the wilted leaves of maples that are toxic, not viable leaves. Differentials are other causes of intravascular hemolysis, nitrate toxicity (methemoglobinemia), and myoglobinuria.

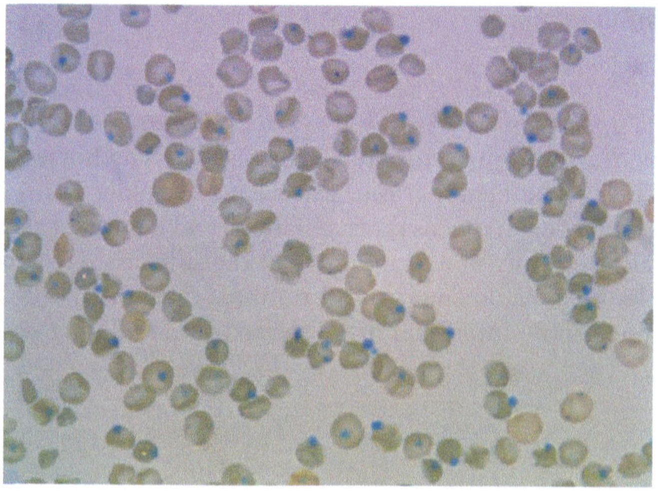

**Figure 15.19.** Horse. Blood Smear. Red Blood Cells. Heinz Bodies. (New methylene blue, Wright-Giemsa) (Courtesy Dr. R. Alleman, University of Florida.)

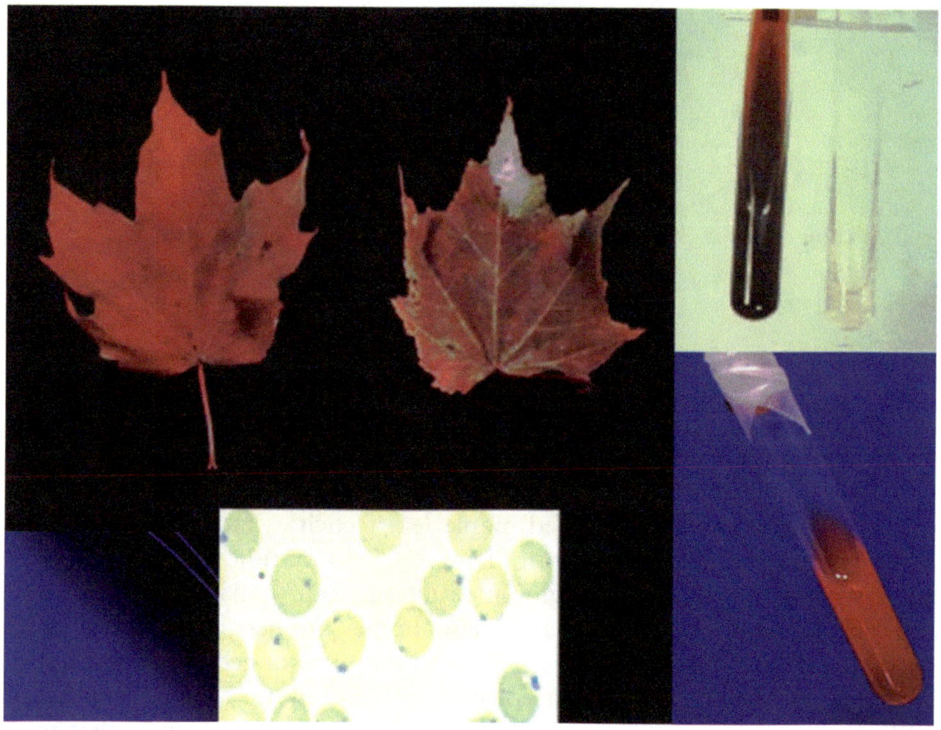

**Figure 15.20.** Horse. Image Composite. Red Maple Toxicity. Two maple leaves, both colored red but the one on the right has scalloped edges that are shallow and helps identify it as a red maple leaf as opposed to the silver maple leaf on the left. Normal yellow urine on right and hemoglobinuria on left. The tube at bottom is plasma with marked hemolysis. When the buffering mechanisms for free hemoglobin in the blood are saturated, the remaining hemoglobin spills into the glomerular filtrate resulting in red-brown urine and probably acute nephrosis. Heinz bodies on smear.

| | Hematuria | Hemoglobinuria | Myoglobinuria |
|---|---|---|---|
| **History** | Dysuria; blister beetles | Recent storm | Postexercise |
| **PCV** | Normal (RR) | Decreased | Normal to increased |
| **Plasma** | Clear | Pink to icteric | Clear to icteric |
| **CPK** | Normal (RR) | Normal, mild increase | Markedly increased 5+ |
| **AST** | Normal (RR) | Normal, mild increase | Markedly increased 5+ |
| **Azotemia** | No | Possible | Likely |
| **Urine** | Red | Red-brown | Red to brown-black |
| **Blood** | 4+ | 4+ | 4+ |
| **RBCS** | TNTC | None, few | None, few |
| **WBCs** | +++ | None, few | None, few |
| **Casts** | None | Variable, many | Variable, many |
| **Urine color postcentrifugation** | Yellow | Pink to red | Red-brown |

AST = aspartate aminotransferase; CPK = creatine phosphokinase; PCV = packed cell volume; RBCs = red blood cells; RR = within reference range; TNTC = too numerous to count; WBCs = white blood cells.

**Table 15.1** Horse: Red brown urine: differentiation of hematuria, hemoglobinuria, and myoglobinuria

## III. Diseases of the thymus

The thymus as a transient organ is mainly susceptible to diseases in juvenile animals where it is undergoing maturation. It functions to establish immune status for adult life and involutes normally with sexual maturity. It may undergo atrophy if an animal is infected with a virus that replicates and causes lysis of lymphocytes such as equine herpesvirus (EHV)-1. The thymus may also atrophy under the stress of a severe disease; a small thymus for the age of an animal may indicate it had a chronic disease. The failure of the thymus to develop maturity is discussed with SCID under bone marrow insufficiency and in Chapter 2, "Diseases of Foals and Juveniles."

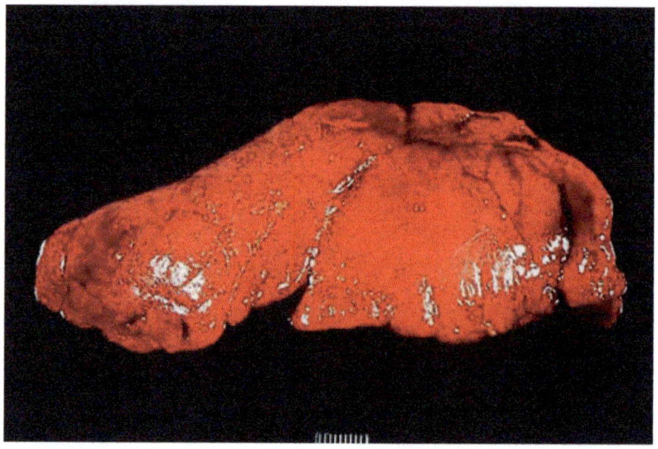

**Figure 15.21.** Juvenile. Thymus. Normal gross appearance.

Occasional cases of cysts of thyroglossal duct remnants, thymoma, and thymic lymphoma have been reported.

## IV. Chylothorax

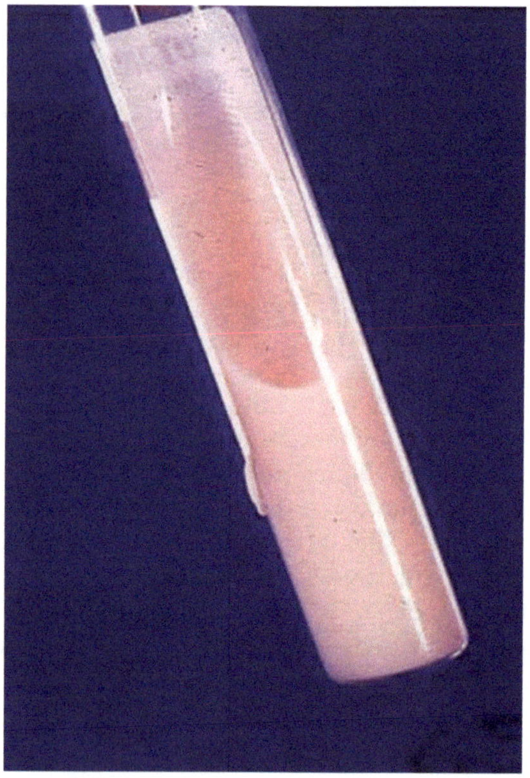

**Figure 15.22.** Foal. Chylothorax. The fluid aspirated of a 5-day-old foal is white. The best way to confirm that an effusion in a body cavity is chyle is biochemistry: compare concentrations of triglycerides in fluid to serum on samples collected concurrently. If fluid triglycerides are greater than serum triglycerides, it is diagnostic for chyle. Also examine the fluid cytologically; if it is lymphocyte rich, the effusion is due to chyle. The concentration of triglyceride and cholesterol can be compared in the fluid, and if triglyceride concentration is higher than cholesterol, this is also diagnostic for chyle. In adult patients it is recommended to examine the cells to determine if lymphoma is present, a common cause of chylothorax in dogs and cats.

Chylous effusions are often idiopathic, but they can be due to trauma, neoplasia, heart failure, or lymphangitis.

## V. Diseases of lymph nodes and lymphangitis

Disease classifications are hypoplasia/atrophy, hyperplasia, inflammation, and neoplasia. Enlarged lymph nodes in a horse are most likely hyperplastic or inflammatory. Etiologic considerations are viral, bacterial, fungal, toxins, and drugs. The most common disease and infectious agent is *Streptococcus equi* subsp. *equi* that produces one or more enlarged lymph nodes often filled with purulent material.

### *1. Lymphoid hypoplasia/atrophy*

Examples of possible etiologies for small lymph nodes were presented previously in the sections on EHV-1 and SCID.

### *2. Reactive lymphoid hyperplasia*

Reactive hyperplasia of draining lymph nodes due to infection in dependent locations is common. Affected lymph nodes contain numerous plasma cells and immature lymphocytes. A generalized lymphoid hyperplasia may be seen with systemic infections such as equine infectious anemia lentivirus.

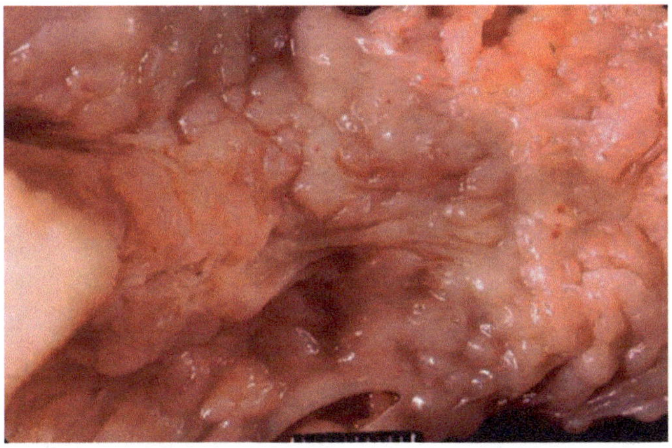

**Figure 15.23.** Horse. Pharynx. Immune Maturation Lymphoid Hyperplasia. In growing horses, tonsils may undergo marked lymphocytic proliferation to cause partial pharyngeal obstruction. Four morphologic grades are distinguished with grade 4 the most severe, inducing clinical signs of dysphagia. Any antigenic stimulation can induce the lymphoid hyperplasia, but EHV-1 is the most likely.

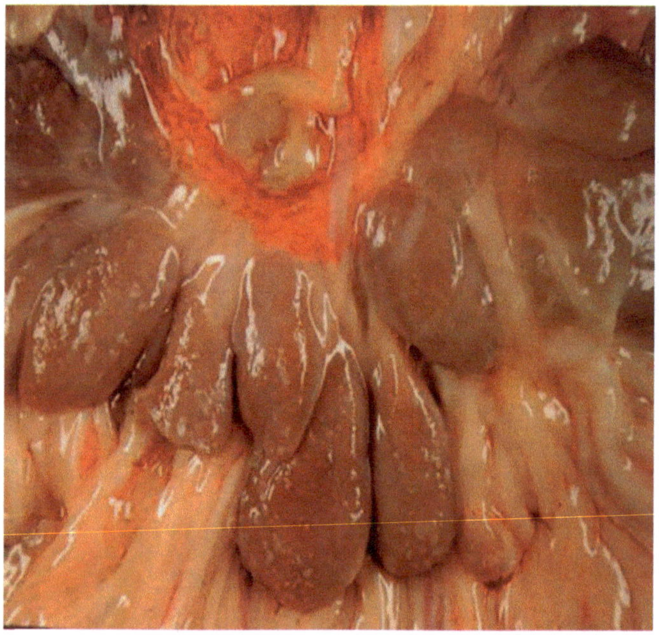

**Figure 15.24.** Horse. Mesenteric Lymph Nodes. Hyperplasia. The lymph nodes have a grapelike configuration and are partially fused. These nodes retain nodal architecture such that cortex and medulla can be recognized.

This scenario occurs as a result of reactive hyperplasia: proliferation of lymphocytes and plasma cells. The response is due to a stimulus that is usually outside of the node, and it is rare to find the antigen in the lymph node. Suppurative inflammation of equine lymph nodes is most commonly associated with *Streptococcus equi* subsp. *equi* and granulomatous inflammation with *Rhodococcus equi*, with the etiologic agents recognizable by special stain within the lymph nodes and other tissues. Morphologic differential diagnoses for enlarged lymph nodes (lymphadenomegaly or lymphadenopathy) are necropurulent lymphadenitis, granulomatous lymphadenitis, myeloproliferative diseases, or lymphoma.

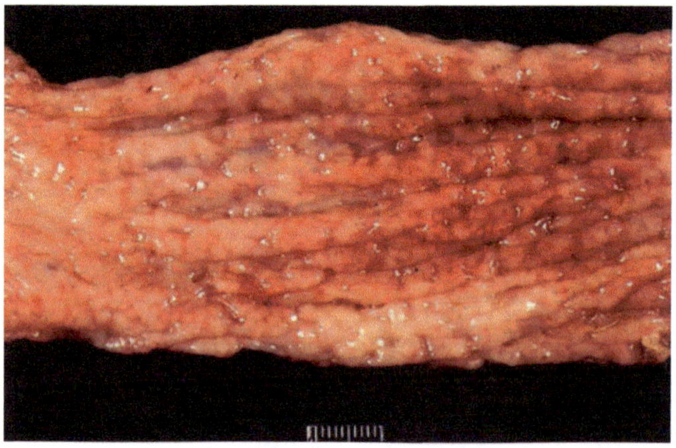

**Figure 15.25.** Horse. Intestine. Alimentary Lymphoid Hyperplasia. Nodular appearance of the mucosa is the result of stimulation of the gut-associated lymphoid tissue (GALT). The reaction occurs in young animals in particular.

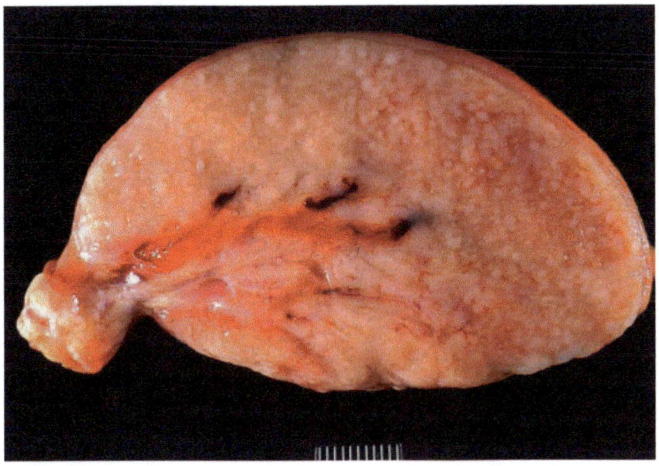

**Figure 15.26.** Horse. Lymph Node. Reactive Lymphoid Hyperplasia. Granular white and hyperplastic changes are featured in the cross section. (Courtesy Dr. Paul Stromberg, Ohio State University.)

### 3. *Lymphadenitis*

#### *a. Streptococcal lymphadenitis*

This highly infectious respiratory disease of horses causes suppurative lymphadenitis, usually in the lymph nodes of the head and neck, especially retropharyngeal and submandibular lymph nodes, but it can be generalized. Tonsillar tissue invasion by *S. equi* subsp. *equi* leads to rapid multiplication of the bacterium. Carriage by tonsillar macrophages to regional retropharyngeal and submandibular lymph nodes results in enlargement due to purulent lymphadenitis with abscess formation.

Rupture of the retropharyngeal lymph node abscess allows internalization of *S. equi* subsp. *equi* into the guttural pouch, which fills with purulent exudate to develop an empyema. The purulent exudate of the guttural pouch may inspissate with time to form chondroids. Chondroids contain viable *S. equi* subsp. *equi* that may persist for several years, thus creating a carrier animal that may transmit the bacterium to naive animals. Clinical signs vary with severity of disease, but coughing and purulent nasal discharges are characteristic features.

Circulatory dissemination of the bacteria may cause purulent lesions in the liver, mesenteric lymph nodes, kidneys, and brain ("ectopic [bastard] strangles"). Deposition of IgA-Streptococcal M protein in vessel walls results in an immune-mediated vasculitis, with subsequent petechial hemorrhage, thrombocytopenia, and peripheral edema, previously discussed as purpura hemorrhagica.

The bacterium produces antiphagocytic factors to evade innate immunity. It evades phagocytosis by neutrophils but may be cleared by macrophages.

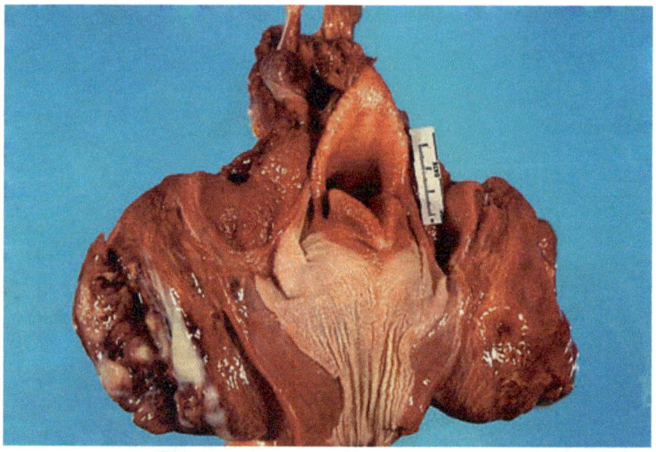

**Figure 15.27.** Horse. Retropharyngeal Lymph Nodes. Bilateral Chronic Suppurative Lymphadenitis. Strangles. Cause: *Streptococcus equi* subsp. *equi*. Enlarged lymph nodes are adhered to the surrounding soft tissue. The lymph node on the left released pus when opened.

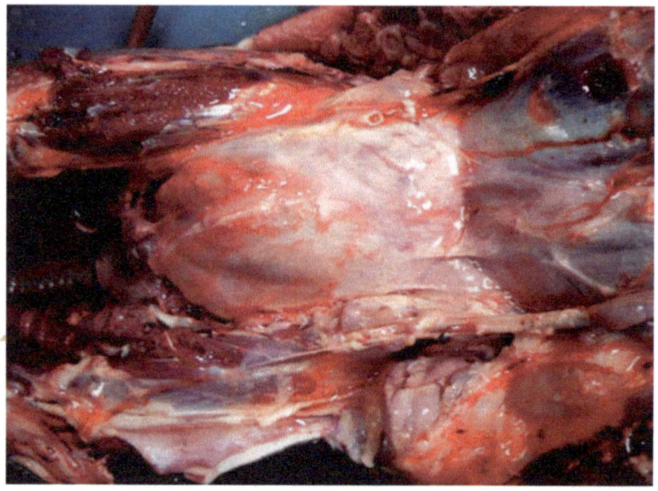

**Figure 15.28.** Horse. Guttural Pouch. Empyema. Strangles. There is a unilateral distension of the pouch containing pus.

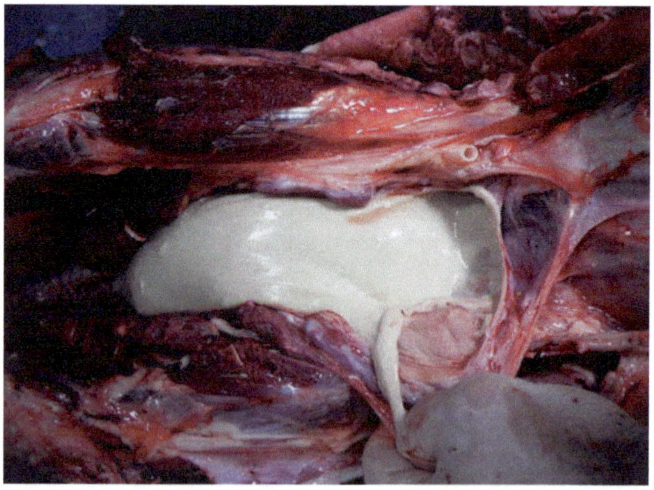

**Figure 15.29.** Horse. Guttural Pouch. Empyema. Strangles. When opened, the pouch contains abundant pus. The exudate may vary from liquid to inspissated.

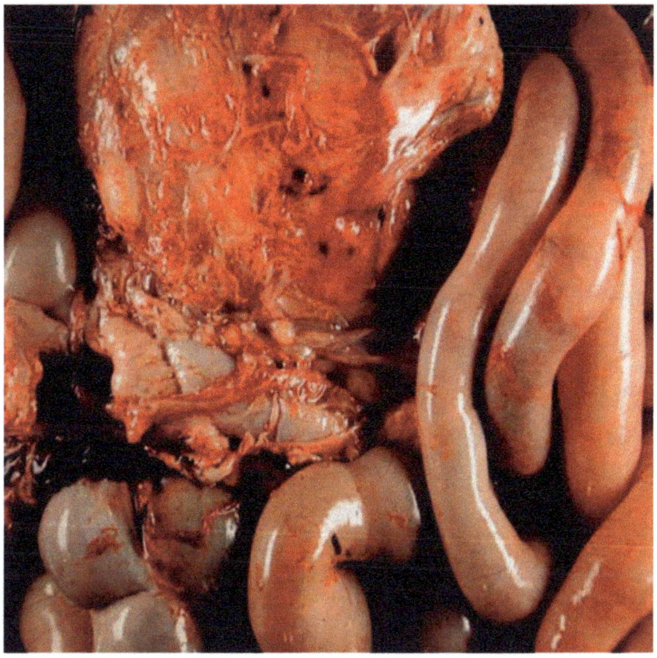

**Figure 15.30.** Horse. Mesenteric Lymph Node. Chronic Fibrosing Suppurative Lymphadenitis with Intestinal Adhesions. Ectopic (Bastard) Strangles. There is evidence of enlargement and fusion of mesenteric lymph nodes between the loops of the small intestine.

## Streptococcal lymphadenitis (strangles) – Fact sheet

**Definition:** Infection of oro-and nasopharynx by *Streptococcus equi* subsp. *equi* with subsequent regional purulent adenitis of retropharyngeal and mandibular lymph nodes.

### Pathogenesis

- Dissemination of cocci to distant sites such as mesenteric lymph nodes, liver, kidneys, brain ("ectopic (bastard) strangles")
- Development of complicating vasculitis from deposition of immune complexes in vascular basement membrane (purpura hemorrhagica)
- Guttural pouch empyema and chondroids in carrier animals
- Clearance by macrophages, but not neutrophils
- Effective protective immunity after recovery

**Pathology:** Purulent lymphadenitis

**Diagnosis:** Culture, PCR, serology

### Differential etiology

- *Corynebacterium pseudotuberculosis*
- *Rhodococcus equi*

### Prevention

- Control of outbreaks through management practices
- Topical and systemic treatment with penicillin
- Vaccination

#### *b. Rhodococcus equi lymphadenitis*

Lymphadenomegaly is pronounced, and on cross section the architecture is effaced by purulent exudate admixed with proliferative tissues. The more solid the lymph node appears on cross section, the more likely the etiology is that of *R. equi* rather than *S. equi* subsp. *equi*. Distinction can be made by the age of the horse, location of enlarged lymph nodes, other gross lesions, cytology, histopathology, and culture. Enlarged lymph nodes of head and neck are most likely *S. equi* subsp. *equi*, and respiratory and abdominal lymphadenomegaly is more likely *R. equi*. Impression films reveal numerous macrophages filled with intracellular coccoid bacteria with a small clear halo if the etiology is *R. equi*.

As the alimentary form, infection with *R. equi* causes necrosis and abscess formation in enlarged mesenteric and colonic lymph nodes in conjunction with enterocolitis. An example of rhodococcal lymphadenitis is presented in Chapter 6, "Diseases of the Gastrointestinal System." Other lesions associated are polyarthritis, hepatitis, encephalitis, uveitis, osteomyelitis, and rarely abortion. The bacterium is a zoonotic agent.

### 4. Lymphangitis

#### *a. Epizootic lymphangitis*

Caused by the fungus *Histoplasma farciminosum*, the primary lesions are fistulous tracts on the limbs. Draining lymph nodes enlarge and become purulent, releasing exudate into adjacent tissue. An example is presented in Chapter 13, "Diseases of the Skin (Integument)." The differential diagnosis is infection with *Corynebacterium pseudotuberculosis*.

#### *b. Sporotrichosis*

Infection with the fungus *Sporothrix schenckii* causes ulcerative lymphangitis. The fungus induces a pyogranulomatous inflammation in lymphatics and lymph nodes of the subcutis. The fungus is considered a zoonotic pathogen.

#### *c. Corynebacterium pseudotuberculosis*

Like in *H. farciminosum* infection, ulcerative lymphangitis in limbs is the pathologic feature, but the disorder is not that common. The infection is more typically characterized by abscess formation in the skin of the ventral midline and pectoral region ("pigeon fever"). Dissemination to other superficial anatomic regions of the body can occur. The infection becomes serious clinically after spread to multiple internal organs. The bacterium can be transmitted by multiple arthropod vectors.

The infectious lymphangitis diseases have to be differentiated from primary chronic progressive lymphedema described in the distal limbs of Clydesdales, Shires, and Belgian draft horses as the result of elastin degradation products causing thick-walled lymphatics with inflammation and fibrosis.

*d. Actinobacillosis*

The principle pathologic changes associated with *A. equuli* in foals has been described in Chapter 2, "Diseases of Foals and Juveniles." Inflammatory changes associated with lymphatics as depicted in Fgure 15.32 are sporadic events in this disease.

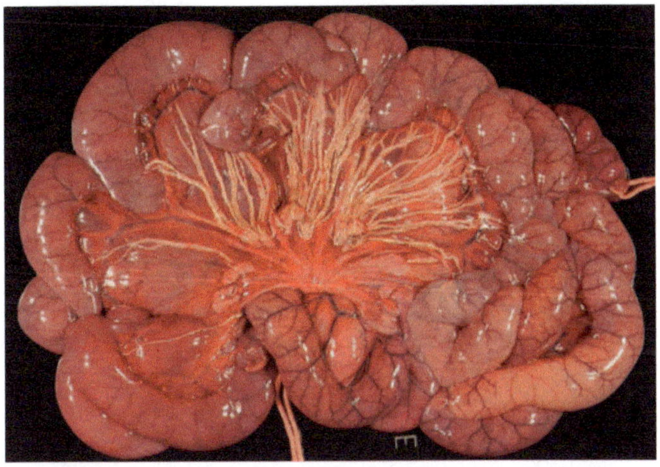

**Figure 15.31.** Foal. Mesentery. Lymphangitis. The lymphatics in this 5-day-old foal form distinct white to yellow lines that fan out from the mesenteric lymph nodes to the surface of the intestines. Differential diagnosis: Postprandial lymphangiectasia.

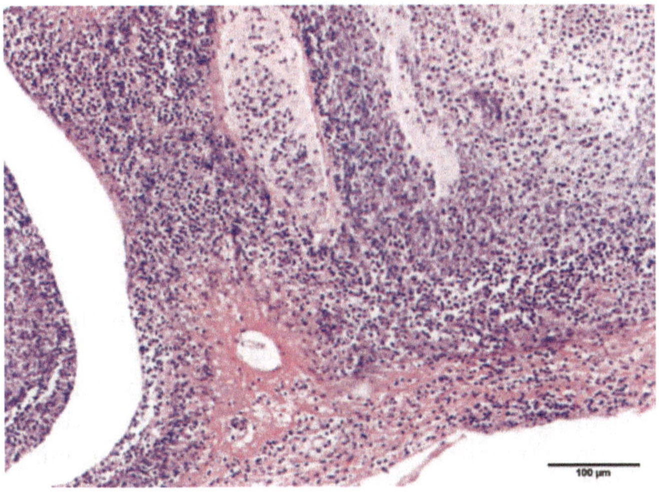


**Figure 15.32.** Horse. Lymph Node. Purulent Lymphangitis. Histologically, degenerative neutrophils have invaded the cortex and are present in sinusoids and the capsule. (H&E) (Courtesy Dr. St. A. Montgomery, North Carolina State University.)

*R. equi*, *S. equi* subsp. *zooepidemicus*, and *Actinobacillus equuli* subsp. *hemolyticus* are additional agents to consider for the morphologic diagnosis of lymphangitis.

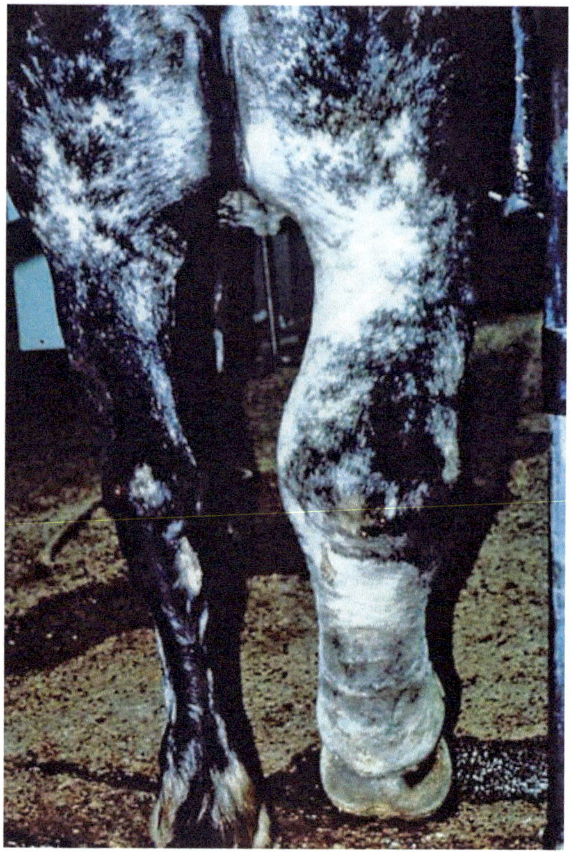

**Figure 15.33.** Horse. Leg. Lymphedema and Lymphangitis. Example of primary chronic progressive lymphedema of draft horses. This Percheron horse has one leg two to three times the size of the opposite limb due to marked lymphangitis and cellulitis.

### *5. Lymphoma*

Lymphoma is the most common malignant tumor in the horse. From a collection of 203 cases of lymphoma, it was concluded that Quarter horses were the breed most frequently affected, followed by Thoroughbreds and Standardbreds. In this study the age of the horses ranged from 2 months to 31 years with a mean of 10.7 years with 13 anatomic tumor sites recorded.

Equine lymphoma is classified into four main categories based on the organ system(s) involved: multicentric (generalized), intestinal (alimentary), mediastinal (thoracic), and cutaneous. Each of these is based on where the predominant clinical signs are coming from or where most of the tumors are located, but lymph nodes are involved in each category. It is extremely rare for lymphoma to be confined to only one system.

Multicentric lymphoma is the most common form. Leukemia rarely accompanies equine lymphoma. Immunotyping has identified 16 subtypes of lymphocytes. T-cell rich large B-cell lymphoma is the most frequent phenotype. T-cell lymphoma is mainly mediastinal; equine B-cell tumors are frequently recognized in the spleen and lymphatic tissues of the head. The cutaneous lymphoma is composed of neoplastic B-cells and nonneoplastic T lymphocytes. Sporadic cases of mycosis fungoides have been described with T-cell lineage of neoplastic lymphocytes.

Depending on the organ involved, different clinical signs may be expected. Paraneoplastic syndromes are uncommon in horses but include hypercalcemia, pruritus, and hypereosinophilia.

Figure 15.34, Figure 15.35, Figure 15.36, Figure 15.37, Figure 15.38, Figure 15.39, Figure 15.40, Figure 15.41, Figure 15.42, and Figure 15.43 are examples of multicentric lymphoma.

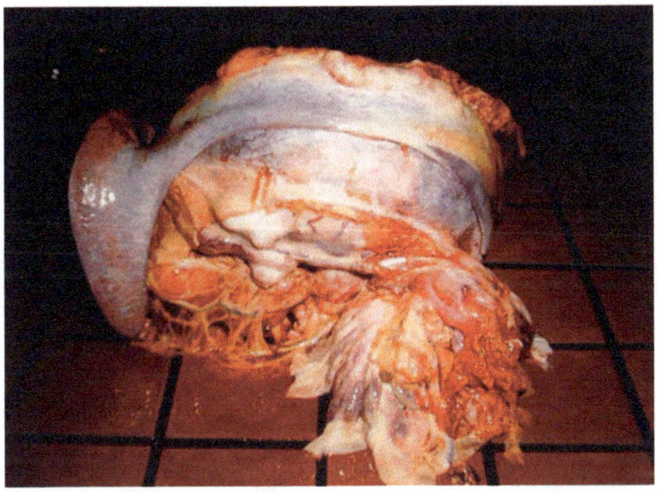

**Figure 15.34.** Horse. Spleen. Lymphoma. A massive growth envelops and compresses the spleen. Adhesions to adjacent omental tissues are present.

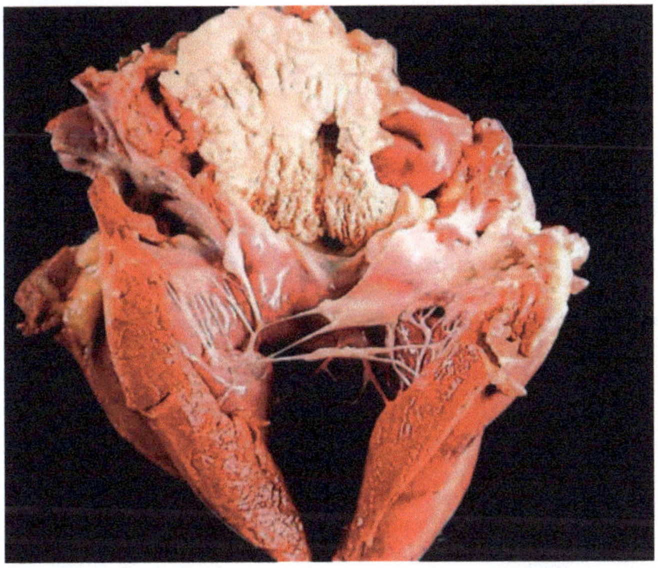

**Figure 15.35.** Horse. Heart. Arial Subendocardial Mineralization. The endocardium of the left atrium is white, crusty, and granular due to paraneoplastic hypercalcemia caused by the lymphoma. Humoral hypercalcemia of malignancy is seen more commonly in horses with gastric squamous cell carcinoma rather than lymphoma.

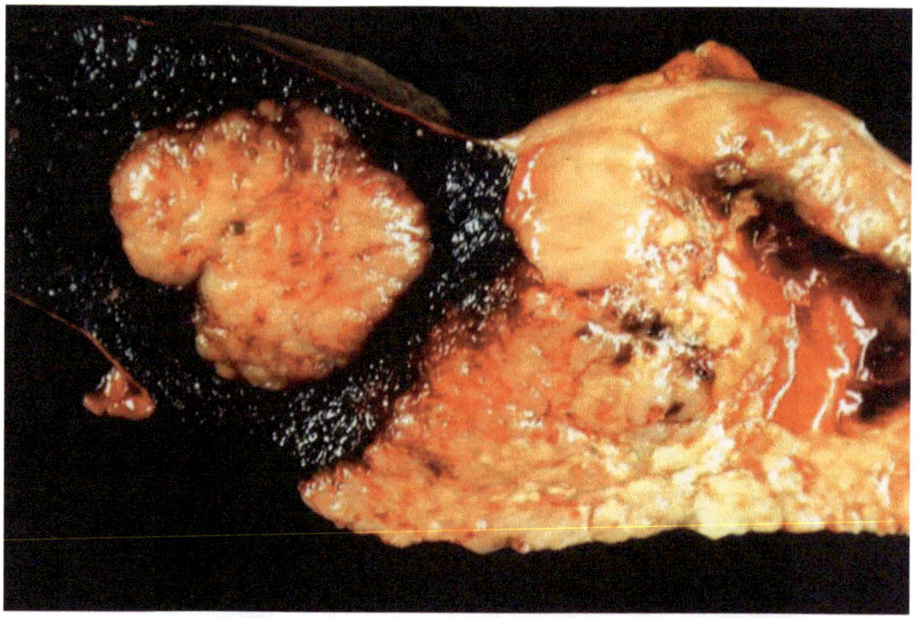

**Figure 15.36.** Horse. Spleen. Lymphoma. A massive white growth has covered the capsular surface and is located within the spleen on cross section. T-cell rich large B-cell lymphomas are the most common subtype. Peripheral T-cell lymphomas and diffuse large B-cell lymphomas are also frequent.

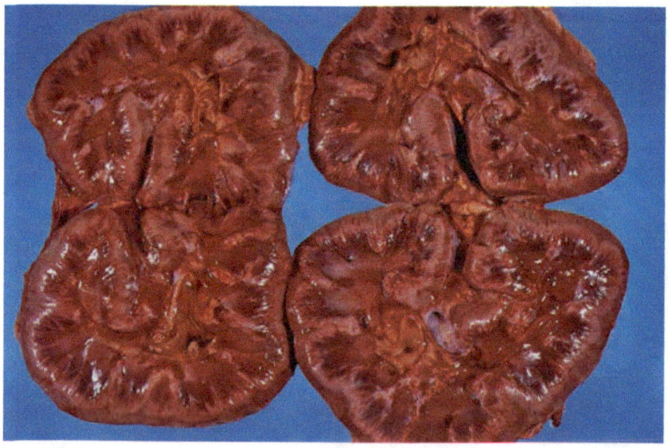

**Figure 15.37.** Horse. Kidney. Lymphoma. The cortices of both kidneys are distorted by white bulging soft tissue that zonally extends into the medulla.

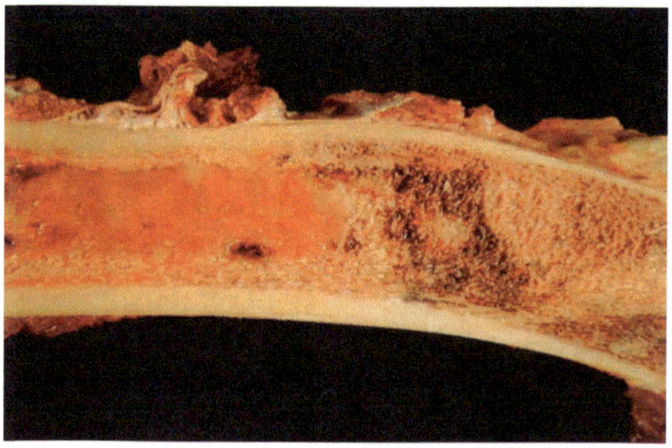

**Figure 15.38.** Horse. Bone Marrow. Lymphoma. A sheet of tan soft tissue has replaced the marrow. The horse suffered from thrombocytopenia due to myelophthisis as evidenced by hemorrhage into the lung.

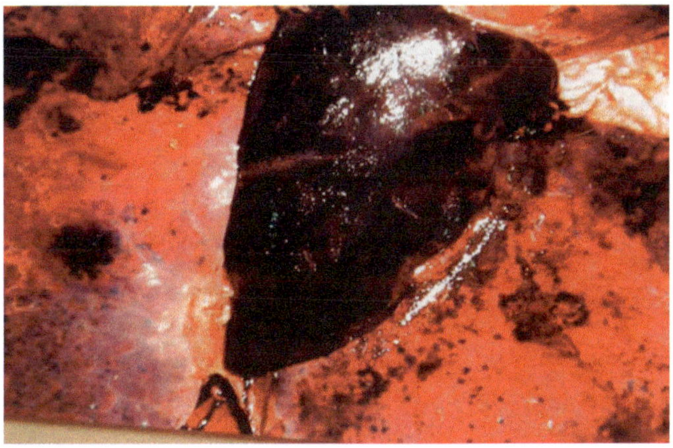

**Figure 15.39.** Horse. Lung. Hemorrhage. The horse with lymphoma suffered from thrombocytopenia due to myelophthisis. Differential diagnosis: lobar torsion.

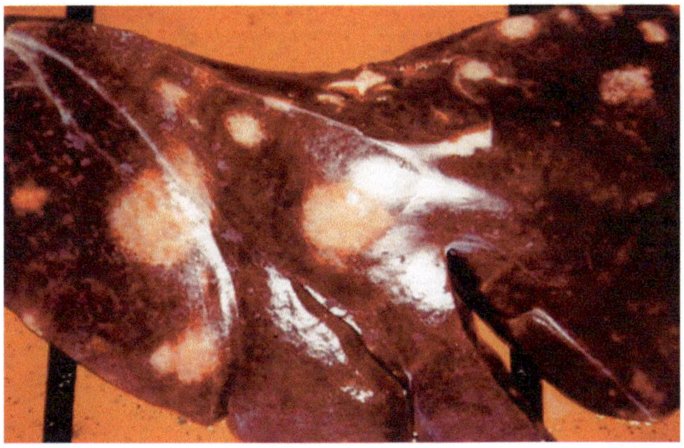

**Figure 15.40.** Horse. Liver. Lymphoma. The neoplasm invaded the organ forming nodules. Although lymphoma can have any distribution, in the horse it tends to develop distinct masses or nodules and therefore looks more like a carcinoma or sarcoma as opposed to dogs and cats in which nodules of lymphoma are much less common and the pattern is usually a diffuse enlargement of the liver.

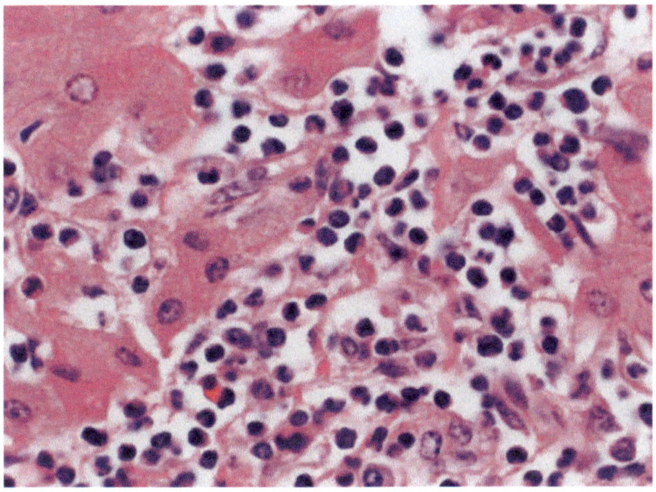

**Figure 15.41.** Horse. Liver. Lymphoma. Neoplastic small T lymphocytes characterized by sometimes irregular nuclei occupy the sinusoids and the Disse's space. (H&E)

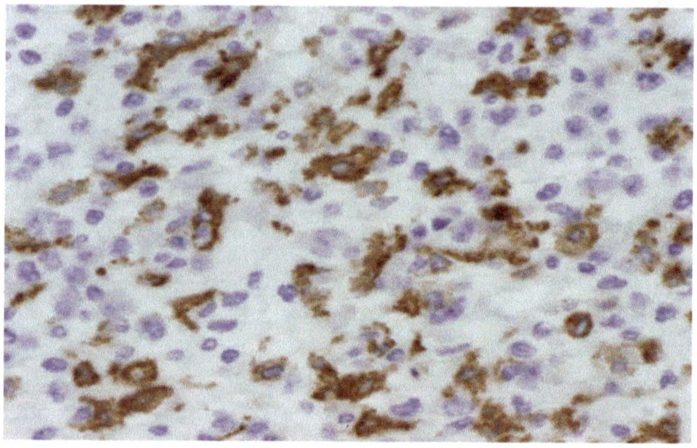

**Figure 15.42.** Horse. Liver. B Cells in Lymphoma. Lymphocytes express B Lymphocyte Antigen (BLA.36), a specific B cell protein localized within the cell membrane. CD20 and CD79A are frequently and effectively used to identify B lymphocytes in mammals. (IHC)

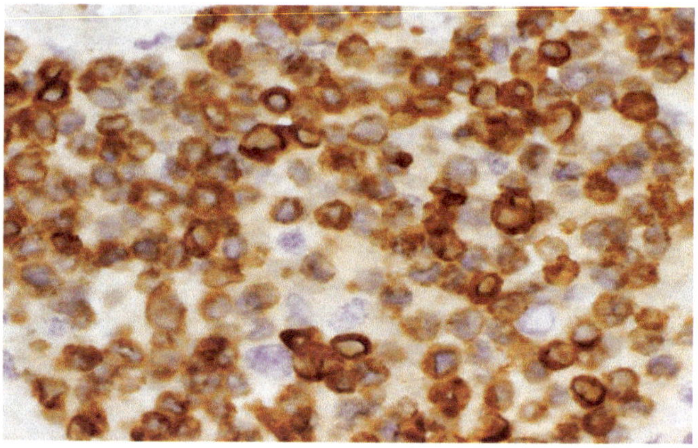

**Figure 15.43.** Horse. Liver. T Cells in Lymphoma. Lymphocytes express CD3, a specific T cell protein localized within the cell membrane. (IHC)

Immunotyping confirmed a T-cell rich, B-cell phenotype of multicentric lymphoma.

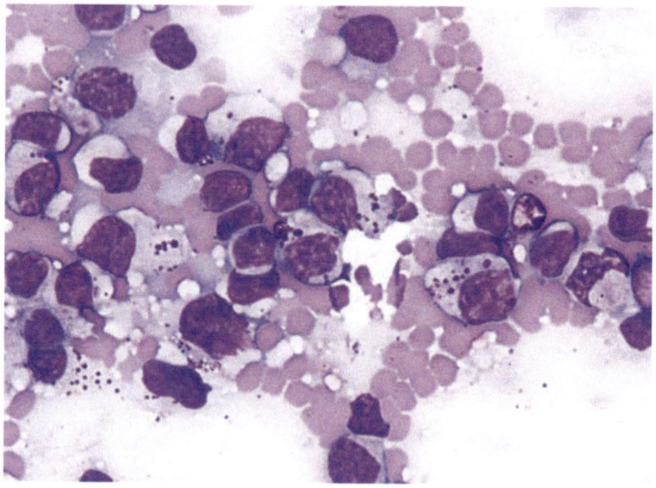

**Figure 15.44.** Horse. Blood Smear. Large Granular Cell Lymphoma (LGL). Cytology. Neoplastic lymphocytes are characterized by slightly irregular and eccentric nuclei and variously sized intracytoplasmic red granules. These are T and NK neoplastic lymphocytes. Granules in LGL are large as compared with dogs. (Diff-Quick) (Courtesy Dr. J. Neel, North Carolina State University.)

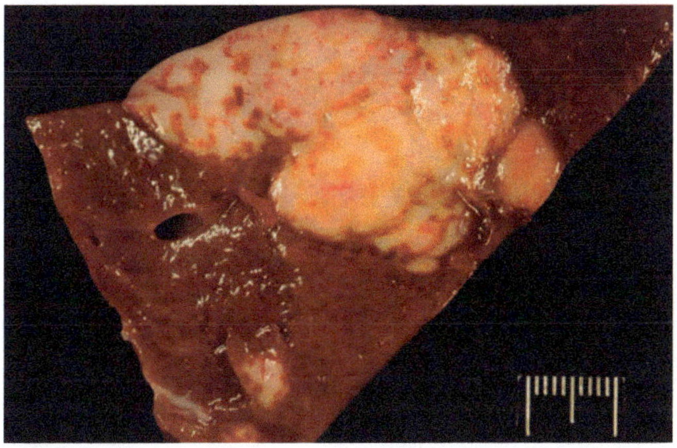

**Figure 15.45.** Horse. Liver. Large Granular Cell Lymphoma (LGL). Variously sized tan nodules with cholestasis occupy the hepatic parenchyma. Differential diagnosis: carcinoma or sarcoma. Occasionally, the hepatic LGL infiltration is subtle and creates a “nutmeg” pattern. (Courtesy Dr. A. Boone, North Carolina State University.)

Figure 15.46 and Figure 15.47 are examples of the alimentary form of lymphoma. It can be difficult grossly to distinguish alimentary lymphoma from granulomatous enteritis.

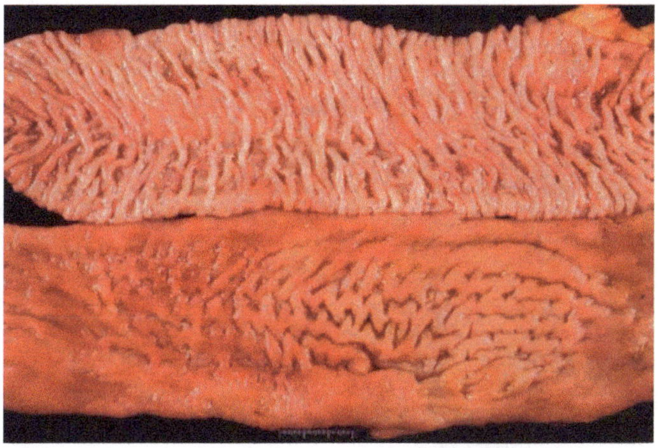

**Figure 15.46.** Horse. Intestine. Alimentary Lymphoma. The opened intestine in the upper part has a normal regular mucosa; the lower segment has glistening thickened lymphoma segments intermixed with unaffected mucosa.

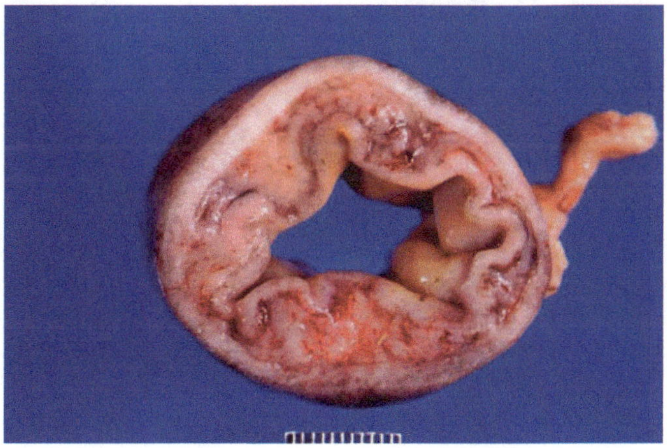

**Figure 15.47.** Horse. Intestine. Alimentary Lymphoma. Cross Section. Mucosa and submucosa are irregular and invaded by tan glistening neoplastic tissue.

Figure 15.48 and Figure 15.49 are examples of mediastinal/thoracic lymphoma.

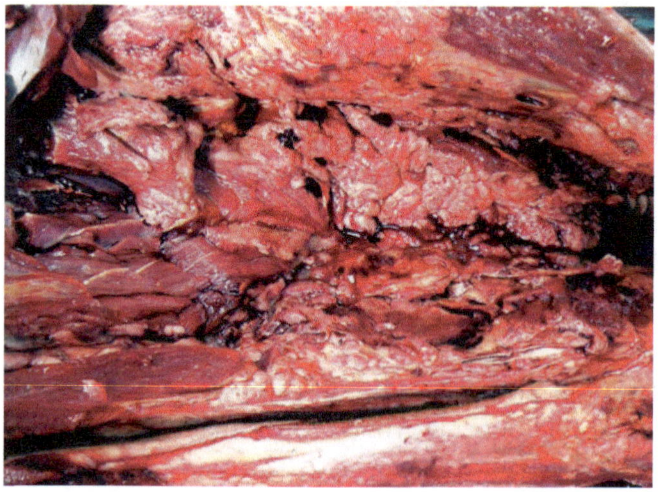

**Figure 15.48.** Horse. Intermandibular Space. Lymphoma. This horse developed a diffusely swollen head and neck suggesting snake bite. It experienced respiratory distress. Necropsy revealed massive cervical edema and a plethora of enlarged lymph nodes of the head, neck, and cranial mediastinum.

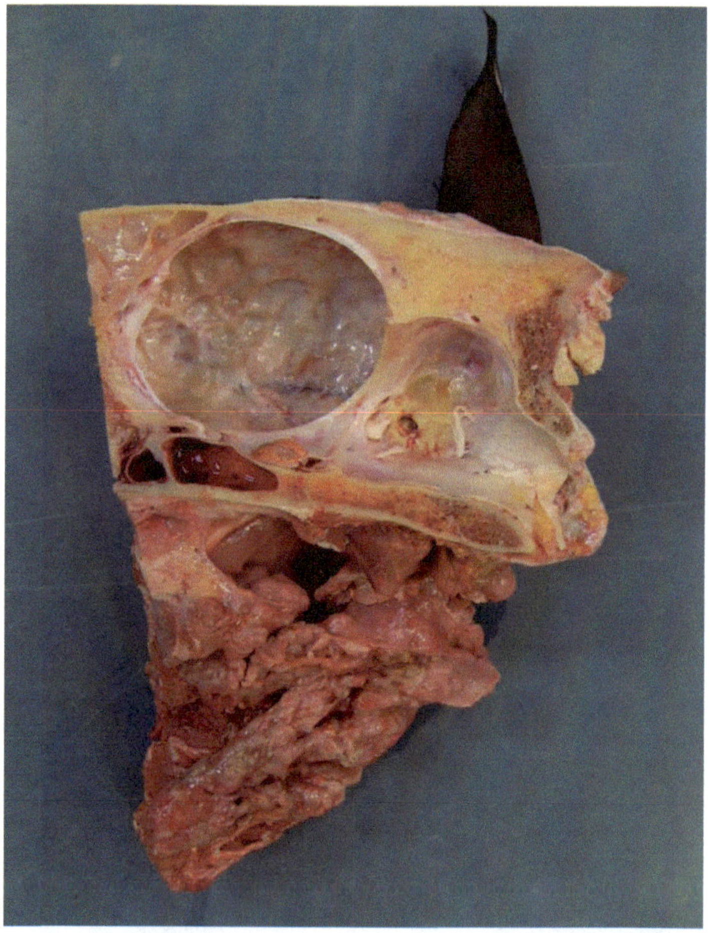

**Figure 15.49.** Horse. Guttural Pouch. Lymphoma. Both guttural pouches were occupied by grapelike nodules diagnosed as lymphoma.

## Equine lymphoma – Fact sheet

**Definition:** Nonviral neoplastic proliferation of lymphocytes

**Breeds:** Quarter horses, Thoroughbreds, Standardbreds

**Age:** 2 months to 31 years (mean: 10.7 years)

### Anatomic sites

Multiple (41%), skin (19%), gastrointestinal (11%), mediastinal (4.5%), nodal (4.5%), ocular/orbital (4%), splenic (2.5%), nasal (2%), CNS (2%), oral cavity (1.5%), hepatic (1%), bone marrow (0.5%), heart (0.5%) (Durham et al., 2013)

### Forms

- Multricentric (generalized)
- Intestinal (alimentary)
- Mediastinal (thoracic)
- Cutaneous

### Phenotypes

- T-cell rich, large B-cell (most common)
- T-cell (mediastinal)
- B-cell (spleen, head lymph nodes)
- B-cell, nonneoplastic T-cell (cutaneous)

Examples of the cutaneous form of equine lymphoma are presented in Chapter 13, "Diseases of the Skin (Integument)."

## VI. Diseases of the spleen

The spleen, fulfilling a variety of protective and eliminating functions, is morphologically divided into white pulp, a reservoir for lymphocytes, and red pulp, a reservoir for blood cells. A network of monocytic and histiocytic cells function as a local particulate removal system via phagocytosis, the mononuclear phagocytic system (MPS). The spleen is prone to splenitis during sepsis.

### *1. Splenomegaly*

The two types of splenic enlargement are due to either an influx of excessive blood resulting in a spongy consistency or to an influx of excessive cells resulting in a firm texture.

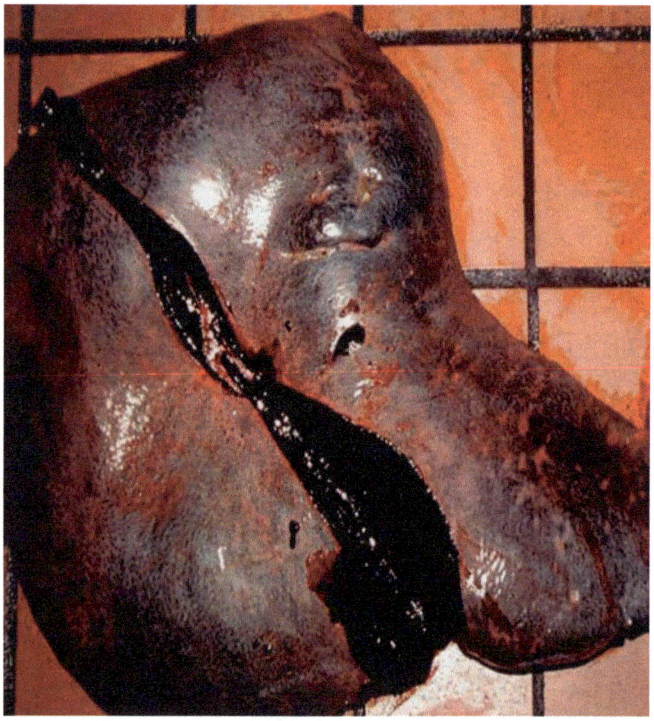

**Figure 15.50.** Horse. Spleen. Splenomegaly. The spleen releases a bloody fluid on cross section. Possible causes include congestion from barbiturate euthanasia, anthrax (rare in horses), EIA, babesiosis, or grass sickness (discussed separately in Chapter 6, "Diseases of the Gastrointestinal Tract").

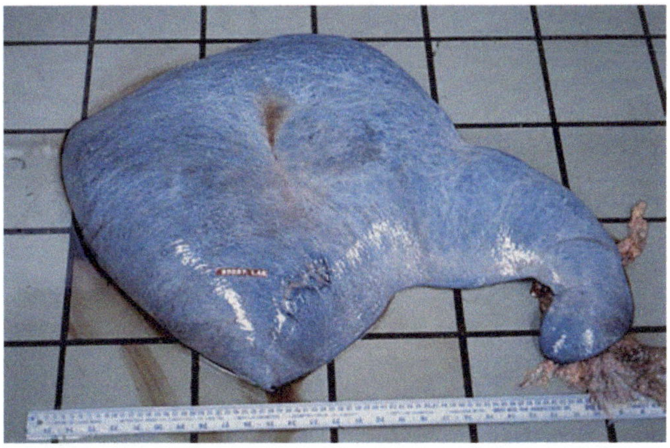

**Figure 15.51.** Horse. Spleen. Splenomegaly. Barbiturate Euthanasia. The spleen is enlarged due to congestion.

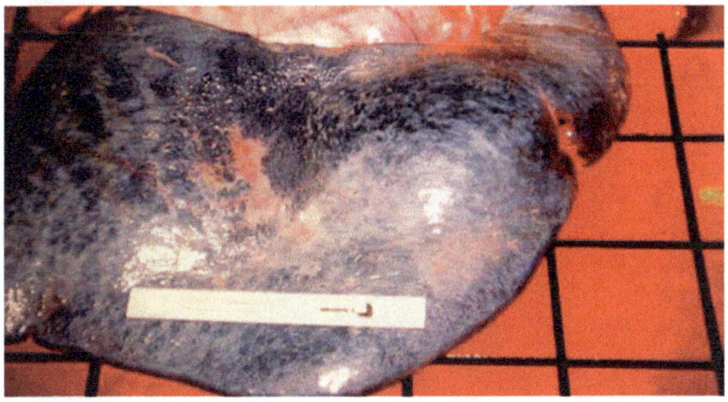

**Figure 15.52.** Horse. Spleen. Splenomegaly. Myeloproliferative Disease. An enlarged firm spleen can result from proliferation of the mononuclear phagocyte system or from influx of preneoplastic or neoplastic circulatory cells (myeloproliferative disorder, lymphoma).

This spleen, enlarged from a lymphoproliferative condition, extended ventrally and to the right of the body at the base of the colon. It weighed 40 kg. The lymphocytes expressed CD3 indicating T cell differentiation. Differential diagnoses should consider lymphoma and EIA.

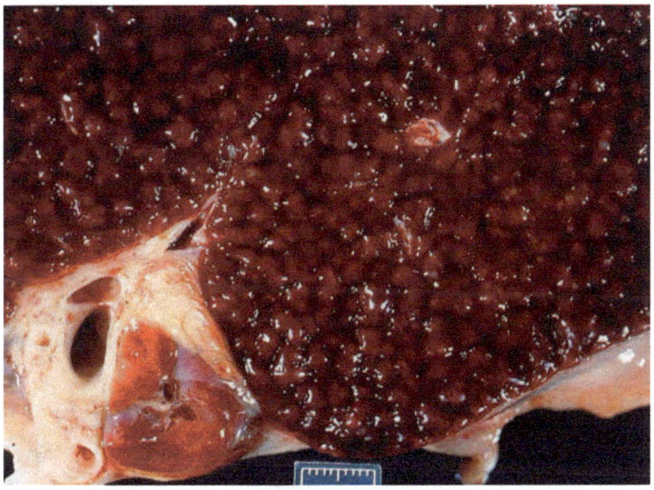

**Figure 15.53.** Horse. Spleen. White Pulp Hyperplasia. The spleen on cross section reveals dense nodular tissue. The adjacent lymph node also appears hyperplastic on cross section. Prominent lymphoid follicles are normal features in fetuses and foals.

### 2. *Inflammation*

Granulomatous splenitis can be caused by fungi or higher structured bacteria, but is it rare in the horse. Abscesses are also rare.

### 3. *Ruptures and tears*

Ruptures and tears are preceded by trauma, such as kicks by other horses or rib fractures. In the case of nontraumatic events, electrocution from lightning might be an alternative cause.

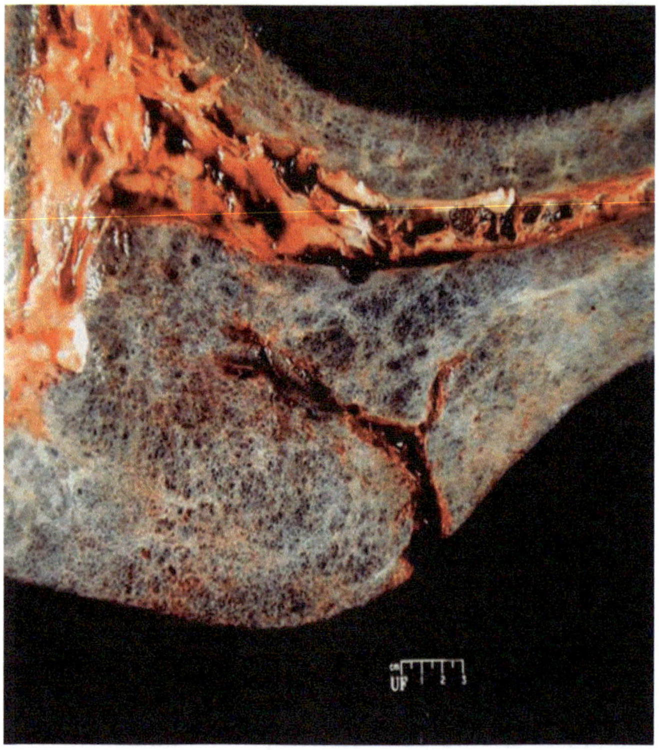

**Figure 15.54.** Horse. Spleen. Focal Rupture. The animal struck by lightning bled to death from a focal splenic tear.

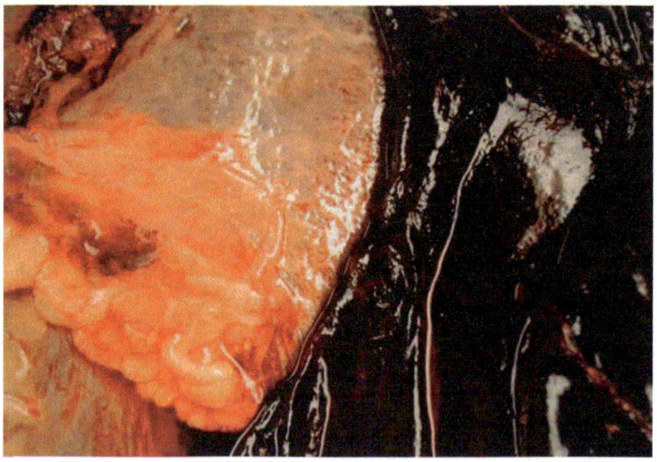

**Figure 15.55.** Foal. Spleen. Hemorrhage. The animal was kicked by the mare and developed fatal hemoabdomen from marked splenic rupture.

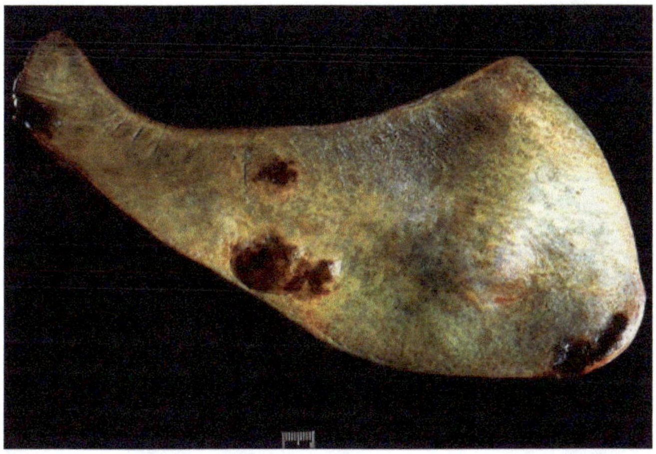

**Figure 15.56.** Horse. Spleen. Capsular Lacerations. Several lacerations are covered by clotted blood. Traumatic tears should be distinguished from normal capsular fissures.

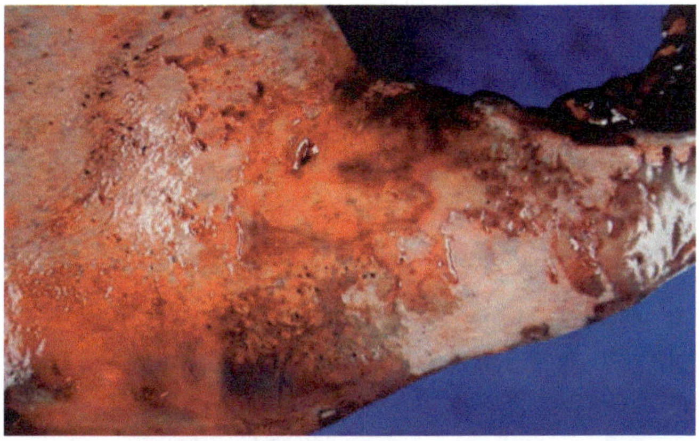

**Figure 15.57.** Horse. Spleen. Chronic Capsular Puncture. The surface is covered by fibrin and fibrous tissue suggesting a chronic sealed surface tear.

### *4. Miscellaneous conditions*

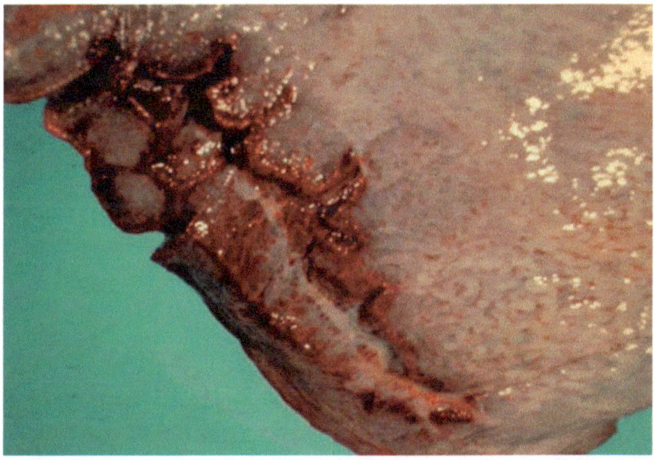

**Figure 15.58.** Horse. Spleen. Normal Fissures. These are normal protrusions of red pulp on the surface. Another pathogenic consideration is that of blocked (thrombosed) capsular veins.

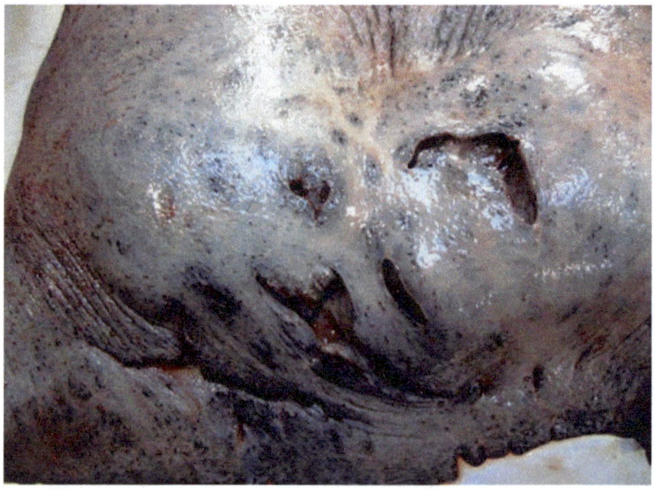

**Figure 15.59.** Horse. Spleen. Folds. These are normal and should not be confused with lacerations.

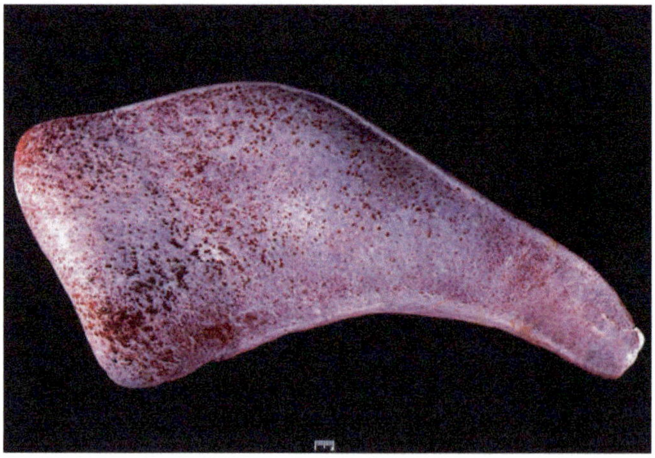

**Figure 15.60.** Horse. Spleen. Red Pulp. The small red blebs represent protruding red pulp tissue.

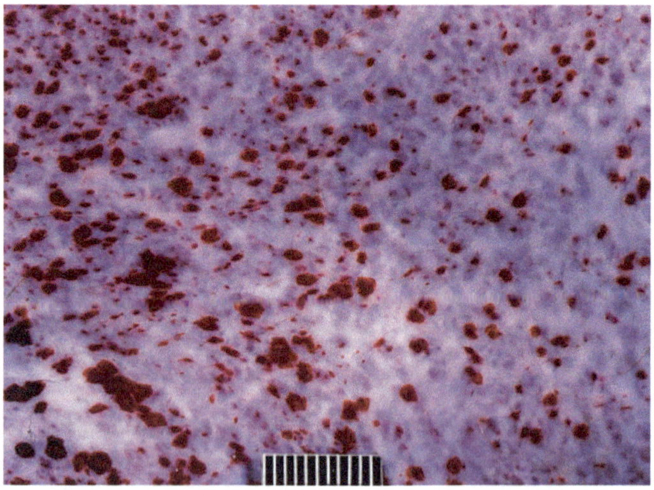

**Figure 15.61.** Horse. Spleen. Red Pulp. The red pulp tissue should not be confused with petechial and ecchymotic hemorrhage from septicemia.

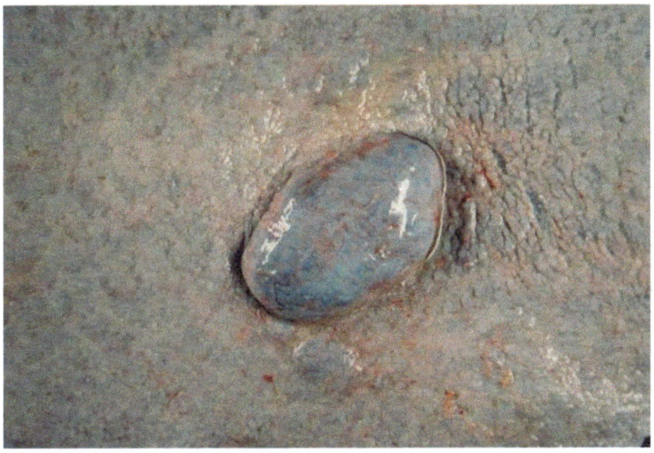

**Figure 15.62.** Horse. Spleen. Accessory Spleen. The oval structure is a miniature spleen tightly adhered to the original spleen. An accessory spleen also can form separately from the regular spleen in adjacent anatomic locations, gaining access to local vascular supply.

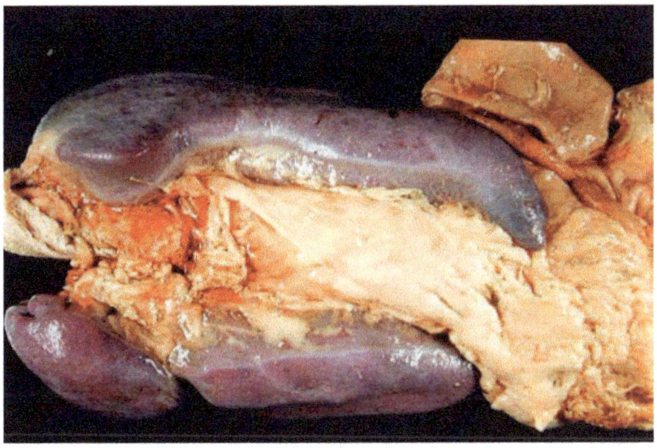

**Figure 15.63.** Horse. Spleen. Duplication. Two identical spleens suggest embryologic duplication or complete separation from a traumatic split.

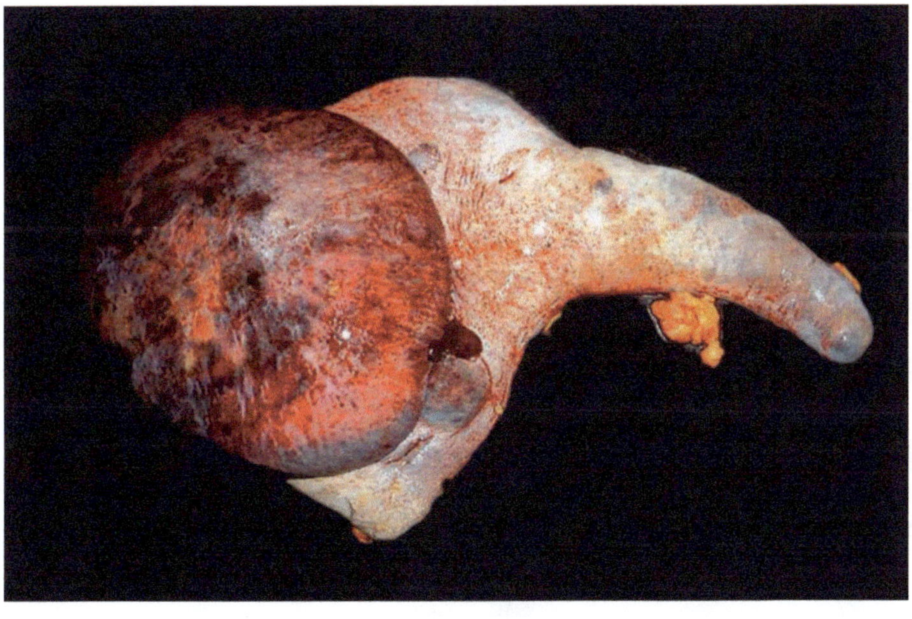

**Figure 15.64.** Horse. Spleen. Hemangiosarcoma. A mushroom-like red growth occupies a large part of the organ and is covered by the capsule.

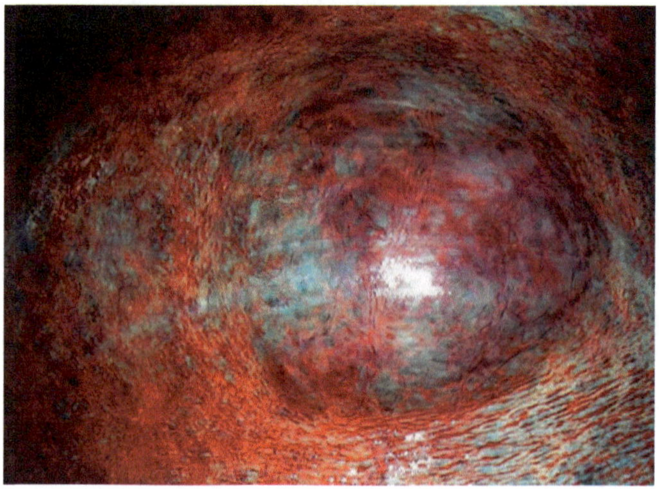

**Figure 15.65.** Horse. Spleen. Hematoma. Traumatic in origin, it should be differentiated from a vascular tumor (e.g., hemangioma or more frequently hemangiosarcoma).

## Selected references


Blue JT, Dinsmore RP, Anderson KL. 1987. Immune-mediated hemolytic anemia induced by penicillin in horses. *Cornell Veterinarian* 77(3):263–278.

De Cock HE, Affolter VK, Wisner ER, Farraro GL, MacLachlan NJ. 2003. Progressive swelling, hyperkeratosis and fibrosis of distal limbs in Clydesdales, Shires and Belgian draft horses, suggestive of primary lymphedema. *Lymphat Res Bio* 1(3):191–199.

Durham AC, Pilitteri CA, Scott F, San Myint M, Valli VE. 2011. 203 cases of equine lymphoma classified according to World Health Organization (WHO) classification criteria [abstract 47]. *ACVP Abstracts.*

Durham AC, Pillitteri CA, San Myint, Valli VE. 2013. Two hundred three cases of equine lymphoma classified according to World Health Organization (WHO) classification criteria. *Vet Pathol* 50(1):86–93.

Golland LC, Hodgson DR, Davis RE, et al. 1995. Retropharyngeal lymph node infection in horses: 46 cases (1977–1992). *Aust Vet J* 72(5):161–164.

Harrold SM, Cook SJ, Cook RF, Rushlow KE, Issel CJ, Montelaro RC. 2000. Tissue site of persistent infection and active replication of equine infectious anemia virus during acute disease and asymptomatic infection in experimentally infected equids. *J Virol* 74(7):3112–3121.

Kelley LC, Mahaffey EA. 1998. Equine malignant lymphomas: morphologic and immunohistochemical classification. *Vet Pathol* 35(4):241–252.

McGuire TC, O'Rourke KL, Perryman LE. 1990. Immunopathogenesis of equine infectious anemia lentivirus disease. *Dev Biol Stand* 72:31–37.

Merant C, Sheoran A, Timoney JF. 2011. Association of *Streptococcus equi* with equine monocytes. *Vet Immunol Immunopathol* 143(1–2):83–86.

Meyer J, DeLay J, Bienzie D. 2006. Clinical, laboratory, and histopathologic features of equine lymphoma. *Vet Pathol* 43(6):914–924.

Newton JR, Wood JL, Dunn KA, DeBrauwere MN, Chanter N. 1997. Naturally occurring persistent and asymptomatic infection of the guttural pouches of horses with *Streptococcus equi*. *Vet Rec* 140(4):84–90.

Short MA, Clark CK, Harvey JW, et al. 2012. Outbreak of equine piroplasmosis in Florida. *J Am Vet Med Assoc* 240(5):588–595.

Sweeney CR, Gilette DM. 1989. Thoracic neoplasia in equids: 35 cases (1967–1987). *J Am Vet Med Assoc* 195(3):374–377.

Timoney JF. 2004. The pathogenic equine streptococci. *Vet Res* 35(4):397–409.

Timoney JF, Kumar P. 2008. Early pathogenesis of equine *Streptococcus equi* infection (strangles). *Equine Vet J* 40(7):637–642.
Waller PS, Paillot R, Timoney JF. 2011. *Streptococcus equi*: a pathogen restricted to one host. *J Med Microbiol* 60(Pt 9):1231–1240.
Weiss DJ, Moritz A. 2003. Equine immune-mediated hemolytic anemia associated with *Clostridium perfringens* infection. *Vet Clin Pathol* 32(1):22–28.

# Appendix A Equine Diseases without Pathology

## I. Botulism

This neuromuscular disorder is caused by *Clostridium botulinum*, a spore-forming bacterium. It produces eight types of potent and lethal neurotoxins. Identification of toxin types is important for antitoxin treatment. Ingestion of contaminated feed, cadaver-contaminated water, ingestion of bird droppings, or contaminated wounds are portals of entry for the bacterium. Toxins interfere with neurotransmitter release at the neuromuscular junction with lower motor neuron dysfunction responsible for clinical signs and death. Clinical signs include, among others, flaccid paralysis, decreased eyelid and tail tone. Death is due to respiratory failure. Other than the pathologic changes seen in grass sickness, with *C. botulinum* implicated to produce a specific toxin inducing neuronal degeneration in autonomic ganglia, no direct pathologic changes are evident at necropsy for botulism. Diagnosis is made from gastric contents, feces, or feed by culturing the spores, by mouse inoculation analyzing for toxins, or by polymerase chain reaction. Protection of infection can be achieved by vaccination.

## II. Tetanus

Tetanus is caused by *Clostridium tetani* producing exotoxins. Soil-contaminated spores of the organism enter through puncture wounds or castration wounds; the produced exotoxins act at neuromuscular junctions to cause tonic muscle spasm and rigidity. Respiratory failure may be responsible for death. The diagnosis is made by looking for clinical signs of muscle rigidity, for wounds or vehicles such as a wire in a wound, and a prolapsed nictitans membrane. Prevention of tetanus is through vaccination.

## III. Japanese yew (Taxus)

Anecdotally, consumption of leaves of Japanese yew (*Taxus cuspidata*), an ornamental shrub, has been cited as one of the quickest causes of sudden death in the horse. Taxane alkaloids are made responsible as toxic principle and can be detected by gas chromatography/mass spectrometry from stomach contents even if the leaves are not detected in the gastric contents. Apparently, there is little pathology to be detected. One necropsy report cites endocardial hemorrhages in both ventricles with mild necrosis of papillary muscle. Best ways for the diagnosis are to find leaves of the plant in the mouth or stomach contents of the dead horse and the history of the plant near the demised horse.

## IV. Selenium toxicity

A recent sudden death scenario in polo ponies receiving an intravenous injection of a performance-enhancing vitamin/mineral supplement containing

*Color Atlas of Equine Pathology*, First Edition. Claus D. Buergelt and Fabio Del Piero.

selenium among other substances resulted in sudden death of those ponies that were administered the drug and not in those that did not receive any. The treated horses exhibited central nervous system disturbances that included ataxia before death. The compound contained toxic levels of selenium due to a mixing error preparing the formulation. Gross lesions of multicentric hemorrhage at necropsy of the demised ponies were inconclusive for being caused by the selenium toxicity as no histologic lesions were identified. Toxicologic analysis revealed 10-fold higher concentrations of blood selenium when compared with the unaffected surviving ponies. Similar increased selenium level observations were made from liver and renal tissue samples.

## Selected references

Desta B, Maldonado G, Reid H, et al. 2011. Acute selenium toxicosis in polo ponies. *J Vet Diagn Invest* 23(3):623–628.

Shi QW,Oritani T, Kiyota H, Murakami R. 2001. Three new taxoids from leaves of the Japanese yew, *Taxus cuspidata*. *Nat Prod Lett* 15(1):55–62.

Tiwary AK, Puschner B, Kinde H, Tor ER. 2005. Diagnosis of Taxus (yew) poisoning in a horse. *J Vet Diag Invest* 17(3):252–255.

# Appendix B List of Equine Neoplasms

Basal cell tumors
Bladder transitional carcinoma
Cementoma associated with incisors
Chondrosarcoma
Epithelioid variant of hemangioma
Fibroma, fibrosarcoma
Gastric adenocarcinoma
Gastric squamous cell carcinoma
Gastrointestinal stromal tumor
Granular cell tumor of the lungs
Hemangiopericytoma (skin)
Hemangiosarcoma
Hepatoblastoma
Intestinal adenocarcinoma
Leiomyosarcoma
Lipoma
Lymphosarcoma
Malignant seminoma
Malignant peripheral nerve sheath tumor
Mammary adenocarcinoma
Mast cell tumor
Melanoma
Meningioma
Mesenteric myofibroblastoma
Mesothelioma
Multiple myeloma
Odontoma
Olfactory neuroma
Osteosarcoma
Ovarian and testicular teratoma
Ovarian granulosa cell tumor
Pancreatic adenocarcinoma
Paraganglioma
Pituitary pars intermedia adenoma
Placental teratocarcinoma
Renal carcinoma
Rhabdomyosarcoma
Sarcoid (skin)
Schwannoma
Sinonasal adenocarcinoma
Squamous cell carcinoma
Suprasellar germ cell tumor
Sweat gland ductal carcinomas
Testicular interstitial cell tumor
Testicular seminoma
Testicular Sertoli cell tumor
Thyroid carcinoma
Thyroid C-cell ademoma
Uterine and intestinal leiomyoma

*Color Atlas of Equine Pathology*, First Edition. Claus D. Buergelt and Fabio Del Piero.

# Appendix C List of Equine Infectious Diseases Foreign to North America

| Disease | Type of Agent | Organs System |
|---|---|---|
| African horse sickness | Orbivirus | Blood vessels of several organ systems |
| Borna disease | RNA virus | CNS, eyes |
| Dourine | *Trypanosoma equiperdum* | CNS, blood, genitalia |
| Equine encephalosis | Orbivirus | CNS |
| Equine torovirus | RNA virus | Intestinal |
| Getah virus | Togavirus | Vessels, lymph nodes, mildly CNS |
| Glanders "Farcy" | *Burkholderia mallei* | Skin, nose, testis, respiratory tract, lymphatics |
| Henipavirus | Paramyxovirus | CNS, lung |
| Japanese B encephalitis | Flavivirus | CNS |
| Kunjin encephalitis | Flavivirus | CNS |
| Louping ill | Flavivirus | CNS |
| Mal de caderas | *T. equinum* | Spleen, lymph node |
| Melioidosis | *B. pseudomallei* | CNS, GI |
| Murray Valley encephalitis | Flavivirus | CNS |
| Nagana | *T. brucei* | Multiple |
| Powassan viral encephalitis | Flavivirus | CNS |
| Ross River virus | Togavirus | Joints, CNS |
| Saint Louis encephalitis | Flavivirus | CNS |
| Surra | *T. evansi* | CNS |
| Tick-borne encephalitis | Flavivirus | CNS |
| Venezuela encephalitis | Togavirus | CNS |
| Vesicular stomatitis | Rhabdovirus | Mouth, coronary band |
| Wallal, Warrego, Eubenangee | Orbiviruses | CNS |

CNS = central nervous system; GI = gastrointestinal.

*Color Atlas of Equine Pathology*, First Edition. Claus D. Buergelt and Fabio Del Piero.

# Index

*Note*: Page numbers in *italics* represent figures; those in **bold**, tables.




*Color Atlas of Equine Pathology*, First Edition. Claus D. Buergelt and Fabio Del Piero.

Printed in the USA/Agawam, MA
September 16, 2026

910661.209